DESIGNED FOR THE MAINTENANCE OF GOOD NUTRITION OF PRACTICALLY ALL HEALTHY PEOPLE IN THE UNITED STATES

Water-Soluble Vitamins							Minerals						
Vitamin C (mg)	Thiamin (mg)	Riboflavin (mg)	Niacin (mg NE)[f]	Vitamin B_6 (mg)	Folate (µg)	Vitamin B_{12} (µg)	Calcium [illegible]	Phos[illegible]	[illegible]	[illegible]	[illegible]	[illegible]	Selenium (µg)
30	0.3	0.4	5	0.3	25	0.3	[illegible]	[illegible]	[illegible]	[illegible]	[illegible]	[illegible]	10
35	0.4	0.5	6	0.6	35	0.5	[illegible]	[illegible]	[illegible]	[illegible]	[illegible]	[illegible]	15
40	0.7	0.8	9	1.0	50	0.7	[illegible]	[illegible]	[illegible]	[illegible]	10	70	20
45	0.9	1.1	12	1.1	75	1.0	[illegible]	[illegible]	120	10	10	90	20
45	1.0	1.2	13	1.4	100	1.4	800	800	170	10	10	120	30
50	1.3	1.5	17	1.7	150	2.0	1,200	1,200	270	12	15	150	40
60	1.5	1.8	20	2.0	200	2.0	1,200	1,200	400	12	15	150	50
60	1.5	1.7	19	2.0	200	2.0	1,200	1,200	350	10	15	150	70
60	1.5	1.7	19	2.0	200	2.0	800	800	350	10	15	150	70
60	1.2	1.4	15	2.0	200	2.0	800	800	350	10	15	150	70
50	1.1	1.3	15	1.4	150	2.0	1,200	1,200	280	15	12	150	45
60	1.1	1.3	15	1.5	180	2.0	1,200	1,200	300	15	12	150	50
60	1.1	1.3	15	1.6	180	2.0	1,200	1,200	280	15	12	150	55
60	1.1	1.3	15	1.6	180	2.0	800	800	280	15	12	150	55
60	1.0	1.2	13	1.6	180	2.0	800	800	280	10	12	150	55
70	1.5	1.6	17	2.2	400	2.2	1,200	1,200	320	30	15	175	65
95	1.6	1.8	20	2.1	280	2.6	1,200	1,200	355	15	19	200	75
90	1.6	1.7	20	2.1	260	2.6	1,200	1,200	340	15	16	200	75

Retinol equivalents. 1 retinol equivalent = 1 µg retinol or 6 µg β-carotene.

[d]As cholecalciferol. 10 µg cholecalciferol = 400 IU of vitamin D.

[c]α-Tocopherol equivalents. 1 mg d-α tocopherol = 1 α-TE.

[f]1 NE (niacin equivalent) is equal to 1 mg of niacin or 60 mg of dietary tryptophan.

ESTIMATED SAFE AND ADEQUATE DAILY DIETARY INTAKES OF SELECTED VITAMINS AND MINERALS[a]

		Vitamins	
Category	Age (years)	Biotin (µg)	Pantothenic Acid (mg)
Infants	0-0.5	10	2
	0.5-1	15	3
Children and adolescents	1-3	20	3
	4-6	25	3-1
	7-10	30	4-5
	11+	30-100	4-7
Adults		30-100	4-7

		Trace Elements[b]				
Category	Age (years)	Copper (mg)	Manganese (mg)	Fluoride (µg)	Chromium (µg)	Molybdenum (mg)
Infants	0-0.5	0.4-0.6	0.3-0.6	0.1-0.5	10-40	15-30
	0.5-1	0.6-0.7	0.6-1.0	0.2-1.0	20-60	20-40
Children and adolescents	1-3	0.7-1.0	1.0-1.5	0.5-1.5	20-80	25-50
	4-6	1.0-1.5	1.5-2.0	1.0-2.5	30-120	30-75
	7-10	1.0-2.0	2.0-3.0	1.5-2.5	50-200	50-150
	11+	1.5-2.5	2.0-5.0	1.5-2.5	50-200	75-250
Adults		1.5-3.0	2.0-5.0	1.5-4.0	50-200	75-250

[a]Because there is less information on which to base allowances, these figures are not given in the main table of RDA and are provided here in the form of ranges of recommended intakes.

[b]Since the toxic levels for many trace elements may be only several times usual intakes, the upper levels for the trace elements given in this table should not be habitually exceeded.

To my Publisher and Editor-in-Chief,
James M. Smith,
who saw a need and filled it

Diet Therapy

Sue Rodwell Williams, *Ph.D., M.P.H., R.D.*

President, SRW Productions, Inc., Clinical Nutrition Consultant, Davis, California;
formerly Chief, Clinical Nutrition Division,
Kaiser-Permanente Medical Center, Oakland, California,
and Regional Metabolic Nutritionist, Kaiser-Permanente Northern California
Regional Newborn Screening and Genetic Program;
and Field Faculty, M.P.H.-Dietetic Internship Program
and Coordinated Undergraduate Program in Dietetics,
University of California, Berkeley, California

with the assistance of

Sara Long Anderson, *Ph.D., R.D.*

Southern Illinois University
Carbondale, Illinois

with 74 *illustrations*

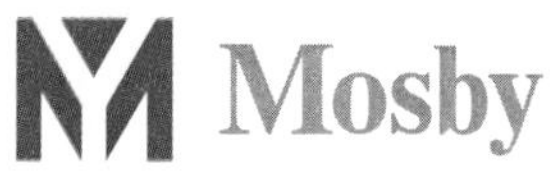

St. Louis Baltimore Berlin Boston Carlsbad Chicago London Madrid
Naples New York Philadelphia Sydney Tokyo Toronto

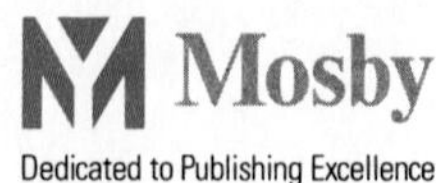
Dedicated to Publishing Excellence

Editor-in-Chief: James M. Smith
Acquisitions Editor: Vicki Malinee
Managing Editor: Terry Eynon
Project Manager: John Rogers
Sr. Production Editor: Kathleen L. Teal
Design Coordinator: Renee Duenow
Manufacturing Supervisor: Theresa Fuchs
Cover art: "Pears by the Porch," WRK, Inc.

Printed in the United States of America
Composition by Graphic World, Inc.
Printing/binding by Von Hoffmann Press, Inc.

Mosby–Year Book, Inc.
11830 Westline Industrial Drive
St. Louis, Missouri 63146

International Standard Book Number 0-8151-9128-6

95 96 97 98 99 / 9 8 7 6 5 4 3 2 1

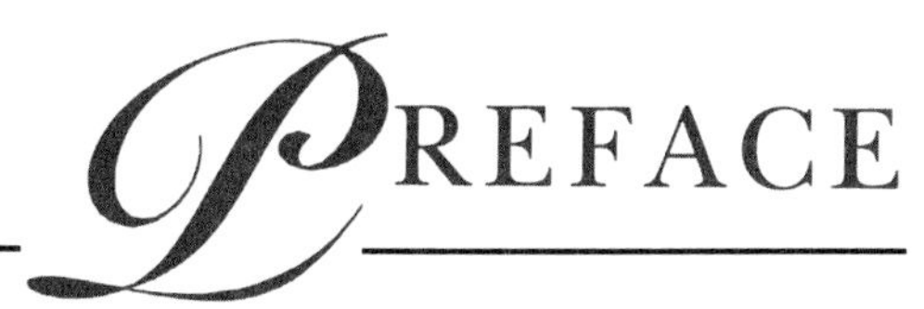

PREFACE

This first edition of *Diet Therapy* emerges as a separate text from its highly successful parent book *Nutrition and Diet Therapy* in response to many requests from users of the main text. This new text maintains the same strong research base and person-centered approach to the study and application of nutrition to human health and disease.

Over the past few years, rapid changes have been occurring in nutrition. New regulations are on the horizon. The science base is expanding. Social problems and structures are changing. Health care systems and practices are changing. Public interest and concern with nutrition in health care and disease are increasing. Nutrition has indeed become more prominent in the marketplace of competing ideas and products. It is natural, then, that all these changes are apparent in the field of nutrition education and professional practice, since nutrition is fundamentally a very human applied science and art.

This first edition of *Diet Therapy* reflects these far-reaching changes. As always, the guiding principle continues to be my own commitment and that of my publisher to the integrity of the parent text. Now in this new offspring our expanded goal is to build on the format introduced in the parent text and produce this completely updated new book, incorporating design and format with sound content to meet the expectations and changing needs of students, faculty, and practitioners in the health professions.

Clinical Nutrition Applied

With the intent of accommodating the demands of a rapidly developing science and society, I have reorganized and updated a large part of the text and made changes, using input from many professors, students, and clinicians, to increase its usefulness. This new book now stands as a separate and specific clinical nutrition text applying principles of medical and nutritional sciences to the modern management and treatment of disease. It fills a need for upperclass courses in Diet Therapy, preparing students for internships, or serving as a concise guide for practitioners in daily medical-nutritional management of disease problems in the care of their patients.

Current content. Each chapter has been painstakingly written and reviewed to meet current practice needs. For instance Chapter 12, *Nutrition and AIDS*, provides substantial coverage of the disease process and the special nutritional needs of the growing number of AIDS patients worldwide. *Enteral and Parenteral Nutrition* are covered in two separate chapters, Chapters 3 and 4, respectively. This distinction provides students and clinicians with more in-depth information on tube feeding and intravenous nutrition support.

The final chapter (Chapter 14) on disabling disease and rehabilitation includes new developments and current discoveries in the fields of musculoskeletal disease, neuromuscular injury and developmental disease, and progressive neurologic disorders. In each case, current knowledge of the disease process and the essential role of nutrition management and rehabilitative care is clarified. Every chapter applies nutrition science and modern technology to meet the expanding needs of practitioners and their clients and patients.

Book format and design. The format has been developed to enhance the book's appeal and encourage its use. The four-color design, along with the two-column format, makes the text interesting and easy to handle.

Learning aids. A number of instructional aids, described in detail later, assist both the student and instructor in the teaching-learning process. These text items will greatly stimulate and facilitate student learning and supply the practitioner with ready clinical reference tools. They apply modern nutritional science to practice needs and a number of current issues and controversies.

Illustrations. Numerous two and four color illustrations—anatomic illustrations, graphic line drawings, and photographs—help students and practitioners better understand the concepts and clinical practices presented.

Enhanced readability and student interest. Much attention has been given to directing this new text to the issues of student interest and clinical comprehension. Every effort has been made to enhance its readability and to enliven it stylistically. Great care was also exercised in the selection of all examples, case studies, models, controversial issues, and illustrations in the interest of ensuring maximal relevance.

Learning Aids Within the Text

As indicated, this new text uses many learning and guiding aids throughout the text.

Chapter openers. To alert students and practitioners to the topic of each chapter and draw them into its study, each chapter opens with a focusing illustration and brief preview text.

Chapter outlines. At the beginning of each chapter, and throughout the chapter text, the major sections are indicated by special type for ease in reading comprehension.

Key terms. Key terms important to the understanding and application of the material in patient care are presented in three steps. They are first identified in the body of the text. Some are particularly pertinent and defined on the right-hand side of each right page. And finally, all terms are collected in a comprehensive glossary, with their root meanings, for easy reference at the end of the book.This three-level approach to vocabulary development greatly improves the overall study and use of the text.

Chapter summaries. To help pull the chapter material together again as a whole, each chapter concludes with a summary of the key concepts presented and their significance or application. The student can then return to any part of the material for repeated study and clarification as needed.

Review questions for testing comprehension. To help the student understand key parts of the chapter or apply it to patient problems, questions are given after each chapter text for review and analysis of the material presented.

Chapter references. A major strength of this book is its current documentation for topics discussed, drawn from a wide selection of pertinent journals. To provide immediate access to all references cited in the chapter text, a full list of these key references is given at the end of each chapter, rather than collected at the end of the book.

Further readings. In addition to referenced material in the text, an annotated list of suggestions for further reading for added interest and study is provided at the end of each chapter. These selections extend or apply the material in the text according to individual needs or areas of special interest. The annotations help identify parts of that reference that may be pertinent to individual interest and extended information.

Issues and answers. A special feature of each chapter is a concluding brief article on nutrition-related issues or controversies based on the text discussion. These interesting and motivating studies help the student see the importance of scientific thinking and develop sound judgment and openness to varied points of view.

Case studies. In many chapters realistic case studies lead the student to apply the text material to related patient care problems. Each case is accompanied by questions for case analysis. These cases also help alert students and practitioners to applications of nutritional therapy for similar patient care needs in their own clinical work.

Diet guides. A variety of diet guides, as well as outlines of medical and nutritional management, are highlighted in each chapter.

Appendices. The appendices include a number of materials for use as reference tools and guides in learning and practice.

Food Value Tables. There are a number of food value tables including major nutrient references and expanded material on amino acids, fiber, sodium, potassium, caffeine, and fast foods.

Water and Electrolyte Balance Problems. Diagrams illustrate the answers to some basic problems in fluid-electrolyte balance encountered in clinical practice.

Nutritional Assessment Tools and Standards. Current growth and development charts, height-weight tables, anthropometric percentiles, and some standard laboratory values for blood and urine are included.

Calculating Aids and Conversion Tables. Tables and background material are provided on the metric and American systems of measurement, with an interconversion table for the two systems. Also, since most U.S. journals are adopting metric SI units for clinical laboratory values, which presents hematologic and clinical chemistry values in molar concentrations with the liter as the reference volume (for example, mol/L, mmol/L), I have inserted this form of reference where appropriate in the text.

Food Guide: Exchange Lists for Meal Planning. The current American Diabetes Association food lists are provided for diet calculations and meal patterns.

Nutritional Management Guides. Current guidelines are provided for nutritional management of cystic fibrosis and food guides for control of renal calculi.

Index. In addition to cross-referencing within the text, a complete summary index of the entire text at the end of the book includes entries made under a variety of headings and subheadings, enabling the reader to easily locate any topic desired.

Supplementary Materials

Several available supplements, designed for the parent text *Nutrition and Diet Therapy*, can also enhance the teaching-learning process with use of this new clinical text. More information on these helpful packages may be obtained from the publisher.

Instructor's manual. This valuable tool features suggested course syllabuses; chapter reviews; behavioral objectives; key terms; chapter outlines with teaching notes on controversial topics; "Nutrition in the News"; additional resources, including slides, films and filmstrips; transparency masters; and an extensive test-item bank of over 1500 questions.

Test bank computer software. Qualified adopters of this text receive a test bank software package. This software is available in versions for both Macintosh and IBM PC-type (DOS) computers. These programs provide a unique combination of user-friendly aids and enables the instructor to select, edit, delete, or add questions, and construct and print tests and answer keys.

Transparency acetates. Illustration of important concepts are available in transparency acetates. These useful tools facilitate learning of key concepts discussed in the text.

Mosby diet simple 2.1 software. This interactive nutrient analysis software includes a unique food list with more than 2250 items, selected activities, and food exchange lists. The program allows students to enter food intake and physical activities to determine total kcaloric intake and energy output over a certain period of time.

A Personal Approach

In the past, users of my major comprehensive parent text have responded very positively to the person-centered approach I have tried to develop. In this new concise clinical offspring I have continued to strengthen this approach.

Personal writing style. In writing the entire book, I have used a fresh and highly readable personal style to reflect the very personal nature of human nutrition and its application in health care and treatment of disease to communicate more directly with the reader. I wish to share my own self and feelings, born of many years of experience in clinical work and teaching, and to create interest and involvement in both learning and sound humanistic practice. In this manner I express my concern for students and their learning, as well as for individuals and clients and their perspectives and needs.

Personal files. Much of the personal application in these pages is drawn from my personal patient/client files and the many varied clinical and personal problems I have encountered in practice as a clinical nutrition specialist and educator. My patients and students have taught me much of what I have attempted to share with you.

Balanced behavioral and physical science base. Along with a strong physiologic and biochemical research base for nutrition science and practice, I have tried to use a balancing emphasis on the behavioral sciences and the psychosocial base of nutritional patterns, health care, and health behaviors. These are twin realities of human life which we must constantly deal with in clinical practice.

Practical application. All the chapters supply expanded practical application of current research in very realistic human terms. There are no "pat" answers to many health care problems, and individual situations often require individual solutions. In every case this approach to individualized care is evident throughout, in the many clinical application boxes, the text itself, and the illustrations.

Acknowledgements

A text of this sort is never the work of one person. It develops into the planned product through the committed hands and hearts of a number of persons. It would be impossible to name all the individuals involved, but several groups deserve special recognition.

First of all, I am grateful to the reviewers who gave their valuable time and skills to strengthen the manuscript:

Sara Long Anderson
Southern Illinois University, Carbondale

Franklin S. Carman III
Western Nevada Community College

Margarette Harden
Texas Tech University

Jean T. Hassell
Youngstown State University

Donna C. Henry
Wabash Valley College

Joan Johnson
University of Wisconsin, Oshkosh

Alice K. Lindeman
Indiana University

Mary C. Mitchell
The Ohio State University

John Orta
California State University, Los Angeles

Noreen B. Schvaneveldt
Utah State University

Barbara Van Droof
Shoreline Community College

Of these reviewers, I also thank Sara Long Anderson for her additional help with a number of the Clinical Application boxes where appropriate, and her input for my writing of Chapters 9, 11, 12, and 13.

Second, I am indebted to Mosby and the many persons there who had a part in this new project. I especially thank my editor-in-chief, James M. Smith, whose insight and considerable talent initiated this new book as a separate clinical nutrition text from my major comprehensive book. I also thank the very capable editorial and book production staffs, including Vicki Malinee, Loren Stevenson, and Suzanne Fannin who worked with me throughout the initial production of my background comprehensive text, and Terry Eynon and Kathleen Teal who managed the development of this new concise diet therapy text to its final pages. To the Mosby marketing and product managers and the many fine Mosby marketing representatives throughout the country, I owe a great deal for their help in guiding the result of my efforts to its ultimate users. I am also grateful for the help of Production Director, Peggy Fagen, and all the associated artists and photographers who participated in this project.

Third, I am very grateful to all those persons who worked with me on my own staff during the various stages of manuscript production, especially to my research assistants, Cindy LeClaire, Mary Herbert, and Mary Ann Lebar, who gathered the comprehensive materials I requested. I also owe a special debt of gratitude to copy editor, business manager and computer systems analyst, Jim Williams, and to Mary Herbert and Ruth Carroll for their sensitive support.

Fourth, my life has been enriched over the years by my many students, interns, colleagues, clients, and patients; their contributions are revealed in all my work. Each one has taught me something about human experience, and I am grateful for those opportunities for personal growth.

And finally, but most of all, I am grateful for the loving support of my family, who always provide refuge in time of need and share both my problems and celebrations throughout my work. All these dear persons close to me stimulate me enormously and never cease to share in all of my writing projects.

Sue Rodwell Williams

CONTENTS IN BRIEF

CONTENTS

CHAPTER 1

Nutritional Assessment and Therapy in Patient Care

CHAPTER OUTLINE

The Therapeutic Process
Nutrition Assessment: Data Base and Analysis
Analysis and Initial Planning
Nutrition Intervention: Food Plan and Management
Evaluation: Quality Patient Care

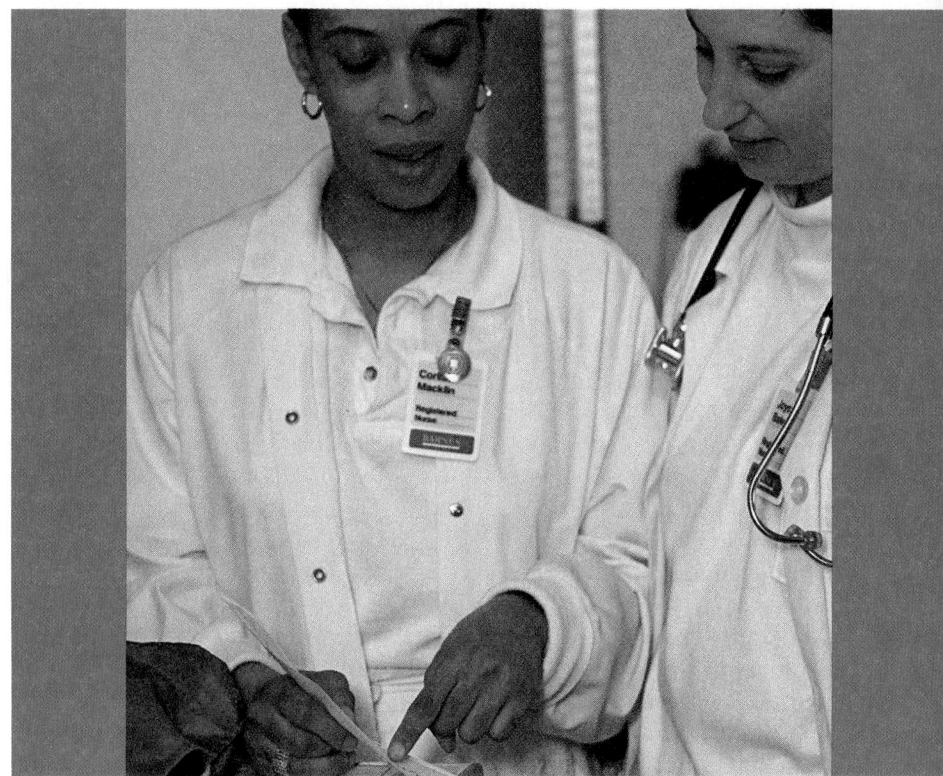

About 2500 years have passed since Hippocrates admonished us to pay closer attention to the significant connection between nutrition and disease, but we are only now, in more modern scientific times, beginning to catch a glimmer of the real depth of his valuable instruction.

This book applies information on nutritional science, community nutrition, and life cycle needs for health maintenance to clinical nutrition needs in disease.

Persons face acute illness or chronic disease and its treatment in a variety of settings: the acute care hospital, the long-term rehabilitation center, the extended care facility, the clinic, the private office, and the home. In all instances, however, nutritional care is fundamental.

It supports any medical treatment being given and frequently provides the primary therapy.

Comprehensive nutritional assessment anchors appropriate nutritional therapy to identified patient needs. Clinical nutritionists with sound clinical judgment and expertise work with an effective clinical care team. Together these professionals provide an essential component for successful medical treatment. They assist the patient's recovery from illness and injury, help the person maintain follow-up care to promote health, and help control health care costs.

This chapter focuses on the essential first step in comprehensive nutritional care: assessing nutritional needs and goals. Wherever the place of care and whatever the need, the health care team of practitioners, patient, and family work together to support the healing process and promote health.

The Therapeutic Process

Stress of the Therapeutic Encounter

The therapeutic encounter between health care providers and their patients occurs under stressful conditions at best. Especially for the hospitalized patient, the nutritional toll is additional. Bed rest itself brings detrimental effects on the body's physiology.[1] For example, after just 3 days lying supine in bed the body begins to lose its resistance to the pull of gravity, and inactivity diminishes muscle tone, bone calcium, plasma volume, and gastric secretions and brings some impairment of glucose tolerance and shifts in body fluids and electrolytes. Also, hospital or **iatrogenic** malnutrition has been widely documented. In addition to the hypermetabolic and physiologic stress of injury or illness, patients may have inadequate nourishment from a number of problems. A fundamental problem is lack of adequate admission nutrition screening or follow-up monitoring to identify patients at malnutrition risk and to provide essential nutritional support immediately.[2] Other problems contributing to lack of adequate nourishment include (1) highly restrictive diets remaining on order and unsupplemented too long, (2) unserved meals because of interference of medical procedures and clinical tests, and (3) unmonitored lack of patient appetite.

An injured or ill patient, a unique person, requires special treatment and care. At the same time, a sometimes formidable array of health care providers seek to determine needs and implement what they perceive to be appropriate care. It is no surprise that the course does not always run smoothly or that patients often feel intimidated and powerless. Sometimes our convoluted system and highly specialized technology get in our way, and we lose sight of our reason for being—to meet individual human needs and personal care. It is at such times we need to remind ourselves of the fundamental ethical principles guiding all our patient care, which should ensure that all we do must (1) *benefit* the patient, (2) do *no harm,* (3) preserve the patient's *autonomy,* (4) *disclose* full and truthful information for patient decisions concerning care, and (5) provide *social justice.*[3] Such ethical behavior is based on the overriding principles of right action found within the Anglo-American law, which emphasizes the basic rights of *privacy* and *free choice.*[4] Constant open and validating communication is essential for such ethical practices, among the health team members and between the health care providers and the patient and family. It is especially important for many stressed elderly patients.[5] In this team effort for quality nutritional care, the clinical dietitian (a clinical nutrition specialist), with the physician, carries the primary responsibility. The nurse and other primary care practitioners provide essential support.

Focus of Care

Patient-Centered Care

The primary basic principle in nutritional practice, too often overlooked in many routine procedures, is evident: to be valid, nutritional care must be *person-centered.* In this renewed "partnership" **paradigm** for patient-centered health care, the patient must be the senior partner.[6,7] It must be based on initial and continuing identified needs and updated constantly with the patient, not only to provide essential physical care but also to support the patient's personal needs for maintaining self-esteem and control as much as possible. Another fundamental fact also needs emphasis: remember that, despite all methods, tools, and technologies described in this text or elsewhere, ***the most therapeutic tool you will ever use is yourself.*** It is to this seemingly simple yet profound healing encounter that you bring yourself.

Health Care Team

In the setting of the individual medical center, with its strengths and despite its shortcomings and within the essential team care provided, the clinical nutritionist or dietitian must care for the patient's nutritional needs in close relationship to the medical and nursing care. Sensitive communication skills are essential for all ages and degrees of health problems. Determining the patient's nutritional care needs is the clinical nutritionist's initial and ongoing responsibility.

Phases of the Care Process

Five distinct yet constantly interacting phases are essential in the therapeutic care process.

Assessment: Data Base

A broad base of relative information about the patient's nutritional status, food habits, and life situations provides the necessary knowledge for making valid initial assessments. Useful background information may come from a variety of sources, such as the patient, the patient's chart, the family or other relatives and friends, oral or written communication with other hospital personnel or staff, and related research. A number of valuable nutritional assessment tools have been developed, some of which are described in detail in this discussion.

Analysis: Problem List

The data collected must be carefully analyzed to determine specific patient needs. Some needs are immediately evident, and others develop as the situation unfolds. On the basis of this analysis, a list of problems may be formed to guide continuing care activities.

Planning Care: Needs and Goals

As problems are identified, valid care is planned. The plan must always be based on personal needs and goals of the individual patient, as well as the identified medical care requirements.

Implementing Care: Actions

The patient care plan is put into action according to realistic and appropriate activities within each situation. In this case nutritional care and education involve decisions and actions concerning an appropriate mode of feeding and the training and education needs for the patient, staff, and family to carry it out.

Evaluating and Recording Care: Results

As every care activity is carried out, results are carefully checked to see whether the identified needs have been met. Then any appropriate revisions of the care plan are made as needed for continuing care. These results are carefully recorded in the patient's medical record. Clear documentation of all activities is essential.

In the following discussion, we look at each of these phases in terms of quality nutritional care. We focus on methods and tools of nutritional assessment, the practical management of nutritional therapy and care, the maintenance of an effective medical record, and the ways of ensuring quality standards of nutritional care.

Nutritional Assessment: Data Base and Analysis

The first step in nutritional assessment, as with assessing any situation to determine needs and actions, is to collect pertinent information—a data base—for use in identifying needs. The basic methods used in clinical nutritional assessment to identify the individual patient's needs may be grouped in four types of activities, often called the *ABCD* approach:

- *A*nthropometrics
- *B*iochemical tests
- *C*linical observations
- *D*ietary and personal histories

Each part of this approach is important because no single parameter alone directly measures individual nutritional status or determines problems and needs. Furthermore, the overall resulting picture must then be interpreted within the context of personal, social, and health factors that may alter nutritional requirements. Only with this type of comprehensive evaluation can nutritional assessment become the real index to the quality of life that it should be.

A broad number of tests may be used for research purposes in a large facility with access to highly sophisticated equipment. However, the procedures outlined next provide a good base in general clinical practice for assessing and monitoring a patient's nutritional status and planning nutritional therapy, maintenance, and rehabilitation. Each assessment tool has strengths and limitations, so careful selection and skillful use of combined methods appropriate to individual patient condition, together with their interpretation according to standard references for age and sex and to personal situation, are all essential for quality nutritional care.

Anthropometrics

Skill gained through careful practice is necessary to minimize the margin of error in making body measurements. Selection and maintenance of proper equipment and attention to careful technique are essential in securing valid data.

Weight

It is necessary to use regular clinic beam scales with nondetachable weights. An additional weight attachment is available for use with obese persons. Metric scales with readings to the nearest 20 g provide specific data; however, the standard clinic scale is satisfactory. All scales should be checked frequently and calibrated

iatrogenic • Caused by treatment of a preexisting condition.

paradigm • A pattern or model serving as an example; a standard or ideal for practice or behavior based on a fundamental value or theme.

every 3 to 4 months for continued accuracy. Hospitalized patients should be weighed at consistent times; for example, before breakfast and after the bladder has been emptied. Clinic patients should be weighed without shoes in light, indoor clothing or an examining gown.

After careful reading and recording of the patient's weight, obtain information about the usual body weight and check standard height-weight tables for comparison. Interpret present weight in terms of percentage of usual and standard body weight for height. Check for any significant weight loss: 1% to 2% in the past week, 5% over the past month, 7.5% during the last 3 months, or 10% in the last 6 months. A check of unexplained weight loss in elderly persons is particularly important, since it may be a clue to depression or cancer and needs to be on record and followed up.[8,9] These amounts of weight loss are significant, however, more than this, the rate of weight loss is severe. Values charted in the patient's record should indicate percentage of weight change.

Body Mass Index

The weight and height measures are used to calculate the patient's body mass index (BMI), a ratio that is used in evaluating obesity states:

$$\text{BMI} = \frac{\text{Weight (kg)}}{\text{Height (m)}^2}$$

The metric conversion factors involved are 1 kg equals 2.2 lb and 1 m equals 39.37 in. The desired health maintenance BMI range for adults is 20 to 25 kg/m^2. Health risks associated with obesity begin in the range of 25 to 30 kg/m^2. Values above 40 kg/m^2 indicate severe obesity.

Elbow Breadth

There has been some question about the arbitrary categories of frame size for height and weight used in the most recent tables of the Metropolitan Life Insurance Company.[10] Thus new standards of weight and body composition by frame size and height have been developed with frame size based on measurement of elbow breadth.[11] With patient's arm extended and forearm bent upward to form a 90° angle and using a specially developed instrument such as the Frameter, measure the distance (cm) between the two outer bony landmarks that indicate elbow breadth, the medial and lateral epicondyles of the humerus. An anthropometric kit containing the reference standards manual and the Frameter, as well as skinfold calipers and metric tapes, is available from the research and development group (Health Products, 2126 Ridge, Ann Arbor, MI 48104).

Ratio of Height to Wrist Circumference

An alternate method of determining body frame size is by calculating the ratio of individual height to wrist circumference.[12] With the patient's right hand extended and using a nonstretchable metric tape, measure the wrist circumference at the joint just distal (toward the fingers) to the bony "wristbone" protrusion, the styloid process. Then calculate the height to wrist circumference ratio:

$$\text{Ratio} = \frac{\text{Height (cm)}}{\text{Wrist circumference (cm)}}$$

Interpret the results by the following standard:

Frame size	Male ratio values	Female ratio values
Small	10.4	11.0
Medium	9.6 to 10.4	10.1 to 11.0
Large	9.6	10.1

Height

If possible, use a fixed measuring stick or tape on a true vertical, flat wall or a rigid, freestanding instrument with a movable block squared at a true right angle against the vertical flat surface that can be moved down to the exact crown of the patient's head. If this device is not available, the movable measuring rod on the platform clinic scales may be used with reasonable accuracy. Have the patient stand as straight as possible, without shoes or cap, heels together, and looking straight ahead. The heels, buttocks, shoulders, and head should be touching the wall or vertical surface of the measuring rod.

Read the measure carefully and compare with previous recordings to detect possible errors or to note growth of children or diminishing height of adults. Metric measures of height in centimeters provide accurate data.

Mid–Upper-Arm Circumference

Use a centimeter tape made of nonstretchable material such as metal, plastic, or fiberglass (not cloth or paper), to locate the midpoint of the upper arm on the nondominant arm, unless it is affected by edema: (1) have the patient bend the arm at the elbow, forming a 90° angle with the palm up; (2) place the tape vertically on the posterior of the arm; and (3) mark the arm midpoint between the acromial process of the scapula (bony protrusion on the posterior of the upper shoulder) and the olecranon process of the elbow (bony part of the elbow). Measure the upper arm circumference at this midpoint, securing the tape snugly but not so tightly as to make an indentation. Read and record the measure accurately to the nearest tenth of a centimeter. Compare the measurement with previous measurements to note possible changes.

Triceps Skinfold Thickness

The triceps skinfold thickness (TSF) measurement provides an estimate of subcutaneous fat reserves. Together with the mid–upper-arm circumference at the same spot, the TSF enables the practitioner to make a good estimate of the mid–upper-arm muscle circumference as a status indicator of the protein compartment of the skeletal muscle mass.

Use a standard millimeter skinfold caliper, such as the Lange, Harpenden, or Holtain. Use your thumb and forefinger to grasp vertically a portion of the patient's skin and subcutaneous fat about 1 to 2 cm above the previously marked mid–upper-arm point. Pull the skinfold gently away from the underlying muscle. Place the caliper jaws over the lifted skinfold at the midpoint mark while maintaining the skinfold grasp. Read the measure of the compressed skinfold to the nearest full or fraction of a millimeter within 2 to 3 seconds after releasing the caliper extender. Avoid excessive pressure or delayed reading. For increased accuracy take three measures and use the mean for comparison with age and sex standards in terms of percentage of the standard and for calculations of mid–upper-arm muscle circumference. Record the results and compare the mean value with the patient's previous measures to note any changes.

Subscapular Skinfold Thickness

Use the back left side of the body to measure the subscapular skinfold thickness (SSF). Locate the subscapular site just below the tip of the scapula (left shoulder blade) and gently grasp a skinfold as before. Place the caliper jaws on a downward and lateral axis. Read and record the measure in the same manner described for the TSF measure.

Mid–Upper-Arm Muscle Circumference

This derived value gives an indirect estimate of the body's skeletal muscle mass. Convert the TSF mean value (millimeters) to centimeters (divide the millimeter value by 10) and then calculate the mid–upper-arm muscle circumference (MAMC) by the following formula:

$$\text{MAMC (cm)} = \text{MAC (cm)} - [3.14 \times \text{TSF (cm)}]$$

If desired, the TSF may be left in millimeters, as measured, and the value of the factor (pi; π) in the formula changed to 0.314.

To interpret these anthropometric measures for monitoring of the patient's nutritional status, compare them as percentages of standards provided in reference tables. Reference standards may come from those based on the classic international nutritional work of Jelliffe or from more recently developed American standards such as those by Frisancho. Some examples of these standards are given in Appendix Q.

Alternate Measures for Nonambulatory Patients

The body measures described previously, except for usual methods of measuring height and weight of ambulatory patients, may be used with nonambulatory patients. Three alternate measures provide values for estimating height and weight of patients confined to bed.

Total arm length. With the patient holding an arm straight down by the side and using a nonstretchable metric tape, measure the arm length from the tip of the acromial process of the scapula at the shoulder to the end of the arm at the styloid process of the ulna at the wrist. The measure of total arm length (TAL) is used as an alternate means of determining body height by comparing results to height equivalent standards.[13] Investigators have also found this method to be a useful alternative to standing body height of ambulatory patients, especially in older persons, in whom a general thinning of weight-bearing cartilages, the "bent knee gait," and a possible **kyphosis** of the spine may make height measurement inaccurate.

Armspan. Armspan has been shown to approximate height at maturity and is relatively independent of aging. Thus it is an alternative to height for adult measures, especially as a reliable and practical measure for height in nonambulatory elderly persons. A reliable body mass index may also be obtained using this alternative height measure. In fact, tests indicate that use of the armspan instead of height in calculating BMI in elderly patients may give a more accurate result.[14] If the patient can stand, the full armspan measure is taken with back against the wall and arms outstretched at right angles to the body with palms facing forward. With the help of an assistant and a flexible steel tape measure marked in centimeters, the full span from fingertip to fingertip is measured, passing in front of the clavicles. This same measure may be taken in the recumbent position, holding the arms

kyphosis • Increased, abnormal convexity of the upper part of the spine; hunchback.

TABLE 1–1

Ideal Weight and Urinary Creatinine Values for Height (Adults)*

Height (cm)	Females		Males	
	Weight (kg)	Creatinine (mg)	Weight (kg)	Creatinine (mg)
140	44.9			
141	45.4			
142	45.9			
143	46.4			
144	47.0			
145	47.5		51.9	
146	48.0		52.4	
147	48.6	828	52.9	
148	49.2		53.5	
149	49.8		54.0	
150	50.4	852	54.5	
151	51.0		55.0	
152	51.5		55.6	
153	52.0	878	56.1	
154	52.5		56.6	
155	53.1	901	57.2	
156	53.7		57.9	
157	54.3	922	58.6	1284
158	54.9		59.3	
159	55.5		59.9	
160	56.2	949	60.5	1325
161	56.9		61.1	
162	57.6		61.7	
163	58.3	979	62.3	1362
164	58.9		62.9	
165	59.5	1005	63.5	1387
166	60.1		64.0	
167	60.7	1040	64.6	1421
168	61.4		65.2	
169	62.1		65.9	
170		1075	66.6	1465
171			67.3	
172			68.0	
173		1111	68.7	1516
174			69.4	
175		1139	70.1	1552
176			70.8	
177		1169	71.6	1589
178			72.4	
179			73.3	
180		1204	74.2	1639
181			75.0	
182			75.8	
183		1241	76.5	1692
184			77.3	
185			78.1	1735
186			78.9	
187				1776
188				
189				
190				1826

Data from Jelliffe DB: *The assessment of the nutritional status of the community,* Geneva, 1966, World Health Organization.
*1959 Metropolitan Life Insurance Company Standards corrected for nude weight without shoe heels.

TABLE 1–2
Clinical Signs of Nutritional Status

Body area	Signs of good nutrition	Signs of poor nutrition
General appearance	Alert, responsive	Listless, apathetic, cachectic
Weight	Normal for height, age, body build	Overweight or underweight (special concern for underweight)
Posture	Erect, arms and legs straight	Sagging shoulders, sunken chest, humped back
Muscles	Well-developed, firm, good tone, some fat under skin	Flaccid, poor tone, undeveloped, tender, "wasted" appearance, cannot walk properly
Nervous control	Good attention span, not irritable or restless, normal reflexes, psychologic stability	Inattentive, irritable, confused, burning and tingling of hands and feet (paresthesia), loss of position and vibratory sense, weakness and tenderness of muscles (may result in inability to walk), decrease or loss of ankle and knee reflexes
Gastrointestinal function	Good appetite and digestion, normal regular elimination, no palpable (perceptible to touch) organs or masses	Anorexia, indigestion, constipation or diarrhea, liver or spleen enlargement
Cardiovascular function	Normal heart rate and rhythm, no murmurs, normal blood pressure for age	Rapid heart rate (above 100 beats/min tachycardia), enlarged heart, abnormal rhythm, elevated blood pressure
General vitality	Endurance, energetic, sleeps well, vigorous	Easily fatigued, no energy, falls asleep easily, looks tired, apathetic
Hair	Shiny, lustrous, firm, not easily plucked, healthy scalp	Stringy, dull, brittle, dry, thin and sparse, depigmented, easily plucked
Skin (general)	Smooth, slightly moist, good color	Rough, dry, scaly, pale, pigmented, irritated, bruises, petechiae
Face and neck	Skin color uniform, smooth, healthy appearance, not swollen	Greasy, discolored, scaly, swollen, skin dark over cheeks and under eyes, lumpiness or flakiness of skin around nose and mouth
Lips	Smooth, good color, moist, not chapped or swollen	Dry, scaly, swollen, redness and swelling (cheilosis), or angular lesions at corners of the mouth or fissures or scars (stomatitis)
Mouth, oral membranes	Reddish pink mucous membranes in oral cavity	Swollen, boggy oral mucous membranes
Gums	Good pink color, healthy, red, no swelling or bleeding	Spongy, bleed easily, marginal redness, inflamed, gums receding
Tongue	Good pink color or deep reddish in appearance, not swollen or smooth, surface papillae present, no lesions	Swelling, scarlet and raw, magenta color, beefy (glossitis), hyperemic and hypertrophic papillae, atrophic papillae
Teeth	No cavities, no pain, bright, straight, no crowding, well-shaped jaw, clean, no discoloration	Unfilled caries, absent teeth, worn surfaces mottled (fluorosis), malpositioned
Eyes	Bright, clear, shiny, no sores at corner of eyelids, membranes moist and healthy pink color, no prominent blood vessels or mount of tissue on sclera, no fatigue circles beneath	Eye membranes pale (pale conjunctivae), redness of membrane (conjunctival infection), dryness of infection, Bitot's spots, redness and fissuring of eyelid corners (angular palpebritis), dryness of eye membrane (conjunctival xerosis), dull appearance of cornea (corneal xerosis), soft cornea (keratomalacia)
Neck (glands)	No enlargement	Thyroid enlarged
Nails	Firm, pink	Spoon-shaped (koilonychia), brittle, ridged
Legs, feet	No tenderness, weakness, or swelling; good color	Edema, tender calf, tingling, weakness
Skeleton	No malformations	Bowlegs, knock-knees, chest deformity at diaphragm, beaded ribs, prominent scapulas

Modified from Williams SR: Nutritional guidance in prenatal care. In Worthington-Roberts BS, Vermeersch J, Williams SR: *Nutrition in pregnancy and lactation,* St Louis, 1985, Mosby.

roughly in line with both shoulders and supporting the elbows if needed in frail persons. For patients with limited movement of the shoulder or elbow because of osteoarthritis or deformities, a recumbent halfspan measure from the center of the sternal notch in the body midline to the fingertip may be measured and doubled to achieve the same result.

Knee height. With the patient lying in the supine position and the left knee and ankle each bent at 90° angles, place the fixed blade of the special sliding broad-blade caliper under the heel of the left foot and the sliding blade on top of the thigh about 2 in from the kneecap. Press the top blade securely and read the measurement to 0.1 cm.[15] A simple comparative measure of knee-to-floor height in the sitting position, from the outside bony point just under the kneecap, indicating the head of the tibia, down to the floor surface, may also be used.[16] Use measurement values as alternate means of calculating body height:

$$\text{Height (women)} = [(1.83 \times \text{knee height}) - (0.24 \times \text{age})] + 84.88$$
$$\text{Height (men)} = [(2.02 \times \text{knee height}) - (0.04 \times \text{age})] + 64.19$$

Calf circumference. With the patient in the same supine position, the left knee bent at a 90° angle, and the use of a nonstretchable metric tape, measure the calf circumference at the largest point by pulling the tape snug but not so tight as to indent tissue. Read the measurement to the nearest 0.1 cm. Use the patient's calf circumference (CC) measure with three previous values—knee height (KH), mid–upper-arm circumference, and subscapular skinfold—as an alternate means of deriving body weight[15,17]:

$$\text{Weight (women)} = (1.27 \times CC) + (0.87 \times KH) + (0.98 \times MAC) + (0.4 \times SSF) - 62.35$$

$$\text{Weight (men)} = (0.98 \times CC) + (1.16 \times KH) + (1.73 \times MAC) + (0.37 \times SSF) - 81.69$$

Biochemical Tests

A number of biochemical tests are available for studying nutritional status. Those most commonly used for assessing and monitoring nutritional status and planning nutritional care in clinical practice are listed in the following discussion. Results of laboratory data should always be interpreted by the standards for normal values established by the individual laboratory and its methods used. General ranges for normal values are given in many standard texts and various reference manuals. Selected examples of normal values are given in Appendix R. Interpretations of results according to risk are discussed in Chapter 4 in relation to parenteral feeding.

Measures of Plasma Protein Compartment

Basic tests measuring plasma protein are the following:

- *Serum albumin.* Serum albumin (ALB) is the body's protector of blood volume and fluid-electrolyte balance. Depletion of ALB is associated with visceral protein impairment, and the test is a basic screen for malnutrition. Normal values range from 3.5 to 5.5 g/dl.
- *Hemoglobin.* The test for hemoglobin (Hg) provides a serum measure of red blood cell. Normal values are for women, 14 g/100 ml, and for men, 16 g/100 ml. The test for hematocrit (Hct) provides a measure of packed red blood cell volume. Normal values are for women, 42 ml/100 ml, and for men, 47 ml/100 ml. Depletions are associated with nutritional anemia.

Additional tests measuring plasma protein are the following:

- *Prealbumin.* Prealbumin (PAB) is a thyroxin-binding protein and provides a sensitive measure of visceral body protein. Normal values range from 15.7 to 29.6 mg/dl.
- *Serum transferrin.* Serum transferrin is the body's chief iron-storage protein and has a normal saturation value of 20% to 55%, or total iron-binding capacity (TIBC) with a normal value range of 250 to 410 μg/100 ml. A newly corrected formula has been developed for deriving the value for either transferrin or TIBC:

$$\text{Transferrin} = (\text{TIBC} \times 0.76) + 18$$

Measures of Immune System Integrity: Anergy

The basic test for immune system integrity measures lymphocytes, the white blood cell components of the body's immune system. An increase in the number of lymphocytes reflects infection or antigen invaders. The normal value is 34% of the blood cell count or a count of $2500/mm^3$. In addition, skin testing provides delayed sensitivity measures of common recall antigens such as mumps, *Candida,* the purified protein derivative of tuberculin (PPD), and streptokinase-streptodornase (SKSD). Skin tests are read at 24 and 48 hours with a wheal greater than 5 mm indicating a positive test and the presence of one positive test indicating intact immunity.

Measures of Protein Metabolism: 24-Hour Urine Tests

Two urine tests that measure protein metabolism are the following:

- *Urinary creatinine.* Total 24-hour excretion is interpreted in terms of ideal creatinine excretion for height—the creatinine-height index (CHI). Some standard adult urinary creatinine values, which reflect normal creatinine excretion from regular tissue turnover, are given in Table 1-1 in relation to height and weight. A patient's results are given as a percentage of this normal value. An elevated creatinine excretion value indicates increased tissue breakdown and loss. Tables of normal urinary creatinine values for age and sex are given in standard reference texts. In general, normal adult creatinine excretion ranges from 1.0 to 1.5 g/24 hr.
- *Urinary urea nitrogen.* Total 24-hour nitrogen excretion is used with calculated dietary nitrogen intake over the same 24-hour period to determine the patient's nitrogen balance:

$$\text{Nitrogen balance} = \frac{\text{Protein intake}}{6.25} - (\text{urinary urea nitrogen} + 4)$$

The formula factor of 4 represents additional nitrogen loss through the feces and skin. Urinary urea nitrogen excretion reflects metabolism of dietary protein, as the nitrogen balance formula indicates, and is a measure of the adequacy of protein nutrition.

Nutritional Assessment: When Being Objective Does Not Always Mean Being Objective

TO PROBE FURTHER

Nutritionists, and other health professionals, like numbers. To identify malnutrition, they monitor serum levels of liver-secreted plasma proteins such as albumin and transferrin, take anthropometric measurements, and determine creatinine-height indexes and cell-mediated immunity response. One study now suggests that these numbers do not add up to the accuracy of the clinical examination in determining a patient's nutritional status.

Researchers from the University of Toronto and Toronto General Hospital suggest that objective measurements may sometimes be inaccurate because they are influenced by several factors: (1) the effects of the disease process itself (rather than the distinct issue of malnutrition) on changes in nutrient levels, (2) delayed response to nutritional depletion (or repletion) because of the relatively long half-lives of indexes such as serum albumin and transferrin, and (3) the wide range of confidence limits in nutritional measurements.

These workers found that two physician clinical evaluators were able to agree on the nutritional status of 81% of 59 surgical patients examined independently. The history—emphasizing weight loss, edema, anorexia, unusual food intakes, and so on—and physical examination—stressing jaundice, muscle wasting, edema, conditions of oral structures, and similar findings—provided enough information for them to come to conclusions that agreed with objective evaluations.

Does this mean that laboratory tests should be placed in "semiretirement," limited to use in epidemiologic surveys instead of evaluating individuals? These researchers think they should, but they do acknowledge that accurate assessment tests do exist, such as total body nitrogen and total body potassium, although these are not generally available. They also suggest the possibility of combining several known indexes to make a more sensitive one, even though this lends itself to the possibility of leaving out one measurement that could have an important effect on the calculations.

However, they do emphasize an important point: nutritional status is as dependent on what you *see* as what you read on a laboratory sheet.

REFERENCES

Baker JP et al: Nutritional assessment: a comparison of clinical judgment and objective measurements, *N Engl J Med* 306(16):969, 1982.

Detsky AS et al: What is subjective global assessment of nutritional status? *J Parenter Enteral Nutr* 11:8, 1987.

Clinical Observations

Careful attention to physical signs of possible malnutrition provides an added dimension to the overall assessment of general nutritional status (see *To Probe Further*, above). A description to guide a general examination for such signs is given in Table 1-2. Make a careful descriptive record of any such observations in the patient's medical record. Other physical data may include pulse rate, respiration, temperature, and blood pressure. A study of the common procedures of a normal physical examination provides useful background orientation.

Dietary and Personal Histories

A careful dietary history provides essential information about the patient's usual food habits. It includes a personal history to relate influences on food behaviors such as family and cultural background, occupation, living situation, and other economic, psychosocial, and personal problems, including extent of alcohol use.[18] These data provide a fundamental base for personal nutritional assessment. However, obtaining accurate information about basic food patterns and dietary intake is difficult at best. We need methods that simplify data collection and analyses and provide information as accurately as possible on the intakes of individuals. A sensitive clinical nutritionist or nurse may obtain useful information using one or more of the basic tools described next.

Specific 24-Hour Food Record

Provide a careful and simple explanation for your patients concerning the purpose of the food record. For example, if a nitrogen balance study and a creatinine-height index is being done, the food record is needed for making the final calculations. During the same 24-hour period of urine collection for the creatinine and urea nitrogen excretion tests, a specific and detailed record of all food intake by the patient is essential for determining total protein and energy values of the diet. The protein value is used to calculate the nitrogen balance by the formula given previously. The kcaloric value gives an indication of how well the patient is meeting goals for energy input. These goals are based on the energy expenditure demands of the patient's illness or health maintenance

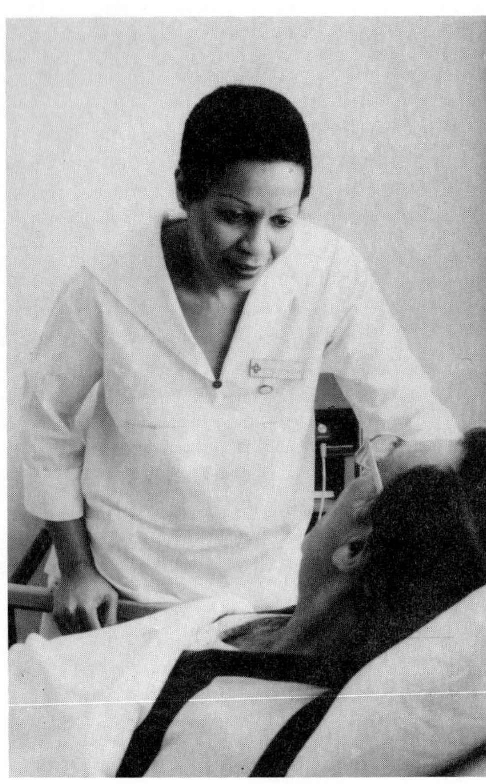

FIG. 1-1 Interviewing of patient to plan personal care.

requirements. At times a full dietary analysis of all nutrient values is needed and is usually done by computer (see *Issues and Answers*, p. 19). But a 24-hour recall or record has limited value in determining basic food habits.

Diet History

General knowledge of the patient's basic eating habits is needed to determine any possible nutritional deficiencies. In conjunction with the patient's usual living situation and related food attitudes and behaviors, medical status, and treatment, the nutrition interview provides an essential base for further personal nutrition counseling and planning of care (Fig. 1-1). For example, an activity-associated day's food intake pattern schedule may guide you in obtaining a fairly valid picture of food habits and eating behaviors. Simple models of portion sizes help determine quantities of food consumed.[19] In addition to food and nutrition information, you need to know about any food intolerances, allergies, or deletions because of religious food laws or personal aversions. Also, drug therapy data from the medical record and the patient or family are essential to determine any possible drug-nutrient interactions involved or any teaching needed by the patient (see Chapter 2).[20] Carefully research all drugs your patient is taking, prescription and over-the-counter, and note any food or nutrient interactions involved.

Food Records

A 3- to 7-day food record is a helpful tool for assessing food patterns, especially when used in conjunction with a comprehensive initial diet history. A 3-day record is generally sufficient for determining overall food and nutrient intake. For validity, careful review of needs and goals and instructions for accurate recordings are necessary. Then a follow-up review with the patient for portion sizes and methods of preparation, as well as brand names of products, prepares the record for nutritional analysis. A number of appropriate software programs are available that make final nutritional computer analysis a simple matter. But, of course, the accuracy of the computer analysis depends entirely on the accuracy of the food record.

Food Frequency Questionnaire

The purpose of the food frequency questionnaire (FFQ) is to help determine food intake over an extended period of time, which provides useful data, especially in combination with specific food records.[21,22] It is useful, for example, when investigating

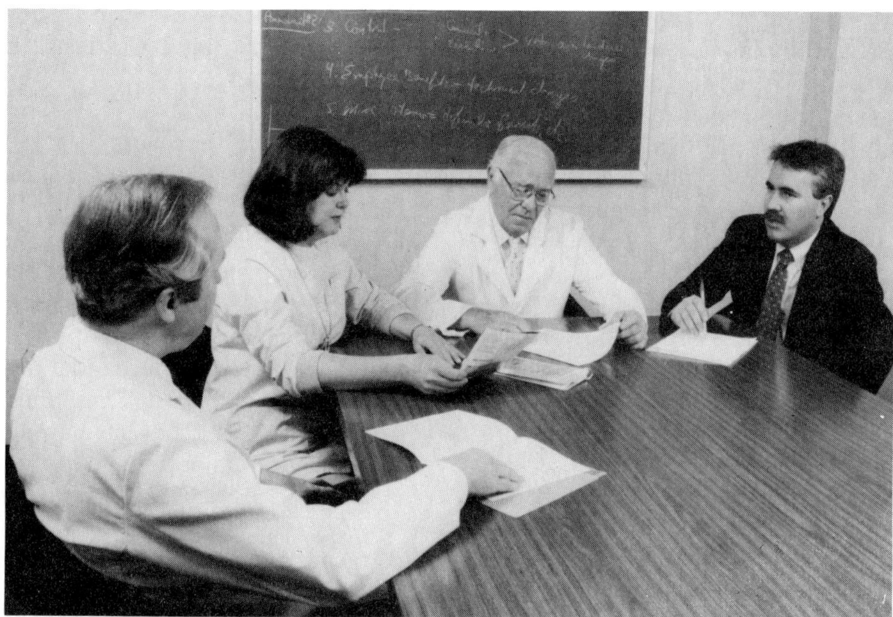

FIG. 1-2 The health team conference for planning patient care. Physician, nurse, clinical nutritionist, and social worker review patient's progress and needs.

possible relations of individual food habits to overall risk of disease such as heart disease or cancer. The FFQ has two basic parts: (1) a list of foods and (2) a scale for checking frequency of use over a given period of time. The food list may be comprehensive to assess overall food habits or a specific selection to focus on use of particular food sources of nutrients related to the disease under study. Quantitative FFQs also include a means of measuring portions of food used.

Analysis and Initial Planning

Data Analysis

All the various nutritional data for each individual patient, collected by the clinical nutritionist and other team members through the broad assessment activities previously described, must be analyzed carefully to make a valid nutritional diagnosis and plan of care. Every health team member participates in this analysis through various communications, discussions, case conferences, records, and reports (Fig. 1-2). The nutritionist serves as coordinator of these activities and carries a major responsibility on the team for interpreting nutrition-related data and making decisions and recommendations concerning any primary or secondary nutritional states. Any nutritional deficiency disease, which may underlie and contribute to the overall illness, may be classified as primary or secondary, depending on the cause. *Primary* deficiency disease results from a lack of an essential nutrient in the diet, for whatever reason. *Secondary* nutrition disease results from one or more barriers to the utilization of the nutrient substances after they are consumed. This inability to utilize a given nutrient may stem from digestive or malabsorption problems such as in lactose intolerance, celiac disease, chemotherapy, radiation treatments (see Chapter 13), or cell metabolism problems such as in genetic disease.

In addition, any related problem with nutritional involvement must be considered, including conditions such as heart disease, hypertension, cancer, liver and renal disease, and surgery. Any quantifiable data collected can be analyzed by computer. Two major nutritional tasks in which the computer excels are (1) baseline screening to identify persons at risk of malnutrition because of their disease, injury, or lifestyle and (2) analysis of intake to monitor effectiveness of ongoing treatment. Laboratory data may be handled in a similar manner, with general patterns of change monitored over time. Careful appraisal of medical and personal data from histories, records, reports, and interviews helps focus on various needs and problems and provides a realistic picture of nutritional and eating difficulties.

In summary, the nutritional diagnosis requires information about all aspects related to the individual patient's needs: nutrient deficiencies, underlying disease requiring a modified nutrient or food plan, and any personal, cultural, ethnic, or economic needs, as well as modes of feeding and dietary management.

Problem List

On the basis of this careful analysis, a problem list is usually developed, around which realistic and relevant care may be planned. Every aspect of the patient's needs is considered. In conference with the patient, family, and health care team, personal goals for care are determined. These establish priorities for immediate care, as well as long-term care.

Problem-Oriented Medical Record

The problem-oriented medical record (POMR) is an example of a well-organized system of data analysis and personal patient care planning that is used in many hospitals and health care settings. It was pioneered by Lawrence Weed in his clinical practice and teaching at Cleveland Metropolitan General Hospital and incorporates a fundamental humanistic philosophy of patient care. A brief summary of this system is included so that you may recognize its parts in the medical records in your facility, if it is used there, and participate in its development. The POMR represents a rather profound change in philosophy from traditional medical care of the past in that it helps to deliver the individual patient's records and thus care from the mystic realm, as one physician put it, of "a private sanctum for the physician with a rigid caste system imposed upon others who might make entries."[22a] Instead POMR provides a far more valid and dynamic vehicle that helps to ensure quality care for all patients by recognizing all patients all the time and by coordinating the activities of all the health team members in this personalized care.

At the initiation of either hospital or clinical care, applying the principles we have just discussed, procedures for establishing a POMR include (1) collection of a data base, (2) construction of a complete problem list with initial plans for each problem, and (3) the use of a continuing care structure for progress notes.

Data Base

A comprehensive data base is collected from the existing records to date by chart review, if the POMR system is being established for the first time. Otherwise it is initiated by introductory information on the following: admission or registration data, such as name, age, sex, race, and referral source; patient's perception of the purpose of the visit or admission (chief complaint); and the place that the patient receives primary care. A brief patient profile from various histories is made at the time of the clinic visit or hospital admission to initiate current care. These important data include information obtained from histories, such as family, marital, social, occupational, educational, living situation, financial status or health insurance coverages or assistance programs, and future plans. These data come from a medical history, physical examinations, laboratory tests, and nutritional and social histories.

Initial Problem List

On the basis of the data base collected, a problem list is constructed that includes the following:

1. *Established problems.* These include any identified problem (medical, nutritional, nursing, psychosocial, behavioral, economic, environmental) that concerns the patient or health care providers and for which an initial plan will be written.
2. *Temporary problems.* These include acute, short-term problems that have predictable resolutions without a major change in the ongoing therapy program; for example, an upper respiratory tract infection.
3. *Status-post problems.* These include any problem resolved before creation of the established problem list but that have left some anatomic, metabolic, or environmental change of concern to the patient or practitioner; for example, a post-gastrectomy state.
4. *Allergy, sensitivity, and intolerance problems.* These include problems involving various allergies, intolerances, or agent interactions; for example, lactose intolerance, specific food allergies, drug allergies, and drug-nutrient reactions. It is obviously imperative that all health care providers on the team have easy access to drug, immunization, nutritional, and diet histories.
5. *Drug and diet problems.* These include any problems related to previous or current drug and diet therapy, with a record of the date on and off the drug or diet therapy, the specific purpose of each therapy, and related patient responses to the therapy (see Chapter 2).

Plans for Each Problem

The initial plans for each problem are constructed according to three specific areas of patient need:

1. *Diagnosis.* Name of the problem with specific definition
2. *Therapy.* Specific treatment plans, including various aspects such as medical, nursing, and nutritional care, outlined by each respective specialist on the health care team
3. *Patient education.* Careful inclusion of discussion, explanation, and educational activities concerning diagnosis and the treatment plan to be conducted with patient or family

Continuing Care

Following the establishment of a comprehensive data base as indicated with construction of a related initial problem list and plans for each problem, the continuing care record includes two important ongoing activities:

1. *Current problem list.* It is particularly important to the successful operation of the system that the problem list be kept up to date. As the patient's care progresses, the problem list is maintained accurately, completely, and currently by adding new problems as they develop and deleting problems as they are resolved, giving data and manner of resolution. This problem list is always kept at the front or back of the chart and serves as a table of contents with cross-reference numbering. A copy of this list may also be kept by each practitioner on the primary care team in a personal office notebook as a constant reminder.
2. *Progress notes.* Rather than having a rambling, disorganized, or biased narrative that leaves health practitioners on the team helplessly leafing through chart pages, the POMR system of continuing care progress notes uses a structured format that succinctly organizes needed information, every element of which forms the easily remembered acronym SOAP:
   - *S*ubjective. Any new information gained from talking with the patient—that is, perceived pain, tolerances, and feelings about health status or care—are charted in "report language" as the patient's statements, descriptions, and reports. This represents subjective data directly from patients as they perceive their problems.
   - *O*bjective. Any specific new data obtained from laboratory or x-ray tests, performance measures, nutritional analyses, physical findings, observations of behavior, and other data are listed in quantified terms.
   - *A*ssessment. Interpretation or significance of these new data provides understanding of the problem as defined.
   - *P*lan. Any continuing or new diagnostic, therapeutic, or patient education activities are indicated as planned for implementation in relation to the data and assessment.

Use of the POMR makes every practitioner on the health care team accountable for quality care and the charting of specific aspects of care that are pertinent to each one's area of expertise and professional responsibility. Health care legislation concerning quality care assessment and assurance monitoring is increasingly mandating that such care be accurately recorded in an organized manner.[23,24] A system such as the POMR helps health care workers provide patient care that is comprehensive and complete rather than fragmented and episodic, responsive and responsible rather than insensitive and impersonal. Furthermore, and perhaps this is a most important ingredient in our increasingly complex and changing world, it communicates our human compassion to the patient by saying simply, "I care."

Nutritional Intervention: Food Plan and Management

Some Basic Concepts

Modified Diets

Special modified diets, as outlined in the remaining chapters of this book and in other resources, are characterized by the following basic principles:

1. *Normal nutritional base.* A therapeutic diet is only a modification of the normal nutritional needs for a particular patient. It is modified only as the specific disease in the individual necessitates. In nutritional care planning and counseling, this is an important initial fact to grasp and impart to patients and clients. For example, it is a great source of encouragement to the mother of a newly diagnosed diabetic child to know that the food plan is based on individual growth and development needs and uses regular foods.
2. *Disease application.* The principles of a special therapeutic diet are based on modification of the nutritional components of the normal diet as a particular disease condition may require. These changes may include the following: (1) *nutrients:* modifications in one or more of the basic nutrients—protein, carbohydrates, fat, minerals, and vitamins; (2) *energy:* modification in energy value, or kcalories; and (3) *texture:* modification in texture or seasoning such as liquid or low residue.
3. *Individual patient adaptation.* A diet may be theoretically correct and contain well-balanced food plans, but if these plans are unacceptable to the patient, they will not be followed. Careful planning *with* the patient based on the comprehensive data base collected is imperative. The diet principles are better understood and motivation is secured to follow through if practitioner and patient work closely together throughout planning the diet. It must be a workable plan adapted to individual needs and desires. Individual tailoring of the diet to personal needs is imperative to successful therapy.

Routine "House" Diets

A schedule of routine "house" diets based on some type of cycle menu is usually followed in hospitals for those patients not requiring a special diet modification. According to general patient need and tolerance, the diet ordered may be liquid (clear liquid or full

CLINICAL APPLICATION

Documenting Nutritional Risk

It is important that progress notes document any nutritional care given to patients along with data (or lack of data) that indicate nutritional status or potential for nutritional problems.

Subjective and objective information

Significant history—historical data that relate to a patient's nutritional status

Patient comments about prescribed diet—information that enables the health care team to relate to the patient's problems as the patient sees them

Contraindicated foods—possible drug-nutrient interactions or food allergies

Anthropometric data—includes diet prescription, measurements of height and weight, and calculations of ideal body weight

Impaired ability to feed self or eat—any physical limitations that prevent intake of nutrients or the inability to masticate or swallow

Assessment of subjective and objective information

Evaluation of pertinent prior intake—summary of the diet history, eating habits, and life-style influences and an evaluation of prior intake and its relationship to the current problem

Evaluation of current dietary intake—food consumed within the preceding 72 hours, usually based on the diet received in the hospital. Generalizations, such as "Pt ate well," should be avoided because they have little or no clinical significance and are open to various interpretations. A more objective statement, "Pt ate all of her meal and consumed 240 cc of whole milk," is more definitive

Evaluation of current nutritional status—evaluation of prior and current diet and of the anthropometric, laboratory, and physical findings

Interpretation of significant laboratory findings—used to support diagnosis of a nutritional problem or to monitor an identified nutritional problem. An assessment of "malnourished" or "nutritionally at risk" usually indicates a diagnosis that nurses and nutrition care specialists cannot make in most states. Consideration of more objective statements, such as "Pt's nutritional status indicators are below acceptable standards," may be warranted

Evaluation of patient's ability to accept and understand nutritional intervention—an important description of how the patient's attitude is assessed and how understanding is demonstrated

Assessment or plan

- Recommendations for consultation or evaluation by nonphysician health professionals
- Implementing, monitoring, and revising the nutritional care plan, including goals and patient-centered objectives for treatment of the nutritional problem
- Disposition indicated, including conclusion about discharge, referral, or follow-up

If available information is inadequate to make a definitive statement about the patient's nutritional status, this lack of information should be noted in the chart. Also, informed refusal of foods or noncompliance with diet orders and nutritional services should be documented. Nutritional care progress notes should adequately document what care is given to the patient. If care is not recorded, it is assumed that care was not given. ◆

REFERENCES

Anderson SL, Green RA: Dietitians, depositions and the law: issues in practice, *Diet Curr* 17(1):1, 1990.

Spencer RA: In defense of dietetics, *Clin Manage* 3(8):29, 1987.

Zeman FJ, Ney DM: *Applications of clinical nutrition,* Englewood Cliffs, NJ, Prentice Hall, 1988.

liquid, with milk used on the full-liquid diet), soft (no raw foods, generally somewhat bland in seasoning), and regular (a full, normal-for-age diet). Occasionally an interval step between soft and regular may be used (a light diet). You may obtain sample menus from your community hospital staff dietitian and compare the differences.

Managing the Mode of Feeding

Depending on the patient's condition, the clinical nutritionist may manage the diet by using any one of the following four feeding modes:

1. *Enteral: oral diet.* Regular enteral feeding, food taken into the gastrointestinal tract by mouth, is preferred for as long as possible. Supplements are added if necessary.
2. *Enteral: tube feeding.* If a patient is unable to eat but the gastrointestinal tract can be used, tube feeding may provide needed nutritional support. A number of commercial formulas are available, or a blended formula may be calculated and prepared (see Chapter 3).
3. *Parenteral: peripheral vein feeding.* If the patient cannot take in food or formula via the gastrointestinal tract, parenteral feeding by vein is needed. These intravenous (IV) feedings contain solutions of dextrose, amino acids, vitamins, and minerals, with intermittent lipid formula. They are fed through peripheral veins when the need is not extensive or long-term.
4. *Parenteral: total parenteral nutrition (TPN).* If the patient's nutritional need is great and support

therapy may be required for a longer time, feeding through a larger central vein is required. This is a special surgical procedure that requires special nutrient solutions prepared by trained pharmacists, and a skilled nutritional support team is essential for successful therapy (see Chapter 4).

Details of all these various modes of feeding are given in Chapters 3 and 4 as they apply to different conditions.

Evaluation: Quality Patient Care

General Considerations

When the nutritional care plan is carried out, the activities require consideration in terms of the nutritional diagnosis and treatment objectives, the extent to which each of the care activities helps to meet the particular goals of the patient and the family. This evaluation is continuous and terminal and requires careful, objective documentation (see the *Clinical Application,* p. 14). It seeks to validate care while it is being given, as well as to determine the effectiveness of a particular course of care. Various areas need to be investigated.

Estimate Achievement of Nutritional Therapy Goals

To estimate the achievement of nutritional therapy goals, the following questions must be answered: What is the effect of the diet or mode of feeding on the illness or the patient's situation? Is there need for any change in the nutrient ratios of the diet as originally calculated in the meal distribution pattern or in the feeding mode?

Judge Accuracy of Intervention Actions

The accuracy of the intervention actions can be judged once the following questions have been answered: Is change needed in any of the nutritional care plan components? For example, is change needed in the type of food or feeding equipment, environment for meals, procedures for counseling, or types of learning activities for nutrition education?

Determine Patient Ability to Follow Prescribed Nutritional Therapy

To determine the ability of a patient to follow the prescribed nutritional therapy, the following questions must be answered: Do any hindrances or disabilities prevent the patient from following the treatment plan? What is the impact of the nutritional therapy action on the patient, family, or staff? Were the necessary nutritional assessment procedures for collecting nutritional data carried out correctly? Do the patient and the family understand the information given for self-care? Have any community resources appropriate for the patient and the family been available or convenient for use? Has any needed food assistance program been sufficient to meet the needs for the patient's care?

Quality Patient Care

Since the establishment of Professional Standards Review Organizations (PSROs) in 1972, emphasis has increased on the setting of standards of practice to ensure the delivery of quality patient care.[23,24] In addition, at present an increased focus on cost control in health care settings requires that mechanisms be developed for effectively evaluating patient care programs on the basis of (1) cost-effectiveness and (2) provision of nutritional services by the most qualified personnel.[25] Within dietetics, standards for professional and support level staff have been developed in a number of medical care settings. These models of quality care have established specific standards for (1) identifying patients who require increased nutritional support or nutrition education, (2) determining patient care priorities and spelling out the degree of care required, and (3) defining role responsibilities for carrying out each part of the care plan. Over the past years since the quality assurance regulations were issued, these models for quality care have been applied to specific patient care needs, such as a standard of practice for quality assurance of nutritional care for patients with cancer.[26,27]

With increasing concerns about health care costs, maintaining a high level of quality patient care requires skill and much human wisdom. Such quality standards as described must also be applied to nutritional care of patients based on specific diagnosis-related groups of disease (DRGs).[28] This management classification scheme was developed in 1981 at Yale University and was based on designated major diagnosis categories (MDCs).[29] This prospective payment control plan was first applied to government funded Medicare patients, but in today's world of economic realities, it is fast becoming a part of practice for the majority of hospitalized patients as well as those in home care and extensive care facilities.[30,31] This increasing emphasis on cost-containment brings a new demand for accountability by all health care professionals and managers.

enteral • A mode of feeding that uses the gastrointestinal tract; oral or tube feeding.

parenteral • A mode of feeding that does not use the gastrointestinal tract but instead provides nutrition by intravenous delivery of nutrient solutions.

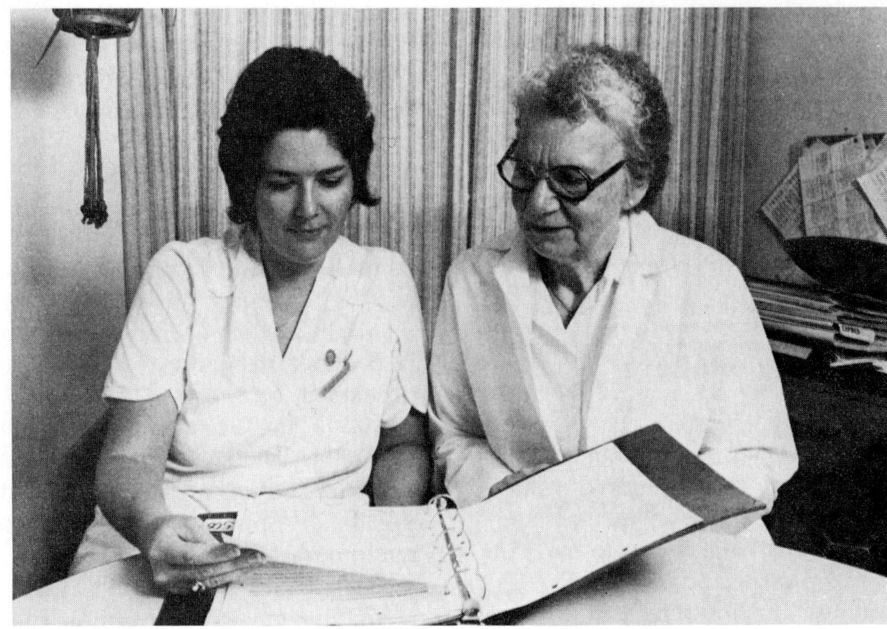

FIG. 1-3 The nurse and nutritionist discuss their patient's care plan.

Collaborative Roles of Nutritionist and Nurse

The clinical dietitian or nutritionist works closely with the nurse in supporting the nutritional care of patients. Skills in consultation and referral are therefore essential. At varying times, depending on need, the nurse may provide valuable nutrition assistance as coordinator, interpreter, or teacher.

Coordinator

Nurses coordinate any special services or treatment required because of their close relationship to patients and their more constant attendance. The nurse may help schedule activities to prevent conflicts or secure needed consultation for the patient with a social worker, dietitian, or other health team member. Sometimes hospital-induced malnutrition exists simply because meals are constantly being interrupted by various procedures, staff interviews, or medical rounds.

Interpreter

Because of a close relationship with the patient, the nurse helps reduce tension by careful, brief, easily understood explanations concerning various treatments and plans of care. This includes basic interpretation of the therapeutic diet from the clinical nutritionist or the physician and of the resulting food selections on the tray. The nurse may sometimes assist the patient in making appropriate selections from the menus provided.

Teacher or Counselor

One of the nurse's most significant roles is that of health care educator and counselor. There are innumerable informal opportunities during daily nursing care for planned conversation about sound nutrition principles to reinforce the counseling of the clinical nutritionist. In addition, according to patient situations, the nurse may work with the clinical nutritionist or dietitian during periods of instruction concerning principles of the patient's modified diet integrated with general health teaching about the disease process (Fig. 1-4). The nurse works in close cooperation with the clinical nutritionist or dietitian and the physician to coordinate medical and nutritional management of the patient's illness into overall nursing care. At all times the nurse works closely with the hospital's clinical dietitians to support and supplement primary nutrition education. The nurse often provides the valuable service of being the key person to ensure that the clinical dietitian has an appropriate uninterrupted environment for inpatient counseling and instruction, as well as discharge planning for follow-up care.[32,33] These dietitians also are excellent resources for teaching materials and needed nutrition information.

It is evident that comprehensive nutritional assessment and learning about the patient's needs should be a continuing activity beginning with hospital admission. Nutritional assessment should follow through and include plans for continuing application in the home environment. Follow-up care may be provided by the hospital's outpatient clinical dietitian, by consultation with clinical nutritionists or registered dietitians in community private practice, by public health nutritionists and nurses, or by referrals to various community resource groups.

To Sum Up

The primary basis of accurate assessment of the patient's nutritional needs is sensitive, continuing communication with the individual patient and family. Physical as well as psychologic, social, economic, and cultural factors in and out of the clinical setting all play roles in estimating the health status and predicting barriers to or enhancers of adherence to nutritional care plans.

Nutritional assessment is based on four basic types of measurements: anthropometric, biochemical, clinical observations, and diet evaluation, as well as the drugs being used. The effectiveness of an assessment based on an analysis of these data depends in turn on effective communication with the patient and family in the development of an appropriate care plan as well as with other members of the health care team.

The patient's medical record is the basic means of communication among health care team members. The problem-oriented medical record (POMR) is an example of such a system of care. It has recommendable qualities, since it "forces" each health care worker to focus on clearly identified problems set in wise order of priority with indications for care in each discipline involved. Problems are constantly updated, and organized, unbiased progress notes are entered in the record.

Nutritional therapy based on a combination of the personal and physiologic needs of the patient requires a close working relationship among nutrition, medical, and nursing staff in the health care facility. Even patients on "house" diets may periodically express a need for a change in texture or kcalories. The nurse's schedule offers many opportunities to teach or reinforce the nutritional principles of the diet. Thus nutritional therapy requires not only an appropriate diet but also in-service activities by the clinical nutritionist for nursing staff regarding the patient's nutritional needs.

Nutritional therapy does not end with the patient's discharge. The clinical nutritionist must be aware of outpatient nutritional services, appropriate social services, and community food resources to which patients can be referred for follow-up needs.

QUESTIONS FOR REVIEW

1. Identify and discuss the possible effects of various psychologic factors on the outcome of nutritional therapy.
2. Outline a general procedure to be followed for assessing nutritional needs and planning care for a 65-year-old widower hospitalized with coronary heart disease (see Chapter 8 if necessary). Include community agencies to which the patient could be referred for follow-up care, services, and information.
3. Describe six anthropometric procedures, five blood tests, and two urine tests commonly used for nutritional status information in terms of significance of the measure or test—what is being measured and what the results tell you.
4. Select six clinical signs used to assess nutritional status and describe what each sign shows in a malnourished person and why.
5. Describe five types of problems usually listed in a POMR. In each case give examples of related nutritional problems.
6. Using the SOAP format, outline a possible progress note for a patient with malnutrition.
7. Describe the nature and purpose of quality assurance plans for standards of patient care.

REFERENCES

1. Rubin M: The physiology of bed rest, *Am J Nurs* 88:50, 1988.
2. Kamath SK et al: Hospital malnutrition: a 33-hospital screening study, *J Am Diet Assoc* 86(2):203, 1986.
3. Bone RC: Ethical principles in critical care, *JAMA* 263(5):696, 1990.
4. Monsen ER et al: Ethics: responsible scientific conduct, *Am J Clin Nutr* 54:1, 1991.
5. Anderson EG: Getting through to elderly patients, *Geriatrics* 46(5):74, 1991.
6. Gilbert J: Partnership: a new paradigm for health care, *Hospitals* 64:72, 1990.
7. Koska MT: Patient-centered care: can your hospital afford not to have it? *Hospitals* 64:48, 1990.
8. Thompson MP, Morris LK: Unexplained weight loss in the ambulatory elderly, *J Am Geriatr Soc* 39:497, 1991.
9. Kubena KS et al: Anthropometry and health in the elderly, *J Am Diet Assoc* 91(11):1402, 1991.
10. Himes JH, Bouchard C: Do the new Metropolitan Life Insurance weight-height tables correctly assess body frame and body fat relationships? *Am J Public Health* 75(9):1076, 1985.
11. Frisancho AR: Nutritional anthropometry, *J Am Diet Assoc* 88(5):553, 1988.
12. Nowak RK, Schulz LO: A comparison of two methods for the determination of body frame size, *J Am Diet Assoc* 87(3):339, 1987.
13. Mitchell CO, Lipschitz DA: Arm length measurement as an alternative to height in nutritional assessment of the elderly, *J Parenter Enteral Nutr* 6(3):226, 1982.
14. Kwok T, Whitelaw MN: The use of armspan in nutritional assessment of the elderly, *J Am Geriatr Soc* 39:492, 1991.

15. Chumlea WC et al: *Nutritional assessment of the elderly through anthropometry,* Columbus, Ohio, 1987, Ross Laboratories.
16. Haboubi NY et al: Measurement of height in the elderly, *J Am Geriatr Soc* 38:1008, 1990.
17. Chumlea WC et al: Prediction of body weight for the nonambulatory elderly from anthropometry, *J Am Diet Assoc* 88(5):564, 1988.
18. Graham AW: Screening for alcoholism by life-style risk assessment in a community hospital, *Arch Intern Med* 151:958, 1991.
19. Posner BM et al: Validation of two-dimensional models for estimation of portion size in nutrition research, *J Am Diet Assoc* 92(6):738, 1992.
20. Trovato A et al: Drug-nutrient interactions, *Am Fam Physician* 44(5):1651, 1991.
21. Zulkifli SN, Yu SM: The food frequency method for dietary assessment, *J Am Diet Assoc* 92(6):681, 1992.
22. Block G et al: Comparison of two dietary questionnaires validated against multiple dietary records collected during a 1-year period, *J Am Diet Assoc* 92(6):686, 1992.
22a. Voytovich AE: The dietitian/nutritionist and the problem-oriented medical record: a physician's viewpoint, *J Am Diet Assoc* 63:639, 1973.
23. Herbelin K: Quality assessment and assurance in a long-term care facility: meeting current federal requirements, *J Am Diet Assoc* 89(10):1499, 1989.
24. Edelstein SF: Using thresholds to monitor dietetic services: the JCAHO 10-step process for quality assurance, *J Am Diet Assoc* 91(10):1261, 1991.
25. Splett PL: Assessing effectiveness of nutrition care: prerequisite for cost-effectiveness analysis, *Top Clin Nutr* 5(2):26, 1990.
26. Ometer JL, Oberfill MS: Quality assurance. I. A level of care model, *J Am Diet Assoc* 82(2):129, 1982.
27. Ometer JL, Oberfill MS: Quality assurance. II. Application of oncology standards against a level of care model, *J Am Diet Assoc* 82(2):132, 1982.
28. Huyck NI, Fairchild MM: Provision of clinical nutrition services by diagnosis-related groups (DRGs) and major diagnostic categories (MCDs), *J Am Diet Assoc* 87(1):69, 1987.
29. Yale University School of Organization and Management: *The new ICD-9-CM diagnosis related groups classification scheme,* New Haven, Conn, 1981, Yale University Press.
30. Sandall MJ, Massey LK: The impact of the diagnosis-related groups/prospective payment system on nutrition needs in home health and extended care facilities, *J Am Diet Assoc* 89(10):1444, 1989.
31. Delhey DM et al: Implications of malnutrition and diagnosis-related groups (DRGs), *J Am Diet Assoc* 89(10):1448, 1989.
32. Picus SS: Evaluation of the nutrient counseling environment of hospitalized patients, *J Am Diet Assoc* 89(3):403, 1989.
33. Weddle DO et al: Inpatient and post-discharge course of the malnourished patient, *J Am Diet Assoc* 91(3):307, 1991.

FURTHER READING

Clay G, Bouchard C, Hemphill K: A comprehensive nutrition case management system, *J Am Diet Assoc* 88(2):196, 1988.

This article describes a proven comprehensive nutritional assessment and case management system developed jointly by nutritionists and nurses in a large southern California county. Its unique features provide a model for (1) decreased charting time, (2) precise documentation, (3) a diagnosis tool for intervention therapy, (4) a standard for consistent quality care, (5) computer adaptation, and (6) quality assurance audits.

Mullenbach V et al: Comparison of 3-day food record and 24-hour recall by telephone for dietary evaluation in adolescents, *J Am Diet Assoc* 92(6):743, 1992.

Posner BM et al: Validation of two-dimensional models for estimation of portion size in nutrition research, *J Am Diet Assoc* 92(6):738, 1992.

These two articles describe nutrition assessment methods and tools developed by research groups that may be applied for practical use in clinical work.

Chumlea WC, Roche AF, Mukherjee D: *Nutritional assessment of the elderly through anthropometry,* Columbus, Ohio, 1987, Ross Laboratories.

Gussler JD, ed: *Nutritional screening and assessment as components of hospital admission,* Eighth Ross Roundtable on Medical Issues, Columbus, Ohio, 1987, Ross Laboratories.

These two manuals continue to provide background for (1) using special alternate techniques and calculations for determining weight and height of nonambulatory elderly patients, complete with illustrations and formulas, and (2) identifying patients at nutritional risk on hospital admission and monitoring their progress on nutritional therapy.

Selecting Computer Nutrient-Calculation Software

In our modern age of electronics, the computer has become a standard tool for rapid calculation procedures. In clinical and community nutrition practices as well as population studies, it saves valuable time and provides a precise nutrient analysis of an individual's reported food intake.

Certainly computerized nutrient analyses are time savers from the previous tedious manual calculations using published food value tables. But just how precise are the results? This depends on the heart of any nutrient-analysis software program—its nutrient data base.

Over the past few years of computer use by clinicians, researchers, and educators, it has become increasingly evident that the quality of the nutrient data base on which all calculations are based determines the quality of the resulting output. Experts in this field at the University of Minnesota Nutrition Coordinating Center have provided important questions that may be used in evaluating the nutrient data base in any software package being considered for purchase.

Does the data base contain all foods and nutrients of interest?

Most data bases contain the most common foods, but you may require particular foods such as ethnic, vegetarian, or fast-food items; brand name products; and infant or nontraditional foods. The number of food items in a data base does not necessarily indicate how comprehensive the system is. And adding your own foods to the data base requires considerable effort.

Is the data base complete for nutrients of interest?

Missing values are common in available software packages and often are not flagged, so you may be unaware of this source of error. Inappropriate patient counseling may result. Such missing value errors in small items such as spices or other condiments may not matter, but a missing value for total saturated fatty acids in a fast-food hamburger because the food manufacturers have not supplied it is not acceptable.

Do foods included in the data base provide sufficient specific data to accurately assess nutrients of interest?

For example, if total fat and fatty acids are of concern, separate data base entries must be included for such items as regular, low-fat, and nonfat dairy products and brand name high-fat items such as margarines and salad dressings. In other cases inclusion of food items according to preparation method or of any dietary supplements for vitamin-mineral calculations may be required.

Is nutrient data base current with changing marketplace and availability of new nutrient data?

The USDA routinely releases updates of the *Agricultural Handbook,* no. 8, the common source of data for nutrient-calculation systems, as new information is available. Information from food manufacturers is also available. A well-maintained software product's data base should include all such data updates, and the vendor should supply information about frequency of updating and sources of data.

Are manufacturers contacted routinely for new information or reformulations of existing products?

This question extends the previous question to emphasize the still too frequent neglect of brand name product updating practices of software developers. *Routine* contact with food manufacturers is essential to maintain an acceptable quality standard.

What quality control procedures are used to ensure data base accuracy?

Because thousands of values for nutrients and nonnutrient information, for example, food-specific serving sizes, the margin for error is great and built-in maintenance procedures for checking such errors should be present.

Vendors of nutrient-calculation software packages should be able to give answers to these important questions. Ask before you buy!

REFERENCES

Buzzard IM et al: Considerations for selecting nutrient-calculation software: evaluation of the nutrient database, *Am J Clin Nutr* 54:7, 1991.

Schakel SF et al: Sources of data for developing and maintaining a nutrient database, *J Am Diet Assoc* 88:1268, 1988.

CHAPTER 2

Drug-Nutrient Interactions

CHAPTER OUTLINE

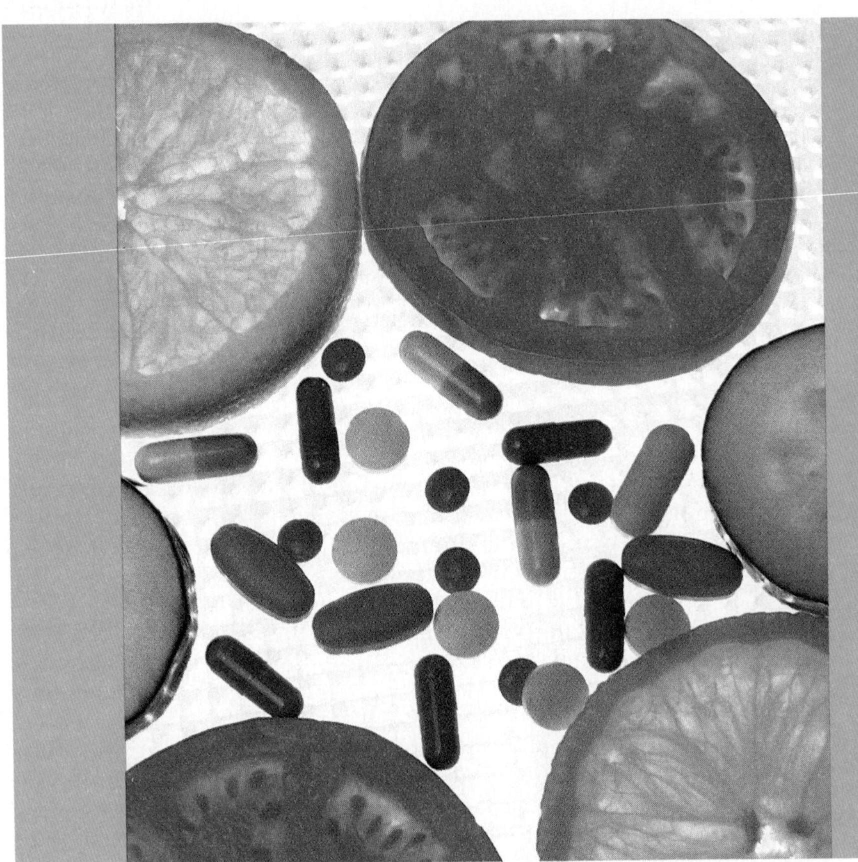

Every year American physicians prescribe and pharmacists dispense a total amount of drugs sufficient to provide seven individual medications for each woman, man, and child in the United States. To this amount we can then add the large volume of nonprescription drugs that Americans purchase over the counter. Some concerned persons have come to view our overmedicated society with alarm. Elderly persons are particularly vulnerable, since they are likely to be on more drugs for longer periods.

Today consumers are generally better informed about drug misuse. However, many are dangerously uninformed or misinformed about the specific drugs they may be taking, especially in relation to the food they eat.

The influence of food and dietary patterns on drug absorption and bioavailability is complex. All members of the health care team must have a basic knowledge of drug actions and nutrition to make the wisest and most effective use of drug and nutritional therapy. This chapter looks briefly at some main effects of combining food and nutrients with drugs and how these interactions affect our nutritional therapy and education for our clients and patients.

Drug-Nutrient Problems in Modern Medicine

Problem Significance: Causes, Extent, Effects

The modern medical world is increasing in complexity and specialization. Every specialty field or discipline easily becomes isolated from many other interacting factors in the care of clients and patients that fall outside its primary area of expertise. Physicians who prescribe medications, pharmacists who fill these prescriptions, or nurses who administer them may not be fully aware of the impact of a particular drug in an individual patient's nutritional state. They may also be unaware of the patient's diet and how it may influence the effects of the medication. Similarly, a clinical nutritionist or dietitian may provide a diet description and food plan and not be fully aware of the client's medication program and its implications for sound nutritional care (see the *Clinical Application* below).

The field of nutrient-drug interaction is indeed complex and confusing. We face a drug-oriented medical environment and a bewildering array of drug items. Some knowledgeable and concerned pharmacologists indicate that outside of extremely serious illness, most general medical problems can be treated with less than 25 drugs. The World Health Organization (WHO) has estimated that only some 150 to 200 drugs are actually needed to take care of almost all ordinary illnesses around the world. Yet on our American market there are about 54,000 drugs, many of them only slight variations of other drugs, the so-called me too drugs.

Elderly Persons at Risk

All of us at any age risk harmful drug or drug-nutrient interactions, but elderly persons have more than their share.[1,2] Several things contribute to this increased risk among the elderly: (1) they are likely to be taking more drugs for longer periods to control chronic diseases; (2) their drugs are likely to be more toxic; (3) they respond to drugs with greater variability; (4) they have less capability to handle drugs efficiently; (5) their nutritional status is more likely to be deficient; and (6) illness, mental confusion, or lack of drug information may increase errors in self-care.[3-6] Concerned physicians, nutritionists, pharmacists, and nurses are increasingly working together as a team to provide drug and nutritional education and therapy on a soun-

CLINICAL APPLICATION — *The Proof of the Pudding. . .*

The senses of taste and smell greatly affect our responses to various foods. The loss of these senses may drive persons to constantly seek elusive satisfaction by overeating, or it may stop them from eating entirely. In either case the pleasure of eating is gone and nutritional status suffers. Patients taking drugs that affect taste and smell need counseling concerning food choices, combinations, and seasonings that can help them overcome this difficulty. Some drugs affecting taste and smell include the following:

- *Anesthetics, local*—benzocaine, cocaine, procaine
- *Antibiotics*—amphotericin B, ampicillin, griseofulvin, lincomycin, streptomycin, tetracyclines
- *Anticoagulant*—phenindione
- *Antihistamine*—chlorpheniramine maleate
- *Antihypertensive agents*—captopril, diazoxide, ethacrynic acid
- *Antiinfectious agent*—metronidazole
- *Cholesterol-lowering agent*—clofibrate
- *Hypoglycemic agent*—glipizide
- *Psychoactive agents*—carbamazepine, lithium carbonate, phenytoin, amphetamines
- *Toothpaste ingredient*—sodium lauryl sulfate

Indeed, the proof of the pudding—our food—*is* in the taste, which is easily affected by a variety of drugs, resulting in diminished appetite and necessary food intake. Patients on these drugs benefit from counseling about these taste effects, along with other effects, and ways of counteracting them in food selection, seasoning, and serving. ◆

REFERENCES

Roe DA: *Diet and drug interactions*, ed 2, New York, 1989, AVI Books.
Powers D, Moore A: *Food-medication interactions*, ed 6, Phoenix, Ariz, 1988, Food-Medication Interactions.
Trovato A et al: Drug-nutrient interactions, *Am Fam Physician* 44(5):1651, 1991.

der basis. The number of possible nutrient-drug interactions demand this type of teamwork in patient care, especially for elderly patients, and a number of team process guides have been developed for various conditions.[3,4] Recent computer-assisted instruction on drug-nutrient interactions—designed for professional and paraprofessional hospital staff in nutrition, pharmacy, nursing, and medicine—has helped to significantly reduce the rate of definite drug-nutrient interactions.[5]

Nutrient-Drug Interaction and Malnutrition

Numerous studies of hospital malnutrition have outlined a number of possible mechanisms of nutrient-drug interaction that relate to malnutrition. Such effects are prevalent especially in hospitalized patients, as well as in persons in deprived situations suffering from protein-energy malnutrition, and require knowledge and attention.[6,7] These nutrient-drug mechanisms include those affecting (1) decreased intestinal absorption; (2) increased renal excretion; (3) direct competition or displacement from carrier protein sites; (4) interference with the synthesis of a necessary enzyme, coenzyme, or carrier; (5) hormonal effects of genetic systems; (6) the drug delivery system; and (7) components in drug formulation. In general, drugs are usually grouped according to primary action. The following discussion reviews briefly various effects of drugs on food and nutrients and effects of food and nutrients on drugs with examples in each case for your reference in patient care.

Drug Effects on Food and Nutrients

Drug Effects on Food Intake

Increased Appetite

The following drugs have an effect of increasing the appetite[1,8]:

1. *Antihistamines.* Cyproheptadine hydrochloride (Periactin), which is an antihistamine and a serotonin antagonist, may cause a sharp increase in appetite and subsequent weight gain.
2. *Psychotropic drugs.* Chlordiazepoxide hydrochloride (Librium), diazepam (Valium), chlorpromazine hydrochloride (Thorazine), meprobamate (Equanil), and some of the mild tranquilizers with antiemetic and antihistaminic properties may lead to *hyperphagia,* or excessive eating (see *Issues and Answers,* p. 31). Tranquilizers that lead to weight gain when given to psychotic patients may have the opposite effect on geriatric patients.

   As with tranquilizers, tricyclic antidepressants such as amitriptyline hydrochloride (Elavil) may promote appetite and lead to significant weight gain.
3. *Steroids.* Nitrogen retention, increased lean body mass, and weight gain are observed with administration of anabolic steroids, including testosterone. Glucocorticoids may increase appetite and lead to weight gain.

Decreased Appetite

The following drugs have the effect of depressing the appetite[1,8]:

1. *Amphetamines.* These drugs act as stimulants to the central nervous system and have the effect of depressing the desire for food and may lead to significant loss of weight. Until recently, these appetite-depressant drugs were used in the treatment of obesity. However, long-term use in such treatment has created problems, since appetite may not be a primary causative factor in the excess weight status. Currently, they are seldom used for this purpose. Children taking amphetamines show dose-dependent growth retardation.
2. *Insulin.* Although general use of insulin in the management of diabetes may bring a feeling of hunger, an insulin-induced drop in blood sugar, *hypoglycemia,* is not marked by hunger but often causes nausea, weakness, and aversion to foods.
3. *Alcohol.* Alcohol abuse leads to anorexia, reduced food intake, major metabolic abnormalities, and malnutrition. Alcoholism requires health risk screening and significant nutritional support in rehabilitation efforts.[9,10] The anorexia stems from gastritis, lactose intolerance, hepatitis, cirrhosis, ketoacidosis, pancreatitis, alcoholic brain syndrome, drunkeness, and withdrawal symptoms. Reduced food intake, which leads to malnutrition, complicates anorexia through deficiencies of thiamin, zinc, or protein.

Taste Changes

The *chelating agent* D-penicillamine is used in the treatment of conditions such as heavy metal poisoning, rheumatoid arthritis, or cystinuria. The use of these agents leads to loss of taste, or *dysgeusia,* caused by induced zinc deficiency from zinc binding. Other drugs affecting taste acuity include *diuretics,* anticancer agents such as methotrexate and doxorubicin hydrochloride (Adriamycin), and agents used to treat Parkinson's disease. Even a 1-g dose of aspirin increases the perception of a bitter taste. A substance often used in toothpaste to improve its cleansing action, sodium lauryl sulfate, makes orange juice taste bitter. A number of other drugs affect taste and smell. Thus when

TABLE 2-1

Drugs Causing Primary Nutrient Malabsorption

Drug	Use	Nutrients lost	Action
Cholestyramine	Holds bile acid; hypocholesterolemic agent	Fat; fat-soluble vitamins A, D, and K; vitamin B_{12}; iron	Binding agent for bile salts and nutrients
Colchicine	Antigout agent	Fat; vitamin B_{12}; provitamin A (carotene); lactose; sodium, potassium	Enzyme damage; inhibits cell division; structural defect
Methyldopa	Antihypertensive agent	Vitamin B_{12}, folic acid; iron	Unclear; possible autoimmune action
Mineral oil	Laxative	Fat-soluble vitamins A, D, and K; provitamin A (carotene)	Nutrients dissolve in oil and are lost in feces
Neomycin	Antibiotic	Fat; vitamin B_{12}; nitrogen; lactose, sucrose; sodium, potassium, iron, calcium	Binds bile salts; lowers pancreatic lipase; structural defect
Para-aminosalicylic acid	Antituberculosis agent	Fat; folic acid, vitamin B_{12}	Blocks mucosal uptake of vitamin B_{12}
Phenolphthalein	Laxative	Calcium, potassium; vitamin D	Rapid intestinal transit; loss of structural tissue integrity
Potassium chloride	Potassium replacement	Vitamin B_{12}	Lowered ileal pH
Salicylazosulfapyridine (Azulfidine)	Anti-inflammatory agent (ulcerative colitis)	Folic acid	Blocks mucosal uptake of folic acid

Adapted from Roe DA: Interactions between drugs and nutrients, *Med Clin North Am* 63:985, 1979; and Roe DA: *Diet and drug interactions,* ed 2, New York, 1989, AVI Books.

any of these drugs are used, discussion of these sensory effects with the patient and use of food seasonings to enhance taste and smell is useful.

Nausea

Many drugs contribute to nausea and vomiting. For example, cardiac glycosides, digitalis, and related drugs produce nausea if they are used in relatively large amounts. A number of the drugs used in cancer chemotherapy (see Chapter 13) have similar effects and also contribute to malnutrition and weight loss.

Bulking Effects

Various bulking agents such as methyl cellulose or other dietary fiber products interfere with absorption of nutrients and contribute to their loss.[11] These agents also contribute to decreased intake of food by creating a sense of fullness and lack of desire for food intake. For this reason they have been used as adjunct therapy in weight management.

Drug Effects on Nutrient Absorption and Metabolism

Increased Absorption

A number of drugs increase nutrient absorption and benefit nutritional status. For example, cimetidine (Tagamet), a gastric antisecretory agent, helps patients with bowel resection. The drug reduces gastric acid and volume output; lowers duodenal acid load and volume; reduces jejunal flow; maintains pH; decreases fecal fat, nitrogen, and volume; and thus improves absorption of protein and carbohydrates. This drug is therefore helpful in the treatment of various gastrointestinal disorders including peptic ulcer disease.

Decreased Absorption

A number of drugs contribute to primary malabsorption. Colchicine, a drug used in the treatment of gout, leads to vitamin B_{12} deficiency, causing megaloblastic anemia. Alcohol abuse provokes malabsorption of thiamin and folic acid with subsequent peripheral neuritis and anemia. Laxatives also produce severe malabsorption, leading to conditions such as osteomalacia. Secondary malabsorption may also be drug induced. Some drugs inhibit vitamin D absorption, leading to malabsorption and consequent deficiency of calcium. For example, the antibiotic neomycin causes tissue changes in the intestinal villi, precipitates bile salts, prevents fat breakdown by inhibiting pancreatic lipase, and decreases bile acid absorption. These effects lead to *steatorrhea* and failure to absorb the fat-soluble vitamins A, D, E, and K. Malabsorption of vitamin D in turn leads to a calcium deficiency. Other drugs cause malabsorption of folic acid or impair its utilization causing malabsorption of still other nutrients. Methotrexate, for example, is used in cancer chemotherapy and is a folic acid antagonist that impairs the intestinal absorption of calcium.

Table 2-1 gives a summary of the causes and consequences of primary drug-induced malabsorption.

TABLE 2-2

Drugs Causing Secondary Malabsorption of Calcium

Drug	Use	Action
Phenytoin, phenobarbital, primidone	Anticonvulsant agents	Accelerated vitamin D metabolism
Diphosphonates	Paget's disease (increased bone resorption and deformity)	Vitamin D hormone [$1,25(OH)_2D_2$] formation decreased
Glucocorticoids, such as prednisone	Collagen disease; allergies	Calcium transport decreased
Glutethimide	Sedative	Impaired calcium transport
Methotrexate	Leukemia	Folic acid antagonist—acute deficiency of the vitamin

Adapted from Roe DA: Interactions between drugs and nutrients, *Med Clin North Am* 63:985, 1979; and Roe DA: *Diet and drug interactions,* ed 2, New York, 1989, AVI Books.

Table 2-2 summarizes drugs causing secondary malabsorption.

Mineral Depletion

Certain drugs lead to mineral depletion, either through induced gastrointestinal losses or through increased renal excretion.[12] For example, *diuretics,* which are intentionally used to reduce levels of excess tissue water and sodium, may also result in loss of other minerals, such as potassium, magnesium, and zinc. Potassium deficiency brings weakness, anorexia, nausea, vomiting, listlessness, apprehension, and sometimes diffuse pain, drowsiness, stupor, and irrational behavior. On the contrary, potassium-retaining diuretics such as spironolactone as well as overuse of potassium supplementation cause the opposite effect of hyperkalemia.

In addition, chelating agents such as penicillamine attach to metals and lead to deficiencies of zinc and copper. Alcohol abuse also leads to diminished levels of potassium, magnesium, and zinc. Antacids, commonly used over-the-counter medications, are of concern because they produce phosphate deficiency with symptoms of anorexia, malaise, **paresthesia,** profound muscle weakness, and convulsions as well as the calcification effects on soft tissue from the prolonged hypercalcemia. Aspirin and other salicylates induce iron deficiency by causing chronic low-level blood loss from erosion in the stomach or intestinal tissue.

Vitamin Deficiency

Drug-induced vitamin effects are antagonistic and cause various deficiencies.

TABLE 2-3

Examples of Drugs That Act as Vitamin Antagonists

Target vitamin	Drugs
Vitamin K	Coumarin anticoagulants
Folic acid	Methotrexate
	Pyrimethamine
	Triamterene
	Trimethoprim
Vitamin B_6	Cycloserine
	Hydralazine
	Isoniazid
	Levodopa

Adapted from Roe DA: Interactions between drugs and nutrients, *Med Clin North Am* 63:985, 1979; and Roe DA: *Diet and drug interactions,* ed 2, New York, 1989, AVI Books.

Vitamin antagonists. Various drugs have successful therapeutic effects through antagonism of certain vitamins. For example, coumarin anticoagulants inhibit regeneration of vitamin K, which is necessary for blood clotting. Also, some cancer chemotherapy drugs such as methotrexate have multiple antagonistic effects on folate metabolism, thus inhibiting the synthesis of deoxyribonucleic and ribonucleic acid (DNA and RNA) and protein. Pyrimethamine, an antimalaria drug, binds to the dihydrofolate reductase enzyme in a manner similar to methotrexate and thus inhibits the action of folate in protein synthesis. Table 2-3 lists vitamin-antagonist drugs.

Hypovitaminosis from use of oral contraceptives. Biochemical analyses have revealed subclinical deficiencies of folate, riboflavin, and vitamins B_6, B_{12}, and C in users of oral contraceptive agents.[13] Table 2-4 includes a list of some of these effects on nutritional status.

Special Adverse Reactions

Several reactions are related to specific drug interactions with particular nutrients.

Monoamine Oxidase Inhibitors

Monoamine oxidase inhibitors (MAOIs) are sometimes used as effective antidepressant medications, probably achieving their effect by increasing the levels of norepinephrine and serotonin in the central nervous system. They also potentiate the cardiovascular effect of simple phenylethylamines such as tyramine, dopamine, and other **vasoactive** amines from food.[14,15] Ordinarily, the mechanism of protective "first pass" metabolism in the gut mucosa and the liver prevents the absorption of these amines. MAOIs evidently inhibit this protective mechanism, allowing the absorp-

TABLE 2-4

Interactions Between Oral Contraceptive Agents (OCA) and Vitamins and Minerals Affecting Nutritional Status

Nutrient affected by OCA	Effect	Clinical result
Vitamins		
Retinol (vitamin A)	Impairs liver storage; increases plasma binding	Unclear
Pyridoxine (vitamin B_6)	Alters metabolism of tryptophan and vitamin B_6	Abnormal protein metabolism; mood changes
Cobalamin (vitamin B_{12})	Reduces vitamin B_{12} serum levels	Unclear
Folic acid	Reduces red cell concentration; increases folate-binding protein	Megaloblastic anemia
Minerals		
Copper	Increases plasma levels of ceruloplasmin	Unclear
Iron	Increases serum levels of transferrin	Unclear
Zinc	Reduces serum levels of zinc	Unclear

Data adapted from Butterworth CE Jr, Weinsier RL: Malnutrition in hospital patients: assessment and treatment. In Goodhart RS, Shilis ME, eds: *Modern nutrition in health and disease,* ed 6, Philadelphia, 1980, Lea & Febiger.

tion of tyramine, the amino acid dopa or its amine derivative dopamine, and other similar amines. MAOIs allow them to escape oxidative deamination, and they enter the systemic circulation causing the release of norepinephrine from local stores in nerve endings and leading to the prolonged action of this catecholamine on adrenergic receptors. This *tyramine syndrome* is marked by headache, pallor, nausea, and restlessness. With increased absorption, symptoms may escalate to apprehension, sweating, palpitations, chest pain, increased blood pressure, and fever. Rarely, blood pressure and confusion increase greatly, even rupturing brain blood vessels, leading to death. One fatality occurs per 100,000 administrations of the most lethal variant of the MAOIs. Chapter 13 contains a low-tyramine food list for use in cases such as these.

Flush Reaction

A variety of drugs react with alcohol to produce a **flushing reaction** along with **dyspnea** and headache (Table 2-5). Central nervous system depressants including hypnotic sedatives, antihistamines, phenothiazines, and narcotic analgesics may potentiate a loss of consciousness when taken in combination with alcohol. Extreme caution must be exercised with these medications, and patients should be alerted to the dangers of mixing them with alcohol.

Hypoglycemia

Drugs such as chlorpropamide (Diabinese) and similar oral medications sometimes used to control non-insulin dependent diabetes mellitus (NIDDM) (see Chapter 9) are hypoglycemic agents. These and other drugs that precipitate a rapid release of insulin may provoke hypoglycemia. This response is especially strong when the drugs are used together with alcohol. The symptoms of hypoglycemia include weakness, mental confusion, and irrational behavior, and if they are not treated, they lead to loss of consciousness.

Disulfiram

Disulfiram (Antabuse) is used to treat alcoholism. Disulfiram is a deterrent to alcohol consumption precisely because of its extremely unpleasant side effects when taken with alcohol. Within 15 minutes, flushing ensues, followed by headache, nausea, vomiting, and chest or abdominal pain. Other drugs may have effects similar to disulfiram including aldehyde dehydrogenase inhibitors.

Food and Nutrient Effects on Drugs

Food Effects on Drug Absorption

The absorption of drugs is a complex matter, and food affects eventual drug absorption in a number of ways.

Solution

An orally administered tablet or capsule must first disintegrate before the drug dissolves. The absorption of the drug from solution in acid gastric juice or in the more alkaline biliary and intestinal secretions may

paresthesia • Abnormal sensations such as prickling, burning, and "crawling" of the skin.

vasoactive • Having an effect on the diameter of blood vessels.

flushing reaction • Short-term reaction resulting in redness of the neck and face.

dyspnea • Labored, difficult breathing.

disulfiram • A white to off-white crystalline antioxidant that inhibits oxidation of the acetaldehyde metabolized from alcohol. It is used in the treatment of alcoholism, producing extremely uncomfortable symptoms when alcohol is ingested following oral administration of the drug.

TABLE 2–5
Adverse Drug Reactions Caused by Alcohol and Specific Foods

Type of reaction	Drugs	Alcohol/foods	Effects
Flushing	Chlorpropamide (diabetes) Griseofulvin Tetrachlorethylene	Alcohol	Dyspnea, headache, flushing
Disulfiram reaction	Aldehyde dehydrogenase inhibitors: Disulfiram (Antabuse) Calcium carbimide Metronidazole Nitrofurantoin Sulfonylureas	Alcohol Foods containing alcohol	Abdominal and chest pain, flushing, headache, nausea and vomiting
Hypoglycemia	Insulin-releasing agents: Oral hypoglycemic drugs	Alcohol Sugar, sweets	Mental confusion, weakness, irrational behavior, unconsciousness
Tyramine reaction	Monoamine oxidase inhibitors (MAOIs): Antidepressants such as phenelzine Procarbazine Isoniazid (isonicotinic acid hydrazide)	Foods containing large amounts of tyramine: Cheese Red wines Chicken liver Broad beans Yeast	Cerebrovascular accident (CVA), flushing, hypertension

Adapted from Roe DA: Interactions between drugs and nutrients, *Med Clin North Am* 63:985, 1979; and Roe DA: *Diet and drug interactions,* ed 2, New York, 1989, AVI Books.

TABLE 2–6
Food Effect on Drug Absorption

Absorption reduced by food	Absorption delayed by food
Amoxicillin	Acetaminophen
Ampicillin	Amoxicillin
Aspirin	Aspirin
Demethylchlortetracycline	Cephalexin
Doxycycline	Cephradine
Isoniazid	Digoxin
Levodopa	Furosemide
Methacycline	Sulfadiazine
Oxytetracycline	Sulfamethoxazole
Penicillin G, V(K)	Sulfamethoxypyridazine
Phenethicillin	Sulfanilamide
Phenobarbital	Sulfisoxazole
Propantheline	
Rifampin	
Tetracycline	

Adapted from Roe DA: Interactions between drugs and nutrients, *Med Clin North Am* 63:985, 1979; and Roe DA: *Diet and drug interactions,* ed 2, New York, 1989, AVI Books.

be more or less complete. The drug then passes through the intestinal mucosa and liver circulation before entering systemic circulation. In systemic circulation it may be subject to metabolism, deactivation, and elimination through the so-called first pass mechanism. Food may affect eventual drug absorption at any of these points.

Stomach Emptying Rate

The rate at which food empties from the stomach is affected by diet composition. Fats, high temperatures, and solid meals prolong the amount of time food stays in the stomach. Food usually increases secretion of bile, acid, and gut enzymes and enhances intestinal mobility and *splanchnic* blood flow. Drugs adsorb to certain food particles.

Clinical Significance

Whether these effects have clinical significance depends on the extent of the effect and the nature of the drug. A small change in absorption is critical for a drug with a steep dose-response curve but perhaps unnoticeable for a drug with a wide range of effective concentrations. In general, the amount of absorption is clinically more important than the rate since it has more impact on the steady-state plasma concentration of the drug after multiple doses. Table 2-6 gives some examples of drugs that are better utilized when taken without food and those that should be taken with food.

Increased Absorption

Various circumstances contribute to the increased absorption of a drug.

Dissolution Characteristics

When a drug has poor *in vitro* dissolution characteristics, prolonging the time it remains in the stomach

The Pain Reliever Doctors Recommend Most

TO PROBE FURTHER

Aspirin has a venerable history. Being a buffered form of salicylic acid, it is a modified version of an ancient folk remedy, willow bark, used for many hundreds of years for fever, aches, and pain. The acetyl group in acetylsalicylic acid makes aspirin easier on the stomach than willow bark.

Aspirin is an analgesic agent, an effect enhanced in combination with caffeine, that is used for relief of minor aches and pains. Its mechanism of action is through inhibition of certain prostaglandins, which have a profound influence on a spectrum of physiologic functions, including blood clotting, blood pressure, the inflammatory process, contraction of voluntary muscles, and transmission of nerve impulses.

Studies implicate aspirin in alleviating many disorders, dangers, and discomforts as indicated in the following examples:

- The risk of repeated *transient ischemic attacks (TIAs)*, little strokes, is reduced by 50% in men (but *not* women) who have already had one.
- Many studies indicate that aspirin is effective in reducing risk for *myocardial infarction*, a heart attack.
- Aspirin is one of the most effective antiinflammatory drugs and is effective in the long-term treatment of *arthritis*.
- Aspirin may play a role in inhibiting the spread of some *cancers* through its action of inhibiting production of prostaglandin E_2.
- Aspirin's effect as an anticoagulant is important in the treatment of *phlebitis* and other clot-related disorders.
- Aspirin may be effective in promoting *sleep*. Many scientists now believe aspirin is as effective as most prescription sedatives, and it has far fewer and less serious side effects.
- Diabetic patients who take aspirin may have a lower risk of developing *retinopathy*.

It is important to remember that aspirin is a *drug*. Many of the benefits of aspirin stem from its systemic, wide-reaching effects on metabolism, which may have unforeseen short- and long-term detrimental results. We do know that aspirin is to be strictly *avoided* by persons with hemophilia. Also, allergic reactions to aspirin can be severe. Aspirin seems to be implicated in asthma. Children are especially vulnerable to side effects and should not be given aspirin without a physician's instructions.

Aspirin is an irritant to the stomach and intestine. Its continuous use is associated with low-level chronic loss of iron caused by mucosal erosion. This leads to iron deficiency anemia.

Aspirin has been linked to birth defects, especially when it is taken later in the course of pregnancy. It increases the risk of infant and neonatal mortality, low birth weight, and intracranial hemorrhage.

The best way to take aspirin is on an empty stomach with a full glass of water. This is important; the absorption of aspirin is facilitated by a large volume of liquid and inhibited by the presence of food. In addition, taking aspirin—especially on an empty stomach—without a large fluid intake invites erosion of the stomach lining. But aspirin should *never* be taken when using alcohol because it increases the bioavailability of alcohol, raises the blood concentration, and thus the effect of alcohol on brain centers.

REFERENCES

Griffith HW: *Complete guide to prescription and non-prescription drugs*, ed 5, Los Angeles, 1988, The Body Press, Price Stern Sloan.

Koch PA et al: Influence of food and fluid ingestion on aspirin bioavailability, *J Pharm Sci* 67(11):1533, 1978.

Roine R et al: Aspirin increases blood alcohol concentrations in humans after ingestion of ethanol, *JAMA* 264(18):2406, 1990.

Schachtel BP et al: Caffeine as an aspirin adjuvant, *Arch Intern Med* 151:733, 1991.

with food may increase its effective dissolution and consequent absorption.

Stomach Emptying Rate

Delayed emptying of food from the stomach has the effect of doling out small portions of a drug, creating more optimal saturation rates on the absorptive sites in the small intestine.

Nutrients

Some nutrients promote absorption of certain drugs. For example, high-fat diets increase absorption of the antifungal drug griseofulvin. This drug is fat soluble, and high-fat diets stimulate the secretion of bile acids, which aid in absorption of the drug. Iron absorption is enhanced by vitamin C and gastric acid. Also, citrus juices increase absorption of the antihypertensive drug nifedipine, as do meals with hydralazine.[16,17]

Blood Flow

Food intake increases splanchnic blood flow, resulting in an increased absorption.

Nutritional Status

In addition to the presence of specific nutrients, nutritional status may also affect bioavailability of certain drugs in different ways. For example, chloramphenicol is absorbed more slowly in children with protein-energy malnutrition (PEM), but elimination of the drug is slower in well-nourished children. In both cases the effect is a net increased bioavailability of the drug.

Decreased Absorption

The absorption of some drugs is delayed or reduced by the presence of food. Absorption of aspirin, for example, is delayed by food, so it should be taken on an empty stomach with ample water, preferably cold (see *To Probe Further,* p. 27). Because aspirin increases the effect of alcohol, however, it should not be taken when using alcohol.[18] In addition, caffeine enhances the analgesic effect of aspirin.[19] Nutritional status may also have an impact on drug absorption. For example, tetracycline absorption is impaired in malnourished individuals. Absorption of this commonly used antibiotic is also hindered when it is taken with antacids, milk, or iron supplements. The tetracycline combines with these to form a new, insoluble compound that the body cannot absorb, causing loss of the minerals involved, calcium or iron.[14,15] The presence of protein inhibits the absorption of phenytoin, whereas carbohydrate increases its absorption. Fat has no impact on the absorption of phenytoin.

Food Effects on Drug Distribution and Metabolism

Carbohydrates and Fat

Dietary carbohydrates and fat, especially their relative quantities, influence hepatic drug-metabolizing enzymes. This effect may occur through alterations in phospholipid composition of the endoplasmic reticulum or by limiting cofactors needed for optimal mixed-function oxidation and configuration. Also, the presence of fats increases the activity of diazepam (Valium). Fat increases the concentration of an unbound, thus active, drug by displacing it from binding to tissue protein sites.

Licorice

Licorice, a sweet-tasting plant extract used in making chewing tobacco, candy, and certain drugs, causes sodium retention and increased hypertension.[20,21] A person being treated for hypertension needs to avoid any licorice-containing product. The active ingredient in licorice is glycyrrhizic acid from the name of its natural plant source, *Glycyrrhiza glabra,* meaning "sweet root," a member of the legume family. An analog of this active part of licorice is marketed under the trade names Biogastrone and Duogasterone, which are widely used to heal gastric ulcers, but hypertension is a side effect.

Indoles

The **indoles** in **cruciferous** vegetables, such as cabbage, brussels sprouts, broccoli, and cauliflower speed up the rate of drug metabolism. They apparently induce mixed-function oxidase enzyme systems in the liver.

Cooking Methods

The method of cooking foods may alter the rate of drug metabolism. Charcoal broiling, for example, increases hepatic drug metabolism through enzyme induction.

Changes in Intestinal Microflora

Changes in dietary protein or fiber, for example, may influence intestinal drug metabolism.

Vitamin Effects on Drug Action

Vitamin Effects on Drug Effectiveness

Pharmacologic doses, large megadoses beyond nutritional need, of vitamins decrease blood levels of drugs when the vitamins interact with the drugs. For example, high folate or vitamin B_6 levels reduce the blood level, and thus efficacy, of phenytoin (Dilantin) or phenobarbital for seizure control. Unwise self-medication with pharmacologic doses of vitamins causes severe toxic complications. On the other hand, vitamins themselves may become medications when used as part of the medical treatment for a secondary vitamin deficiency induced by a childhood genetic or metabolic disease, for example, the use of biotin in certain organic acidemias or of riboflavin in certain defects of fatty acid metabolism.

Control of Drug Intoxication

Riboflavin is useful in treating boric acid poisoning. Boric acid combines with the ribityl side chain of riboflavin and is excreted in the urine. Vitamin E combats pulmonary oxygen toxicity. Premature human infants at risk for development of bronchopulmonary dysplasia by oxygen treatment have been protected by vitamin E administration during the acute phase of respiratory distress requiring oxygen treatment.

indole • A compound produced in the intestines by the decomposition of tryptophan; also found in the oils of jasmine and clove.

cruciferous • Belonging to the botanical family *Cruciferae* or *Brassica,* whose members have crosslike, four-petaled flowers—broccoli, cabbage, brussels sprouts, and cauliflower.

Nutrition-Pharmacy Team

Decades of Change

A decade or so ago hospitalized patients as a whole were less severely ill than they are today. Now, however, reflecting our more complex medical system and economic reform efforts, patients that are hospitalized are more acutely ill, more at risk for nutritional deficits, and more likely to develop malnutrition, which leads to increased lengths of stay and higher costs. In the 1960s and 1970s hospitals were beginning to develop multidisciplinary nutrition support committees to administer special enteral and parenteral feeding plans for more seriously ill persons, a form of nutritional care that required key roles of the clinical pharmacist and clinical dietitian.[22] At the same time, as the body of scientific knowledge advanced and more drugs were developed to match this advance, the task of monitoring food and drug interactions also became more complex and required team responsibilities. It was soon recognized that coordinating pharmacy, food service, and clinical nutrition minimized adverse drug-nutrient interactions.

Current Trends

The movement in hospitals and other health care facilities today is a shift in focus toward key processes and functions such as drug-nutrient interactions in this case, rather than the strictly compartmentalized tasks of departments. Current standards focus on departmental or service roles. But this is changing because of economic necessity as well as philosophy of care. This changing focus is being shaped, for example, in the work of the Joint Commission on the Accreditation of Healthcare Organizations (JCAHO).[22] By 1994 JCAHO's accreditation manual will reflect this philosophy that key functions often involve different disciplines coming together, partners with clearly defined responsibilities. The team of clinical nutritionist and clinical pharmacologist is clearly one of these partnerships.[23] The current JCAHO guideline, Standard 6.18, mandates the monitoring of drug therapy by clinical dietitians responsible for diet therapy and counseling with patients about adverse drug-nutrient interactions.[24] In fact, programs are already being developed in medical centers such as the comprehensive program initiated by the clinical nutrition staff at the University of Maryland Medical System in Baltimore.[25] In this program the departments of clinical nutrition, pharmacy, and nursing have coordinated responsibilities in the process of monitoring and counseling on potential drug-food-nutrient interactions. As computer capabilities are expanded into the twenty-first century, computer-generated flagging, monitoring systems, and printouts provide more commonly used tools as rapid communication. Then, as the Baltimore group has shown, partnerships of clinical nutrition-pharmacy-nursing professions and their patients in relation to drug-nutrient interactions will become routine. Further JCAHO directives will *require* such specific responsibilities.

To Sum Up

The field of nutrient-drug interaction is in its infancy but is healthy and growing fast. Continuing research is leading to fundamental change in hospital organization and operation of services to provide improved care in a more cost-effective manner. The new nutrition-pharmacy team reflects these changes, a natural partnership to intervene and prevent costly malnutrition.

Drugs have multiple effects on the body's absorption, metabolism, retention, and status of nutrients. Drugs provoke adverse reactions in combination with certain foods. Among these reactions are flushing, hypoglycemia, the disulfiram effect, and the influence of monoamine oxidase inhibitors (MAOIs) on the metabolism of vasoactive amines, which is serious. Antidepressant MAOIs combined with food or drinks high in tyramine, dopamine, or related amines lead to a hypertensive crisis. Drugs also influence appetite, either repressing it or artificially stimulating it. Drugs either increase an individual's absorption of nutrients, or more commonly decrease absorption, sometimes leading to clinical deficiencies. Drugs also induce mineral and vitamin deficiencies.

Just as drugs affect our utilization of food, food affects our utilization of drugs. Food affects the absorption of drugs in a variety of ways: by changing the amount of time the drug stays in the stomach, by influencing the digestive system, by increasing splanchnic blood flow, or by regulating the release of drugs into the systemic circulation. Foods also have an effect on the subsequent distribution and metabolism of drugs. Certain foods, notably the cruciferous vegetables (brussels sprouts, broccoli, cabbage, and cauliflower), affect hepatic metabolism via enzyme induction. A related effect is seen from charcoal-broiled foods.

Vitamins may interfere with drug effectiveness especially if they are taken in pharmacologic doses. On the other hand, large doses of vitamins are effective in countering certain drug toxicity conditions.

QUESTIONS FOR REVIEW

1. Name four ways food may affect drug use, and give examples of each.

2. If your patient were using a prescribed MAOI such as tranylcypromine sulfate (Parnate), what foods would you instruct him to avoid?
3. What is the most effective way to take aspirin? With what type of liquid? With or without food?
4. What foods would you suggest to a hypersensitive patient on the diuretic hydrochlorothiazide (HCTZ) as good sources of potassium replacement?
5. Outline suggestions you would discuss with a patient experiencing a drug-induced taste loss. How would you explain the cause of the taste loss?
6. How does cimetidine help to improve the nutritional status of persons with gastrointestinal disease?

REFERENCES

1. Roe DA: Diet nutrition and drug reactions. In Shils ME, Young VR, eds: *Modern nutrition in health and disease,* ed 7, Philadelphia, 1988, Lea & Febiger.
2. Roe DA: *Diet and drug interactions,* ed 2, New York, 1989, AVI Books.
3. Roe DA: Process guides on drug and nutrient interactions for health care providers and patients. I. An overview, *Drug-Nutrient Interactions* 5(3):131, 1987.
4. Roe DA: Process guides on drug and nutrient interactions in arthritics, *Drug-Nutrient Interactions* 5(3):135, 1987.
5. Magnus MH, Roe DA: Computer-assisted instruction on drug-nutrient interactions for long-term caregivers, *J Nutr Educ* 23(1):10, 1991.
6. Kamath SK et al: Hospital malnutrition: a 33-hospital screening study, *J Am Diet Assoc* 86(2):203, 1986.
7. Torum B, Viteri FE: Protein-energy malnutrition. In Shils ME, Young VR, eds: *Modern nutrition in health and disease,* ed 7, Philadelphia, 1988, Lea & Febiger.
8. Griffith HW: *Complete guide to prescription and non-prescription drugs,* Los Angeles, 1988, The Body Press, Price Stern Sloan.
9. Graham AW: Screening for alcoholism by life-style risk assessment in a community hospital, *Arch Intern Med* 151:958, 1991.
10. Biery JR et al: Alcohol craving in rehabilitation: assessment of nutrition therapy, *J Am Diet Assoc* 91(4):463, 1991.
11. Roe DA et al: Effect of fiber supplements on the apparent absorption of pharmacologic doses of riboflavin, *J Am Diet Assoc* 88(2):212, 1988.
12. Murray JJ, Healy MD: Drug-mineral interactions: a new responsibility for the hospital dietitian, *J Am Diet Assoc* 91(1):66, 1991.
13. Masse PG: Nutrient intakes of women who use oral contraceptives, *J Am Diet Assoc* 91(9):1118, 1991.
14. Trovato A et al: Drug-nutrient interactions, *Am Fam Physician* 44(5):1651, 1991.
15. Farrington E, Litteral J: Pediatric drug monitoring: clinically important drug-nutrient reactions, *Pediatr Nurs* 16(6):594, 1990.
16. Bailey DG et al: Interaction of citrus juices with felodipine and nifedipine, *Lancet* 337:268, 1991.
17. Semple HA et al: Interactions between hydralazine and oral nutrients in humans, *Ther Drug Monit* 13:304, 1991.
18. Roine R et al: Aspirin increases blood alcohol concentration in humans after ingestion of ethanol, *JAMA* 264(18):2406, 1990.
19. Schachtel BP et al: Caffeine as an analgesic adjuvant, *Arch Intern Med* 151:733, 1991.
20. Morris DJ et al: Licorice, tobacco chewing, and hypertension, *N Engl J Med* 322:849, 1990.
21. Baker ME, Fanestil DD: Liquorice as a regulator of steroid and prostaglandin metabolism, *Lancet* 337:428, 1991.
22. Hard R: Food service, pharmacy team up for nutrition, *Hospitals* 65:46, 1991.
23. Kessler DA: Communicating with patients about their medications, *N Engl J Med* 325(23):1650, 1991.
24. Joint Commission on the Accreditation of Healthcare Organizations: *Accreditation manual for hospitals,* Oakbrook, Ill 1990, JCAHO.
25. Lasswell AB, Loreck ES: Development of a program in accord with JCAHO standards for counseling on potential drug-food interactions, *J Am Diet Assoc* 92(9):1124, 1992.

FURTHER READING

Ahmed FE: Effect of nutrition on the health of the elderly, *J Am Diet Assoc* 92(9):1102, 1992.

Kerstetter JE et al: Malnutrition in the institutionalized older adult, *J Am Diet Assoc* 92(9):1109, 1992.

These excellent companion articles in a single issue of the Journal of the American Dietetic Association speak to the twin problems of malnutrition and "polypharmacy"—multiple drug use among elderly persons.

Beckley-Barrett LM, Mutch PB: Position of the American Dietetic Association: nutrition intervention in treatment and recovery from chemical dependency, *J Am Diet Assoc* 90(9):1274, 1990.

Mohs ME et al: Nutritional effects of marijuana, heroin, cocaine, and nicotine, *J Am Diet Assoc* 90(9):1261, 1990.

These experienced authors provide important background relating the staggering problem of addiction to social drugs, including alcohol, and the nutrition and health impact calling for professional nutrition intervention.

Clayman CB, ed: *Know your drugs and medications,* The American Medical Association Home Medical Library Series, Pleasantville, NY, 1991, Dorling Kindersley and Reader's Digest.

This clearly written and illustrated book helps consumers know more about drugs in common use so they understand their effects and use them safely. It is a helpful reference for patient education programs.

The Calming of America?

American medicine has many names for its psychoactive drugs that act on the mind to dull its reactions. These drugs interact dangerously with alcohol and in some cases with common foods. Perhaps the name that best fits the effect of these drugs is *tranquilizer,* from a Latin root meaning "calm, quiet, stillness." This meaning signifies the escape many persons seek from a turbulent, confusing world.

We live in an age of stress, often called the "Era of Anxiety." We also live in a culture committed to "instant cures" and the avoidance of discomfort. Often instead of probing the causes of our problems and striving to alter the conditions that develop them, we believe that somehow we must never feel uncomfortable. If we do, we take something for it. We seek the "magic potion" to ease the pain and often the symptoms.

To what extent do we actually use such antianxiety drugs in our search for relief? According to the National Academy of Sciences, some 8.5 million Americans take prescription sleeping pills at least once a year. Two million Americans take them every night for at least 2 months at a time. A study conducted by the National Institute on Drug Abuse indicated that 17 million Americans have used stimulants, 28 million have taken sedatives, and 51 million, nearly one out of every four Americans, have taken tranquilizers.

America's single most widely prescribed tranquilizer drug is *diazepam* (Valium). For example, in one recent year, 3.2 billion pills were sold legally, up 50% from the year before and enough to provide every man, woman, and child in the United States with 145 pills a year. It is still widely prescribed for depression along with others such as chlorpromazine and lithium. It is difficult to explain just why Valium has been such a frequently prescribed psychoactive drug in the United States. Certainly from a scientific or a pharmacologic viewpoint no superior effectiveness has been proved. Its popularity probably can be explained by an aggressive marketing program, leading increased number of physicians to prescribe it and increased quantities of the drug to be manufactured. In turn the increased amount of the drug available has led to increased black market exposure and easy street usage.

Valium belongs to a group of psychoactive drugs first introduced in 1960 called *benzodiazepines.* These antianxiety drugs bind to specific receptor sites in the brain. Their clinical effects are mediated through the central nervous system. For some time scientists have sought the identity of the body's natural compound that occupies these receptor sites in the brain. Now pharmacologists report purification of this natural substance. Paradoxically, they have discovered that this new 104-amino acid brain peptide not only blocks the receptor binding action of the antianxiety drugs but also appears to induce anxiety, indicating that it is not a natural tranquilizer but has just the opposite effect. This newly identified compound has been named *diazepam-binding inhibitor (DBI)* peptide. These scientists suggest that the naturally occurring DBI acts to trigger anxiety-associated behavior. Apparently, drugs such as Valium achieve their antianxiety effect by getting in the way of this naturally occurring, anxiety-producing brain peptide.

Along with its desired effect, a drug usually causes some unwanted side effects. In the case of antianxiety drugs such as Valium, several interactions and side effects relate to nutrition counseling needs.

Alcohol

Tranquilizers and alcohol do not mix. These drugs enhance the effects of alcohol and other central nervous system (CNS) depressant drugs that slow down the nervous system. In addition to alcohol, other CNS depressant drugs include over-the-counter antihistamines or medicine for hay fever, other allergies, or colds, as well as prescribed anticonvulsants such as Dilantin, pain medications, and narcotics. Long-term use of alcohol also induces liver enzyme changes, leading to more rapid metabolism and reducing the effect of drugs that are detoxified by the liver. Thus in the alcoholic person benzodiazepines may be metabolized more rapidly, and the person may use increasingly larger doses to achieve the desired effect.

Weight gain

Persons taking these antianxiety drugs often experience a great increase in appetite with subsequent weight gain. This may bring added concern and require general weight management counseling.

Gastrointestinal problems

Some general side effects interfere with food intake and utilization. These problems range from heartburn, nausea, and vomiting to constipation and diarrhea. Individual counseling relating to food choice, combinations, and forms may be needed.

Pregnancy and lactation

Some cases of birth defects from benzodiazepine use during the first 3 months of pregnancy have been reported. In addition, continued use during pregnancy may cause fetal dependency with withdrawal side effects after birth. During lactation these drugs may pass into the breast milk and cause unwanted side effects in the infant.

A more recently introduced antidepressant drug with the trade name Prozac has widespread positive use, primarily because it is relatively free of side effects. However, such widespread use of tranquilizers means that we

Continued.

frequently encounter them in clinical practice and that nutrition counseling must cover their interactions with food and other drugs, including alcohol.

Current research at the National Institute of Mental Health is encouraging. The studies of psychiatrist Robert Post seem to indicate that repeated severe depressive episodes affect gene-modulated brain changes more permanently so that preventive drug therapy should be used more in recurrent illness. Early maintenance therapy may provide the double service of preventing not only the painful recurrences but also the more lasting brain cell changes. Post indicates that the key thing now is to match the patient with the right type of medication, and in the long run there will be better medications to match with patients.

REFERENCES

Griffith HW: *Complete guide to prescription and non-prescription drugs* ed 5, Los Angeles, 1988, The Body Press, Price Stern Sloan.

Holden C: Depression: the news isn't depressing, *Science* 254:1450, 1991.

CHAPTER 3

Enteral Nutrition

CHAPTER OUTLINE

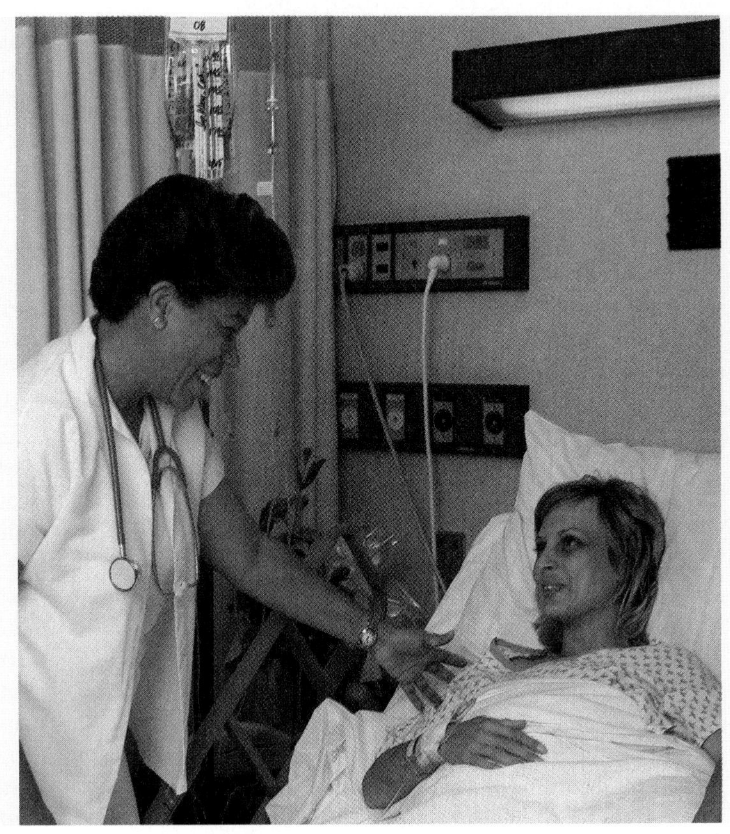

*This chapter begins a two-chapter sequence on alternate modes of feeding to provide nutritional support for patients with special needs. We first examine ways of feeding when the gastrointestinal tract can still be used—**enteral** nutrition. Then in the chapter following, we review the alternative of nutrient feeding directly into the vein when the gastrointestinal tract cannot be used—**parenteral** nutrition.*

In hospitalized patients, especially those with hypermetabolic illness or injury, protein-energy malnutrition is a serious concern. Often a highly personalized aggressive nutritional program provided by the skilled hospital nutritional support team is lifesaving. Many patients who require nutritional support over an extended time can continue this therapy at home with continuous follow-up care and monitoring and reduced costs.

In this chapter, then, we look at the process of enteral nutrition and its various components, starting with its role in clinical nutrition and the vital role of the support team from medicine, clinical nutrition, pharmacy, and nursing that administer enteral nutrition in the hospital and in the home.

Enteral Feeding in Clinical Nutrition

Nutritional Support Needs

Malnutrition is the common enemy health professionals face in many hospitalized patients as well as in home care patients. Persons with hypermetabolic demands, such as those with underlying chronic disease or traumatic injury, are particularly at risk. Elderly persons are especially vulnerable. The lack of adequate nutrition to meet metabolic demands is increasingly recognized as a serious concern in medical and surgical patients. A number of surveys have shown that as many as 50% of surgical patients and 44% of medical patients suffer significant protein-energy malnutrition.[1] These patients range widely from those with sudden severe burns or other critical injury to those developing illness of alcoholic hepatitis or with a malignant cancer. In all such cases with the gastrointestinal tract functioning, enteral nutrition support may provide a front line of restoring or, in the case of sudden injury, maintaining an optimal state of nutrition.

Questions do not center on the effectiveness of enteral nutrition support, even feeding by tube if needed, for this has been proved. Rather, current questions center on the most appropriate formula for each patient's specific disease state, the preferred method of formula delivery, and in the case of tube-feeding, the causes and extent of any tube-related complications involved.[1]

Modes of Enteral Nutrition Support

Some patients cannot maintain or restore a good nutritional status because they are unable to eat enough regular food to sustain themselves, even though they have a functioning gastrointestinal tract. They need to take in more nutrient-dense nourishment. Two modes of enteral nutrition support are possible. First, depending on the patient's condition the initial option may be to add an oral, general energy-nutrient food supplement such as Ensure (Ross) with or between regular meals. Second, if sufficient oral intake of food and supplemental formula is not possible, then the second option is enteral nutrition by tube feeding either as a supplement or as the complete diet.

TABLE 3-1

Questions Guiding Choice of Enteral Nutrition Tube-Feeding Route

Question	Answer	Action
Can the gastrointestinal tract be used safely?		
	No	Use parenteral nutrition.
	Yes	Proceed with enteral nutrition.
Is there adequate intestinal absorption?		
	No	Use defined formula diet.
	Yes	Use protein isolate diet.
Will nutritional support last longer than 4 to 6 weeks?		
	No	Use nasoenteric tube-feeding.
	Yes	Use enterostomy tube-feeding.
Is the patient at risk for aspiration?		
	No	Use shorter nasogastric or gastrostomy tube.
	Yes	Use longer duodenal or jejunal tube.
Is nutritional support providing adequate nutrient delivery?		
	No	Add small vein peripheral parenteral nutrition.
	Yes	Continue present formula tube-feeding and route.

Assessment and Patient Selection

An assessment of nutritional status (see Chapter 1) is needed to identify malnourished persons at risk for medical and surgical problems. A general assessment program at hospital admission should be routine procedure to identify those already in states of malnutrition as well as those with risk of potential malnutrition because of the nature of their disease or injury. Clinical experience has shown that underlying malnutrition carries its own substantial risk of illness and death *above and beyond* that associated with the patient's primary disease.[2]

Thus baseline nutritional assessment is always the first step in identifying patients in need of nutritional support and the choice of feeding mode required. Table 3-1 provides guidelines for these decisions. The baseline nutritional assessment for nutritional support and the schedule of regular follow-up assessments to monitor results and progress are done according to the precise protocol written and developed by the nutritional support team. Metabolic activity factors (MAFs) have been recognized and coded according to their added stress on the clinical state—factors such as disease, trauma, surgery, or sepsis (see Chapter 11). Also, the clinical dietitian who is the primary practitioner of nutritional care in the hospital discovers and evaluates a number of additional personal risk factors. These risks may include eating problems associated with loss of appetite, restricted eating in continuous weight cycling, or the extreme eating disorders of anorexia nervosa and bulimia nervosa, highly limited or fad diets, cultural or religious dietary restrictions, excess alcohol intake, depressed sense of taste and smell, oral problems with chewing and swallowing, or adverse food or nutrient interactions with drugs (see Chapter 2). Other malnutrition risks in the current hospitalization and medical-surgical treatment are the inability to eat for more than 7 to 10 days or maintenance on low kcalorie intravenous fluids for 10 days or more.

After patients in need of nutritional support have been identified and the indicated mode of feeding to be used is enteral nutrition, the choices of formula and delivery system follow.

Complete Enteral Formulas

Blender Mixed or Commercial

Our current age of advanced nutritional science and technology has brought the development of a variety of commercial formulas and smaller, safer feeding tubes. Only a few decades ago, however, medical and infant formulas were prepared in special hospital formula rooms using sterile techniques and autoclaving of bottled formula. Formulas for oral or nasogastric tube feeding were blended mixtures of regular cooked foods such as cereal, meat, vegetables, and fruits, along with juices, milk, egg, vegetable oil, corn syrup, and additions of early protein powders made from casein. Now with a wide range of commercial formulas available, this question seldom arises.

However, in some instances of home enteral nutrition, the patient or family may want to explore the possible use of a home blender-mixed diet and needs to know the problems involved. The use of familiar foods may bring emotional comfort to some persons, especially elderly patients cared for at home, and such home formulas are certainly less costly, but there are problems with preparation and administration.

Problems with blender-mixed formulas involve its physical form, safety, and digestion and absorption. First, foods broken down and mixed in a blender generally yield a viscous solution that is difficult to feed through a tube. Thus because of particle size and tendency to stick to the tube, a large-bore feeding tube that is more uncomfortable is required. Second, such blender-mixed formulas carry problems of bacterial growth and inconsistent nutrient composition from settling out of solid components. Third, the blended food formula requires a fully functioning digestion and absorption system to digest the food and absorb its released nutrients. Some patients have gastrointestinal deficits that require nutrients with varying degrees of predigestion or smaller molecular structure. In overall comparison, then, commercial formulas provide a sterile, homogenized solution suitable for more comfortable small-bore feeding tubes and ensure a fixed profile of nutrients in intact or predigested form.

TABLE 3-2

Common Carbohydrate Forms in Commercial Enteral Nutrition Formulas

Starch—polysaccharides

Modified food starch
Hydrolyzed cereal solids
Tapioca starch
Pureed vegetables: green beans, peas, carrots

Glucose polymers*

Glucose polysaccharides
Glucose polymers
Glucose oligosaccharides
Maltodextrins
Corn syrup, corn syrup solids

Disaccharides

Sucrose—from starch hydrolysis
Lactose—from milk
Maltose—from starch and oligosaccharide hydrolysis

Monosaccharides

Glucose (dextrose)
Fructose

*From partial hydrolysis of cornstarch.

Nutrient Components

Carbohydrates

About half of the kcalories in the American diet come from carbohydrates, the body's primary energy source. In modern commercial formulas, with the exception of lactose, carbohydrates are the most easily digested and absorbed nutrient component. The two main carbohydrate differences among the various formulas are in form and concentration (Table 3-2). The form ranges from large starch molecules (polysaccharides) to small single sugar units (monosaccharides). These differences in form contribute to varying degrees of sweetness, osmolality, and digestibility. The larger forms of carbohydrate molecules (1) taste less sweet; (2) exert less osmotic pressure, which depends

viscous (viscid) • Physical property of a substance dependent on the friction of its component molecules as they slide by one another; viscosity.

TABLE 3-3

Classes of Lactose Deficiency

Primary: inherited

Racial, ethnic
Genetic

Secondary: enzyme deficiency, mucosal damage

Fasting
Malnutrition
Inflammatory bowel disease
Infections (gastroenteritis, cholera)
Medications (colchicine, neomycin)
Radiation

Relative deficiency

Gastric surgery
Short bowel syndrome

on the number of particles in solution, not particle molecular size; and (3) require more digestion. Although the large starch molecules are well tolerated and easily digested by most patients, their relative insolubility creates problems for use in most formulas. Thus the smaller saccharides formed by partial or complete hydrolysis of corn starch are common formula components. In addition to the simple sugars composed of one and two saccharide units, mainly glucose and sucrose, the carbohydrate formula components include intermediate glucose polymers with varying chain lengths of glucose units. These intermediate products of hydrolysis may be glucose polysaccharides of more than 10 glucose units or glucose oligosaccharides of only a few, about 2 to 10 glucose units (Table 3-2).

The disaccharide lactose is often deleted in the manufacture of nutritional support formulas because of primary and secondary lactose intolerance in many malnourished individuals. A *primary* lactase deficiency is inherent in particular racial groups, whereas a *secondary* deficiency is the result of mucosal tissue loss from absorbing surfaces of the small intestine, including much of the microvilli brush border where lactase is located. A *relative* deficiency, depending on the extent of remaining gastrointestinal tissue, follows surgical resections of the stomach and small intestine, which leaves a decreased available absorbing surface area. Some of these various causes of lactase deficiency indicating use of a lactose-free formula are shown in Table 3-3.

Protein

The protein content of standard enteral formulas is most critical because it maintains the body cell mass and all its major functions. The biologic quality of dietary protein depends on its amino acid profile, especially its relative proportions of essential amino acids. The nutritive value of a protein is expressed in terms of its *chemical score,* which is derived from its amino acid content in relation to the amino acid pattern of a high-quality reference protein food such as egg white. The essential amino acid with the greatest deficit limits the body's utilization of that food protein and is thus called its *limiting amino acid.* The percentage of that limiting amino acid in the dietary food in comparison with the high quality standard protein egg white provides the chemical score. Studies of standard and special enteral formulas have indicated that the limiting amino acids are either methionine (plus its metabolic product cysteine) or phenylalanine (plus its metabolic product tyrosine).[3] Investigators recommend that support nutrition clinical dietitians use the chemical score to assess the protein quality of complete enteral and parenteral formula diets.

Research indicates that traumatized, catabolic, or seriously undernourished patients require at least 40% of the total amino acid intake as essential amino acids to restore and maintain desired nutritional status.[3] To supply these needs, three major forms of protein are used in nutritional support enteral formulas: intact proteins, hydrolyzed proteins, and crystalline amino acids.

Intact proteins. Intact proteins are the complete and original forms as found in foods, although some *protein isolates* such as lactalbumin and casein from milk are intact proteins that have been separated from their original food source. Intact proteins do not add much to the formula's osmotic effect, but they do require normal secretion of pancreatic protein-splitting enzymes for complete digestion.

Hydrolyzed proteins. Hydrolyzed proteins are those protein sources that have been broken down by enzymes into smaller protein fragments and amino acids. The smaller products—tripeptides, dipeptides, and free amino acids—are absorbed more easily into the blood circulation, but the larger peptides must be broken down further before they are absorbed.

Crystalline amino acids. Pure crystalline amino acids are easily absorbed, but because of their small size they increase the osmotic effect of the formula. They adversely affect the formula taste and, if used as an oral supplement, require flavoring aids or different forms—for example, liquid beverage, pudding, frozen "slush," or popsicle—to improve palatability.

Table 3-4 shows some common sources of protein

TABLE 3-4

Common Protein Forms in Commercial Enteral Nutrition Formulas and Examples of Conditions for Use

Intact protein	
Milk protein: casein isolates, lactalbumin, whey Sodium and calcium caseinates Soy protein isolates Pureed beef Egg white solids	Normal pancreatic enzymes and normal small intestine absorption
Hydrolyzed protein	
Casein, lactalbumin, whey Soy protein Meat protein, collagen	Reduced absorptive surface, disorders of amino acid transport, and pancreatic insufficiency
Crystalline amino acids	
L-Amino acids	Renal failure and hepatic failure

in standard commercial formulas and examples of conditions for which they are used.

Fat

The major role of fat in a nutritional support enteral formula is to supply a concentrated energy source. The major forms of fat in standard formulas are butterfat in milk-based mixtures; vegetable oils from corn, soy, safflower, or sunflower; the specially produced medium-chain triglycerides (MCTs), monoglycerides, and diglycerides; and lecithin. The vegetable oils provide a rich source of essential fatty acids, especially linoleic acid. Current research is leading to the development of alternate structured lipids from various combinations of short-chain fatty acids, medium-chain fatty acids, and omega-3 fatty acids.[4,5]

Vitamins and Minerals

To provide complete nutrition, standard whole diet commercial formulas include sufficient vitamins and minerals for nutrient requirements when energy needs are fully met. Low kcaloric intakes and the use of diluted formulas require evaluation and the supplementation of deficient formulas with liquid vitamin and mineral preparations. Vitamin K is usually not added to commercial formulas because it is synthesized by intestinal bacteria and a deficiency is rare. However, a general weekly supplement as a precaution is recommended by some clinicians, and specific vitamin K supplementation is usually indicated in conditions relating to fat malabsorption; for example, short bowel syndrome or biliary obstruction.[2] On the other hand, patients receiving anticoagulant drugs require vitamin K assessment to carefully monitor supplement needs (see Chapter 8).

Physical Properties

After the initial choice of a formula according to nutritional requirements and individual gastrointestinal function, certain physical properties of formulas may affect tolerance. Individual intolerance is reflected in *gastric retention* with abdominal distention and pain and diarrhea or constipation. These problems, of which diarrhea is the most common, are often unrelated to the formula itself but may result from inappropriate tube-feeding techniques or drug interactions (see *Issues and Answers,* p. 47). Physical properties of the formula that may cause intolerance include factors such as osmolality, kcalorie-nutrient density, and residue.

Osmolality

A formula's osmolality is one of its most important physical characteristics because of its direct effect on the body's water balance and thus state of hydration. To understand this effect, recall your study of water balance and apply it. Body water and some solutes pass freely across body membranes that are semipermeable. The force of *osmosis* moves water and its *solvent* molecules across a semipermeable membrane. To equalize solute concentrations on both sides of the membrane, the solvent (water) moves from the side of low solute concentration to the side of high solute concentration. The basic *osmotic pressure* that pulls water through the membrane is directly proportional to the *number* of particles in the solution, not their size according to their molecular weight. In the body's water-based system, the osmotic pressure of a solution is measured in *milliosmoles (mOsm).* One millimole (mmol) of a substance such as glucose that does not dissociate in solution exerts an osmotic pressure of 1 mOsm. One millimole of a substance such as sodium chloride that dissociates into two particles has an osmotic pressure of 2 mOsm, and so on. In clinical practice the commonly used term is *osmolality,* which is defined as the number of osmotic particles per *kilogram* of solvent, which in the body is water. A rarely used related term is *osmolarity,* which is defined as the number of osmotic particles per *liter* of solution. In tissue fluids that are very dilute, the difference in the two measures is small and can be ignored. However, in enteral nutrition feeding solutions, which contain large concentrated amounts of nutrient solutes to restore and maintain optimal nutritional status, the two

osmolality • Property of a solution that depends on the concentration of the solute per unit of the solvent.

values are significantly different. Thus for more precise and realistic measure for liquid solutions of nutritional support formulas, the term *osmolality* is preferred.

The osmolality of the enteral nutrition formula affects the solute load and hence water requirements within the body. The protein's metabolic product *urea,* along with the major tissue electrolytes sodium (Na^+), potassium (K^+), and chloride (Cl^-), collectively contribute most of the solute load presented to the kidney for excretion. This excretion load is commonly called the *renal solute load (RSL).* Carbohydrates normally make no contribution because they are metabolized and do not appear in the urine. Fat also makes no contribution because it is not excreted in the urine. The greater this RSL is, the more water is required for its excretion.

To calculate the RSL of a formula (mOsm), an important consideration in nutritional support management, the values for protein and electrolyte contributions are used. In adults, each gram of protein (or amino acids) yields an RSL of 5.7 mOsm. In children, each gram of protein yields only 4.0 mOsm because more protein is being stored during growth. Any anabolic patient excretes less urea, whereas a catabolic patient loses more urea because of tissue breakdown. In all patients, each milliequivalent of electrolyte yields 1 mOsm. Thus the RSL from a tube feeding may easily be calculated by the following formula, using the protein metabolic factor of 5.7 mOsm for adults and 4.0 mOsm for children:

$$\text{RSL of formula (mOsm)} = (\text{g protein} \times 5.7) + \text{mEq (Na} + \text{K} + \text{Cl)}$$

For children and anabolic patients, substitute the protein metabolic factor of 4.0 for the general adult factor of 5.7. The total RSL is calculated as mOsm per day. All values refer to an amount per day.

Nutrient-Kcalorie Density

Malnourished ill or injured persons on tube-fed nutritional support formula diets require increased nutrient and energy intakes. Adequate protein and kcalories are required within the limits of patient toleration to restore and maintain optimal nutritional status. Too dense a formula, however, produces a high renal solute load with the danger of dehydration. Most tube-feedings contain about 1 kcal/ml, but some for more debilitated patients may be more concentrated—1.5 to 2.0 kcal/ml. As formula density increases with more protein and electrolytes, the patient requires more water. Also nutrient density affects gastrointestinal function. High intakes of fat-containing formula delay gastric emptying. In addition, if a patient's gastrointestinal tract has not been used for an extended period or has mucosal damage or disease, gradual initiation of a diluted or less dense formula and building to a desired nutrient-kcalorie intake may be indicated. This process allows time for restoration of mucosal tissue growth and enzyme function.

Intestinal Fuels

To help prevent intestinal mucosal deterioration from disuse or disease, current studies are evaluating new special formulas that use forms of nutrients that the intestine uses as rapid fuels to maintain surface epithelial cells. These special fuels include the following[6]:

- *Glutamine.* This plentiful amino acid provides vital fuel for rapidly developing enteric cells on the surface of the intestinal mucosa.
- *Short-chain fatty acids.* Two-, three-, and four-carbon chain fatty acids—*acetate, propionate,* and *butyrate,* respectively—are water soluble, easily absorbed, and supply an average of 4.4 kcal/g.
- *Dietary fiber.* Soy polysaccharide, for example, not only serves as intestinal fuel but has low viscosity and helps prevent diarrhea in critically ill tube-fed patients.

Residue

General consideration of residue content of enteral nutrition support formulas has been receiving increased attention. Many tube-feeding formulas are low in residue because less residue may be desirable when an underlying intestinal disorder such as inflammatory bowel disease is present. However, when constipation occurs, a formula with added residue may be needed but must be monitored for its potential turnaround effect of diarrhea.[7]

Medical Foods for Specific Needs

Certain formulas designed for special nutritional therapy are called medical foods. The U.S. Food and Drug Administration (FDA) first recognized the concept of medical foods as distinct from drugs in 1972, when the formula Lofenalac (Mead Johnson) was developed for treatment of the genetic disease phenylketonuria in newborns (see Chapter 5). During these early years as medical research and development produced an increasing number of the special formulas, the precise definition of "medical foods" remained in a rather murky territory between labels of food or drug. In 1988 Congress amended the Orphan Drug Act to include medical foods, defining them as food specifically formulated for use under medical supervision for primary treatment of metabolic-genetic disease having distinctive nutritional requirements based on recognized scientific principles (21 U.S. Code 360ee).[8] This defining statement extended the concept of orphan drugs to encompass the concept of orphan medical foods, that is, enteral formula products for specific metabolic-genetic conditions that occur so rarely that developing and marketing them requires some subsidy, as with orphan drugs. The Orphan Drug Act Amendment to include and define medical foods has now been incorporated into the reformed Nutrition Labeling and Education Act of 1990. From a legal perspective, this action identifies medical foods as a subcategory of foods for special dietary uses, and orphan medical foods are identified as a special subset of medical foods. These concepts are now becoming part of the international Codex Alimentarius Commission of the Food and Agriculture Organization (FAO) of the World Health Organization (WHO), divisions of the United Nations (UN).[8] At the request of the FDA, the Life Sciences Research Office (LSRO) of the Federation of American Societies for Experimental Biology (FASEB) has provided guidelines for appropriate use of other special medical foods for enteral nutrition therapy in four categories of specified diseases or disorders: (1) end-stage renal disease, (2) hepatic disease, (3) pulmonary disease, and (4) hypermetabolic stress states.[8]

Modular Enteral Formulas

Basic Modules for Individual Needs

The commercial complete enteral formula products for tube-feeding are designed with a fixed ratio of nutrients to meet general standards for nutritional needs. Some patients' particular needs are not met by these standard fixed-ratio formulas, and they require an individualized *modular formula*. Such an individual formula is planned, calculated, prepared, and administered with the combined expertise of the nutritional support team, with the clinical dietitian on the team having the major responsibility. The modules vary from a single nutrient to a combination of several nutrients. For example, they may be single modules of carbohydrates, fat, and protein or either combined or single vitamins and minerals.

Carbohydrate Modules

Four carbohydrate modules are commonly used: (1) polysaccharides and oligosaccharides, (2) glucose polymers, (3) disaccharides, and (4) monosaccharides (Table 3-2). Generally, carbohydrate modules combine easily with liquid formulas and are digested without problem. Glucose polymers are used often because they have two advantages over smaller carbohydrate molecules such as glucose or dextrose: (1) lower osmolality contribution and (2) higher kcaloric density. Also, compared with other nutrient modules, carbohydrate units cost less. An example of a commonly used carbohydrate module composed of glucose polymers is Polycose (Ross), which is produced in liquid and powdered forms.

Protein Modules

The three main forms of protein modules are the same forms used in standard complete formulas: (1) intact proteins, (2) hydrolyzed proteins, and (3) crystalline amino acids. The protein form affects the formula osmolality and palatability. The larger intact proteins contribute the least osmolality and are generally more palatable. Conversely, the smaller molecular size of the synthetic amino acids contributes more osmolality to the formula, but they have a more unpleasant odor and taste so are usually used in tube-fed formulas. Examples of protein modules include Casec (Mead Johnson), made from calcium caseinate, a major milk protein; Promix (Navaco), made from a protein in milk whey; EMF (Control Drugs), a hydrolyzed protein made from collagen; and Aminess (Cutter), crystalline amino acids in tablet form. Compared to carbohydrate and fat modules, protein modules are more expensive because they require more processing.

Fat Modules

Various forms of fat modules are available, with fat molecules varying in chain length and degree of saturation of the constituent fatty acids. Butterfat, vegetable oils, and fat emulsions are the major sources of fat used. All of these are polyunsaturated long-chain (more than 12 carbons) triglycerides. An alternate form is produced from shorter, medium-chain (6 to 12 carbons) triglycerides, which are more water soluble and hence more easily absorbed. Attention to essential fatty acids is important. The long-chain triglycerides in vegetable oils are rich sources of essential fatty acids but medium-chain triglycerides have none because they are made from fractionated coconut oil. Fat modules contribute little to the formula osmolality but are high density sources of concentrated energy. Examples of fat modules include Lipomul (Upjohn), a corn oil emulsion; Microlipid (Organon), a safflower oil emulsion; and MCT (Mead Johnson), a fractionated form of coconut oil. Because MCT is more water soluble and easily absorbed, it is useful in malabsorption conditions. Also, like carbohydrate modules, fat

medical foods • Specially formulated nutrient mixtures for use under medical supervision for treatment of various metabolic diseases.

modules are relatively inexpensive, except for MCT, which is a manufactured oil not occurring naturally and thus requiring more extensive processing.

Vitamin and Mineral Modules

Generally, vitamin modules contain 100% of the RDAs. Mineral modules contain standard electrolytes such as calcium, sodium, and potassium as well as the essential trace elements, all in recommended allowances. Special mineral modules with different electrolyte compositions are made for particular conditions. For example, a mineral module restricted in sodium and potassium may be indicated for use in formulas for patients with renal insufficiency and congestive heart failure.

Uses of Special Modular Formulas

The advances in support nutrition formula products have made possible more specific nutrient-energy combinations to tailor an individual formula to meet underlying disease needs such as in diabetes, congestive heart failure, renal failure, or liver disease.[2]

Diabetes

Patients with underlying diabetes who require nutritional support feeding achieve better management of their diabetes with a modular formula that can be adjusted from day to day in response to their blood glucose levels. Also, using a complex carbohydrate module of glucose polymers instead of the simple sugars of monosaccharides or disaccharides helps maintain more steady, appropriate blood glucose levels. For example, the formula may combine modules of Polycose (Ross), Microlipid (Organon), and Casec (Mead Johnson) in a water base with amounts calculated to supply the necessary total kcalories and relative kcaloric percentages of carbohydrates, fat, and protein for individual blood glucose control (see Chapter 9).

Congestive Heart Failure

Patients with congestive heart failure may become cachectic with loss of lean body tissue and fat, resulting in poor nutrient digestion and absorption. These patients may benefit from a special nutrition support formula. Such a formula should provide about 1.0 g of protein/kg body weight, 0.5 ml of water/kcal of formula given (1000 to 1500 ml), and sodium restricted to 0.5 to 1.5 g/day (see Chapter 8).[9] It should provide easily digested and absorbed forms of protein and fat. An appropriate nutritional support formula can be developed by combining a standard formula for malabsorption with an added fat module of MCTs. For example, Vital HN (Ross) is a high-nitrogen formula with hydrolyzed protein from soy, whey, and meat; fat from safflower oil and MCTs; and carbohydrates from glucose oligosaccharides; and a relatively low sodium content. It may be combined with an added fat module of water-soluble MCT (Mead Johnson) for an easily absorbed and protein-sparing energy source. Such a combination provides the needed nutrients and energy to help build a more positive nutritional status and to meet special dietary modifications required by the underlying heart disease.

Renal Failure

Patients with renal failure need minimal urea formation for a decreased renal solute load, and if fluid output is low, they may need to restrict total intake (see Chapter 10). Formulas enriched with essential amino acids help reduce urea formation. High-kcalorie formulas help control fluid intake. Also, patients with renal failure may benefit from formulas with increased kcalorie/nitrogen ratios and reduced levels of potassium. An example of a formula for temporary use, such as during short-term acute renal failure, is Amin-Aid (McGaw), which has carbohydrates as maltodextrins and sucrose, protein as essential crystalline amino acids, and fat as soy oil and provides a formula high in kcalories (2.0 kcal/ml) and low in sodium and potassium in an essential amino acid base. Also, a low-protein modular formula can be made using as a base the support formula Osmolite (Ross), which has carbohydrates as corn syrup solids; protein as caseinate and soy isolate; and fat as corn oil, soy oil, and MCT (Mead Johnson) oil. This base can then be combined with a carbohydrate module of Polycose (Ross) and a fat module of Microlipid (Organon) to increase nonprotein kcalories.

Hepatic Insufficiency

Patients with liver disease may need restriction of protein, sodium, and fluid. Standard high density enteral nutrition support formulas have an excess of protein when used alone. However, a relatively low protein formula may be made by combining a high density formula with added modules of carbohydrates and fat. For example, a high density formula such as Amin Aid (McGaw) mixed with a carbohydrate module of Polycose (Ross), composed of complex glucose polymers, and a fat module of MCT (Mead Johnson), composed of easily absorbed medium-chain triglycerides, produces a modular formula low in protein, sodium, and free water with sufficient nonprotein energy sources to spare protein for tissue repletion.

Enteral Nutrition Delivery Systems

Feeding Equipment

Feeding Tubes

Feeding liquids into the esophagus and stomach of patients unable to eat has a long history stretching

CLINICAL APPLICATION

Preventing Complications in Patients Receiving Enteral Nutrition by Nasoenteric Tube

Most complications of enteral alimentation are easily treated and prevented through proper monitoring. Complications are metabolic, gastrointestinal, or mechanical in nature.

Tube obstruction or clogging

Use liquid medications when possible. Flush the tube before and after administration of medication. Flush the tube (20 to 50 cc of water) before and after each feeding or every 4 hours during continuous feeding.

Gastric retention and aspiration pneumonia

Elevate the head of the bed 30° to 45° during and for 2 hours after infusion of food. Monitor and confirm tube placement before feeding.

Tube discomfort

Consider using soft, small-bore feeding tubes. Keep the mouth and lips moist. Allow chewing of sugarless gum, gargling, or sucking on anesthetic lozenges, if appropriate.

Nausea, vomiting, cramping, and distention

Return to a slower infusion rate, and increase it by smaller increments. Dilute the formula to isotonic strength if gastric residuals are consistently high. Increase the concentration over several days. Consider changing to isotonic formula. Check gastric residuals every 4 to 6 hours in continuously fed patients or before each bolus.

Constipation

Monitor intake and output. Add free water if the intake is not greater than the output by 500 to 1,000 ml/day. Use a formula with added fiber. Evaluate medication side effects. Increase patient activity if possible.

Diarrhea

Diarrhea is defined as passage of more than 200 g of stool per 24 hours or the passage of liquid stools. Use an isotonic or elemental formula at a slow rate initially. Check for infections with stool, blood, or formula cultures. Review tube-feeding handling and infection control procedures. If bolus feeding, change to continuous feeding or decrease the bolus volume and increase the frequency of feeding.

Hyperosmolar dehydration

Initiate hypertonic feedings at reduced rates, dilute the formula, or consider using an isotonic formula.

Fluid overload or overhydration

Restrict fluids, and use a concentrated formula.

Serum electrolyte or mineral abnormalities

Monitor electrolytes daily making individualized adjustments as needed.

Glucose intolerance

Monitor blood sugar levels frequently making adjustments in insulin dose. Avoid formulas high in simple sugars.

Increased respiratory quotient, excess carbon dioxide production, and respiratory insufficiency

Reduce the respiratory quotient by balancing the kcalories provided from fat, protein, and carbohydrates. Increase the percentage of kcalories provided from fat. ◆

REFERENCE

American Dietetic Association: *Handbook of clinical dietetics*, ed 2, New Haven, 1992, Yale University Press.

back beyond the Renaissance. Over the years early physicians used various forms of "gravity drip" methods and then large-bore stiff tubing with the nasogastric tube being introduced over a hundred years ago.[2] But it was not until more recent years that advances in science and technology have made possible the enteral nutrition delivery systems used today. Modern small-bore nasoenteric feeding tubes are made of softer, more flexible polyurethane and silicone materials that make them more comfortable for patients (see the *Clinical Application* above). These tubes easily carry the variety of nutrient solutions now available in enteral nutrition support formulas. These nasoenteric tubes can also be inserted not only into the stomach but also beyond the pyloric valve into the small intestine, duodenum, or jejunum (Fig. 3-1). These lower placements are used to avoid dangers of vomiting and aspiration by patients on ventilators or for those who are restrained, have a depressed gag reflex, or are comatose. These longer tubes have weighted tips to hold them in place. Insertion and correct placement are guided by radiographic visualization.[10,11]

Containers and Pumps

Additional parts of the enteral nutrition support tube-feeding system are the formula container and often a

cachexia • A specific profound effect caused by malnutrition and a disturbance in glucose metabolism usually seen in patients with terminal cancer or heart failure; general poor health and malnutrition indicated by an emaciated appearance.

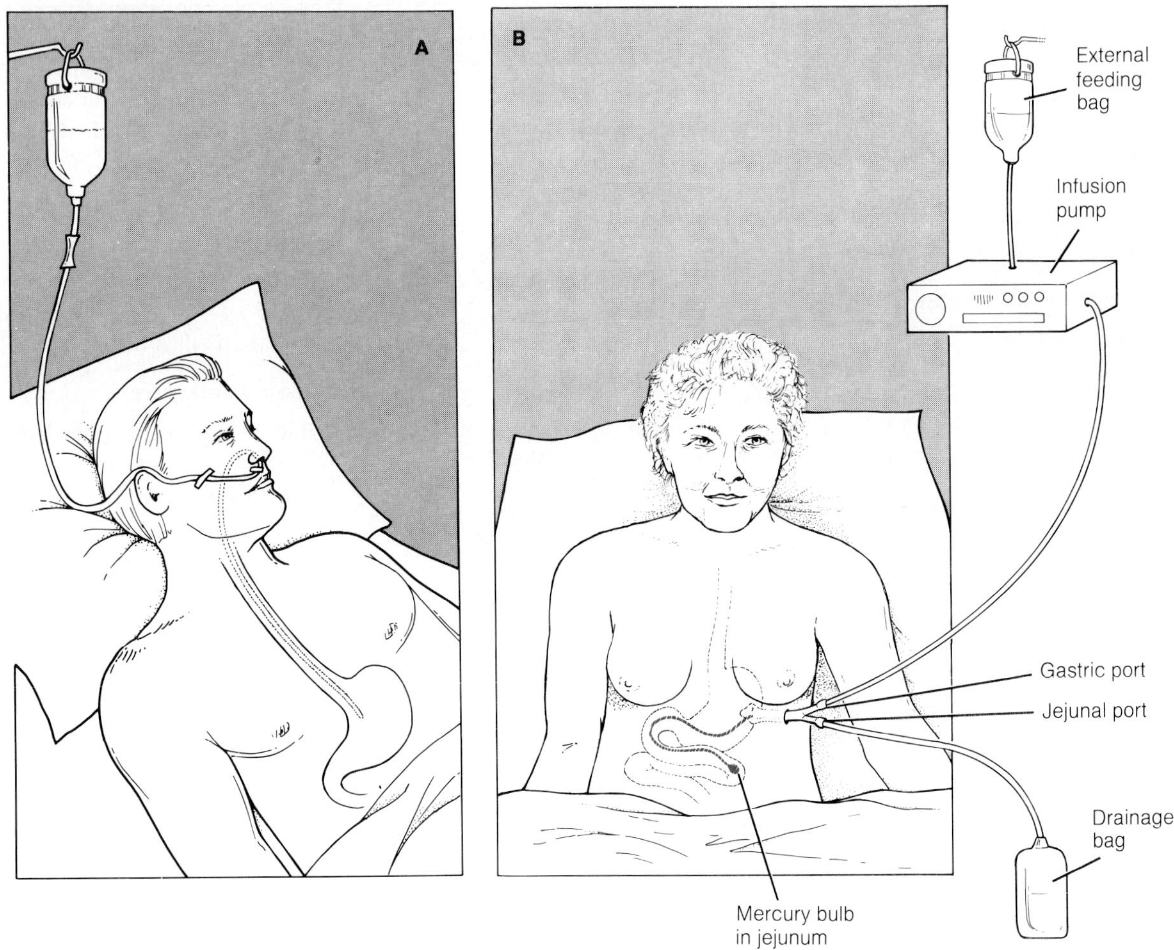

FIG. 3-1 Types of tube feeding. **A,** Common nasogastric feeding tube. **B,** Gastrostomy-jejunal enteral feeding tube.

pump. A number of containers and feeding sets are available, and the clinical dietitian and nurse need to know details of their comparative advantages and limitations. For example, containers that hold a large volume of formula, as much as 1 L, may be convenient for the nursing staff, but if they are not used within a limited time they are subject to bacterial contamination. Sets that attach to the manufacturer's container reduce contamination. Also, an accurate flow rate must be controlled. A pump may be needed for more accurate control, which is essential for feedings that go directly into the small intestine or for more viscous formulas.

In the final analysis, whatever the type of formula and equipment used, it is essential that microbiologic quality control programs with stringent standards be maintained by enteral nutrition support services at all institutions.[12,13] Such quality standards of practice reduce bacterial counts significantly, thus improving patient tolerance to enteral feeding and reducing complications of infection, diarrhea, and sepsis.

Alternate Routes of Formula Delivery

The nasoenteric route described previously is indicated for short-term therapy in many clinical situations. However, for long-term feedings, *enterostomies*—surgical placement of the tube at progressive points along the gastrointestinal tract—are the preferred route.[10] At the level of the cervical spine to the side of the neck, a cervical *esophagostomy* is often placed after head and neck surgeries for cancer or traumatic injury. This removes the discomfort of the nasal route and the entry point can be concealed easily under clothing. If the patient is not at risk for aspiration, a *gastrostomy* tube may be surgically placed into the stomach. Otherwise, a *jejunostomy* tube is surgically placed into the jejunum, the middle section of the small intestine. This procedure is indicated for patients who

Problem-Solving Tips for Patients Receiving Enteral Nutrition by Nasoenteric Tube Feedings

TO PROBE FURTHER

- *Thirst, oral dryness.* Lubricate lips, chew sugarless gum, brush teeth, rinse mouth frequently with water, suck lemon drops occasionally.
- *Tube discomfort.* Gargle with a mixture of warm water and mouth wash, gently blow nose, clean tube regularly with water or water-soluble lubricant. If persistent, pull tube out gently, clean it, and reinsert the tube. (Many long-term users of tube feeding have learned to pass their own nasogastric tubes.) Request a smaller tube.
- *Tension, fullness.* Relax and breathe deeply after each feeding.
- *Loud stomach noises.* Take feedings in private.
- *Limited mobility.* Change positions in bed or chair, and walk around the house or hospital corridor.
- *General gustatory distress with feeding.* Warm or chill feedings, but avoid having formula too cold because that causes diarrhea, and check about occasional use of blender-mixed "regular" foods.
- *Persistent hunger.* Chew a favorite food, then spit it out; chew gum; suck lemon drops.
- *Inability to drink.* Rinse mouth frequently with water and other liquids.

lack a competent gag reflex or functional gastric emptying or who have gastric cancer or gastric ulcerative disease.[10]

Monitoring the Tube-Fed Patient

The nutritional support team carefully monitors all patients who are being nourished by tube-feeding. The nursing staff administering the formula to the patient checks for gastric residuals or gastric emptying rate, noting any signs of abdominal distention or bloating, and monitors usual vital signs—temperature, pulse, and respiration. Attending nurses also monitor the formula flow rate and record the intake and output of formula and fluid. The nutritional support clinical dietitian monitors tolerance for the formula, state of hydration, and nutritional status response following laboratory test panels commonly included in nutritional support assessment protocols (see Chapter 4). Also monitored are any other special test results related to the patient's disease status or metabolic complications, such as insulin-dependent diabetes mellitus (IDDM), traumatic injury, or sepsis.

Formula Tolerance

Gastrointestinal signs such as vomiting, abdominal distention or bloating, and stool frequency and consistency are noted (see *To Probe Further* above). If these occur, the feeding may need to be adjusted to a less concentrated formula that feeds the patient more slowly with continuous rather than intermittent bolus feeding until tolerance improves and symptoms subside.

Daily urine tests for glucose and acetone for the first week or so, according to protocol, reflect carbohydrate tolerance. If test results continue to be negative in the nondiabetic patient, these tests may be discontinued. Blood glucose monitoring may be used instead of urine testing. Patients who are diabetic or those who are severely stressed with sepsis may have difficulty metabolizing carbohydrates.[14,15] Rather than reducing the formula carbohydrate needed for energy, sometimes insulin is given.

Hydration Status

Daily weights, compared with a baseline weight before starting the formula, help indicate hydration status. Daily *separate* input and output measures and records of formula and water are essential.[14] Sudden weight changes indicate hydration imbalance and need to be investigated. Signs of dehydration include weight loss; poor skin turgor; dry mucous membranes; low blood pressure from decreased blood volume; and increased levels of serum protein, blood cells, and hematocrit. Signs of overhydration include weight gain, edema, jugular vein distention, and elevated blood pressure. Regular protocol monitoring includes serum tests for glucose, potassium, sodium, chloride, albumin, complete blood cell counts, and blood urea nitrogen along with periodic tests for urine specific gravity. Dehydration indicators include elevated blood levels of sodium, chloride, glucose, and urea and elevated levels of hematocrit and urine specific gravity. Severe dehydration is critical and life-threatening. It can be prevented by careful monitoring and supplying the patient's daily fluid requirements with needed water given through the tube. If it does occur, the feeding is stopped and intravenous rehydration with a 5% glucose solution usually follows.

Nutritional Response

In addition to body weights and selected laboratory values described previously, usual protocol of enteral nutrition support programs includes the following basic monitoring assessments of patient response.[14,15]

- *Kcalorie calculation.* Daily during the first week then weekly thereafter, compute the kcalories in the amount of formula actually taken in by the patient and compare with kcalories in the amount of formula ordered.
- *Nitrogen balance study.* Using laboratory tests of urinary urea nitrogen and urine creatinine for initial baseline assessment, take measurements daily for the first week and weekly thereafter, together with calculations of dietary (formula) nitrogen intake.
- *Energy expenditure.* Estimate energy expenditure initially and repeat the estimate when a change in patient situation occurs.
- *Serum albumin.* With a 21-day half-life, serum albumin is a basic indicator of general body protein status to be measured every 2 weeks. Serum *prealbumin,* with a rapid 2-day half-life, thus reflecting current status, is increasingly being used also.
- *Serum iron and transferrin or total iron-binding capacity.* Measure these basic indicators of iron status and nutritional anemia risk every 2 weeks.
- *Serum magnesium.* Measure serum magnesium, an indicator of the degree of malnutrition, every week, or more frequently in severe malnutrition.

Documentation of the Enteral Nutrition Tube-Feeding

The patient's medical record is one of the most essential means of communication among the members of any health care team (see Chapter 1). It is especially necessary for nutritional support teams in monitoring each tube-fed patient and responding rapidly to individual reactions and needs. Divisions of team responsibilities vary, but the nutritional support clinical dietitian is involved in documenting (1) all ongoing nutritional analyses of the actual formula intake, (2) tolerance of the formula and any complications, (3) recommendations for corrective actions in formula changes, tubing, method and rate of delivery, and (4) education for patient and family.

Home Enteral Nutrition

Patient Selection

Home enteral nutrition tube-feeding is not useful to all patients, but for those who require continued tube-feeding to meet clinical and nutritional needs, it provides a physiologic, safe, and relatively simple and less costly method of replenishing and maintaining nutritional support. With the recent rapid developments in enteral formulas and tube-feeding equipment, the process of home feeding has been simplified and is now easier to manage. Thus the numbers of patients on home tube-feeding is increasing. Over the past decade of development, for example, during a mid-1980s 2-year period alone, the number of patients using tube-feeding for home enteral nutrition jumped from 7500 to 52,000, and the number continues to increase.[16] Also, since enactment of Public Law 99-457 in 1986, which provided for mainstream public school education for disabled children, surgical placement of gastrointestinal feeding tubes has allowed children with feeding problems to attend school through the team care of nutritional support clinical dietitian and nurse, special education teachers, and the family.[17]

Teaching Plan

Educating the patient and family for home care is usually a team responsibility of the nutritional support clinical dietitian and nurse. Standards of practice for nutritional support dietitians require a level of expertise and experience that includes teaching skills and responsibilities, not only for hospital patients and staff but also for patient and family when home care is indicated.[18,19] This home care teaching plan includes the following topics and related tasks in preparing patients and families for discharge on home enteral feeding[16]:

- Determining the patient's nutrient and fluid requirements
- Selecting the formula, complete or modular, and computing amounts
- Determining the feeding schedule
- Teaching the patient/family formula nature, rationale, and preparation
- Teaching the patient/family the feeding process, equipment, and pump function
- Teaching the patient/family how to flush the tube and care for the tube site
- Teaching the patient/family how to recognize formula intolerance
- Teaching the patient/family how to avoid complications
- Teaching the patient/family how to give medications with feeding

The nutritional support clinical dietitian is responsible for the first four tasks that assess needs and determine the formula components and their preparation. The nurse is usually responsible for the next two tasks related to feeding process and equipment care. Depending on the hospital staffing pattern and comparative levels of expertise, the clinical dietitian and the nurse may share the three final teaching tasks.[20,21] The nutritional support team pharmacist may share in the final task. A teaching manual with illustrations and detailed information and instructions for all topics is prepared and reviewed by the nutritional support team for use in the initial teaching periods and for continuing guidance at home. The teaching plan should start as soon as the decision for home feeding is made. A social worker should join the team and schedule a separate counseling visit to determine any personal, psychosocial, or economic problems with the care and to confer with the nutritional support team to help work them out. Finally, the teaching plan should allow 2 full days before discharge for the patient and family to practice with the support nurse and for the clinical dietitian to observe the patient (1) administer the formula and (2) record all necessary information about formula and fluid intake, formula tolerance, and complications. Directions for this record are included in the home care manual. The registered dietitian observes and reinforces as needed the patient's skill and learning. Records are reviewed by nutritional support team specialists providing follow-up care at home or clinic visits.

Follow-up Monitoring

The plan for follow-up monitoring should follow the specific protocol schedule developed by the nutritional support team for laboratory, clinical, and nutritional assessments. In early home visits the clinical dietitian and nurse team check progress and troubleshoot any problems that need to be worked out or that require adjustments in the formula or feeding plan.

To Sum Up

For patients with functioning gastrointestinal tracts, enteral nutrition support has proved to be a potent tool against present or potential malnutrition. This nutritional support is achieved by a regular oral diet with nutrient-energy supplementation or alternately by tube-feeding when the patient cannot, will not, or should not eat.

An increasing variety of commercial enteral nutrition products have largely replaced the previous nasogastric tube use or blender-mixed food formulas making possible a simpler and safer, though more costly, tube-feeding process. Modern commercial products provide complete formulas or separate nutrient modules for individualizing a formula mixture to meet special needs. Companion advances in tube-feeding technology have provided extended tube-feeding systems of two types: (1) longer nasoenteric tubes reaching the duodenum and jejunum of the small intestine and placed by x-ray visualization and (2) surgical enterostomies in which tubes are placed in a cervical esophagostomy, gastrostomy, or jejunostomy. Electric pumps control the rate of formula flow.

Based on the new systems of formulas, tubing and container systems, and electric pumps, home enteral nutrition support is increasing rapidly. A detailed teaching plan for patient and family, developed by the nutritional support team and taught by the team's clinical dietitian, nurse, and pharmacist, along with a 2-day supervised practice period, prepares the patient for discharge. Follow-up monitoring includes continuing assessment and therapy adjustments as needed through home and clinic visits.

REFERENCES

1. Benya R, Morbarhan S: Enteral alimentation: administration and complications, *J Am Coll Nutr* 10(3):209, 1991.
2. Rombeau JL, Caldwell MD: *Enteral and tube feeding,* Philadelphia, 1990, WB Saunders.
3. Bell SJ et al: A chemical score to evaluate the protein quality of commercial parenteral and enteral formulas: emphasis on formulas for patients with liver failure, *J Am Diet Assoc* 91(5):586, 1991.
4. Bell SJ et al: Alternate lipid sources for enteral and parenteral nutrition: long- and medium-chain triglycerides, structured triglycerides, and fish oils, *J Am Diet Assoc* 91(1):74, 1991.
5. Gottschlich MM: Selection of optimal lipid sources in enteral and parenteral nutrition, *Nutr Clin Prac* 7(4):152, 1992.
6. Evans MA, Shronts EP: Intestinal fuels: glutamine, short-chain fatty acids, and dietary fiber, *J Am Diet Assoc* 92(10):1239, 1992.
7. Frankenfield DC, Beyer PL: Dietary fiber and bowel function in tube-fed patients, *J Am Diet Assoc* 91(5):590, 1991.
8. Talbot JM: Guidelines for the scientific review of enteral food products for special medical purposes, *J Parenter Enteral Nutr* 15(suppl3):100S, 1991.
9. Heymsfield SB et al: Nutritional support in cardiac failure, *Surg Clin North Am* 61:635, 1981.
10. Monturo CA: Enteral access device selection, *Nutr Clin Prac* 5(5):207, 1990.
11. Caulfield KA et al: Technique for intraduodenal placement of transnasal enteral feeding catheters, *Nutr Clin Prac* 6(1):23, 1991.
12. Fagerman KE: Limiting bacterial contamination of enteral nutrient solutions: six-year history with reduction of contamination at two institutions, *Nutr Clin Prac* 7(1):35, 1991.
13. Fagerman KE: Microbiologic standards for enteral nutrient solutions overdue in the United States, *J Am Diet Assoc* 92(3):336, 1992.

14. Zeman FJ, Ney DM: *Applications of clinical nutrition*, Englewood Cliffs, NJ, 1988, Prentice Hall.
15. Bernstein LH: Monitoring quality of nutrition support, *Diet Curr* 19(2):1, 1992.
16. Skipper A, Rotman N: A survey of the role of the dietitian in preparing patients for home enteral feeding, *J Am Diet Assoc* 90(7):939, 1990.
17. Isaacs JS et al: Transitioning the child fed by gastrostomy into school, *J Am Diet Assoc* 90(7):982, 1990.
18. American Society for Parenteral and Enteral Nutrition: Standards of practice for nutrition support dietitians, *Nutr Clin Prac* 5:74, 1990.
19. Bradford S et al: Position of the American Dietetic Association: the role of the registered dietitian in enteral and parenteral nutrition support, *J Am Diet Assoc* 91(10):1440, 1991.
20. Skipper A, Feitelson M: The changing role of the dietitian in clinical practice, *Nutr Clin Prac* 7(suppl3):5, 1992.
21. Compher C, Colaizzo T: Staffing patterns in hospital clinical dietetics and nutrition support: a survey conducted by the Dietitians in Nutrition Support dietetic practice group, *J Am Diet Assoc* 92(7):807, 1992.

FURTHER READING

Bower RH: Nutritional and metabolic support of critically ill patients, *J Parenter Enteral Nutr* 14(suppl5):257S, 1990.

Morales E et al: Dietary management of malnourished children with a new enteral feeding, *J Am Diet Assoc* 91(10):1233, 1991.

These two articles provide interesting background about the research and development that prepares a commercial nutritional support formula for market. Dr. Bower describes the clinical studies of Impact (Sandoz), a new high-protein nutritional support formula for patients with suppressed immune function from hypermetabolic illness or injury, which in these studies also reduced the number of days study subjects with sepsis spent in intensive care units (ICU) thus reducing costs that range upward from $1400 per day. Dr. Morales' group describe their studies of PediaSure (Ross), the new concentrated formula for children ages 1 to 6 years who are recovering from protein-energy malnutrition.

Frankenfield DC, Beyer PL: Dietary fiber and bowel function in tube-fed patients, *J Am Diet Assoc* 91(5):590, 1991.

These authors provide an excellent review of the metabolism and function of fiber in conjunction with tube-feedings and the use of fiber in enteral formulas to treat constipation and diarrhea in tube-fed patients.

Troubleshooting Diarrhea in Tube-Fed Patients: A Costly Chase

Clinicians seem to agree generally that diarrhea is one of the most common complications associated with tube-feeding, yet the reported incidence ranges widely from as little as 2% to as much as 63% in general patient populations and as high as 68% in intensive care patients. Questions that relate to this wide variance and that plague investigators apparently center on definition and cause. But the ultimate bottom line for patient and family and their health insurers if they have any is the price of the clinical search for the culprit. As we shall see, it is in fact a costly chase.

Problem of definition

It appears on the surface that the question of what diarrhea is, is easy to answer. We've all had some experience, more or less. However, a valid clinical research study demands more—a precise operational definition on which to establish a research design and evaluate results. And judging from reports, investigators have not been able to agree on a definition, methods of reporting the extent of the diarrhea, the length of time tube-fed patients were monitored, and the sample of patients studied.

In fact, a current report of a 3-month study clearly indicates that the messy state of defining and reporting diarrhea in tube-fed patients resembles that of the disorder itself. These investigators—using the usual diarrhea criteria of frequency, consistency, and quantity—found as many as 14 different definitions in their review of studies in the scientific literature, no doubt accounting for the varying incidence reported. Of course the tube-fed patients, if asked, could have easily defined their diarrhea in terms of the psychologic and physical discomfort involved, as could their nurses in terms of increased cleanup work and concern for the patient.

Problem of cause

Reported causes of diarrhea in tube-fed patients also vary. These concerns usually center first on the formula itself, often followed by numerous adjustments in components and concentrations that only cloud the picture further and make the search for the actual culprit more difficult. A variety of conflicting causes associated with the complication of diarrhea have been reported, including not only the formula itself but also medications or some aspect of the patient's condition.

Formula. Possible formula factors relate to osmolality or concentration and to rate of delivery. However, conflicting reports have shown no increase in the incidence of diarrhea when the formula concentration varied widely from 145 to 430 mOsm, and no significant association has been made between malabsorption and formula osmolality or rate of delivery. Formulas providing 30% or more of total kcalories as fat have been associated with a higher incidence of diarrhea, whereas those providing 20% fat rarely were involved. Further study of fat composition is needed, specifically comparing medium- versus long-chain triglycerides and omega-3 versus omega-6 fatty acids. Studies of the role of fiber in tube feedings have also been conflicting. Reviewers have found that the studies thus far have been few, the models used variable, the limitations substantial, and the conclusions of the investigators mixed.

Bacterial contamination. Studies have demonstrated that the problem of diarrhea does not lie in the quick assumption that the formula as such was at fault but in the reality that bacterial contamination, frequently *Clostridium difficile* toxin, of the formula or feeding equipment was the cause. This problem may result from lack of careful aseptic technique in handling the formula and equipment or from failing to follow manufacturers' guidelines for appropriate hang times for formulas—usually no longer than 8 hours for systems set up by the nursing staff and 24 hours for systems prefilled with formula by the manufacturer and attached by connections. The less any system is handled and opened, the less chance there is for contamination. Bacteria are easily introduced where the delivery tubing connects with the patient's feeding tube and whenever the system is open.

Patient's condition. Malnourished or critically ill patients are more susceptible to mucosal tissue breakdown, depressed serum albumin levels, and malabsorption leading to diarrhea. The hypoalbuminemia contributes to reduced colloidal osmotic pressure within blood vessels. This loss of osmotic pressure in turn, leads to edema of the intestinal mucosa, malabsorption, and diarrhea. Use of an easily absorbed elemental enteral formula is probably helpful, at least until the nutritional status improves sufficiently to progress to a standard intact protein formula. Albumin may be given intravenously, but unless there is adequate nutritional support the body uses the infused albumin for energy rather than tissue rebuilding. In addition, periods of stress, including sepsis and central nervous system insults, result in decreased motility of the gastrointestinal tract, including ileus. Such decreased motility contributes to bacterial overgrowth.

Medications. Multiple medications routinely given to hospitalized patients have been related to diarrhea. Antibiotics are most often associated, but this practice coexists with poor patient condition, multiple organ failure, and therefore with diarrhea. In general, drug reactions may relate to the metabolically active agent or to another ingredient added for its physical properties in the form of the drug, for example, tablet or liquid as the following case illustrates.

Continued.

Case of the costly chase

A recently reported case of unexplained diarrhea in a tube-fed patient illustrates the difficult, and often costly, search for the cause. A 55-year-old man, whom we call "Max," suffered an aortic aneurysm and had emergency surgery to repair it. In the intensive care unit, the postoperative course was complicated by respiratory problems requiring ventilator assistance. He was given a bronchodilator drug, theophylline, in tablet form, crushed and given by nasogastric tube with water. When Max was able to take nourishment, an isotonic formula given by enteral tube-feeding was started, and the crushed theophylline tablets were changed to a sugar-free theophylline solution. Within a day, Max began to have progressive abdominal distention and continuous liquid diarrhea. To rule out an abdominal catastrophe related to the aneurysm or surgery, a computed abdominal tomography scan, an aortogram, and a colonoscopy were done, but all of these studies were normal.

Despite stopping the enteral feeding, the distention and diarrhea continued. Stool specimens were tested for fecal leukocytes, parasites, and *Clostridium difficile* toxin, and an enteric pathogen culture was prepared. All were nondiagnostic. Extensive additional serum and urine tests as well as a sigmoidoscopy with rectal biopsy gave no clue. Then stool electrolytes and osmolality measure suggested an osmotic diarrhea. Because Max was not receiving enteral feedings, his physicians thought a secretory bacterial toxin was probably causing the continuing diarrhea, so the previous studies were repeated to confirm the osmotic nature of the diarrhea. In addition, all the medications were reviewed, but none appeared to be the cause.

At this point because the continued diarrhea prohibited enteral feeding and Max needed nourishment, total parenteral nutrition (TPN) was ordered. This move immediately brought an automatic Nutrition Support Service consultation, which included further assessment of medications. This evaluation revealed that the sugar-free theophylline solution was 65% *sorbitol.* Sorbitol is a polyhydric alcohol used as a sweetener in many sugar-free products such as dietetic foods and chewing gum. There was no information about sorbitol on the label or package insert of the drug for the physicians to know these facts, and because it was not thought to be an active agent, this information could be obtained only by contacting the manufacturer.

Fortunately for Max, however, the nutrition support team did know and found the hidden culprit in his medication. After calculations of the regular daily amount of the theophylline Max was taking, he was receiving nearly 300 g of sorbitol daily when the usual laxative dose was only 20 to 50 g. The nutritional support team immediately recommended that this sorbitol-sweetened solution of theophylline be discontinued and that a sorbitol-free form of the medication be used instead. Almost immediately the diarrhea began to decrease and in 3 days was gone.

The extent of this costly chase was revealed in Max's hospital bill. He had continued to receive the faulty drug for almost half of his 3-month hospital stay, during which time the diarrhea prevented enteral feeding and he had to have the more expensive TPN. The TPN cost $4860 more than the enteral feedings would have cost for the same period. In addition, all the extensive investigations to find the cause of the diarrhea cost $4250, which together with all the indirect costs for extra days of care and supplies made a total hospital bill of about $170,000.

The causes of diarrhea in tube-fed patients are many, but in the hands of a skilled nutritional support team, the formula is seldom one of them. It is often found in the medications. Just remember what this medication's hidden ingredient—sorbitol—cost Max.

REFERENCES

Benya R, Mobarhan S: Enteral alimentation administration and complications, *J Am Coll Nutr* 10(3):209, 1991.

Bliss DZ et al: Defining and reporting diarrhea in tube-fed patients—what a mess! *Am J Clin Nutr* 55:753, 1992.

Bokus S: Troubleshooting your tube feedings, *Am J Nurs* 91:24, 1991.

Frankenfield DC, Beyer PL: Dietary fiber and bowel function in tube-fed patients, *J Am Diet Assoc* 91(5):590, 1991.

Guenter PA et al: Tube feeding-related diarrhea in acutely ill patients, *J Parenter Enteral Nutr* 15(3):277, 1991.

Hill DB et al: Osmotic diarrhea induced by sugar-free theophylline solution in critically ill patients, *J Parenter Enteral Nutr* 15(3):332, 1991.

CHAPTER 4

Parenteral Nutrition

CHAPTER OUTLINE

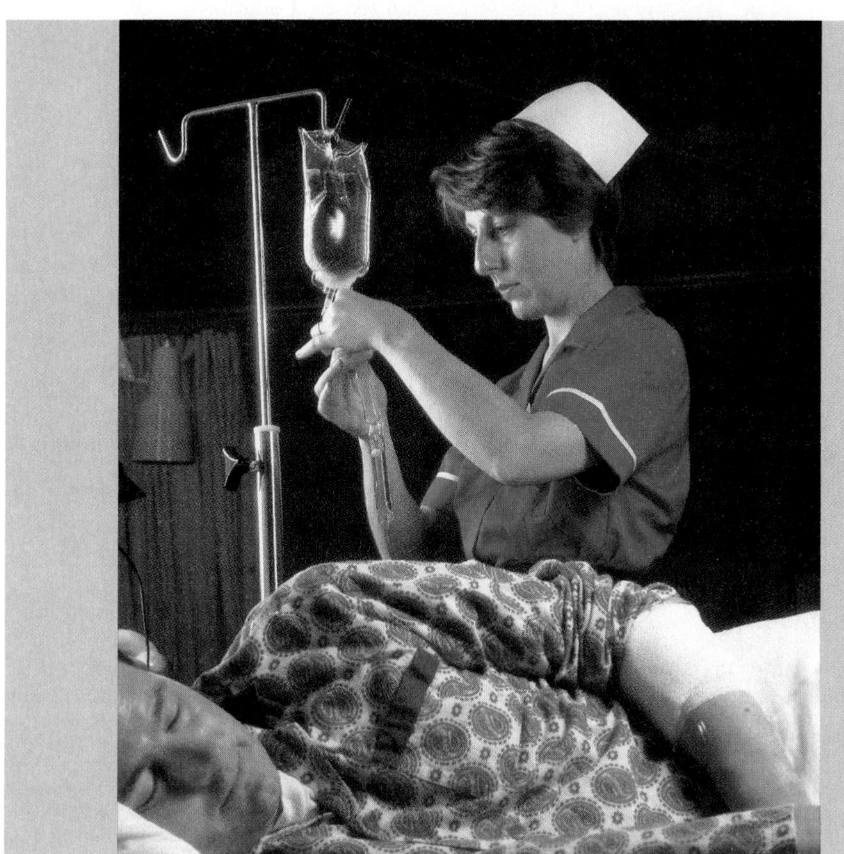

*After reviewing in the previous chapter the many formulas and processes of administering enteral nutrition support, we turn now to the second chapter in this two-part sequence on special nutrition support. We look at the remaining nutrition support alternative when the gastrointestinal tract cannot be used—*parenteral *nutrition—feeding directly into the veins.*

The story of parenteral nutrition support is a remarkable one of American medical discovery three decades ago and an expanding technologic development of formula solutions and delivery systems since those early beginnings. Now experienced nutritional support teams have sharpened their skills and techniques, developed detailed protocols, and advanced their expertise in hospitals of all the world's developed countries. Wise nutritional support clinicians have learned much since those early, exciting days about what they can and cannot do. Parenteral nutrition has matured and is still evolving.

Over the years, total parenteral nutrition has provided not only for brief periods of nutrition rehabilitation but also an ongoing life support system, a veritable "artificial gut," for some individuals on a continuing basis. In this chapter, we look at parenteral feeding and its uses.

Parenteral Feeding in Clinical Nutrition

Basic Technique

Applied to nutritional therapy, parenteral nutrition refers to any feeding methods other than by the normal gastrointestinal route. Specifically, in current medical and nutritional usage, it refers to the special feeding method of infusing basic "predigested" nutrient elements directly into the blood circulation through certain veins when the gastrointestinal tract cannot be used. Depending on the nutrition support need, two routes are available: (1) *central parenteral nutrition (CPN)*—the use of a large central vein to deliver concentrated solutions that supply full nutritional support for longer periods of time (Fig. 4-1)

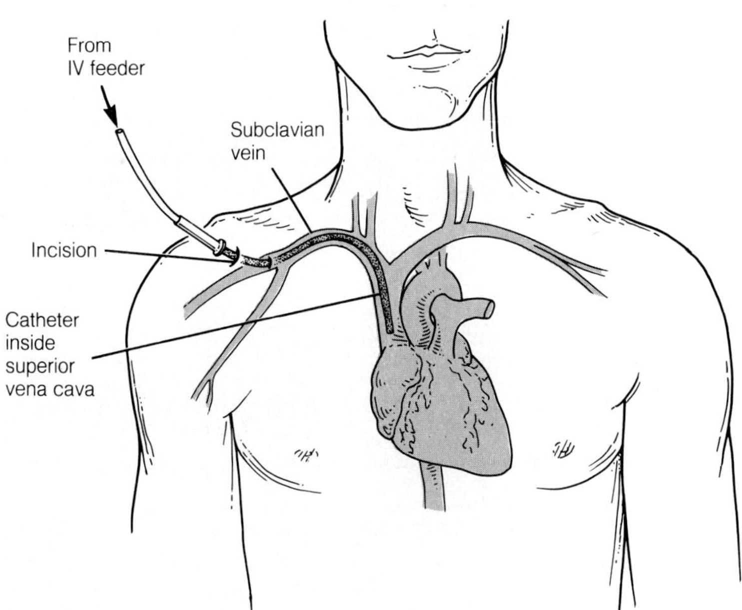

FIG. 4-1 Catheter placement for total parenteral nutrition (TPN) made for feeding via subclavian vein to superior vena cava.

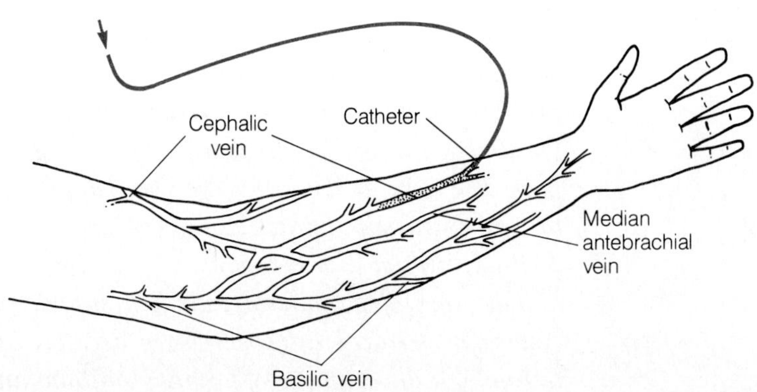

FIG. 4-2 Peripheral parenteral nutrition feeding into small veins in the arm.

and (2) *peripheral parenteral nutrition (PPN)*—the alternate use of a smaller peripheral vein, usually in the arm, to deliver less concentrated solutions for brief periods (Fig. 4-2).

Since the development over the past two decades of this basic surgical technique of inserting venous catheters in specific veins for feeding basic nutrients, parenteral nutrition has provided a major advance in critical patient care. Major illness from traumatic injury or extensive debilitating disease creates actual or potential malnutrition and hypermetabolic nutritional demands. If the patient's condition is further complicated by inability to eat or take enteral tube feedings, nutritional status can be improved and maintained over extended periods solely through intravenous feeding. Hypertonic solutions of essential nutrients can be fed into a large central vein. Vascular inflammation and thrombosis are avoided, and individually required amounts of life-sustaining nourishment, which is otherwise not available, are delivered. This complete sustaining of individual nutritional requirements through intravenous feeding has been termed *total parenteral nutrition (TPN).*

TPN Development

Largely through the pioneering work of Dudrick and his associates,[1,2] the current era of parenteral nutrition found its direction in the early 1970s. Surgeons were able to develop and successfully demonstrate a technique for introducing highly concentrated nutrient solutions into larger blood vessels capable of handling its osmotic density by rapidly diluting it into central circulation. This early technique involved the feeding of a solution of protein hydrolysates (solutions now use amino acids) and concentrated glucose with added vitamins and minerals. It was fed through an indwelling catheter into the superior vena cava leading directly to the heart by way of a large central vein, usually the subclavian vein. In the 1970s and 1980s development of the surgical technique, equipment, and nutrient solutions to meet the increased nutritional requirements of catabolic illness has lead to its current widespread use.[3,4]

TPN has helped prevent complications of malnutrition, sepsis, and general tissue breakdown in patients denied the normal use of gastrointestinal feeding pathways by critical illness or injury. It has also helped to meet added kcalorie and protein needs imposed by hypermetabolic conditions. Many studies in the past few years have substantiated the effectiveness of carefully administered TPN by a highly skilled nutritional support team to wisely selected patients. Also, experience has shown that peripheral vein parenteral nutrition is used in many cases as a viable alternative, or it may be used in conjunction with oral intake or tube feeding. This is frequently the case in transition feeding. The nutritional support team's clinical dietitian who has special advanced training is responsible for assessing the patient's nutritional status, calculating nutritional needs, and then designing an appropriate parenteral solution to be recommended to the physician.[5,6] Now the nutritional support clinical dietitian and physician have a wide spectrum of nutrient solutions and delivery systems from which to plan individual nutritional therapy according to the clinical problems presented. Nutritional support pharmacists mix each individual patient solution, and nutritional support nurses administer it to the patient.

Indications for Parenteral Nutrition Support

Three basic considerations govern decisions concerning the use of parenteral nutrition: (1) the availability of the gastrointestinal tract, (2) the degree of malnutrition, and (3) the degree of hypermetabolism or catabolism.[7] Since risks are involved as well as considerable increase in costs, assessment of each of these factors is imperative.

Availability of the Gastrointestinal Tract

A long-standing medical adage certainly applies: "If the gut works, use it!" However, if the gut has been rendered totally unavailable for use by major abdominal injury, for example, an alternative means of sustaining nutrition is an obvious necessity. In other cases the gut may be unavailable because of obstruction, **fistulas,** or malignant disease. In still other cases the patient may be unable to eat because of coma, severe anorexia and self-starvation, or mental disturbance.

Degree of Malnutrition

If a patient is malnourished, any medical treatment attempted has less chance of success. Studies in the past few years have indicated that far more general malnutrition exists among hospitalized patients than was previously assumed. In addition, it is now clear that disease imposes an even greater threat to positive nutritional status. Thus the assessment of nutritional status becomes an important part of overall care, especially for hospitalized patients (see Chapter 1). For the severely malnourished patient, especially those facing problems such as major organ failure or extensive surgery, serious consideration of TPN is indicated (Table 4-1).

fistula • Abnormal passageway usually between two internal organs or leading from an internal organ to the surface of the body.

TABLE 4–1

Patient Situations Imposing Need for TPN

Patient with limited or impossible use of gut	Metabolic rate, degree of catabolism (nitrogen loss per 24 hr)	Degree of malnutrition*
Situation 1	Normal (0-8 g)	Normal
Situation 2	Moderate (8-15 g)	Moderate
Situation 3	Severe (15 g)	Severe

*In terms of percent of normal standards by nutritional assessment.

Degree of Hypermetabolism or Catabolism

If a patient is suffering from major trauma or severe sepsis or from radiation or chemotherapy enteritis in the treatment for malignant disease (see Chapter 13), the rate of catabolism, or inability to absorb nutrients, may take a devastating toll on the body's resources. This toll may be measured in nitrogen balance studies with a loss ranging up to 15 g of nitrogen over 24 hours. In some patients such as athletes with large lean body masses and extensive injuries, the loss may be even more severe. Catabolic periods seem inevitable following surgery, with more extensive surgery bringing the greatest losses of body resources. The extent of these increased demands is seen in the increased nutritional requirements, especially in energy demand.

Basic Rules for TPN Use

Using the three basic considerations, most clinicians have formed general rules to guide the choice of TPN as the preferred means of therapy. Some combinations of these factors indicating the need for TPN are illustrated in Table 4-1. Two basic rules form the basis for choice of TPN.

The "Rule of Five"

If a patient has had no food for *5 days* and is likely not to be able to eat for at least another 5 days, TPN must be considered *then* rather than waiting until malnutrition has developed. It is an easier task to *maintain* positive nutrition than to *replenish* body stores from malnutrition losses. Starvation effects on the body, even during relatively brief periods, are well documented.[3] The 50 to 75 g of glucose stored in the liver as hepatic glycogen is a small but crucial energy source able to maintain the body's normal blood sugar levels for only about 12 hours. During the early days of starvation, amino acids of the body's tissue proteins are deaminated to provide blood glucose (gluconeogenesis) and substrate for needed metabolic functions with a urinary nitrogen loss of 10 to 15 g/day. Also, fatty acids are mobilized from the body's adipose tissues to provide keto acids as the principal fuel for the heart, brain, and other vital organs.

Weight Loss Rule

Any patient who has lost 7% of their usual body weight over 2 months and who is deprived of oral nutrition for 5 to 7 days or longer is a candidate for TPN.

Patient Candidates for TPN

On the basis of the following general considerations, a number of patient situations suggest a need for vigorous TPN support:

- *Preoperative preparation of severely malnourished patients.* These cases include congenital anomalies causing gastrointestinal disorders, stricture or cancer of the esophagus and swallowing difficulties, cancer of the stomach, and severe peptic ulcer disease or gastric obstruction.
- *Postoperative surgical complications.* These cases include prolonged ileus and obstruction; stomal dysfunction; short bowel syndrome; enterocutaneous, biliary, or pancreatic fistulas; and peritoneal sepsis.
- *Inflammatory bowel disease.* These cases include intractable gastroenteritis, regional enteritis, acute regional enteritis (Crohn's disease), ulcerative colitis, extensive diverticulitis, and radiation enteritis.
- *Inadequate oral intake or malabsorption.* These cases include malignant neoplasms and chemotherapy or radiation treatment; acute and chronic relapsing pancreatitis; hypermetabolic states, major trauma, and massive burns; coma, hepatic insufficiency, or encephalopathy; and chronic malnutrition or anorexia nervosa.

Generally, decisions to use PPN instead of TPN are based on comparative energy needs and anticipated time of use. PPN is usually the choice in the following situations:

- No more than 2000 kcal/day is required.
- No more than 10 days of therapy are needed.

Nutritional Assessment

Initial individual nutritional assessment provides the necessary basis for (1) identifying patients requiring special therapy, (2) calculating their nutritional requirements, and (3) determining the specific nutrient formulas to meet these requirements. This is the responsibility of the nutritional support team's clinical dietitian. Once therapy begins, careful monitoring of nutritional and metabolic parameters is essential for maintaining optimal therapy and avoiding metabolic complications.

TABLE 4-2

Indication of Severe Protein–Kcalorie Malnutrition According to Percentage of Recent Weight Loss

Body weight loss (%)	Time period
2	1 week
5	1 month
7.5	3 months
10	6 months

TABLE 4-3

Determination of Protein-Kcalorie Malnutrition by Plasma Values

Laboratory data	Normal values	Degree of malnutrtion: Moderate	Degree of malnutrtion: Severe
Serum albumin (g/dl)	3.5	2.1-3	<2.1
Serum transferrin (mg/dl)	180-260	100-150	<100
Total lymphocyte count per mm^3	1500-4000	800-1200	<800
% WBC	20-53		

Guidelines for Nutritional Assessment

Necessary assessment of patients on parenteral nutrition support is done by the standard ABCD approach—*A*nthropometrics, *B*iochemical laboratory data, *C*linical observations, *D*ietary evaluations—together with a comprehensive detailed history. These general assessment methods are described in detail in Chapter 1. According to individual patient needs and clinical situations, specific guidelines for parenteral nutrition support assessment include the following six procedures.

Classify degree of weight loss. Use measures of current body weight and height. Interpret current actual body weight (ABW) in terms of desirable body weight for height (DBW), usual body weight (UBW), and amount of recent weight change:

Percent desirable weight = ABW ÷ DBW × 100
Percent usual body weight = ABW ÷ UBW × 100
Percent weight change = UBW − [ABW ÷ UBW] × 100

Compare the patient's amount of recent weight change with the values indicating malnutrition as given in Table 4-2.

Estimate body fat stores and skeletal muscle mass. Using caliper measures of the triceps skinfold (TSF) and standard reference tables (see Appendix Q) for TSF data, estimate the patient's body fat stores. Using the mid–upper arm circumference measure (MAC), calculate the mid–upper arm muscle circumference (MAMC) and compare it with the standard references for MAMC data. This gives an estimate of the patient's muscle mass interpreted as a percentage of the standard:

MAMC (cm) = MAC (cm) − [0.314 × TSF (mm)]

Estimate lean body mass. Use the creatinine-height index (CHI) as an estimate of overall lean body mass. Compute the patient's CHI by using the daily urinary creatinine excretion value determined by laboratory analysis of a 24-hour urine collection. Compare this value with the ideal creatinine value for the patient's height in centimeters from standard tables (see Chapter 1). This gives an effective index of the patient's overall muscle mass and total lean body mass.

Calculate degree of catabolism. Measure the degree of catabolism by calculating the daily nitrogen balance. Using an accurate record of the patient's protein intake for the day (food or formula) and the laboratory analysis of the urinary urea nitrogen in a careful 24-hour collection of urinary output, calculate the nitrogen (N) balance for that day:

$$\text{N balance} = \text{N intake}\left(\frac{\text{protein intake}}{6.25}\right) - \text{N loss (urinary urea N + 4)}$$

To monitor the effectiveness of continuous TPN therapy and provide faster response time to meet indicated needs, some clinicians use two consecutive 12-hour urine collections to calculate nitrogen balance over a 24-hour period.[8]

Estimate immune function. Use the total lymphocyte count or the percentage of lymphocytes in the total white blood cell (WBC) count to determine general function of the patient's immune system. Compare this with the values in Table 4-3.

$$\text{Total lymphocyte count} = \text{Percent lymphocytes} \times \frac{\text{WBC}}{100}$$

Skin testing for sensitivity to common recall antigens such as purified protein derivative of tuberculin (PPD) and streptokinase-streptodornase (SKSD) provides additional immune function data. Delayed hypersensitivity skin testing is occasionally used with hospitalized patients at risk for **anergy** as a means for detecting cellular immune status. Protocols for its use have been standardized.

Measure plasma protein compartment. Measure serum transferrin directly, or using laboratory analysis of total iron-binding capacity (TIBC), calculate the value for transferrin, the body's iron transport protein compound:

$$\text{Transferrin (mg/dl)} = [\text{TIBC } (\mu g/dl) \times 0.8] - 43$$

The serum albumin measure (half-life of 21 days) provides additional long-term data concerning the body's visceral protein mass. However, a decreased transferrin value is a more sensitive marker of recent malnutrition than serum albumin because transferrin has a shorter half-life (10 days) and is depleted faster. Compare these serum protein values obtained for the patient with the values in Table 4-3.

Baseline and Monitoring Assessment for TPN

At the initiation of TPN, a broad base of nutritional and metabolic data is gathered as a baseline by which to measure progress. Then at designated periods during therapy, repetition of certain tests is used to monitor the patient's course and to avoid metabolic complications. Specific protocols vary in different medical centers. However, a general guide for such standard monitoring data is summarized in Table 4-4. All the baseline and monitoring data are recorded in the patient's chart, along with all TPN solution orders.

Clinical Recommendations

As nutritional support teams have gained experience with TPN, clinicians have a broader base for evaluating the various measures of nutritional status to determine the effectiveness of the nutritional support therapy in meeting individual patient care objectives. Basically, the metabolic aim of nutritional support in malnourished patients is to reverse the malnutrition or prevent it by reversing energy and protein catabolism, and of course, no one test reflects how well the nutritional support is achieving this basic aim. However, a battery of tests that includes sensitive markers of short-term nutritional status, together with careful clinical observations, which some clinicians have wisely called a "subjective global clinical assessment," helps the nutritional support team make appropriate decisions concerning adequacy of the TPN.[9,10]

Generally, clinicians give primary importance to two major monitoring procedures: (1) constant evaluation of *kcaloric intake* to ensure adequacy of the energy base to meet metabolic demands and (2) regular measure of *protein-nitrogen* adequacy to meet tissue rebuilding needs. Nutritional support teams are increasingly using the laboratory test for **prealbumin (PAB)** as the most sensitive rapid plasma protein marker of current malnutrition status and response to nutritional support because of its rapid turnover and half-life of only 2 days.[11,12] An imperative role in assessing nutritional care has been assigned by the Joint Commission on the Accreditation of Healthcare Organizations (JCAHO) to the nutritional support clinical dietitian, and these assessments are being included in quality assurance programs submitted to the JCAHO for approval.[13,14] Thus quality assurance protocols for hospital nutritional support programs are including not

TABLE 4-4

Monitoring Protocol for TPN

Baseline tests

CBC: Hb	Nitrogen balance	SGOT
Hct	Fe and TIBC	Alkaline phosphatase
RBC indexes	FBS	Serum osmolality
WBC differential count	BUN	Cholesterol
Platelets	Creatinine	Triglycerides
Na^+ Ca^{++}	Uric acid	Urinalysis
K^+ PO_4	PT	Chest x-ray film
Cl^- Mg^{++}	PTT	ECG
CO_2	Prealbumin	Body weight (kg)
Skin tests (PPD, mumps, cocci)	Albumin	Height (cm)
	Total protein	
	Bilirubin	

Stabilization tests (daily for first 5-7 days)

Fractional urines (sugar and acetone) every 6 hours; simultaneous blood sugars first and second days
Body weight
Intake and output record
Nitrogen balance
Serum electrolytes
Blood glucose
Prealbumin

Follow-up routine

Daily	Fractional urines (sugar and acetone) Body weight Intake and output
Three times a week	Electrolytes (Na^+, K^+, Cl^-, CO_2) Prealbumin
Once a week	CBC: Platelets, RBC indexes; PT; Ca^{++}; PO_4; Mg^{++} Creatinine BUN
Once a month	Repeat baseline tests Add serum vitamin B_{12}, folate, Zn^{++}

CBC, Complete blood cell count; *HB,* hemoglobin; *Hct,* hematocrit; *RBC,* red blood cell; *WBC,* white blood cell; *PPD,* purified protein derivative of tuberculin; *TIBC,* total iron-binding capacity; *FBS,* fasting blood sugar; *BUN,* blood urea nitrogen; *PT,* prothrombin time; *PTT,* partial thromboplastin time; *SGOT,* serum glutamic oxalocetic transaminate; *ECG,* electrocardiogram.

TABLE 4–5

Example of Basic TPN Formula Components

Components	Amounts
Basic solution	
Crystalline amino acids	2.75%
Dextrose	25%
Additives	
Electrolytes	
Na	50 mEq/L
Cl	50 mEq/L
K	40 mEq/L
HPO_4	25 mEq/L
Ca	5 mEq/L
Mg	8 mEq/L
Vitamins	
Multiple (MVI)	1.7 ml conc./L
Vitamin C (per day)	500 mg
Trace elements solution (per day)	
Zn	3 mg
Cu	1.6 mg
Cr	2 μg
Se	120 μg
Mn	2 μg
I	120 μg
Fe	1.5 μg
Other additives (as needed)	
Regular insulin	0-25 U/L
Heparin	1000 U/L

only these energy and protein intake evaluations but also a regular rapid feedback prealbumin marker to indicate effectiveness of the nutritional support, for example, a PAB rate of increase of at least 2.0 mg/dl weekly and serum concentration increases to greater than 11.0 mg/dl toward a normal value of 15.7 to 29.6 mg/dl.[11,12]

Nutritional Requirements: the TPN Prescription

The TPN prescription and plan of care are based on the calculation of basic nutritional requirements plus additional needs resulting from the patient's degree of catabolism, malnutrition, and any activity. An example of a basic TPN formula plan is shown in Table 4-5. This same principle guides nutritional therapy in any feeding mode. Nutritional needs are fundamental—energy (kcalories), protein, electrolytes, minerals, and vitamins.

Energy Requirements

The energy needs of critically ill patients are great, even as high as twice the normal basal rates in the case of major trauma such as massive burns.[15] It is necessary to meet the following kcalorie requirements: (1) basal energy expenditures (BEE), (2) additional needs to cover the energy cost of catabolism, fever, and malnutrition—the *metabolic activity factor (MAF)* (see Chapter 11), and (3) any physical activity.

Basal Energy Expenditure

An estimate of the adult patient's energy needs for basal tissue metabolism may be calculated by the following commonly used classic Harris-Benedict equations, which involves measures of weight in kilograms, height in centimeters, and age in years[16]:

$$\text{Women: BEE} = 655 + [9.6 \times \text{Weight (kg)}] + [1.7 \times \text{Height (cm)}] - [4.7 \times \text{Age (years)}]$$

$$\text{Men: BEE} = 66 + [13.7 \times \text{Weight (kg)}] + [5.0 \times \text{Height (cm)}] - [6.8 \times \text{Age (years)}]$$

The term *resting energy expenditure (REE)* is often used interchangeably with BEE in discussing basal energy needs of hospitalized patients, and for practical purposes they are synonymous and are calculated by the same equations. Both are based on data from indirect calorimetry under fairly similar patient situations, and both help define the metabolic behavior of the patient.[17,18] Measurements of basal metabolic rate (BMR), or BEE, are made early in the morning in a darkened room immediately after the patient awakes and before any movements are made. More practically, REE is measured more than 2 hours after a light meal and after the patient has rested in the supine position for more than 30 minutes.[3,19] When using the equations previously given to estimate basal energy needs in obese patients, Ireton-Jones and Turner[20] recommend that the actual weight be used instead of the "ideal" weight, because the actual weight more accurately predicts energy expenditure. Also, advancing age in patients on TPN influences kcaloric needs. Recent studies by Shizgal et al.[21] of the effect of age on response to TPN reinforce the fact that depleted body composition in malnourished older patients over age 65 is restored more slowly than in younger adults and requires a greater kcaloric intake.

Additional Energy Requirements

In addition to basal energy needs, total kcalorie requirements reflect the large energy drain of the illness

anergy • Diminished immunologic reactivity to specific antigens.

prealbumin (PAB) • Plasma protein with a short half-life (2 days) used as a biochemical measure for assessing current nutritional status.

A 50% Solution to Protein Loss in Trauma Victims

TO PROBE FURTHER

The need for protein in patients suffering from trauma such as severe injuries, sepsis, severe burns, or major surgery is accentuated by the high stress metabolic response to injury and the acute catabolism that this stress triggers. These patients often require TPN to supply needed nutritional support. The metabolic stress effect is indicated by elevated amino acid levels in the blood from the increased gluconeogenesis and catabolism. High levels of the branched-chain amino acids (BCAAs) valine, leucine, and isoleucine have been seen. These are known to help slow down protein catabolism in the body. They also take part in gluconeogenesis and are easily used as energy substrates in muscle. With all these health-promoting activities, do BCAAs have a therapeutic effect when added to the diet?

Some researchers seem to think so. They have tried different concentrations of BCAAs in infused solutions used in patients recovering from major abdominal surgery to see which was most helpful in achieving or preserving nitrogen balance. Of the three concentrations—15.6%, 50%, and 100%—the 50% solution, when given as part of the formula feeding, seemed most effective in preserving nitrogen balance without elevating any amino acids to abnormally high levels. However, before this solution becomes standard therapy, any adverse effects need to be avoided by careful analysis of plasma amino acid levels and evaluation of clinical outcome.

Recent studies, using 19% and 44% solutions of BCAAs with admixtures of dextrose and lipid emulsion as nonnitrogen kcalories for a fuel base, found little difference in nitrogen retention and no significant clinical advantage over use of a standard amino acid formulation. As yet, continuing study has not been promising enough to justify the much greater cost of the BCAA-enriched formula, which is about five times that of a standard amino acid solution. For the present, BCAA supplementation is being used as a tool for research study, but not yet for nutritional support in stressed, critically ill patients.

So the question remains.

REFERENCES

Bonau RA et al: Muscle amino acid flux in patients receiving branched-chain amino acid solutions after surgery, *Surgery* 101:400, 1987.

Desai SP et al: Plasma amino acid concentrations during branched-chain amino acid infusions in stressed patients, *J Trauma* 22:747, 1982.

Heyman MB: General and specialized parenteral amino acid formulations for nutritional support, *J Am Diet Assoc* 90(3):401, 1990.

Scholten DJ et al: Failure of BCAA supplementation to promote nitrogen retention in injured patients, *J Am Coll Nutr* 9(2):101, 1990.

or injury. Physiologic stress demands sufficient kcalories to combat the hypermetabolism and its resulting catabolic state and weight loss. If any large degree of malnutrition exists, even more kcalorie input may be necessary. Total kcalorie requirements must also include any muscular or physical activity, which varies considerably depending on the patient's condition, respiratory status, fever or sepsis, and extent of mobility. In comparison with normal needs, the general range of energy requirements for hospitalized patients on parenteral nutrition support varies with the degree of added metabolic stress:

- Normal needs—25 to 30 kcal/kg/day
- Elective surgery—28 to 30 kcal/kg/day
- Severe injury—30 to 40 kcal/kg/day
- Extensive trauma or burns—45 to 55 kcal/kg/day

Protein Requirements

Nitrogen Balance

The function of protein in health is to sustain tissue growth and maintenance. In healthy adults this ideal state is reflected in nitrogen equilibrium. In illness, however, catabolism is reflected by a state of *negative nitrogen balance,* that is, more nitrogen loss than intake, indicating wasting of tissue protein. Therefore, the goal of nutritional therapy in illness is to maintain a state of positive nitrogen balance constantly monitored by accurate nitrogen balance studies to counteract the catabolic deterioration.[8,22]

Essential Amino Acids

The quality of the protein intake in terms of equivalent essential amino acids is fundamental to tissue synthesis (see *To Probe Further* above). The essential amino acids must be present in the optimal ratio for best use of individual amino acids. One amino acid, methionine, is even toxic in large amounts.[23]

Ratio of Nitrogen to Nonprotein Kcalories

To protect the nitrogen sources (the amino acids) and make them available for tissue synthesis, sufficient nonprotein energy sources must be present to meet the increased kcalorie need. Carbohydrates are necessary to promote incorporation of plasma amino acids into muscle tissue protein. For optimal use, the normal adult diet sustains a ratio of 150 nonprotein kcal/1 g of nitrogen. To meet the metabolic stress of critical illness with minimal activity, this ratio should be 150 to 200 kcal/1 g of nitrogen. In terms of protein, the requirements in illness reflect these increased needs:

Catabolic state: Weight (kg) × 1.2 to 1.5 g protein
Healthy state: Weight (kg) × 0.8 to 1.0 g protein

Electrolyte Requirements

Special electrolyte profiles are required in intracellular and extracellular fluid for all tissues to maintain normal water balances throughout the body. These balances must be maintained during illness in the face of metabolic imbalances. For example, active tissue synthesis requires phosphate and potassium and is also influenced by available sodium and chloride ions. Monitoring of individual electrolyte status supplies the data needed to determine daily electrolyte requirements. In general, the basic electrolyte needs for a 3000 kcal intake (3 L solution) are approximately the following: 120 to 150 mEq of sodium (Na), 120 mEq of potassium (K), 150 mEq of chloride (Cl), 24 to 36 mEq of magnesium (Mg), 6 to 15 mEq of calcium (Ca), and 60 to 75 mEq of phosphate (HPO_4). This pattern varies according to metabolic needs of individual patients.

Vitamin and Mineral Requirements

The need for vitamins and minerals is based on normal standards (see the current RDAs listed inside the front cover). These needs are increased in hypermetabolic states. Individual nutrients may be added as needed to cover increased metabolism and depletion states. Attention to necessary trace minerals is especially important. Observations of patients on long-term TPN have confirmed risks of iron, zinc, and copper deficiencies and have provided new evidence for clinically significant deficiencies of selenium, chromium, and molybdenum.[24] Trace element supplements of zinc and copper are needed especially by patients with severe burns because of their essential roles in wound healing during the acute recovery period.[25] The prescribed TPN solution reflects these needs and additions.

Preparation of TPN Solution

With the development of the TPN technique, products for use in TPN nutrient solutions have also been developing. A number of nutrients in differing strength solutions are available for use by the TPN team in formulating individual nutritional needs for each patient based on the nutritional requirements for protein, nonprotein energy, electrolytes, vitamins, and minerals.

Protein-Nitrogen Source

Remember that 6.25 g of protein equals 1 g of nitrogen. In the TPN solution, this protein-nitrogen need is supplied by essential and nonessential crystalline amino acids. We have come through two previous generations in the development of amino acid solutions: (1) the initial use of protein hydrolysates through the 1970s, which had problems of inconsistent amino acid content, since the protein being hydrolyzed determined the amino acid composition, and of contamination; and (2) the early crystalline amino acid solutions, which had problems of acidosis and of structure. They were mixtures of D-amino acid (D stands for **dextrorotatory (dextro-; R-)** meaning right, the molecular configurations of which the human body cannot use, so they were excreted, and "mirror image" L-amino acids (L stands for **levorotatory (levo-; L-),** meaning left, the molecular configurations of which the body recognizes, so they are used. All amino acids occurring naturally in proteins belong to the L-configurational family. Now in their third generation, crystalline solutions of all pure L-amino acids are used. A fourth generation of tailor-made amino acid solutions being researched and tested for use in specific conditions—such as liver or kidney failure, sepsis, severe trauma, or immature or abnormal metabolic pathways—is becoming the next stage.[26] A number of general and specialized parenteral amino acid formulations are available.

General Standard Solutions

Commercial amino acid solutions range in concentration from 3% to 11.4%, four of which provide a general standard product of 8.5%—Aminosyn (Abbott), FreAmine II (McGaw), Novamine (Cutter), and Travasol (Travenol).[26,27] They vary only slightly in comparative essential and nonessential amino acids, with no clinically significant differences among them.

Specialized Solutions

Currently, two types of specialized amino acid solutions have been formulated, although they are more expensive than standard formulations and their superiority remains unclear. Five modular solutions, all to be mixed with modules of 50% to 70% dextrose,

dextrorotatory (dextro-; R-) • Physics term; molecular structure or configuration of a chemical compound that turns the plane of polarized light to the right.

levorotatory (levo-; L-) • Physics term; molecular structure of configuration of a chemical compound that turns the plane of polarized light to the left.

as well as with electrolytes, vitamins, and trace elements, illustrate these special formulas. Two are enriched with the three BCAAs isoleucine, leucine, and valine, and three are enriched with increased amounts of essential amino acids (EAAs)[27]:

1. *BCAA-enriched solutions:* FreAmine HBC 6.9% (McGaw) is for patients with extensive trauma and severe catabolic stress, who have shown large urinary nitrogen losses and low plasma levels of these three amino acids, and Hepatamine 8% (McGaw) is for patients with deteriorating liver disease, especially cirrhosis, who have also shown decreased levels of BCAAs.
2. *EAA-enriched solutions:* Aminosyn 5.2% (Abbott), Nephramine 5.4% (McGaw), and Renamin (Travenol) prevent the development of hyperuremia in patients with acute renal failure.

With careful aseptic technique and protective equipment confined under a laminar air-flow hood, the pharmacist on the nutritional support team is responsible for mixing the individual patient's formula according to the TPN prescription determined by the physician with recommendations from the special nutritional support team clinical dietitian based on initial nutritional status assessments and constant monitoring. However, all team members must know about these various solutions and keep up with the commercial product changes. For example, a usual amino acid need is supplied by a 3.5% or 4.25% dilution achieved by use of 1 L of standard 7% or 8.5% amino acid solution mixed with 1 L of dextrose solution.

Nonprotein Energy Source (Kcalories)

Nonprotein kcalories to protect protein (amino acids) for tissue synthesis demands are supplied by glucose and lipid solutions.

Glucose (Dextrose)

Glucose is the most common and least expensive source of kcalories used for parenteral nutrition support. Available solutions range from the 5% solution used traditionally in peripheral intravenous support of fluid and electrolytes after general surgery, to the hypertonic 50% to 70% solutions used for TPN formulations. Glucose for parenteral nutrition support is commercially available as dextrose monohydrate ($C_6H_{12}O_6H_2O$), which has an energy value of 3.4 kcal/g, not the energy value of 4 kcal/g of the regular dietary glucose form ($C_6H_{12}O_6$).

Lipids

Lipid emulsions provide a concentrated energy source, 9 kcal/g, as well as the essential fatty acid, linoleic acid. Lipids also have practical values associated with their effects on respiratory gas (carbon dioxide and oxygen) exchange, autoimmune disease, and vascular disease.[27] About 4% to 10% of the daily kcalorie intake should consist of fat emulsion to prevent fatty acid deficiency.[28] A 500-ml bottle of 10% or 20% fat emulsion provides 555 kcal (1.1 kcal/ml) or 1000 kcal (2.0 kcal/ml), respectively. These solutions are made isotonic by the addition of glycerin, which allows them to be fed by parenteral infusion, and are stabilized by the addition of egg phospholipids. Three commercial products currently available for TPN use lipid emulsions of soybean oil and safflower oil combined—Liposyn II (Abbott)—or soybean oil alone—Intralipid (Kabi Vitrum) and Soyacal (Alpha Therapeutic).

Traditionally, lipid emulsions were fed separately from the dextrose–amino acid base solution. More recently, however, with improved solutions and equipment, in some cases lipids have been combined with the dextrose and amino acid base and called a 3-in-1 **admixture.**[29] With the additional modules of electrolytes and vitamins and adequate fluid, the whole feeding is identified as a *total nutrient admixture (TNA).* Stable TNAs have also been prepared successfully for pediatric use.[30] Current refinements in products and technique have allowed various admixtures of lipids, carbohydrates, and protein in a common bag, complete with adequate fluid and electrolytes and either single or multiple forms of vitamins and trace elements. Such standardized formulations both ease administration and lessen cost. Newer alternate lipid sources include forms such as short-chain fatty acids, medium-chain fatty acids, omega-3 fatty acids, and blended or structured lipids.[31]

Electrolytes

The formulation of electrolytes is based on the usual requirements for normal electrolyte balance with adjustments according to individual patient monitoring. Most commercial amino acid formulations are available with or without added electrolytes. If electrolytes are present in the amino acid solution, they must be taken into account when calculating additions for a specific patient requirement. Three basic considerations in determining individual patient requirements include the following actions: (1) correct any preexisting deficits immediately, (2) recognize and replace excessive fluid and electrolyte losses to prevent chronic deficits, and (3) monitor and determine electrolyte needs daily.[32]

Vitamins

The Nutrition Advisory Group of the American Medical Association has established guidelines for parenteral administration of 12 vitamins: A, D, E, thiamin, riboflavin, niacin, pantothenic acid, pyridoxine, folic

Clinical Application: Administration of TPN Formula

Careful administration of TPN formula is essential. Specific protocols vary somewhat, but they usually include the following points:

Start slowly. The patient needs time to adapt to the increased glucose concentration and osmolality of the solution.

Schedule carefully. During the first 24 hours give 1 to 2 L by continuous drip. The slow rate should be regulated by an infusion pump.

Monitor closely. Note metabolic effects of glucose (blood glucose level should not exceed 200 mg/dl) and electrolytes.

Increase volume gradually. After the first day increase by 1 L/day to reach the desired daily volume.

Make changes cautiously. Watch the effect of all changes and proceed slowly.

Maintain a constant rate. Keep to the correct hourly infusion rate, with no "catch-up" or "slow-down" effort to meet the original volume order.

Discontinue slowly. It is critical that TPN feeding be discontinued gradually, reducing the rate and daily volume about 1 L/day. ◆

acid, biotin, B_{12}, and ascorbic acid. Based on these recommendations, four essentially identical multivitamin preparations are currently available: MVI-12 (Armour), MCV 9 + 3 (Lymphomed), Multivitamin Additive (Abbott), and Berocca Parenteral Nutrition (Roche). Vitamin K is not a component of any formulation for adults. If it is needed for individual maintenance, it is added to the solution. Any larger deficit is treated by periodic intramuscular injection as needed.

Trace Elements

The American Medical Association has also set guidelines for the addition of four trace elements in parenteral solutions: zinc, copper, manganese, and chromium. Three commercial products supply these four elements: Multiple Trace Element Additives (Abbott), Multiple Trace Metal Additives (IMS), and Multiple Trace Element Solution (American Quinine). Two additional manufacturers also supply a separate product with selenium added: Multe-Pak-4 and Multe-Pak-5 (Solo Pak) and MTE-4 and MTE-5 (Lymphomed). Single mineral products are also available for each of these trace elements. Iron is not routinely added. If it is needed by an individual patient, it is administered apart from the parenteral nutrition admixture.[32] Caution is needed in adding minerals to the TPN solution. Incompatibilities of certain electrolytes and other components may form insoluble substances that separate out, depending on ion concentration and solution pH.

Administration of TPN Solution

Equipment

Throughout the entire TPN administration process, strict aseptic technique by all the special nutritional support team members involved is essential, including the solution preparation by the pharmacist, the surgical placement of the venous catheter by the physician, and the care of the catheter site and all external equipment and administration of the formula by the nurse. At every step of the TPN process, strict infection control is one of the primary team responsibilities.[33,34]

Venous Catheter

Surgical placement of the venous catheter is done by the physician at the bedside. Strict aseptic technique is aided by a variety of commercially prepared kits containing all the necessary equipment items to gain access to a large central vein for feeding the nutritional support solution directly into the central blood circulation.[35] Flexible silicone catheters are available in different lengths and calibers. Smaller, shorter catheters (15 to 25 cm) are designed for use in the hospital. Larger, longer catheters such as the 1.6 mm caliber Hickman catheter are designed for long-term intermediate or home use. The catheter entry is usually by way of large outlying veins in the neck area, such as the subclavian, cephalic, or internal jugular that feed directly into the larger central venous system. The catheter is passed through the outer vein into the central superior vena cava, which leads directly into the heart (Fig. 4-1). In the vena cava the catheter tip lies so that concentrated TPN solutions of 1500 mOsm/L, five times the concentration of blood plasma, can

admixture • A mixture resulting from adding or mingling another ingredient; a combination of two or more substances that are not chemically united or that exist in no fixed proportion to each other.

be infused at a rate of 2 to 3 ml/min and can be immediately diluted by a large blood flow of 2 to 5 L/min, a dilution factor of at least a thousand.[36] Over the past years of TPN development, new catheters and insertion techniques have greatly reduced catheter-related complications. Commercial sterile dressing kits for continuing nursing care have also aided aseptic technique and infection control.

Infusion Devices

Various infusion devices control the solution flow rate, maintaining an accurate flow range. Infusion pumps may be used to deliver the solution at a constant rate to prevent metabolic complications. Strict asepsis throughout the delivery system is essential. Protocols for external delivery system tubing changes guided by infection control monitoring include maintenance of sterility of the catheter hub and tubing junction.[37]

Solution Administration

The nutritional support nurse checks frequently to see that the entire TPN delivery system is operating accurately (see the *Clinical Application,* p. 59). Careful administration of the TPN formula is essential. Specific protocols vary somewhat, but they usually include the following points:

- *Start slowly.* Give the patient time to adapt to the increased glucose concentration and osmolality of the solution.
- *Schedule carefully.* During the first 24 hours give 1 to 2 L by continuous drip. The slow rate is usually regulated by an infusion pump.
- *Monitor closely.* Note metabolic effects of glucose (blood glucose levels should not exceed 200 mg/dl) and electrolytes.
- *Increase volume gradually.* After the first day, increase the volume by 1 L/day to reach the desired daily volume.
- *Make changes cautiously.* Watch the effect of all changes and proceed slowly.
- *Maintain a constant rate.* Keep to the correct hourly infusion rate, with no catch-up or slow-down effort to meet the original volume order.
- *Discontinue slowly.* Discontinue TPN feeding gradually, reducing rate and daily volume about 1 L/day.

Monitoring

In the hands of a well-trained TPN team, risks have been minimized and complications controlled by constant team effort. Specific protocols guide continuing assessment and monitoring with related solution adjustments by the nutritional support team according to metabolic and nutritional needs.

Home Parenteral Nutrition

Experience from home use of other long-term medical care equipment, such as that for renal dialysis, has led to the concept of self-infusion of parenteral nutrients at home. Following the pattern given in the preceding chapter for home enteral nutrition, a full patient and family TPN education plan with supervised practice is essential. In the hands of these selected, well-trained patients and their families, home TPN allows mobility and travel, but there are problems (see *Issues and Answers,* p. 63). It has offered special promise in long-term management of conditions such as severe abdominal injury or chronic severe inflammatory bowel disease. Special equipment, solutions, and guidelines for training selected patients and families have been developed and are successfully being used in a number of cases.

To Sum Up

For patients with critical hypermetabolic injury or illness or obstruction that makes the gastrointestinal tract unavailable for supplying their large nutritional demands, parenteral nutrition support acts as an "artificial gut," an alternate lifeline. This alternate lifeline depends heavily on biomedical technology for the development of tubes, bags, pumps, and other equipment to facilitate the feeding of nutrients directly into veins for blood circulation to the cells. The route of entry may be a large central vein capable of receiving a concentrated nutrient solution over a long period of time or a smaller peripheral vein in the arm capable of receiving a less concentrated solution over a shorter period of time.

Total parenteral nutrition (TPN) may be supplied for an indefinite time through a large catheter surgically placed through the subclavian vein reaching into the superior vena cava, a large central vessel leading to the heart. In this large volume of rapidly moving blood, the concentrated nutrient solution is quickly diluted and carried to cells throughout the body. Following an individual assessment of needs, the TPN prescription reflects basic demands for energy, protein, minerals, and vitamins.

The solution order for dextrose and lipids to supply nonprotein energy, crystalline amino acids to provide a protein-nitrogen source, together with vitamin and electrolyte modules, is mixed by the nutritional support pharmacist and administered by the nurse, both tasks requiring strict aseptic technique to control infection. The nutritional support clinical dietitian and nurse are key team members to help the patient cope with this altered feeding method, and if TPN is to be continued at home after hospital discharge, to help the patient and family learn the necessary skills and aid in the recovery.

QUESTIONS FOR REVIEW

1. You are caring for a 45-year-old man, a previously healthy truck driver who suffered an accident in which he sustained a severe abdominal injury requiring extensive surgical repair and leaving the gastrointestinal tract unavailable for use for an undetermined period of time. He is referred to the nutritional support team for follow-up TPN. Early in this care he asks you how this feeding works. How would you describe and explain the TPN feeding process?
2. What nutritional status assessment procedures would be done to the truck driver, and how would you explain the nature and purpose of each measure to him?
3. From your study of this chapter, outline your estimate of the truck driver's basic nutritional needs to serve as a basis for determining his TPN therapy.
4. List the typical components of a basic TPN formula that the truck driver may require, and describe the purpose of each to help reassure him of its adequacy and importance.
5. Sufficient energy (kcalorie) intake is essential to immediately meet the truck driver's metabolic needs after surgery. Assume his normal preinjury weight and height and an added metabolic activity factor (MAF) for stress of 1.5 times his basal energy expenditure (BEE). Calculate his total kcalorie need, using the Harris-Benedict equation for BEE and adding the MAF stress need.
6. Define *prealbumin* and describe why it is a primary test for monitoring the effectiveness of the TPN formula in meeting the truck driver's nutritional support needs for recovery.

REFERENCES

1. Dudrick SJ et al: Can intravenous feeding as the sole means of nutrition support growth in the child and restore weight loss in an adult? *Ann Surg* 169:974, 1969.
2. Dudrick SJ: A clinical review of nutritional support of the patient, *Am J Clin Nutr* 33(suppl):1191, 1982.
3. Rhoads JE, Dudrick SJ: History of intravenous nutrition. In Rombeau JL, Caldwell MD, eds: *Parenteral nutrition, clinical nutrition,* vol 2, Philadelphia, 1986, WB Saunders.
4. Fischer JE, ed: *Total parenteral nutrition,* Boston, 1991, Little, Brown.
5. Zemen FJ, Ney DM: *Applications of clinical nutrition,* Englewood Cliffs, NJ, 1988, Prentice Hall.
6. Zeman FJ: *Clinical nutrition and dietetics,* ed 2, New York, 1991, Macmillan Publishing.
7. DeChicco RS, Matarese LE: Selection of nutrition support regimens, *Nutr Clin Prac* 7(5):239, 1992.
8. Candio JA et al: Estimation of nitrogen excretion based on abbreviated urinary collections in patients on continuous parenteral nutrition, *J Parenter Enteral Nutr* 15(2):148, 1991.
9. Barbul A: Measurements of relevant nutrition data for determining efficacy of nutritional support. In Fischer JE, ed: *Total parenteral nutrition,* ed 2, Boston, 1991, Little, Brown.
10. Jeejeebhoy KN et al: Assessment of nutritional status, *J Parenter Enteral Nutr* 14(suppl 5):193, 1990.
11. Bernstein LH: Monitoring quality of nutrition support: a chemical marker, *Diet Curr* 19(2):1, 1992.
12. Sawicky CP et al: Adequate energy intake and improved prealbumin concentration as indicators of the response to total parenteral nutrition, *J Am Diet Assoc* 92(10): 1266, 1992.
13. Geibig CB et al: Quality assurance for a nutritional support service, *Nutr Clin Prac* 6(4):147, 1991.
14. Powers T et al: A nutrition team quality assurance plan, *Nutr Clin Prac* 6(4):151, 1991.
15. Ireton-Jones CS, Baxter CR: Nutrition for adult burn patients: a review, *Nutr Clin Prac* 6(1):3, 1991.
16. Harris JA, Benedict FG: *A biometric study of basal metabolism,* Washington, DC, 1919, Carnegie Institution of Washington.
17. Kinney J: Indirect calorimetry: the search for clinical relevance, *Nutr Clin Prac* 7(5):203, 1992.
18. McClave SA, Snider HL: Use of indirect calorimetry in clinical nutrition, *Nutr Clin Prac* 7(5):207, 1992.
19. Stokes MA, Hill GL: A single, accurate measurement of resting metabolic expenditure, *J Parenter Enteral Nutr* 15(3):281, 1991.
20. Ireton-Jones CS, Turner WW: Actual or ideal body weight: which should be used to predict energy expenditure? *J Am Diet Assoc* 91(2):193, 1991.
21. Shizgal HM et al: The effect of age on the caloric requirements of malnourished individuals, *Am J Clin Nutr* 55:783, 1992.
22. Konstantinides FN: Nitrogen balance studies in clinical nutrition, *Nutr Clin Prac* 7(5):231, 1992.
23. Anderson SA, Raiten DJ, eds: *Safety of amino acids used as dietary supplements,* Life Science Research Office, Federation of American Societies for Experimental Biology, Bethesda, Md, 1992, US Government Printing Office.
24. Fleming CR: Trace element metabolism in adult patients requiring total parenteral nutrition, *Am J Clin Nutr* 49:573, 1989.
25. Cunningham JJ et al: Zinc and copper status of severely burned children, *J Am Coll Nutr* 10(1):57, 1991.
26. Heyman MB: General and specialized parenteral amino acid formulations for nutritional support, *J Am Diet Assoc* 90(3):401, 1990.
27. Sax HC: Practicalities of lipids: ICU patient, autoimmune disease, and vascular disease, *J Parenter Enteral Nutr* 14(suppl 5):223, 1990.
28. Torosian MH, Daly JM: Solutions available. In Fischer JE, ed: *Total parenteral nutrition,* ed 2, Boston, 1991, Little, Brown.
29. Warshawsky KY: Intravenous fat emulsions in clinical practice, *Nutr Clin Prac* 7(4):187, 1992.

30. Bullock L et al: Emulsion stability in total nutrient admixtures containing a pediatric amino acid formulation, *J Parenter Enteral Nutr* 16(1):64, 1992.
31. Gottschlich MM: Selection of optimal lipid sources in enteral and parenteral nutrition, *Nutr Clin Prac* 7(4):152, 1992.
32. LaFrance RJ, Miyagawa CI: Pharmaceutical considerations in total parenteral nutrition. In Fischer JE, ed: *Total parenteral nutrition,* ed 2, Boston, 1991, Little, Brown.
33. Cahill SL, Benotti PN: Catheter infection control in parenteral nutrition, *Nutr Clin Prac* 6(2):65, 1991.
34. Thompson B, Robinson LA: Infection control of parenteral nutrition solutions, *Nutr Clin Prac* 6(2):49, 1991.
35. Seltzer MH et al: Parenteral nutrition equipment. In Rombeau JL, Caldwell MD, eds: *Parenteral nutrition, clinical nutrition,* vol 2, Philadelphia, 1986, WB Saunders.
36. Flowers JF et al: Catheter-related complications of total parenteral nutrition. In Fischer JE, ed: *Total parenteral nutrition,* ed 2, Boston, 1991, Little, Brown.
37. Davis CL: Nursing care of total parenteral and enteral nutrition. In Fischer JE, ed: *Total parenteral nutrition,* ed 2, Boston, 1991, Little, Brown.

FURTHER READING

DeChicco RS, Matarese LE: Selection of nutrition support regimens, *Nutr Clin Prac* 7(5):239, 1992.

These experienced nutritional support clinical dietitians provide an excellent review of the process used to determine whether a patient needs nutritional support, what type of feeding access and techniques should be used, and how and when to make the transition back to oral feedings.

Heyman MB: General and specialized parenteral amino acid formulations for nutritional support, *J Am Diet Assoc* 90(3):401, 1990.

This gastroenterologist's comprehensive review of the "state of the art" in amino acid formulations, especially for pediatric nutritional support, provides a clearer understanding of evolving special amino acid solutions and why their use should be approached with caution. Standard solutions, he concludes, provide adequate protein for most adults and children.

Nuutinen LS et al: Nutrition during ten-week life support with successful fetal outcome in a case with fatal maternal brain damage, *J Parenter Enteral Nutr* 13(4):432, 1989.

Watson LA et al: Total peripheral parenteral nutrition in pregnancy, *J Parenter Enteral Nutr* 14(5):485, 1990.

These two articles describe cases in which parenteral nutrition support was used in pregnancy. In the first case a mother sustained a sudden severe brain hemorrhage at her twenty-first week of pregnancy and remained in deep coma, but successful nutritional support provided for fetal growth and development, with the healthy infant delivered by cesarean section at 32 weeks. The second article describes the use of peripheral parenteral nutrition support for 20 pregnant women who were unable to eat for various reasons and who were totally supplied their kcaloric and metabolic needs by use of a 3-in-1 admixture of standard formula with added lipid emulsion for concentrated energy needs.

Sawicky CP et al: Adequate energy intake and improved prealbumin concentration as indicators of the response to total parenteral nutrition, *J Am Diet Assoc* 92(10):1266, 1992.

This article illustrates the monitoring focus on total intake of kcalories and the rapid feedback rise of serum prealbumin as a primary focus for determining effectiveness of TPN therapy.

The Challenge of Long-Term TPN Therapy

The purpose of any nonoral feeding method is to restore the patient, if possible, to the oral feeding state. How long this takes varies with the original nutritional and health status of the patient and the extent of the illness. Persons with inflammatory bowel disease (see Chapter 6) have been known to require 2 to 3 months to achieve the benefits of TPN, and at least one individual with "no bowel" syndrome is known to have done well on TPN for more than a decade. Although this makes TPN's potential for long-term use seem tremendous, it is not without its drawbacks.

Hazards of gastrointestinal disuse syndrome

Failure of intestinal barrier-immune function. The intestinal mucosa forms an extraordinarily efficient barrier between the body's interior and exterior environments. It guards against infectious agents entering from the outside, and from *translocation* of the more than 500 species of bacteria that normally colonize the intestine into the normally sterile surrounding body tissues such as the lymph nodes of the mesentery and other internal organs. Any break in this barrier from injury or perforating ulceration or from tissue breakdown from disuse or atrophy allows bacteria and toxins to pass through the denuded area. In addition, the intestinal mucosa forms an integral part of the body's overall *immune system.* This gut-associated lymphatic tissue consists of B cells and T cells, macrophages, and the **mesenteric** lymph nodes (see Chapters 12 and 13) that help kill invading disease-causing agents. TPN indirectly contributes to this mucosal breakdown process from disuse of normal gastrointestinal functioning and breaching the integrity of the gut-barrier.

Decreased secretions. The intestinal effects of TPN suggest additional potential hazards with long-term use. The lack of food in the alimentary canal depresses normal secretions that the presence of food stimulates, thus maintaining a functioning mucosal tissue surface for digestion and absorption. For example, lack of food results in the following:

- Reduced secretion of hormones and enzymes into the gastrointestinal tract
- Suppression or stoppage of bile flow caused by an increased viscosity of bile that is *not* secreted into the gastrointestinal tract
- Mucosal atrophy *hypoplasia,* probably resulting from reduced levels of cholecystokinin
- Less insulin secreted in response to the same amount of glucose obtained orally

These difficulties do not interfere with the ability to digest foods for 2 to 3 months. But what if the patient graduates to oral or tube feedings after that length of time? Are there difficulties with (1) undigested foods, (2) a higher risk of gallstones, (3) impaired nutrient absorption across an atrophied mucosa, or (4) a risk of hyperglycemia? These questions may indicate the need for careful monitoring, and *gradual* refeeding for such patients; however, such concerns still must be verified and measured.

Problems associated with formula solution

Other problems regarding long-term TPN *have* been verified and measured. These difficulties have more to do with the nature of the formula solutions rather than the intestine. Their potential for malnutrition warrants careful control and prevention on the part of the nutritional support team, especially the clinical dietitian. The TPN process uses solutions of glucose, fats, and amino acids, as well as vitamin and mineral supplements. The nature of these nutrients is discussed in the text.

Nonprotein energy sources. During use of these energy solutions, glucose levels must be carefully monitored because excess amounts may result in the following:

- Hyperglycemia
- Respiratory distress, especially in critically ill patients (excessive glucose intake raises the respiratory quotient [carbon dioxide/oxygen] by increasing carbon dioxide production)
- Lipogenesis

These problems may not be desirable in individual patients. The best defense against them is a solution that derives about half of its nonprotein energy from fats and half from glucose.

Amino acid solutions. These solutions have been associated with several nutritional imbalances, including deficiencies in the following:

- *Carnitine.* Carnitine is an amino acid that helps incorporate fatty acids into the cell for energy use. Patients on long-term TPN have developed muscle weakness, high bilirubin levels, and hypoglycemia; and carnitine levels have been found to be low. Symptoms subside after carnitine supplementation.
- *Calcium.* Amino acid solutions provide extra *sulfur* from the amino acids methionine and cystine, which binds with calcium and promotes its excretion. As a result, premature infants on TPN have been known to develop a painful bone disease characterized by osteomalacia and associated with the resulting calcium deficiency.

Amino acid solutions have also been known to induce *metabolic acidosis,* a condition that may be symptomless or marked by irritability, hypoxia, neuromuscular hyperexcitability, impaired gastrointestinal motility, polyuria, tetany, and other symptoms. It is associated with loss of endogenous acids such as gastric hydrochloric acid (HCl), which occurs in several conditions for which TPN is in-

Continued.

dicated, for example, chronic vomiting and fistulas. Ironically, this loss is aggravated by TPN, specifically by the lactate or acetate that is added to amino acid solutions to *prevent* this condition's counterpart, *metabolic alkalosis.* Since acetate is added to all commercial solutions, the nutritional support team must be prepared to correct its pH by adding water or HCl. Arginine HCl and ammonium chloride can be used, although with caution if renal or hepatic insufficiency is suspected. Sodium chloride and potassium chloride have also been used, but they are not as effective as HCl.

Vitamin and mineral supplements. Vitamin and mineral additions to TPN solutions may create a problem because of the difficulty that is connected with their release from solution or because of the variability in requirements among patients, as in the example of iron. Iron dextran, the supplement sometimes used in TPN solutions, does not release iron as easily as desired. Ferrous citrate has been used in some instances. Because of these problems, some clinicians prefer to use iron apart from the parenteral nutrition admixture.

Thus for maximal promotion of the nutritional status of patients requiring long-term TPN, skilled professionals on the nutritional support team do the following:

- Carefully monitor a *gradual* refeeding program to avoid problems created by reduced gastrointestinal secretions and mucosal atrophy.
- Provide sufficient fats, that is, half of the nonprotein kcalories to prevent respiratory distress in very ill patients and to spare protein for tissue repair and rebuilding.
- Remain aware of deficiency symptoms and potential effects of "undesirable" additives, such as sulfur and ammonia, and be prepared to adjust the solution accordingly.
- Adjust vitamin and mineral levels to suit individual needs.
- Select solutions from which nutrients are readily available.

Actually, the concept of the artificial gut and the transfer of TPN to long-term home use is a relatively new therapy covering only two decades of sophisticated medical technology developments. It has allowed many patients to survive, but problems with chronic fluid, electrolyte, and micronutrient deficiencies; catheter sepsis; and insurance coverage often restrict optimal rehabilitation and quality of life. And for short-term use in terminal cases, its limited effectiveness may not justify its large cost. It is one of the most expensive new home therapies, usually costing $75,000 to $150,000 per year.

Recent data from large medical centers and the relatively new North American Registry for home parenteral nutrition outcome, which started monitoring results in 1984, have begun to provide the first step in baseline information. On this basis more guidance for developing clinical outcome standards can emerge. Such consensus is needed for the proper use of this valuable but expensive therapy.

REFERENCES

Alexander JW: Nutrition and translocation, *J Parenter Enteral Nutr* 14(suppl 5):170, 1990.

Burnes JU et al: Home parenteral nutrition—a 3-year analysis of clinical and laboratory monitoring, *J Parenter Enteral Nutr* 16(4):327, 1992.

Detsky AS: Parenteral nutrition—is it helpful? *N Engl J Med* 325(8):573, 1991.

Evans MA, Shronts EP: Intestinal fuels: glutamine, short-chain fatty acids, and dietary fiber, *J Am Diet Assoc* 92(10):1239, 1992.

Howard L et al: Four years of North American Registry home parenteral nutrition outcome data and their implications for patient management, *J Parenter Enteral Nutr* 15(4):384, 1991.

CHAPTER 5

Nutritional Therapy in Diseases of Infancy and Childhood

CHAPTER OUTLINE

Hospitalized Infants and Children
Gastrointestinal Problems
Malabsorption Problems
Genetic Diseases
Food Allergies
Weight Management
Dental Caries

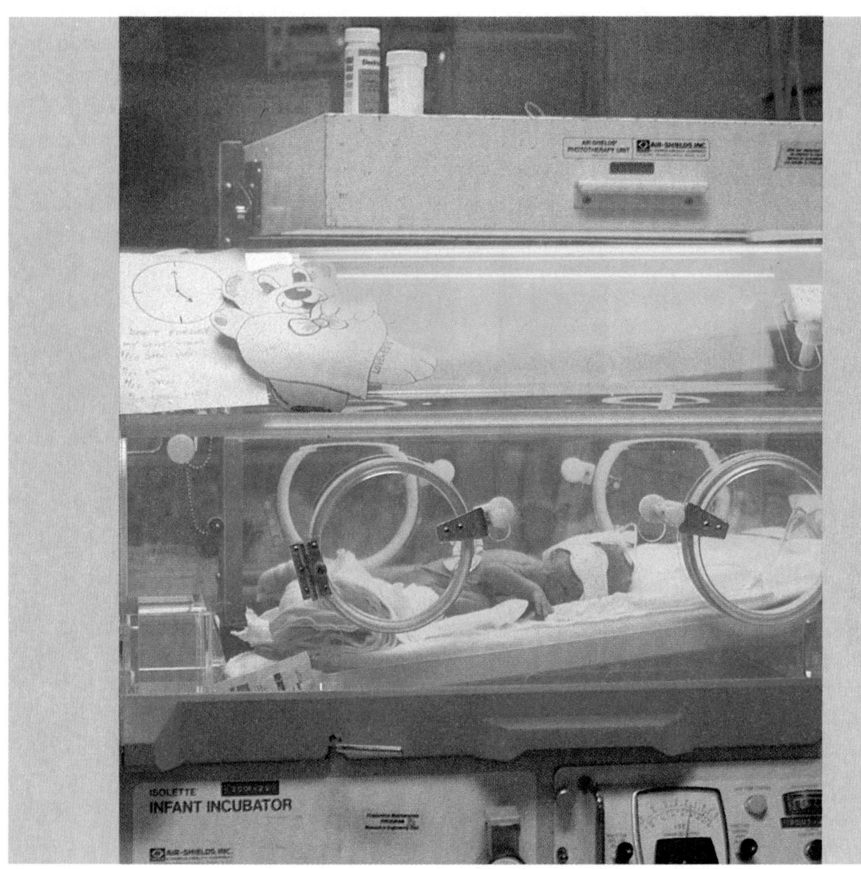

This chapter begins our final sequence on clinical nutrition, the study of nutritional therapy in disease. First we look at the beginning of the life cycle and special health problems of children. Then, in the remaining nine chapters, we examine major medical conditions occurring at various times throughout the life span that require special nutritional therapy.

This chapter examines the general needs of the hospitalized child and pediatric conditions that require special nutritional care. Sick or well, all infants and children struggle to accomplish the universal tasks of "growing up" physically and emotionally. During the stress of illness, some degree of regression occurs. Thus in exploring patient needs and planning care, we are concerned not only with the treatment needs of the disease but also with the child's particular response to the experience of illness.

The first consideration is the hospitalization experience of the child and the individual support needs it brings. Then some of the conditions that require modification of normal nutritional needs or feeding modes are reviewed.

Hospitalized Infants and Children

Stress of Childhood Illness

Ill infants and children have special needs. High-risk, low-birth-weight babies struggle to survive. Children face pain and fear during disease and its treatment, and their reaction to illness is conditioned by past experiences and the common growth and development patterns of childhood.

Nutritional therapy plays a fundamental role in the care of a growing child. The normal nutritional needs of a particular growth period take on added significance in meeting the physiologic stress of disease. Specific nutrients must be ensured in the diet, yet feeding problems often intervene. In some cases, dietary modifications need to be made to accommodate a particular disease condition. Throughout this special care process, observant and sensitive practitioners find many opportunities to provide support and positive health care learning experiences for children and their parents. A primary part of this health care is always good nutrition.

Good patient care essentially centers on two factors: (1) determining the needs of the patient and (2) planning wise action to meet those needs. Many health care practices considered helpful in themselves are not necessarily helpful to a particular patient and a particular situation. This is especially true with children, to whom we have an added responsibility. We must be able to communicate with the children we care for and adapt this care to their special needs. A child perceives the world, thinks, reasons, and uses language in different ways at different age levels. The ability to care for children requires this knowledge and understanding of childhood mental development to

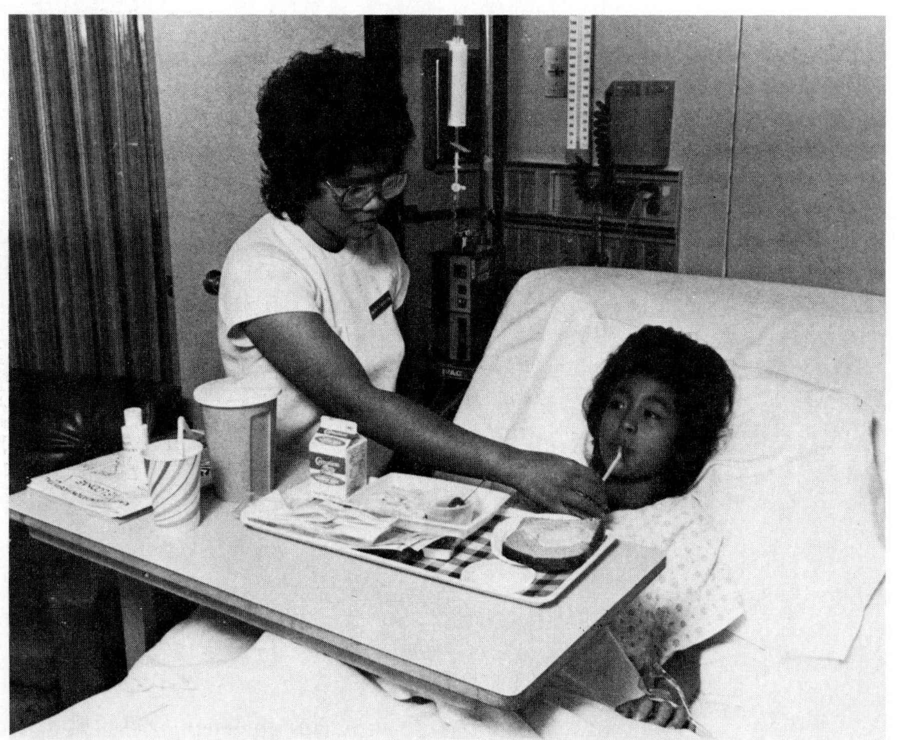

FIG. 5-1 Adequate fluid intake is essential for children, especially during illness.

communicate with children more effectively and to help them understand their care. This ability comes from knowing children and caring about *their* concerns and helps us to establish contact with a child who is often inarticulate, emotionally disturbed, and physically ill. Then we can plan for nutritional care as an integral part of total care.

Basic Needs of Hospitalized Children

Physical Care

Often it is the high quality of physical care by sensitive and skilled nurses and nutritionists that makes a difference in the child's illness and aids in the recovery process. A major part of this care is nutritional: close observation of the child's food attitudes and food and fluid intake and careful recording of these observations for analysis by the health care team (Fig. 5-1).

Emotional Support

Hospitalized children usually have anxieties and fears that may stem from family separations and from the illness and its treatment. A number of factors influencing a child's adjustment to hospitalization include the child's age, the nature of the illness, the kind of care provided, and inner personal resources developed from the past experiences that help in coping with the present situation. Particular life experiences may have provided few resources to meet this added crisis. There may be malnutrition or lack of emotional strength and control. Understanding the child's emotional needs and providing wise ways of meeting them are necessary to deal with such situations.

Nutritional Support

Food is essential in physical and emotional recovery from illness. It is a fundamental means of metabolic return to health, even in this age of "miracle" drugs and treatments. Sometimes this simple fact is forgotten. The biochemical base of health functions at the cellular level through the media of many chemical nutrients and their metabolic interactions. These nutrients or their precursors must be obtained in food. The necessary food must be provided, and the food must be eaten. Usually in a hospital setting, the administration and trained personnel are adequately equipped to accomplish the first aim. The crux of the problem is more often the second need, the child's acceptance of the food. This aspect of the problem becomes the responsibility mainly of the clinical dietitian and the nurse.

Plans for Nutritional Care of Hospitalized Children

In planning for the nutritional care of the hospitalized child, personal needs must be considered; for example, general age-group needs, any necessary diet modifications, the individual child and family, and nutritional assessment findings.

Age-Group Needs

What age and in what stage of growth is the child? What related developmental age-group needs is the child struggling to meet? How are these in any way related to the child's feeding, food, and fluid intake?

Diet Modification

What is the illness? Is it related to the child's living environment (see *To Probe Further,* p. 68)? Is it long- or short-term? Is it serious or even terminal, or is it a simple disorder? Does it hinder eating ability in any way? Does it require any dietary modifications? If so, what changes are required and why? Have these needs been discussed by the nutritionist or the nurse with the health care team?

Family Involvement

Explore the child's home eating habits with a parent or other family member. Discuss general ways the child's food is prepared and served. This gives helpful background information for planning the child's nutritional care during the hospital experience. Also, allow parents to express their own anxieties about the child. Help lead them to mutual learning concerning normal growth and development needs of children. If the child requires any special diet modifications, discuss these needs with the parents. Help them explore ways to make the child's needs compatible with the family eating habits if there is need for continuing the modification after hospitalization.

Food Acceptance

Illnesses and the anxieties they bring may contribute to children's poor appetites or refusal of food. Sometimes they are too ill or too weak to eat. Some may have a physical intolerance for the food, whereas others may require liquid or soft food, food substitutions, or gentle help in feeding. Children who are ill are often tense and frightened in the strange and unfamiliar hospital surroundings. They may be concerned about the illness and about its outcome.

Involve the parents in plans for care and help make arrangements for mother or father to be with the child to provide needed security and support. Help the child talk about particular fears, and understand and accept these fears. Provide simple, brief explanations of needed care and treatment to help reduce anxiety, gain the child's confidence, and provide added resources with which to cope.

A warm atmosphere at mealtime is a major in-

Lead in Children's Diets

TO PROBE FURTHER

Lead poisoning has been a major public health problem for centuries, with a not-so-glowing record of its damaging social effects. Now we are finding from new studies that it not only poisons our air and soil but also contaminates the food we eat, the dust in our homes, and the water that 42 million of us drink. And most disturbing of all is its danger to our children, especially during the first 6 years of life.

In the United States more than 250,000 children, most of them between the ages of 2 and 3 years, are found to have absorbed excessive amounts of lead each year. Most health workers assume that these children obtained most of the excess lead from lead-based paint chips or contaminated dirt or dust. However, at least one researcher has estimated that 55% to 85% of our daily lead intake is provided by food.

A recent 7-day food consumption survey of 371 children from birth to 5 years of age indicated that they ingested approximately 15 to 234 μg of lead from foods each day. The average dietary intake was 62 μg, almost two thirds of the 100-μg level considered safe by the Food and Drug Administration. Canned vegetables, fruits, and juices contributed 23.8% of the lead, plus lead pigments in labels on bread wrappers, which leaches into the food when the wrappers are turned inside-out for storing food. This suggests a strong "environmental" influence, that is, the lead from cans and bread wrappers.

Lead poisoning is associated with anemia, fatigue, poor learning ability, and ultimately death. It is a silent, relentless destroyer of brain cells and affects multiple organ systems in children and adults who are exposed to it in their environments. This should not occur. It can and should be eradicated if all persons involved have the vision and will to do so. At least some beginning public awareness is seen in developing environmental surveillance registries and lowering levels of lead in public water. The U.S. Environmental Protection Agency's new lead rules for water require municipal water suppliers to monitor lead levels beginning in 1992 and 1993 and to keep them under 15 parts per billion (ppb), whereas the prior standard had allowed a level of 50 ppb.

REFERENCES

Baser ME: The development of registries for surveillance of adult lead exposure, 1981 to 1992, *Am J Public Health* 82(8):1113, 1992.

Needleman HL: Childhood lead poisoning: a disease for the history books, *Am J Public Health* 81(6):685, 1991.

Neggers YH, Stitt KR: Effects of high lead intake in children, *J Am Diet Assoc* 86(7):938, 1986.

New lead rules for water, *Science News* 139(20):308, 1991.

Sciarillo WG et al: Lead exposure and child behavior, *Am J Public Health* 82(10):1356, 1992.

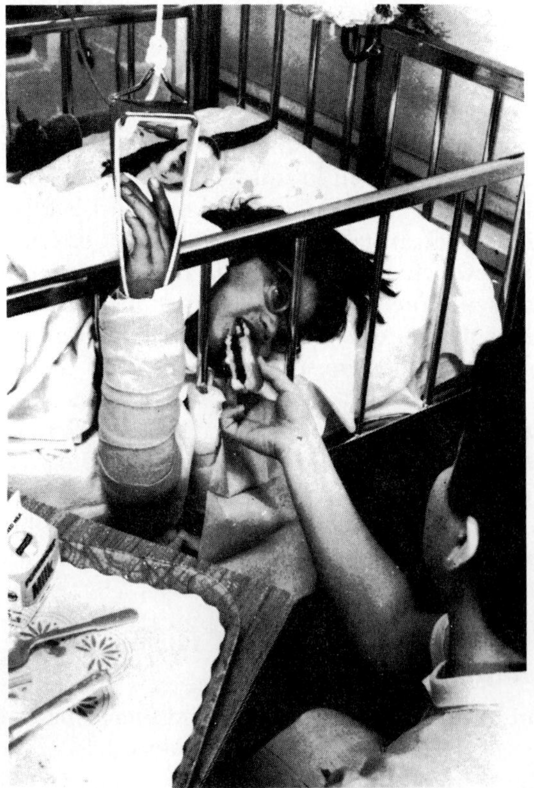

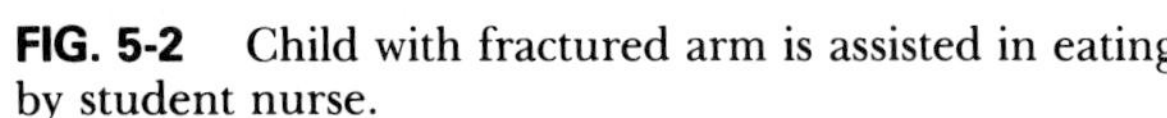

FIG. 5-2 Child with fractured arm is assisted in eating by student nurse.

fluence on the child's reaction. The following factors may help to build this environment in the pediatric ward:

Self-selection. Wherever possible, provide a selective menu and guide the child in making personal food choices. Consider a child's likes and dislikes and encourage new tastes in foods. A cycle menu for pediatric patients can be developed that includes the necessary flexibility to meet the needs of the individual child.

Staff involvement. Provide a warm, supportive food environment. Serve food attractively in proper-sized, small portions and use correct, child-sized dishes and utensils. Make bed patients as comfortable as possible, and assist them in eating as needed (Fig. 5-2).

Group eating. Have ambulatory patients eat together at small tables whenever possible. Interest is heightened if the children can be involved in the preparation. For example, some may be able to help arrange the table and chairs and serve as host or hostess.

Festive days. Observe holidays and birthdays with special food, favors, or decorations, which help to interest children and provide support.

Familiar food. Consider providing special ethnic or family foods. Sometimes a familiar food or dish from home that is not contraindicated by the child's illness stimulates the appetite and interest in eating. It secures not only needed nourishment but also provides emotional support, especially during an extended illness.

Special Infant Needs

Low Birth Weight

Over the past decade, tremendous strides have been made in the care of low-birth-weight infants. Improved nutritional management and feeding techniques, together with other aspects of care, such as attention to respiratory and environmental conditions, have helped improve survival rates. Some of these tiny babies do well on breast milk, although its protective features may be lost if it is pasteurized or stored, especially frozen, for any period while holding it in a "breast milk bank." Some clinicians believe that the potential advantages of human milk may outweigh some of its disadvantages for low-birth-weight infants, at least for a brief, initial period of use. Other infants require and thrive on special newly developed commercial formulas. Nutrition management includes changes such as earlier feedings and more use of enteral nutrition support through nasoenteric or surgically placed enterostomy tubes (see Chapter 3). Some low-birth-weight infants are started on regular strength formulas (67 kcal/dl), building to early use of higher-energy, special premature infant formulas (80kcal/dl), although some clinicians think this excess nutrient load is unnecessary (see *Issues and Answers,* p. 94). Parenteral nutrition support (see Chapter 4) may be provided in cases of special need.

Failure to Thrive

The general term *failure to thrive* has been used in pediatrics to describe any child who does not measure up to usual growth and development standards.[1] Fomon's[2] initial more specific definition helps identify special children at risk: "a rate of gain in length and/or weight less than the value or corresponding to two standard deviations below the mean during an interval of at least 56 days for infants less than five months of age, and during an interval of at least three months for older infants." Sometimes a pediatrician uses a brief hospital stay to classify infants who fail to thrive, during which the nurse and the nutritionist play important roles. Careful nutritional assessment is required to identify underlying causes of feeding problems so that the appropriate care can be planned. The following factors may be involved in failure to thrive:

Clinical disease. There may be central nervous system disorders, endocrine disease, congenital defects, or partial intestinal obstruction.

Neuromotor problems. There may be problems associated with poor sucking, abnormal postural tone, and the retention of primitive reflexes that should have faded at an earlier age. Eating, chewing, and swallowing problems may be so severe in some children as to compromise their nutrient intake.

Dietary practices. Some infants may have suffered from parental misconceptions and health beliefs about what constitutes a "normal" diet for infants. Others may have been deprived of needed energy and nutrients from inappropriate formula feeding, use of improper dilutions in mixing, or other poor practices that result in an inadequate kcaloric intake.

Unusual nutrient needs or losses. Other infants may receive an adequate diet to promote growth but suffer from inadequate nutrient absorption and therefore excessive fecal loss. In other cases a hypermetabolic state may require increased kcaloric intake that is not being met.

Psychosocial problems. Early feeding problems during infancy may have psychosocial causes within the family environment and relationships that result in emotional deprivation of the child. Nutritional-medical intervention is essential. Similar problems may also occur later, between 2 and 4 years of age, when parents and children have conflicts concerning food patterns, food jags, erratic appetite, reduced milk intake, and disinterest in eating many foods such as vegetables. In such cases normal transient behavior in toddlers and preschoolers may turn into severe parent-child conflicts.

Often failure to thrive results from a complex of factors; there are no easy solutions. Careful history taking, supportive nutritional guidance, and much warm care are required to influence growth patterns. Rehabilitation of these infants and children requires not only full nutritional support but also careful and sensitive correction of social and environmental issues surrounding the problem.

Gastrointestinal Problems

General Functional Disturbances

Infantile Colic

Intermittent periods of long, continuous crying by an infant are generally attributed to colic.[3,4] This is not uncommon and affects about 20% of infants during the first 3 to 4 months of life. It is a self-limiting difficulty, ending spontaneously without any effect on normal growth and development. To young, tense parents, however, this brief interval may seem an eternity. Treatment usually involves careful history taking to discover attitudes and feeding practices. The infant may be underfed and simply screaming from hunger or may be overfed and have abdominal discomfort. At times the newborn's immature nervous system may be responding to sensory input load and overstimulation from musical toys, voices, lights, faces, television noise, and excessive holding or handling.[3] Usually treatment involves explanation and moral support to the parents, with continued reassurance that their child is growing normally.

Functional Infantile Vomiting

Regurgitation, or "spitting up," is common in most infants. Its cause is usually gastric distention from overfeeding or from air swallowed during feeding or crying. Related factors may be ineffective burping and leaving the baby in a supine rather than a prone or side position after feeding. Also, overactivity and semiacrobatics soon after feeding from doting fathers, grandparents, and other relatives may stimulate regurgitation. Temperature may be a factor, since feedings that are too hot may induce vomiting. Milk at room temperature or even cold feedings usually cause no difficulty. Simple attention to possible causative factors and reassurance to young parents provide support.

Infantile Constipation

Occasional, simple physiologic constipation is little cause for concern. It is aided by moderately reducing the milk intake, increasing the carbohydrate intake, increasing fruits and vegetables, and increasing the water intake. Dietary manipulation is often not a fundamental cure but simply a helpful adjunct.

Infantile Diarrhea

Fluid and Electrolyte Losses

Diarrhea in infants is a much more serious problem, especially if it is prolonged and associated with infection. Because of the infant's relatively high water content and large area of intestinal mucosa in proportion to body surface area, fluid and electrolyte reserves may be rapidly depleted.

Oral versus Intravenous Therapy

In acute diarrhea, pediatricians trained in the Western nations have usually relied on intravenous feeding of fluid and electrolytes, withholding oral feedings of solid foods, and have achieved successful results. However, numerous studies and experiences of pediatricians in the United States, as well as in underdeveloped countries, have shown that oral rehydration therapy for infantile diarrhea with earlier solid feedings achieves equally successful results with no intravenous therapy in infants and young children. The World Health Organization (WHO) and the Nutrition Committee of the American Academy of Pediatrics (AAP) have advocated and approved essential, simple oral rehydration solutions.[5-7] The AAP recommends a solution comprised of the following ingredients[8]:

- 75 to 90 mmol/L sodium
- 20 mmol/L potassium
- 20% to 30% of anions as base (acetate, citrate, lactate, or bicarbonate)
- Remainder as chloride, with 2% to 2.5% glucose

The WHO and the United Nations International Children's Emergency Fund (UNICEF) formula, used throughout the world in hundreds of clinical trials over the past 20 years, is dispensed for financial and shelf-life reasons as a dry packet of salts and glucose to be mixed with a liter of clean or boiled water. This solution contains the following ingredients[9]:

- 90 mmol/L sodium
- 20 mmol/L potassium
- 80 mmol/L chloride
- 30 mmol/L base bicarbonate
- 111 mmol/L glucose

With these oral rehydration solutions, immediate early refeeding within 24 hours is recommended by the WHO and AAP, using breast-feeding or diluted formula in younger infants and in older infants added foods such as rice cereal, bananas, potatoes, and other nonlactose carbohydrates.[10,11]

The glucose in these oral rehydration solutions, either as glucose or glucose polymers (two to nine glucose units) from rice-based solutions, is added because glucose acts as an active cotransport agent for absorbing the electrolytes, especially sodium, as well as providing kcalories.[12] These glucose-electrolyte oral solutions may completely replace intravenous fluids, which are more costly, in the majority of well-nourished children. They have shown that oral rehydration is a successful means of treating acute diarrheal illnesses in medical centers of the Western world and in underdeveloped areas when the affected children receive not only oral rehydration therapy but also critical kcalories from appropriate semisolid or solid foods within a few hours.

Cleft Lip and Palate

Infant feeding problems may also result from upper gastrointestinal tract anatomic abnormalities such as cleft lip and palate. Normal sucking and swallowing, as well as respiration, are hindered.

Incidence and Cause

Cleft lip and palate occur in about one in every 700 to 800 live births.[13] Although the precise cause is unclear, it is thought to have genetic and environmental roots, because it recurs in families and it increases among mothers continuing to use alcohol, tobacco, or heroin during their pregnancies.

Prenatal Development

Early in the course of a normal pregnancy, at about 4 to 6 weeks of embryonic development, the upper lip forms from two side flaps and a central flap that grow together and fuse. If this normal fusion does not occur, the infant is born with an unclosed, open lip—a *cleft lip.* It may be only a small incomplete notch on the upper lip, or it may be a complete cleft extending up into the nostril. In addition, the infant may have a *cleft palate.* The normal palate forms the roof of the mouth. It consists of two parts: (1) the *hard palate,* a bony shelf immediately behind the upper front teeth, and (2) the *soft palate,* soft tissue continuing on toward the back of the mouth, dividing the oral pharynx from the nasal cavity. As early embryonic development continues, at about 7 to 8 weeks of gestation, this palate structure has grown in from the sides and joins in the middle. If this normal fusion does not occur, an opening remains between the mouth and the nose. This remaining cleft may be only in the rear soft palate or it may extend forward into the hard palate, where it may be partial or total and of varying width. The incompletely fused lip or palate may occur separately or together, but bilateral cleft palate is usually accompanied by a cleft lip.[14] The open abnormal mouth structure contributes to breathing problems and frequent respiratory infections that spread into the *eustachian tube,* which connects the middle ear with the back of the nose and throat. Constant ear infections affect hearing and lead to speech development problems.

Surgical Repair

Corrective reconstruction of the abnormal oral structures in two stages is now started at an earlier age to avoid advancing feeding and speech problems. First, the cleft lip is repaired when the infant achieves a weight gain of 4.5 kg (10 lb) or at 10 weeks of age. Then the cleft palate is repaired later, usually at 12 to 14 months of age, before speech patterns develop. Nutritional care of the infant relates to the surgery schedule.

Nutritional Care

Nutritional care is based on the extent of the infant's oral physical abnormalities and resulting feeding problems, normal growth needs, resistance to infection, and weight gain to prepare for surgery. Normal sucking is difficult or impossible, especially with a separation of both the hard and soft palates, because the infant cannot create the necessary airtight seal in the mouth. Because of this lack of suction, special equipment for bottle feeding is necessary: (1) the *Breck feeder,* a bulb-type syringe with plastic tube, or (2) the *Beniflex feeder,* a soft bag with a cross-cut nipple. In place of sucking, the infant learns to chew or squeeze the nipple to obtain milk. If the mother wishes, breast milk may be expressed and fed in a bottle instead of a standard formula. If it is necessary to increase nutritive value and needed weight gain in preparation for surgery, a more concentrated formula yielding 24 kcal/oz may be used rather than the standard formula that provides 20 kcal/oz. Feeding is slow and often tiring, so the frequency of feeding may need to be increased to about every 2 hours. To aid the feeding process, hold the infant in a more upright position with frequent burping, and direct the flow toward the cheek. Then later, as the infant learns a suck-swallow-breathe rhythm, the nipple may be changed to a firmer one with regular, smaller openings to help develop facial muscles for chewing and speech. When the child is weaned from the feeder to using a cup and spoon at about 4 to 6 months, solid foods are added, beginning with soft, nonacidic foods and gradually increasing texture with age. Foods that are hard to chew or may form a sticky plug are avoided. Some foods reported to cause difficulty by getting caught in the cleft and slipping into the trachea include leafy vegetables, peelings of raw fruit, grapes, weiners, biscuits, creamed foods, and peanut butter as well as nuts, jelly beans, hard candies, popcorn, and chewing gum.[15]

The second surgery, for repairing the cleft palate, comes when the child is about 1 year old, before speech patterns are set. Postoperatively, the child is fed only by cup, with no spoon or straw to injure the repair site, gradually advancing from clear liquids the first week to full liquids for the next 2 or 3 weeks. Then soft, pureed or mashed foods are used, finally resuming a regular diet for age but avoiding hard foods such as crackers or toast. For some time, until full healing has occurred and the repair site tissue has strengthened, no objects such as silverware, straws, nipples, pacifiers, or toothbrushes are allowed in the mouth. In some cases of extensive surgical reconstruction, the surgeon may elect to use gastrostomy tube-feedings for a period of time to protect the oral tissues from harm and to ensure adequate enteral nutrition support for healing.[16]

Malabsorption Problems

Celiac Sprue

In 1889 a London physician named Gee observed a number of malnourished children having diarrhea and distended abdomens. He gave the name "celiac" to the general clinical condition from the Greek word *kolia,* meaning "belly" or "abdomen." For several decades afterward the cause remained unknown, although the clinical symptoms, all of which indicated some form of intestinal malabsorption, were clearly described: (1) general malnutrition; (2) multiple, foul, foamy, greasy stools; (3) distended abdomen caused by an accumulation of improperly digested food material and inadequate absorption, as well as abnormal gas accumulations; and (4) secondary vitamin deficiencies.

Metabolic Defect

In the early 1950s, the Dutch pediatrician Dicke observed that children with this disease had an increase in their symptoms from eating certain cereal grains, including wheat and rye. Shortly afterward, he and his associates demonstrated that the *gliadin* fraction of the protein *gluten* in wheat produced fat malabsorption in patients with celiac sprue. In the mid-1950s a definitive diagnostic technique of peroral biopsy was developed. Using a flexible tube with a suction-guillotine tip, small tissue samples of the intestinal mucosa could be obtained for microscopic study. These tissue studies confirmed that what had been termed celiac disease in children and nontropical sprue in adults was a single disease, thus called now *celiac sprue.*[17] As currently used, the alternate terms *celiac disease* and *gluten-sensitive enteropathy* are synonymous with celiac sprue. Electron micrographs of such diseased tissues have consistently shown an eroded mucosal surface lacking the number or form of villi normally seen and having only sparse microvilli. This erosion effectively reduces the absorbing surface area by as much as 95%.

Although studies thus far clearly show that gluten somehow interacts with and damages the intestinal mucosa, the primary host defect that causes celiac sprue remains obscure.[17] Several mechanisms are under study, including an enzyme deficiency and a genetic base. Whatever the underlying mechanism, celiac sprue is associated with a metabolic defect in the intestinal mucosal cells brought out by the gliadin fraction of wheat or rye gluten, and in the process of the disease, the villi of the intestinal mucosa atrophy, greatly reducing the absorptive and secretory surface. Tissue changes occur in the mucosal cells bringing on pathologic lesions. About 47% of the weight of the wheat gliadin has been identified as the amino acid *glutamine.* Studies of this amino acid implicate it in the biochemical defect. It is now apparent that the steatorrhea is a secondary manifestation caused by the primary biochemical reaction to gliadin in sensitive patients.

Clinical Symptoms

In children who develop gluten-sensitive celiac disease, the onset usually occurs between the ages of 6 and 18 months, with symptoms appearing later in those who are breast-fed. It usually begins with a chronic course but may suddenly be worsened by a celiac crisis, usually triggered by an infection. This is a severe episode of dehydration and acidosis in which there are large, watery stools and copious vomiting. It is an acute medical emergency. The chronic diarrhea continues with passage of characteristic foul, foamy, bulky, greasy stools. About 80% of the ingested fat appears in the stools, usually in the form of soaps and fatty acids. There is progressive malnutrition with signs of deficiency states secondary to the malabsorption—anemia, rickets, and an increasing bleeding tendency. The abdomen is grossly distended. There is loss of subcutaneous fat tissue, leaving the buttocks flattened and wrinkled with folds of skin. The child takes on the emaciated, apathetic, and fretful appearance of malnutrition.

Dietary management. Nutritional therapy for celiac sprue is better defined as *low-gluten* rather than gluten-free, since it is impossible to remove all the gluten completely, and usually a small amount of gluten is tolerated by most patients. Wheat and rye are the main sources of gluten; it is also present in oats and barley. Therefore these four grains (wheat, rye, oats, and barley) are eliminated from the diet. Corn and rice are the substitute grains used. The offending grains are obvious in their cereal form, but they are

TABLE 5–1

Low-Gluten Diet for Children with Celiac Disease

Dietary principles

- Kcalories—high, usually about 20% above normal requirement, to compensate for fecal loss
- Protein—high, usually 6 to 8 g/kg body weight
- Fat—low, but not fat-free, because of impaired absorption
- Carbodydrates—simple, easily digested sugars (fruits, vegetables) should provide about one half of the kcalories
- Feedings—small, frequent feedings during ill periods; afternoon snack for older children
- Texture—smooth, soft, avoiding irritating roughage initially, using strained foods longer than usual for age, adding whole foods as tolerated and according to age of child
- Vitamins—supplements of B vitamins, vitamins A and B in water-miscible forms, and vitamin C
- Minerals—iron supplements if anemia is present

Food groups	Foods included	Foods excluded
Milk	Milk (plain or flavored with chocolate or cocoa) Buttermilk	Malted milk; preparations such as Cocomalt, Hemo, Postum, Nestle's chocolate
Meat or substitute	Lean meat, trimmed well of fat Eggs, cheese Poultry, fish Creamy peanut butter (if tolerated)	Fat meats (sausage, pork) Luncheon meats, corned beef, frankfurters, all common prepared meat products with any possible wheat filler Duck, goose Smoked salmon Meat prepared with bread, crackers, or flour
Fruits and juices	All cooked and canned fruits and juices Frozen or fresh fruits as tolerated, avoiding skins and seeds	Prunes, plums (unless tolerated)
Vegetables	All cooked, frozen, canned as tolerated (prepared *without* wheat, rye, oat, or barley products); raw as tolerated	Any causing individual discomfort All prepared with wheat, rye, oat, or barley products
Cereals	Corn or rice	Wheat, rye, oat, barley; any product containing these cereals
Breads, flours, cereal products	Breads, pancakes, or waffles made with suggested flours (cornmeal, cornstarch; rice, soybean, lima bean, potato, buckwheat)	All bread or cracker products made with gluten; wheat, rye, oat, barley, macaroni, noodles, spaghetti; any sauces, soups, or gravies prepared with gluten flour, wheat, rye, oat, or barley
Soups	Broth, bouillon (no fat or cream; no thickening with wheat, rye, oat, or barley products); soups and sauces may be thickened with cornstarch	All soups containing wheat, rye, oat, or barley products

also used as ingredients (thickeners or fillers) in many commercial products. The child's parents need specific instructions about products to avoid in each main food group, what constitutes a basic meal pattern, and recipes for food preparation. Commercial products using gluten and careful label-reading habits should be discussed, since parents' knowledge of gluten-containing food products is highly variable and influences the child's attitudes toward dietary compliance.[18] With an increasing number of processed foods being marketed, as well as increasing use of ethnic foods in Western society, it is difficult to detect all foods containing gluten, so a home test kit for gluten has been developed.[19] Good dietary management varies according to the child's age, the clinical status, and pathologic conditions. Generally, a dietary program based on the low-gluten diet guide given in Table 5-1 may be followed.

In a small subgroup of patients with celiac sprue, the symptoms persist despite strict adherence to a gluten-free diet. In rare instances, persons with such a "refractory" form of the disease respond only to parenteral nutrition support.[17]

Cystic Fibrosis

Cystic fibrosis is inherited as an autosomal recessive trait mainly in Caucasian populations in which 1 in 20 is a carrier and now 1 in 2500 newborns is affected.[20] It is the most common fatal genetic disease in North America. Although cystic fibrosis is mainly a Caucasian disease, it does occur rarely in other population groups: 1 in 17,000 black live births and 1 in 90,000 Oriental live births.[15] In past years, children carrying the disease have generally lived to about age 10, dying from complications such as pulmonary disease with progressive damage to airway epithelial cells and pancreatic insufficiency from fibrosis. Improved management of the disease based on increasing scientific knowledge has helped push the life expectancy up into the 30s.

Currently, a screening test for newborns helps detect the disease early.[21,22] This blood test is an assay procedure for *immunoreactive trypsinogen (IRT).* The diagnosis is confirmed by two positive sweat tests done on different days that measure the concentration of the electrolyte chloride in the body perspiration according to methods approved by the Cystic Fibrosis Foundation.[23] In this test, the drug *pilocarpine,* which has cholinergic activity, is given to stimulate perspiration. Perspiration is collected during a 30-minute period on preweighed gauze or filter paper and measured for concentration of electrolytes. A positive test result is a chloride measurement above 60 mmol/L in the perspiration. An early diagnosis allows earlier intervention and support by a skilled cystic fibrosis team of health care professionals who can accurately assess physical and emotional status, help families cope with the impact of the diagnosis, and develop an appropriate therapeutic plan.[22,23] Early aggressive nutritional therapy and monitoring, as well as better basic care routines, help control malabsorption and infection and prevent malnutrition.[22]

Metabolic Defect

In the summer of 1989, the gene responsible for cystic fibrosis was discovered on the long arm of chromosome 7, following a highly competitive race among research groups in Canada, the United States, and England.[24] Now continuing studies have disclosed the underlying biochemical defect. It lies in the mutant gene's inability to code for, and thus transcribe correctly, the amino acid sequence of the normal gene's protein product. Scientists have named this product for its function, *cystic fibrosis transmembrane conductance regulator (CFTR).*[25] This large protein product, composed of 1480 amino acids in 5 domains, controls the opening and closing of ion channels that actively transport chloride ions across epithelial cell membranes. Because of this defective epithelial ion transport, chloride is trapped in the cells and excess sodium is also absorbed. This imbalance leads to the thickened mucus formation and effects in the various organ systems involved.

The next two logical research steps to control cystic fibrosis are (1) to identify carriers of the gene and (2), once the disease is detected in newborns, to prevent its development by gene therapy. The first step, widespread screening for carriers, has been delayed by scientists' discovery of a number of different mutations of the cystic fibrosis gene, thus allowing their present test to detect only about 75% to 85% of the carriers.[20] They are striving for a higher percentage of coverage, but the demand for testing is growing and the perfect test may never be a reality. Thus pilot testing programs are already underway in various genetic centers, such as the large testing program currently being conducted by the Kaiser-Permanente health maintenance organization in California.[26] The second step, gene therapy, is an even more difficult problem because it involves the task of inserting the normal gene into defective cells.[27,28] This has already been done in the laboratory, but achieving this transfer in a living human body is far more difficult. Nonetheless, the scientific foundation has been laid. The gene responsible for cystic fibrosis has been identified, cloned for laboratory cell study, and its structure identified. Continuing research is intense and answers for clinical practice will follow.

Clinical Symptoms

The classic clinical symptoms of cystic fibrosis include the following[15,23,29]:

1. *Thick mucus in the lungs* that accumulates and clogs air passages, damages the epithelial tissue of these airways, and leads to *chronic obstructive pulmonary disease (COPD)* and frequent *respiratory infections,* both contributing to increased metabolism and in turn increased energy-nutrient needs.
2. *Pancreatic insufficiency* caused by progressive clogging of pancreatic ducts and functional tissue degeneration, resulting in *lack of normal pancreatic enzymes:* protein-splitting trypsin, chymotrypsin, carboxypeptidase, fat-splitting lipase, and starch-splitting amylase; progressive loss of functional insulin-producing beta cells in the islets of Langerhans, resulting in *insulin-dependent diabetes mellitus (IDDM).*
3. *Malabsorption* of undigested food nutrients and extensive *diarrheal nutrient loss* leading to *malnutrition* and stunted growth.
4. *Biliary cirrhosis* caused by progressive clogging of bile ducts producing biliary obstruction and functional liver tissue degeneration.
5. *Salt (NaCl) concentration* increased in the body perspiration, resulting in salt depletion.

Dietary Management

Current nutritional management of cystic fibrosis follows new guidelines developed by a consensus committee of the U.S. Cystic Fibrosis Foundation (CFF).[30] Increased knowledge of the disease process, early diagnosis and intervention, and improved therapeutic products such as pancreatic enzymes have led to a more aggressive nutritional management program in all of its cystic fibrosis centers throughout the country. The overall goal is to support normal nutrition and growth for patients of all ages. This management program is based on an initial and ongoing schedule for assessment of nutritional status, including anthropometry, laboratory studies, and nutritional evaluation (Table 5-2). Related therapy is then outlined in five levels according to individual assessment results and nutritional care needs and actions (Table 5-3).

TABLE 5–2

Basic Nutritional Assessment for Nutritional Management of Cystic Fibrosis

Key assessments	Monitoring schedule and indications
Anthropometry	
Weight	Every 3 months or as needed for growth evaluation and routine care
Height (length)	
Head circumference (until age 2)	
Midarm circumference	
Triceps skinfold	
Midarm muscle circumference (derived)*	
Biochemical data	
CBC† TIBC,† serum iron, ferritin Plasma/serum retinol, alpha-tocopherol	Yearly routine care, interim as needed to detect deficiencies, iron status
Albumin, prealbumin	As indicated, weight loss, growth failure, clinical deterioration
Electrolytes, acid-base balance	Summer heat, prolonged fever
Dietary evaluation	
Dietary intake	As indicated, history and food records, full energy-nutrient analysis
3-day fat balance study‡	As indicated, weight loss, growth failure, clinical deterioration
Anticipatory guidance	Yearly, interim as needed according to growth or situational needs

Adapted from CFF consensus report; Ramsey B et al: Nutrition assessment and management in cystic fibrosis: a consensus report, *Am J Clin Nutr* 55:108, 1992.
*See Chapter 19 for equations.
† *CBC,* Complete blood count; *TIBC,* total iron-binding capacity.
‡Three day food records for analysis of fat intake; stool collections for analysis of fat content and degree of malabsorption.

TABLE 5–3

Levels of Nutritional Care for Management of Cystic Fibrosis

Levels of care	Patient groups	Nutrition actions
Level I—Routine care	All	Diet counseling, food plans, enzyme replacement, vitamin supplements, nutrition education, exploration of problems
Level II—Anticipatory guidance	Above 90% ideal weight-height index, but at risk of energy imbalance; severe pancreatic insufficiency, frequent pulmonary infections, normal periods of rapid growth	Increased monitoring of dietary intake, complete energy-nutrient analysis, increased kcaloric density as needed; assess behavioral needs; provide counseling, nutrition education
Level III—Supportive intervention	85%-90% ideal weight-height index, decreased weight-growth velocity	Reinforce all the above actions, add energy-nutrient dense oral supplements
Level IV—Rehabilitative care	Consistently below 85% ideal weight-height index, nutritional and growth failure	All of the above plus enteral nutrition support by nasoenteric or enterostomy tube feeding (see Chapter 3)
Level V—Resuscitative or palliative care	Below 75% ideal weight-height index, progressive nutritional failure	All of the above plus continuous enteral tube feedings or TPN (see Chapter 4)

Adapted from CFF consensus report: Ramsey B et al: Nutrition assessment and management in cystic fibrosis: a consensus report, *Am J Clin Nutr* 55:108, 1992.

Level I—*Routine management* for all cystic fibrosis patients:

- *Food plan.* Provide a normal diet pattern with increased energy-nutrient values, varying to about 120% to 150% of the RDA depending on the energy-nutrient loss from malabsorption. Current dietary recommendations, to maintain an ideal weight-height index and normal growth while enzyme therapy controls malabsorption, are for high-protein and normal to high-fat dietary content, with the total increased kcalories divided approximately 20% as protein, 40% as carbohydrates, and 40% as fat.[31] Until recently, the "traditional" cystic fibrosis diet was low in fat because of its poor digestion and the older less effective nonenteric coated enzymes available. Now a nonrestricted fat diet with adequate enzyme replacement therapy is much more effective in meeting nutritional goals.[32] Infants may be breast-fed or given a hydrolyzed formula such as Pregestimil (Mead-Johnson).[22,33,34] If assistance is needed, infants with cystic fibrosis can be referred to Women, Infants, and Children (WIC) programs in each state for provision of the predigested formula.
- *Pancreatic enzyme replacement.* New capsule-encased enteric coated microspheres—"beads"—of pancreatic enzymes correct maldigestion in cystic fibrosis patients and help support energy-nutrient growth needs. These **pancreatic enzyme preparations** replace normal enzymes lost from pancreatic insufficiency, which occurs in 90% of cystic fibrosis patients. Current products such as Pancrease (McNeil Pharmaceutical) are in large enough doses to normalize fat excretion. Children under 10 years of age benefit from taking the enteric coated enzymes before meals, but timing before or during meals is not as significant for older children. The pH-sensitive enteric coating protects the enzyme microspheres from acid breakdown in the stomach (pH 2). The coating dissolves only at an alkaline pH of 6 or greater, which is the normal pH of the upper small intestine.[31] Pancrease and the similar products Cotazyme and Viokase are substances made from hog pancreas, which contains the pancreatic enzymes amylase, peptidases, and lipase and differs mainly in the relative amount of lipase present.
- *Vitamin supplementation.* Supplements of fat-soluble vitamins A and E particularly, with vitamins D and K as needed, are given. Fat-soluble vitamins are best absorbed when taken in the morning with fat-containing meals and pancreatic enzymes. B-complex supplements also replace losses.
- *Nutrition counseling and education.* Individual counseling and education for parents of infants and young children and increased teaching of self-management skills and personal counseling for older children and adolescents are required.[35,36] Many new materials are being developed, including programmed instruction in a series of small steps designed for preadolescent children.[37]

The remaining four levels of nutritional care relate to increasing risk of malnutrition and progressive nutritional failure (Table 5-3):

- Level II—*Anticipatory guidance:* Proactive education anticipates increased needs, such as the rapid growth periods of infancy and adolescence, closer monitoring of intake, ways of increasing kcaloric density, and exploring problems.
- Level III—*Supportive intervention:* This includes the addition of homemade or commercial oral supplements, with focus on increasing frequency and density of meals, achieving optimal enzyme therapy, and identifying stress factors.
- Level IV—*Rehabilitative care:* This includes the addition of enteral nutrition support by feeding through nasoenteric or enterostomy tubes (see Chapter 3).[38]
- Level V—*Resuscitative or palliative care:* This includes the addition of parenteral nutrition support (see Chapter 4).[39]

Directions with equations for calculating energy needs for cystic fibrosis patients, basal metabolic rate (BMR) and daily energy requirements (DER), accounting for physical activity and disease status, are included in Appendix V.

A primary concern in gastrointestinal problems of children is preventing malnutrition and supporting growth. A summary of some of these conditions with a variety of feeding modes for nutritional support is given in Table 5-4.

Genetic Diseases

Genetic Inheritance Concept

The concept of "inborn errors of metabolism" was first introduced by Sir Archibald Garrod in 1908. Although he probably had no clear conception of enzyme action, he pointed the way to a large number of conditions known today as genetic diseases that result from an inherited mutant gene. The science of genetics has advanced rapidly in recent years, with many

pancreatic enzyme preparations • Commercial preparations of pancreatic enzymes—protease, lipase, and amylase—that have the same action as do the human enzymes from the pancreas; used in the treatment of pancreatic insufficiency.

TABLE 5–4

Guidelines for Preventing Malnutrition in Hospitalized Infants and Children with Primary and Secondary Gastrointestinal Problems

Problem	Barriers to care	Nutritional therapy	Additional information
Prematurity— Less than 32 weeks' gestation	Immature gut and kidney Poor suck-swallow coordination Tendency to develop necrotizing enterocolitis with tube feedings Tendency to develop respiratory distress and heart problems	Delay oral feeding for 2 weeks Intermittent gavage feeding with nasogastric tube Continuous intragastric feedings via indwelling catheter Continuous intragastric feedings via gastrostomy tube Continuous transpyloric (nasojejunal) feedings TPN, peripheral or central vein; usually given in addition to nipple or gavage feedings of breast milk or formula	Does not prevent reflux; requires small feedings Slow rate minimizes distention and osmolar intolerance Used for infants with congenital gastrointestinal anomalies; *not recommended* for routine use with premature infants Minimizes reflux *Complications:* intestinal perforation, necrotizing enterocolitis, and decreased nutrient assimilation Limit glucose in central vein infusions to prevent hyperglycemia *Complication:* cholestatic liver disease
Short-bowel syndrome Follows intestinal resection, usually to treat necrotizing colitis, jejunoileal atresia, and Crohn's disease	Length of remaining bowel Gastric hypersecretion Malabsorption of bile acid Abnormal intestinal motility Massive diarrhea; nutrient and fluid loss	*Stage 1* (immediately to 3 weeks after surgery) Parenteral supply of fluids and electrolytes *Stage 2* (1-3 weeks after surgery) Slow reintroduction of oral feedings Some patients require months of intragastric feedings before advancing to stage 3 *Stage 3* (3 or more weeks after surgery) Oral feedings Replace long-chain with medium-chain triglycerides to reduce stool losses of stages 1 and 2	Continue until diarrhea stops, and hydration and electrolyte levels are adequate Continue parental nutrition support until oral intake is adequate Parenteral nutrition is not required for fluid and electrolyte balance High-fat therapy is associated with greater loss of calcium and magnesium
Intractable diarrhea of infancy Diarrhea lasting longer than 2 weeks; occurs mainly in infants less than 3 months old; 45% mortality	Decreased nutrient absorption Progressive protein-energy malnutrition Milk (cow or soy) intolerance Colitis	Intravenous fluids, 24-48 hours Peripheral parenteral nutrition Continuous nasogastric drip, beginning with 0.33 kcal/ml elemental or semielemental formula Remove nasogastric tube; begin oral feedings	Until rehydrated Until stool volume is less than 10-20 ml/kg body weight/day Stool volume closely monitored; formula concentration adjusted to account for volume changes Continue until weight gain is steady and feedings are tolerated every hour Discharge after infant shows steady weight gain

Continued.

TABLE 5-4

Guidelines for Preventing Malnutrition in Hospitalized Infants and Children with Primary and Secondary Gastrointestinal Problems—cont'd

Problem	Barriers to care	Nutritional therapy	Additional information
Inflammatory bowel disease Crohn's disease Ulcerative colitis	*General* Anorexia Abdominal pain Malabsorption (fat-soluble vitamins, fats) Diarrhea (fluids, electrolytes) Blood loss (anemia) Toxic effects on bone marrow (low folate levels)	*General* Nasogastric infusions of elemental diets *Ulcerative colitis* Mild Lactose-free diet, if indicated Adequate kcalories, protein, vitamins, and minerals	
	Crohn's disease Growth failure Delayed puberty	TPN and gut rest	Requires longer therapy than for colitis Children and adolescents may receive infusions for 10-12 hours/day at home for 1-6 months
Cancer Effects caused by disease or treatment	Increased BMR (especially with solid tumors, lymphomas, leukemia) Altered taste perception Anorexia Increased protein turnover, muscle wasting Enlarged liver Nausea, vomiting Stomatitis Diarrhea Anergy	Must be *individualized* May include central vein parenteral nutrition—most reliable method for nourishing cancer patients with malnutrition	Parenteral nutrition facilitates nutrient retention by tumor as well as host tissue Recommended for periods of antitumor therapy or in preparation for therapy or surgery
		For advanced malignancy Reduce glucose infusion rate Provide base in solution	Vigorous nutritional therapy may lengthen survival time
		During abdominal radiation therapy Include hydrolyzed protein Provide low-residue, low-fat, gluten- or casein-free diet	Protects against enteritis Protects against diarrhea and malnutrition

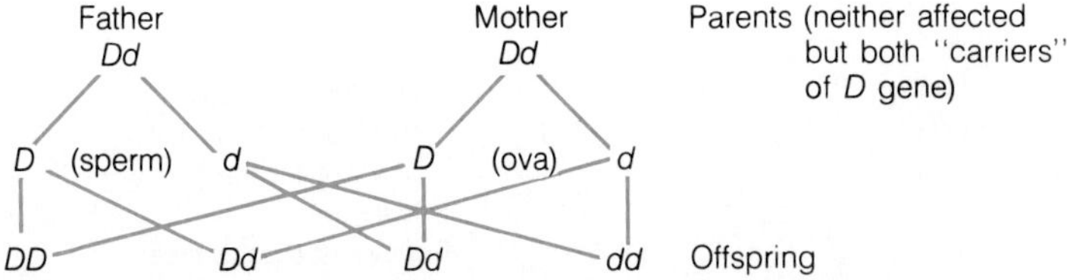

FIG. 5-3 Diagram of genetic disease inheritance showing transmission of involved genes and formation of controlling gene pairs (alleles). *D,* Gene for disease state (metabolic defect); *d,* gene for the normal state (absence of metabolic defect); *DD,* homozygote (has overt disease); *dd,* homozygote (normal, does not have the disease or carry the trait); *Dd,* heterozygote (outwardly normal, does not have the disease but does carry the trait). Autosomal dominant inheritance: by *DD* or *Dd;* autosomal recessive inheritance: by *dd.*

applications to clinical medicine. This section focuses only briefly on metabolic disease and its genetic transmission.

An understanding of a simple diagram (Fig. 5-3) and several key terms may help clarify the basic concept of genetic disease.

1. *Chromosomes* are complex rod-shaped bodies composed of thousands of genes. They are formed in the cell nucleus. Each human cell contains 46 chromosomes arranged in 23 pairs. One pair forms the sex chromosomes, which carry the sex trait and other genetic information. The remaining 22 pairs of chromosomes control the various other characteristics of the cell and of the individual.
2. *Autosomes* are any of the chromosomes other than the pair responsible for sex characteristics. Pairs of autosomes are *homologous,* that is, each member of a pair has the same configuration and genetic material as the other member of the pair. Conversely, pairs of sex chromosomes (XX in female; XY in male) are *heterologous,* that is, the X and Y chromosomes differ in size and function. The X chromosome is about five times as large and carries more extensive genetic information than does the Y chromosome.
3. *Genes* (from Greek verb *gennan,* to produce) are self-producing particles in the cells, and genes are located at definite individual points (loci) on chromosomes. They are the basic units of heredity. Each gene is a long, double-stranded molecule (helix) of *deoxyribonucleic acid (DNA),* with a special arrangement of its components, its so-called genetic code (see Chapter 13). This DNA molecule is the chemical basis of heredity.
4. *Alleles* (from the Greek *allelon,* of one another) are genes that occupy homologous loci, or partner genes. Therefore each individual has two of each kind of gene from each chromosome of a pair.
5. *Mutant gene* (from the Latin verb *mutare,* to change) is an altered form of a gene. Usually genes remain stable over generations, but they can change or mutate and thereby transmit a new or altered trait to future generations. Genes may mutate spontaneously or by environmental agents such as radiation, drugs, or viral infection.
6. *Inheritance* is either *autosomal* or *X-linked (sex-linked),* depending on the location of the gene on the chromosome. It is also either *dominant* or *recessive,* depending on the nature of the gene pairs required for the trait or disease to be manifest. The gene is dominant when the related disease or condition is present, if *D* is one gene of a pair of genes *(Dd)* or is both genes *(DD).* The gene is recessive when the disease is present, only if *d* is both genes *(dd)* (Fig. 5-3).
7. *Autosomal recessive inheritance,* such as in phenylketonuria, involves a gene trait that does not manifest itself unless both alleles are identical. The recessive gene must be carried by both parents to cause a defect.

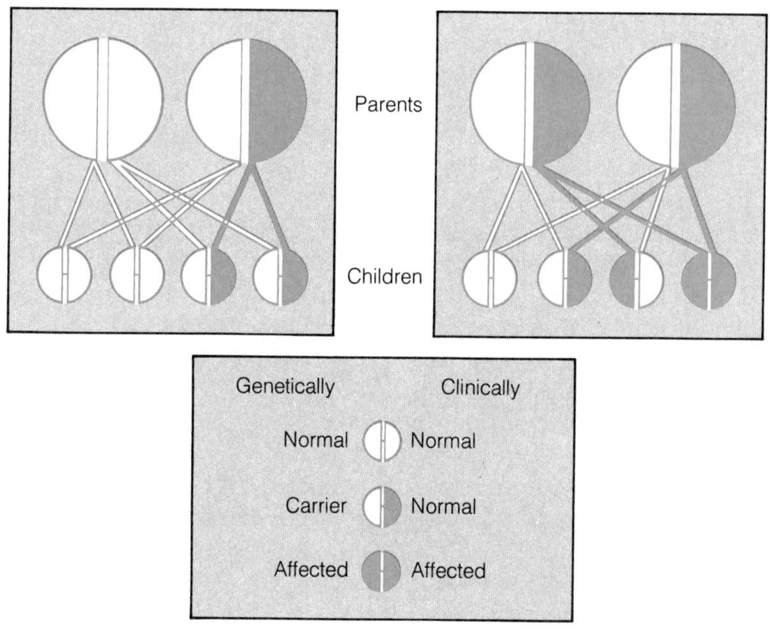

FIG. 5-4 Pattern of genetic disease. Transmission of recessive traits follows Mendel's law. If two carriers marry, the chances are that one child will be normal, one child will manifest the trait, and two children will be carriers.

8. *Heterozygote* is an individual in whom the members of one or more gene pairs are unlike. Such a person is sometimes called a "carrier" of that trait *(Dd)* but does not manifest its symptoms *(dd)*. Transmission of recessive traits to successive generations follows the pattern established by **Gregor Johann Mendel** (Fig. 5-4). If two carriers have children, the risk for each birth is 25% to manifest the trait, 50% to be a carrier, and 25% to be normal. However, geneticists have recently learned that this exact Mendelian pattern does not always happen when some traits do not obey these rules. A phenomenon called parental *imprinting* of genes occurs in which a bit of DNA marks the gene according to which parent it came from, so that a child may receive both genes for a given trait from the mother and none from the father.[40,41] This has been the case, for example, in at least five known babies who "could not" inherit cystic fibrosis because the father was not a carrier but who were born with it.[41]

Genetic Control

Control of Heredity

As indicated, when the human ovum (female sex cell) is fertilized by the sperm (male sex cell), the fertilized ovum from which the new individual develops contains 46 chromosomes, 23 contributed by the sperm cell from the father and 23 contributed by the ovum from the mother. These 46 chromosomes align themselves in 23 pairs in the fertilized ovum. With each successive cell division (mitosis), these same pairs of chromosomes are duplicated in the nucleus and become a part of the new cell. The gene pattern of the original chromosomes received at conception from the parents remains to determine the offspring's inherited physical traits or genetic disease pattern.

Control of Cell Function

The genes control not only common hereditary characteristics but also the metabolic functions of the cell. They regulate the synthesis of some 1000 or more specific cell enzymes. Each one of these enzymes is a specific protein synthesized by a specific DNA pattern in a specific gene. When a specific gene is abnormal (mutant), the enzyme whose synthesis it controls cannot be made. In turn, the metabolic reaction controlled by that enzyme cannot take place. A genetic disease manifests symptoms relative to those reaction products.

Although some 1500 to 2000 single mutant-gene errors are known, in only about 200 of these has the precise biochemical problem been identified.[42] The specific genetic defect affects metabolism of certain amino acids, carbohydrates, or lipids. Now that nutritional therapy—indeed the main therapy—based on use of special formula products as basic medical food has been developed for a number of these genetic diseases, the profound neurologic results of the untreated condition have been prevented. Thus the clinical significance of these genetic-metabolic conditions far exceeds their relatively rare incidence. As primary examples, we look at two such genetic diseases in more detail: (1) *phenylketonuria,* which affects amino acid metabolism, and (2) *galactosemia,* which affects carbohydrate metabolism. Phenylketonuria and galactosemia are detected early by newborn screening, and the controlling diet therapy is begun immediately to ensure normal growth and development. Several other metabolic defects involving amino acids and carbohydrates are also examined.

Phenylketonuria

Metabolic Defect

Phenylketonuria (PKU) was first observed in 1934 by the Norwegian physician Asbjorn Folling. This genetic disease results from a mutant autosomal recessive gene. The normal gene controls the synthesis of the liver enzyme *phenylalanine hydroxylase,* which oxidizes *phenylalanine,* an essential amino acid, to *tyrosine,* another amino acid. Since the controlling gene is defective, the enzyme cannot be produced, and the reaction does not proceed normally (Fig. 5-5). As a result, phenylalanine accumulates in the blood, and its alternate metabolites, the phenyl acids, are excreted in the urine. One of these acids, *phenylpyruvic acid,* is a phenylketone, hence the term *phenylketonuria.* The condition may exist as classic PKU or as one of several *hyperphenylalaninemia variants.* Work over the past decade has shown that phenylalanine hydroxylase is not a single enzyme but a mixture of three isozymes, one or more of which may be active. Ongoing work indicates that phenylalanine hydroxylase may be controlled by more than one gene.

Clinical Symptoms

In the past years, before current newborn screening and treatment practices, the most profound effect observed in *untreated* PKU was mental retardation. The IQ of affected persons was usually below 50 and most frequently less than 20. The central nervous system damage caused increased motor irritability, hyperactivity, convulsive seizures, and bizarre behavior. Also, because tyrosine, the amino acid normally produced from phenylalanine, is used in the production of the pigment material *melanin,* the untreated PKU children usually had blond or light brown hair and blue eyes and fair skin. Tyrosine is also involved in the production of the hormones epinephrine (adrenalin) by the adrenal gland and thyroxin by the thyroid gland.

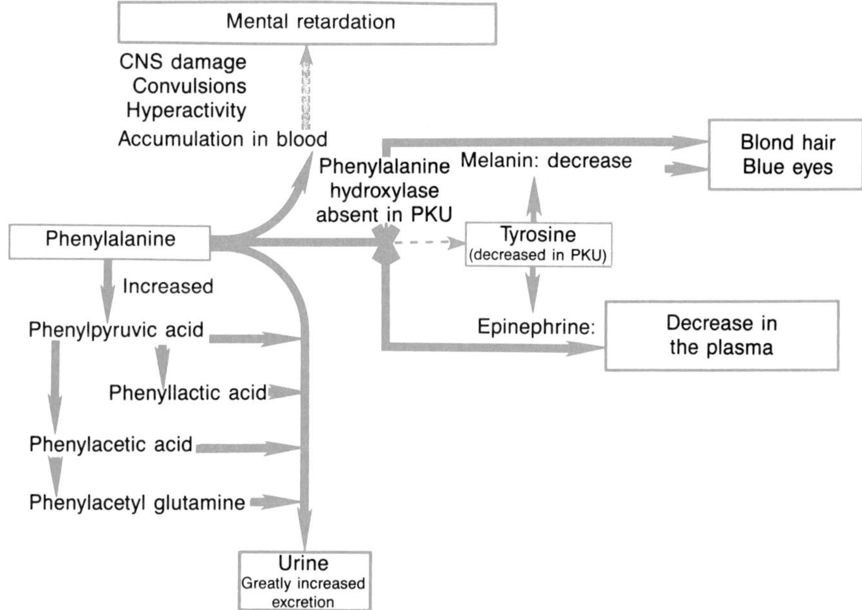

FIG. 5-5 The metabolic error in phenylketonuria. Because of the absence of the enzyme phenylalanine hydroxylase, the essential amino acid phenylalanine cannot be converted to tyrosine.

Dietary Management

Now, however, PKU is controlled well by dietary means. Newborn screening is done on day 3 (day 5 in European countries) with a serum phenylalanine diagnostic cut-off point of 240 μmol/L (4 mg/dl).[43] The special low-phenylalanine diet is begun immediately. It effectively controls the serum phenylalanine levels to maintain them at appropriate amounts to prevent clinical symptoms, especially central nervous system damage. The low-phenylalanine diet consists of a special low-phenylalanine or phenylalanine-free formula product, such as Lofenalac (Mead Johnson); the age-related product series of Analog, Maxamaid, and Maximum (Scientific Hospital Supplies); and a new 1993 Metabolic Formula System (Ross Laboratories). These products are classified as medical foods (see Chapter 2) started in infancy and continued as a basic beverage replacing milk. Low-phenylalanine food lists then serve as the guide for food choices as the child grows older. The individual child's diet begins immediately after newborn diagnosis and is monitored carefully and recalculated regularly based on body weight and serum phenylalanine levels. There is no known age at which the diet can safely be discontinued. Studies indicate that developmental problems, such as poor bone growth and impaired mental capacities, still occur in older children and young adults who have not followed the diet carefully.[44,45]

Thus the current practice is long-term dietary management, and families are counseled accordingly. This need for continued dietary therapy creates a difficult challenge as these children grow into adolescence. It becomes especially critical in young women who face the potential high-risk pregnancy.[46] To study the effects of maternal PKU on pregnancy outcome, the National Institute of Child Health and Human Development of the National Institutes of Health has recently conducted a collaborative study involving all 50 states and the District of Columbia and all the Canadian provinces. This PKU Collaborative Study demonstrates the effectiveness of a phenylalanine-restricted diet in reducing the poor reproductive outcome generally associated with maternal PKU.[46,47]

Since phenylalanine is an essential amino acid necessary for growth, it cannot be totally removed from the diet. Blood levels of phenylalanine are constantly monitored by the clinical nutritionist or the physician on the metabolic team, and the nutritionist calculates

Mendel, Gregor Johann (1822-1884) • Austrian monk and naturalist; discovered natural laws governing direct inheritance by offspring of certain traits or characteristics from one or the other parent. The modern study of genetics derives from his work.

the diet to allow the limited amount of phenylalanine tolerated by the individual child to maintain the acceptable goal for serum phenylalanine levels of approximately 121 to 484 μmol/L (2 to 8 mg/dl). (Normally, only a trace of phenylalanine is in the blood, about 4 to 9.8 μmol/L [0.6 to 1.5 mg/dl].) These monitored blood tests are used as guidelines for ongoing dietary management.

As indicated, dietary management is built on the two basic components of a milk substitute and guidelines for adding solid foods[48]:

1. *Milk-substitute formula.* Milk has a relatively high phenylalanine content, so a special modified formula is necessary. In the United States several special formulas are available. Some are casein hydrolysate products, and others are formulated using elemental crystalline amino acids. Some have a small amount of phenylalanine and others are phenylalanine free. All are balanced with fat, carbohydrates, vitamins, and minerals. The nutritionist arranges with the parents for an appropriate product selection for each child, calculates the individual formula, instructs the parents in its preparation, monitors serum phenylalanine responses, and adjusts the formula as needed for growth and control of serum levels. A small, designated measure of milk or regular infant formula is added to the special formula to adjust the essential phenylalanine content as tolerated. The mother who wishes to breast-feed her baby may do so with careful guidance and support from the clinical nutritionist and the other metabolic program team members. Other special medical beverage products formulated for growing children and free of phenylalanine are used for older children, along with a number of available low-protein food products, to allow a greater variety of foods to take up the limited phenylalanine allowance in the diet.
2. *Expanded low-phenylalanine diet.* When the infant is about 6 months of age, solid foods are added to the diet, calculated according to their phenylalanine content. These food additions are selected from a list of phenylalanine food exchange groups or equivalents. A widely used current expansion of original low-protein food lists has been developed by nutritionists and is available, along with a newly revised low-protein cookbook, to guide food selections and preparation.[49] The individual child's diet is prescribed by the clinical nutritionist or physician according to the child's blood phenylalanine test, age, and weight. The nutritionist then calculates the nutrient and energy levels and outlines the food plan in terms of special formula and numbers of food choices for the child.

Family Counseling

Since dietary management of PKU is the only known effective method of treatment, initial education of the parents is essential. Studies have indicated that the dietary control during the first year of life is directly related to three factors: (1) the parents' understanding of the diet; (2) the appropriateness of the dietary prescription to the needs of the individual infant; and (3) the frequency of infection (the metabolic effect of infection increases blood phenylalanine levels). A number of teaching guides and materials are available to help in family counseling and education. Parents must understand and accept the absolute necessity of following the diet carefully. This requires patience, understanding, and continued reinforcement. Frequent home visits by the nutritionist and nurse may be a source of guidance and support as the child grows older. Other family members and any subsequent siblings should also be tested for PKU.

PKU Team

The physician, the clinical nutritionist, and the nurse carry primary responsibilities on the clinical care team, with supportive care by social services and various behavioral therapists provided as needed. Together with wise parents, who have formed supportive parents' groups in many places, this team provides initial and continuing care so that the PKU child grows and develops normally (Fig. 5-6).[50] Such a child, diagnosed at birth by widespread screening programs, has a healthy and happy adulthood ahead, instead of the profound disease consequences that have been experienced only a few years ago.

Public Health Implications

Continuing PKU screening surveys indicate an incidence of about 1 in every 13,000 births. The possibilities of severe mental retardation from undiagnosed and untreated PKU make public health responsibilities obvious. Several blood serum tests used in such screening procedures are given in Table 5-5.

Other Disorders of Amino Acid Metabolism

Tyrosinosis

A genetic disease similar to PKU, tyrosinosis, with high genetic frequency among people of French Canadian descent, is characterized by elevated plasma and urinary levels of tyrosine and by an increase in urinary levels of phenolic acids. Tyrosinosis is caused by the missing liver enzyme *parahydroxyphenylpyruvic acid oxidase,* which converts parahydroxyphenylpyruvic acid (HPPA), a metabolic product in the normal pathway of tyrosine oxidation, to *homogentisic acid.* The resulting increase in tyrosine and its metabolites in

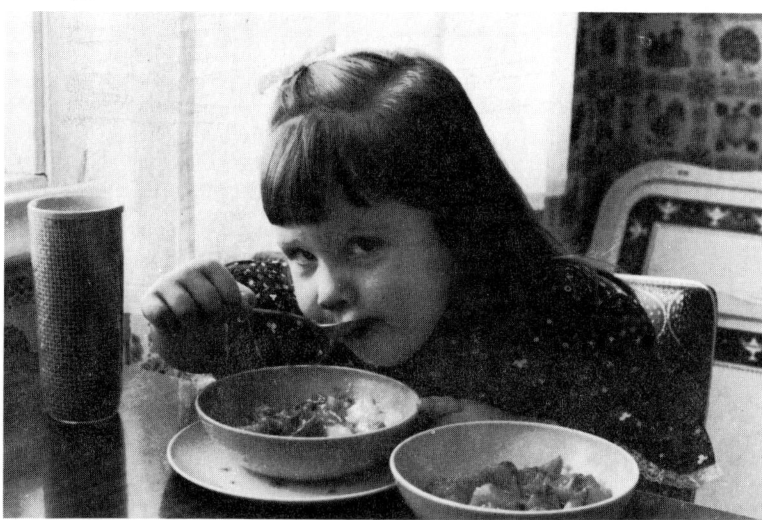

FIG. 5-6 PKU. This child is a delightful, perfectly developed 3-year-old. Screened and diagnosed at birth, she has eaten a carefully controlled low-phenylalanine diet and is growing normally.

TABLE 5-5

Blood Tests Used for PKU Screening and Monitoring

Test	Method	Use
Guthrie inhibition assay test	Drops of blood placed on filter paper Laboratory uses a bacterial growth inhibition test Phenylalanine level greater than 8 mg/dl blood is diagnostic of PKU	Effective in newborn period; used also to monitor PKU diet Blood easily obtained by heel or finger prick Inexpensive, used for wide-scale screening
McCaman and Robins fluorometric methods	About 5 ml blood is drawn, with serum separated and tested for phenylalanine Level greater than 8 mg/dl indicates PKU or loss of dietary control	Diagnostic and diet-monitoring tool; laboratory procedure simpler than LaDu-Michael method Test not available in many laboratories
LaDu-Michael method	About 5 ml blood is drawn, with serum separated and tested for phenylalanine Level greater than 8 mg/dl indicates PKU In PKU patients, levels above 8-12 mg/dl indicate loss of dietary control	Useful diagnostic and diet monitoring tool Requires blood drawn from the patient Laboratory method more difficult than the others, and test not available in many laboratories

body fluids and tissues accounts for the clinical symptoms, which include cirrhosis of the liver, hypophosphatemia, rickets, renal tubular damage, and mental retardation. Management by nutritional therapy is designed to control tyrosine and its precursor phenylalanine, as well as methonine, in the diet.

Principles such as those used in the treatment of PKU are followed: (1) use of milk substitutes, commercial products made from casein hydrolysate from which most of the phenylalanine and tyrosine have been removed, and (2) addition of selected foods from carefully calculated food lists according to the content of these amino acids. Clinical experience with several patients showing elevated serum methionine levels has led some practitioners to restrict this amino acid also. Food lists reflecting restriction of these amino acids—phenylalanine, tyrosine, and methionine—are provided for the clinical nutritionist and the other metabolic team members.

Maple Syrup Urine Disease

Another rare genetic disease of amino acid metabolism is maple syrup urine disease (MSUD), so called because of the sensory and physical characteristics of

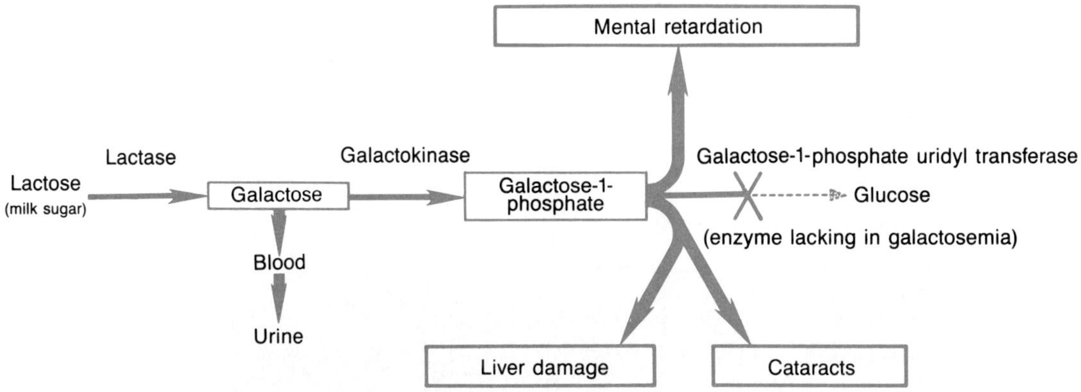

FIG. 5-7 Metabolic error in galactosemia. Because of the absence of the enzyme galactose-1-phosphate uridyl transferase, galactose cannot be converted to glucose.

the urine. It is an autosomal recessive disease involving a deficiency of the oxidative decarboxylation of the branched-chain amino acids (BCAAs) leucine, isoleucine, and valine. The only treatment is dietary restriction of these amino acids, but this is no small task.[51] Helpful food guides for this difficult diet, along with tabulated food lists, are available to provide more variety in food choices.

Homocystinuria

This rare aminoaciduria, only 1 in every 160,000 births, is caused by a recessive gene. Homocystinuria is a defect of methionine metabolism caused by the impaired activity of the enzyme *cystathionine synthase,* which participates in the conversion of homocystine, a metabolite of methionine, one of the essential amino acids.[52,53] In these cases plasma methionine levels are elevated, and homocystine is excreted in the urine. Clinical symptoms include various skeletal deformations such as **scoliosis,** dislocated lenses in the eyes, and frequently mental retardation. Two forms of the disease are known; one responds to vitamin B_6 therapy and the other does not. Dietary management is based on a low-methionine diet (see Chapter 10), curtailing additional cystine. However, such a diet must be carefully administered, since there is a risk of malnutrition with severe methionine restriction.

Galactosemia

Metabolic Defect

Galactosemia is a genetic disease caused by a missing enzyme, which in this case affects carbohydrate metabolism. The incidence of galactosemia is lower than that of PKU, about 1 in every 25,000 to 50,000 births. The metabolic defect, transmitted by a single autosomal recessive gene, is illustrated in Fig. 5-7. The missing enzyme is *galactose-1-phosphate uridyl transferase (G-1-PUT).* This is one of the three enzymes that controls steps in the conversion of galactose to glucose. Milk, the infant's first food, contains a large amount of the disaccharide lactose (milk sugar), which is acted on by the intestinal digestive enzyme *lactase* to produce the monosaccharides glucose and galactose. After galactose is initially combined with phosphate to begin the metabolic conversion to glucose, it cannot be metabolized further in the galactosemic infant. Galactose rapidly accumulates in the blood and in various body tissues.

Clinical Symptoms

In the past the excess tissue accumulations of galactose caused rapid damage to the untreated infant. The child failed to thrive, and clinical symptoms were apparent soon after birth. Continued liver damage brought jaundice, enlarged and failing liver and spleen, and fluid accumulation in the abdominal cavity. Without treatment, death usually resulted from liver failure. If the infant survived, the continuing tissue damage and accompanying hypoglycemia in the optic lens and the brain caused cataracts and mental retardation. Now, however, with newborn screening programs, these infants are detected immediately and provided with special dietary management. With this vital nutritional therapy, they continue to grow and develop normally.

scoliosis • Lateral curvature of the spine; an appreciable deviation of the normally straight vertical line of the spine.

TABLE 5–6

Foods that May Be Included or Excluded in a Galactose-Free Diet

Food groups	Foods included	Foods excluded
Milk and milk substitutes	Milk substitutes—Isomil, Neomullsoy, Nutramigen, Prosobee, Soyalac Meat-base formula	Breast milk Animal milk (cow, goat)—whole, low-fat or nonfat, dried or evaporated Imitation or filled milk Cream Cottage cheese, hard cheeses Yogurt Ice cream, ice milk, sherbet Milk by-products—casein, whey, curds, lactose, whey solids, nonfat dry milk solids
Protein foods	Plain meats, poultry, fish, eggs, nuts, legumes (if monitored for erythrocyte galactose-1-phosphate)	Organ meats (liver, pancreas, kidney, sweetbreads, brains) Foods prepared in cream sauce or breaded (unless milk-free) Processed meats (unless milk-free)
Breads and cereals	Many are made with milk; contact local bakeries for list of breads safe to use Rice, noodles, spaghetti, macaroni	Prepared mixes (muffins, biscuits, waffles, pancakes); unverified breads, cereals (cooked and dry) Foods that are creamed, breaded, buttered Foods processed with lactose or other unsafe ingredients
Fruits	All fresh, frozen, canned, dried, except those in excluded list	Fruits processed with unsafe ingredients, such as milk and milk products or by-products
Vegetables	All fresh, frozen, canned, dried, except those in excluded list	Vegetables processed with unsafe ingredients Foods that are creamed, buttered, breaded (unless milk-free) French fries, instant mashed potatoes containing lactose or other unsafe ingredients
Fats	Vegetable oils, shortening lard, margarines made with safe ingredients, bacon, mayonnaise, olives, salad dressings made with safe ingredients	Butter Cream Margarine containing lactose Salad dressing made with butter, milk, lactose
Soups, sauces, and gravies	Clear soups (bouillon, broth, consomme) Vegetable soups using allowed vegetables Homemade cream soups, sauces, gravies made with milk substitutes Water-base gravies	Cream soups, chowders, dried or canned soups made with unsafe ingredients Cream sauces made with milk or lactose Gravy made with butter, milk, cream, margarine Dehydrated gravy mixes made with unsafe ingredients
Desserts and sweets	Angel food cake Homemade products made with milk substitutes, water, vegetable oils Flavored gelatin and puddings with water Water and fruit ices	Commercial products made with unsafe ingredients Sweet rolls Custard, regular puddings Ice cream, ice milk, sherbet
	Beverages—cocoa powder, carbonated punch-base and fruit drinks without lactose	Hot or cold chocolate drinks, cocoa mix, Ovaltine, malted milk, powdered soft drinks
	Candy—sugar-free and regular chewing gum made with safe ingredients, plain sugar, rock candy, marshmallows without lactose	Butterscotch, caramels, milk chocolate, peppermint, toffee
	Sweeteners—brown sugar, molasses, white sugar, corn syrup, carob powder, honey, jams, jellies, marmalades (made without lactose), unsweetened bittersweet and semisweet chocolate	Milk chocolate made with unsafe ingredients Chocolate syrup made with unsafe ingredients
Miscellaneous	Artificial sweeteners made with safe ingredients Catsup, mustard Olives, pickles Nuts, nut butters Nondairy creamers, (Cremora, Mocha Mix), in limited amounts Popcorn, plain; corn, potato chips Instant coffee (lactose-free) Pure spices, seasonings	Artificial sweeteners made with unsafe ingredients Dietetic, diabetic preparations Chips made with unsafe ingredients Nondairy creamer made with unsafe ingredients Dried, shredded coconut Drugs or food coloring made with lactose Syrups, fats, margarines containing lactose

Dietary Management

The main indirect source of dietary galactose is milk. Therefore *all* forms of milk and lactose must be removed from the diet. In this instance a *galactose-free diet* is used. Although galactose is part of certain body structures, the needed amount can be synthesized by the body. Milk-substitute formulas, usually with a soy base, are used. They are complete protein hydrolysate products free of galactose, such as Nutramigen (Mead Johnson), Isomil (Ross), and Prosobee (Mead Johnson). Breast-feeding, of course, cannot be used. As solid foods are added to the infant's diet at about 6 months of age, careful attention must be given to avoid lactose from other food sources. A general outline of foods to use and to avoid is given in Table 5-6. Parents are carefully instructed to check labels on all commercial products to detect any lactose or lactose-containing substances.

Public Health Implications

There is some evidence that galactosemia may not be quite as rare as originally thought. Asymptomatic carriers have been detected in families of galactosemic children and other individuals. Early detection at birth and immediate, careful treatment with a galactose-free diet are essential to prevent the profound effects on body organs and tissues, especially the brain. Tests have been developed for such immediate screening and are used in most states. Cord blood may be used immediately after birth to establish a diagnosis, using a simple test for G-1-PUT activity in erythrocytes. Infants who are detected to have high G-1-PUT activity are carefully observed with continuing blood tests periodically to monitor the effects of the diet. Because a carrier can also be identified by a lowered enzyme level in the red blood cells, it is advisable to eliminate lactose from the prenatal diet of a mother detected as a carrier.

Lactose and Fructose Intolerances

A deficiency of any one of the disaccharidases in the intestine—lactase, sucrase, or maltase—may produce a wide range of gastrointestinal problems and abdominal pain because the specific sugar involved cannot be digested. Of these, a lactase deficiency causing lactose intolerance is perhaps the most common. A diet similar to that used for galactosemia is required, although the underlying cause of the difficulty is quite different. Milk and products containing lactose are avoided or used only to limited tolerance, and soy milk products are substituted.

In hereditary fructose intolerance, another enzyme defect affects metabolism of the monosaccharide fructose. The basic metabolic defect is in the gene controlling synthesis of the enzyme *aldolase B*, which is found only in the intestinal mucosa, liver, and kidney, where it catalyzes the cleavage of fructose-1-phosphate or fructose-1,6-diphosphate into two 3-carbon fragments.[54] Symptoms may be acute or chronic, resulting from tissue accumulation of fructose-1-phosphate, and include gastrointestinal problems, hepatic enlargement and failure, renal dysfunction, hypoglycemia, and hypophosphatemia. Nutritional therapy centers on a diet eliminating fructose, either as such in food products or as a constituent of its precursor sugar sucrose. Most U.S. infant formulas are fructose-free. But several, including Isomil (Ross) and Nutramigen (Mead Johnson), do contain sucrose and thus yield fructose on digestion.

Insulin-Dependent Diabetes Mellitus

The care of children with the genetic disease diabetes mellitus is discussed in Chapter 9. Included in that chapter is a detailed discussion of sound dietary management. Comprehensive care is based on normal nutrition for growth and development and regular habits, with support of a continuing teaching-counseling program.

Food Allergies

Underlying Etiology

Allergic Response

The word *allergy* is from the Greek *allos* (other) and *ergon* (work). Thus the name implies an unusual or inappropriate response to a stimulus. An allergic condition results from a disorder of the immune system (see Chapter 12). It is immunity gone wrong.

Food Allergy

The term *food allergy* should be used only for hypersensitivity that is caused by a normal immunologic reaction to specific constituents of food or their digestion products. Food allergy is distinct from food intolerances, which are caused by nonimmunologic mechanisms; for example, cow's milk intolerance resulting from lactase deficiency. In general, there are three basic approaches to the diagnosis and treatment of adverse reactions to foods: (1) clinical assessment, (2) dietary manipulation, and (3) laboratory tests. Appropriate dietary counseling is essential.

Common Food Allergens

The care of an allergic child is often frustrating and formidable for the child and the parents. A wide variety of environmental, emotional, and physical factors influence the child's reaction, and a suitable regimen is sometimes difficult to find. Since sensitivity to protein substances is a common basis of food allergy, the early foods of infants and children are frequent offenders. However, children tend to become less allergic to food sources as they grow older.

Milk

Cow's milk has long been a common cause of allergic disease in infants.[55] In sensitive children it causes gastrointestinal difficulties such as vomiting, diarrhea, and colic. The problem is generally identified by clinical symptoms, family history, and a trial on a milk-free diet, using a substitute *hypoallergenic* formula such as the casein hydrolysate formulas Nutramigen and Pregestimil (both from Mead Johnson) or the special hydrolysate formula Alimentum (Ross).[56] A remission of symptoms on a milk-free diet is usually followed by a retrial on milk to determine if it does indeed cause the symptoms to reappear. Only then is the diagnosis of milk allergy established.

Eggs, Wheat, and Other Foods

Among the dominant food allergens in infants are chicken eggs, cow's milk, and wheat. The specific biochemical sensitivity to gluten (a protein found in wheat) in the child with gluten-induced celiac sprue is caused by a specific biochemical defect in the mucosal cell in celiac disease and represents a different sensitivity mechanism from the immunophysiology causing a true food allergy. Other true food allergens among children, some continuing through adulthood, include peanuts, soy, tree nuts, other cereal grains, and shellfish.[57]

Dietary Management

In an allergic child's diet, solid foods are usually added slowly to the original formula, with common offenders being excluded in early feedings. The following basic list of most frequently offending food allergens must be avoided[57,58]:

- Chicken eggs
- Cow's milk
- Wheat
- Peanuts
- Tree nuts
- Soy products
- Fish, shellfish

Citrus fruits, berries, and tomatoes may cause skin rash, but this is a local reaction and not the immunologic response that identifies true allergy.[57]

In some cases a series of diagnostic food elimination diets may be used to identify offending food allergens. A core of less-often offending foods is used initially, with gradual addition of other single foods one at a time to test the child's response. If a given food causes the return of the allergy, the food is then identified as an offending allergen and is eliminated from use. It may be retested subsequently to determine if it is still an allergen. Guidance in the substitution of special food products and in the use of special recipes can be provided for the child's parents. Most food allergies tend to weaken as the child grows older. However, serious allergic reactions to a few key foods, especially peanuts, may continue into adulthood and require constant monitoring of food products and dishes to avoid severe attacks.[58] These attacks of severe *anaphylactic shock* are marked by sudden bronchial spasms, vomiting, dropping blood pressure, and irregular heart rhythm.

Family Education

The education of the parents and family of an allergic child should include a knowledge and understanding of the allergic state and the many factors that influence it. If specific foods have been definitely identified as offenders, careful guidance to eliminate these from the child's diet must follow. The food's common use in daily meal patterns and its occurrence in a number of commercial products and other hidden sources are discussed. Label reading and recipe adaptation are important. As the child grows older and the allergic reaction to a given food wanes, it may be gradually reinstated to the diet.

Weight Management

Background Concerns

Individual Needs

Great variations in weight and height occur among normal, healthy children; therefore it is somewhat difficult to establish criteria for a definition of obesity in children. In some cases the state of obesity may be an important resolution in the child's personality or deep-seated psychiatric problems. However, the appreciable amount of obesity among American children is related to general health problems of a chronic nature in later years.

Preventive Aspects

Obesity is the factor most often identified as contributing to chronic conditions of hypertension and cardiovascular problems involving lipid disorders. Especially in high-risk families in which familial essential hypertension and lipid disorders such as hypercholesterolemia are present, establishing prudent family food patterns that control sodium, fat, and cholesterol is now recommended by pediatricians.[59,60] In studies of children and adults, body weight is usually the factor that relates most strongly to elevated levels of blood pressure and blood cholesterol.[61] From the point of view of preventive medicine, the control of childhood obesity is a significant factor in avoiding such problems later. The mechanism by which obesity contrib-

CLINICAL APPLICATION

Hypertension: Stopping It Before It Starts

"You get old, you get high blood pressure."

This may be true in the United States. The average infant with a "normal" blood pressure of 70/50 mm Hg usually grows up to be a teenager (age 17 to 18) with a "normal" blood pressure of 120/80, although more frequently this figure rises to 140/90 or more by age 16. However, the existence of cultures in which blood pressures rarely rise beyond childhood levels suggests that this old axiom should only be taken with a grain of salt.

These "low blood pressure cultures" usually include far less sodium in their diets than the amount found in countries like the United States or Japan. The hypertensive effect of sodium is nothing new, of course. But recent speculation of the possibility that some people are more sensitive to this effect than others *is* new. Also, speculation that this effect is greatest in those exposed to high-sodium diets for longer periods has spurred researchers to investigate sodium levels in the diets of children from infancy through adolescence. These efforts may lead to the development of strategies for reducing the risk of future generations becoming "high blood pressure cultures." These researchers have discovered the following:

- Table, canned, and other foods with added salt are the main sources of excess sodium in the American child's diet, especially after 6 months of age. Milk and milk products, as commonly used in infancy, are adequate for supplying sodium to meet children's needs.
- Excess sodium "sneaks" into snacks commonly served to children. This is especially true of most microwave meals and snacks marketed to children. When flavors in foods do not have the chance to blend together and be enhanced by standard cooking procedures, manufacturers add flavor enhancers (usually sodium-based) to "spice" things up. It has been estimated that a whole generation of children will be "addicted" to sodium because of these foods.
- Even the most conscientious parents have a difficult time figuring out the sodium content of foods. Presently, less than half of all snack product labels indicate the *amount* of sodium provided. Parents can only guess by reading the order of ingredients or the number of times the word *sodium* appears in the product ingredient list, neither of which usually correlates well with the actual amount. New food labeling regulations should change this situation.
- Children who eat breakfast tend to have lower blood pressures. The validity of this finding is limited, however, since obese children are the ones who skip breakfast most often, and obesity is strongly associated with elevated blood pressures. On the other hand, children who skip breakfast at home may snack on salty foods purchased on the way to school.
- Children who gained weight as they grew older showed a similar gain in their blood pressures. Body weight did not relate to kcaloric intake, an observation consistent with findings in other studies on obesity. It was suspected that the overweight teenagers simply consumed more salt, rather than kcalories, and that being overweight was possibly more a result of inactivity.

These findings suggest that high blood pressure control in infancy and childhood is associated with, among other things, a reduced sodium intake. They also suggest the roles that many of us can play in reducing the risk for high blood pressure among children. Parents can (1) wait until their babies are 4 to 6 months old before serving solid foods, (2) serve baby foods made with no salt added, and (3) encourage regular meals for school-age children to discourage their eating high-sodium snack foods. Nutrition counselors can (1) help parents identify foods with "hidden" sodium to avoid, especially in processed foods and prepared breakfast cereals, and (2) identify other risk factors for hypertension in the child or family.

If everyone makes an honest effort, perhaps our children will change the opening axiom to something like this: "So you get old. At least without hypertension, you can enjoy it more." ◆

REFERENCES

Ballew C et al: Comparison of three weight-for-height indices in blood pressure studies in children, *Am J Epidemiol* 131(3):532, 1990.

Faulkner B: Management of hypertension in children and adolescents, *Am Fam Physician* 34:101, 1986.

Gutin B et al: Blood pressure, fitness, and fatness in 5- and 6-year-old children, *JAMA* 264(9):1123, 1990.

Liebman B: What are they feeding our children? *Nutrition Action Health Letter* 16(1):10, 1989.

Luger SW: Breakfast of champions or of hypertension, *N Engl J Med* 314:1052, 1986.

Schmidt SB: Hawking food to kids, *Nutrition Action Health Letter* 16(1):1, 1989.

utes to higher blood pressure is unclear. The increased sodium inherent in a higher kcaloric diet with many salty snack foods consumed by obese individuals may be the main reason, and the increasing taste for salt is a learned one (see Chapter 8).

Various lines of investigation have focused on childhood metabolic predictors of obesity-related degenerative diseases. In a study of weight management in obese boys ages 9 to 12, even moderate dietary control in combination with appropriate physical activities tailored to the home environment in a practical approach was sufficient to stop the weight gain pattern and to normalize key metabolic response patterns that were predictive of vascular disease, hypertension, and diabetes (see the *Clinical Application*, p. 88). Childhood obesity results in the development of a greatly increased number of fat cells. Thus its prevention could have a major impact on obesity later in life and potentially play a large role in preventing hypertension and cardiovascular lipid disease in adults.[61]

Causes of Excessive Weight

Cultural Factors

Many cultural factors condition food intake. Meal patterns and foods are different in different cultures. The three-meals-a-day pattern is a cultural one, not a biologic necessity. Some indications exist that eating less food more often may be better to control weight than eating larger meals less frequently. However, there needs to be some consideration of the type and frequency of snacks. Too often among children, snack foods tend to be rich in sugar and fat, as well as salt, and relatively low in other nutrients, serving only to provide excess kcalories and salt.

Excessive Parental Concern with Appetite

The normal slowed and erratic childhood growth pattern follows a period of rapid growth during the first year. As a result, there is a normal decrease in food intake and an irregular eating pattern during the latent childhood years. Frequently during these periods, parents worry unnecessarily about the amount of food their children eat. Thus they may tend to overfeed them, pushing food at times when such an intake is not needed. Behavioral, family-based treatment studies for obese children, in which the parents participated along with their children, have had positive results as shown in a 10-year follow-up survey.[62-64]

Decreased Physical Activity

Much evidence shows that in this age of automation, the amount of physical activity among growing children is decreasing. Frequently, the underlying cause of a child's obesity may be not so much an excess kcalorie intake as a lower level of physical activity and spending more time in passive activities such as watching television.

Food Practices during Growth Years

Infant Feeding

Breast-feeding is recommended for infants for at least the first 6 months of life, with additions of solid food beginning only at about 4 to 6 months of age. Before that age the infant does not need solid foods and cannot handle them very well. Most of the attempts at early feeding are culturally derived or are based on attitudes of rapid growth progress rather than on biologic needs.[65]

Sex Differences in Early Years

If the sex differences in kcalorie expenditure at the early age of 2 or 3 years are considered, it is evident that all toddlers are not going to eat the same amount of food. The basal metabolic rate is higher in boys than in girls during the second and third years of life. Therefore parents should be prepared for early differences among young boys and young girls. Also, cultural attitudes based on sex stereotyping sometimes appear early. For example, a boy may be expected to eat more and a girl may be admonished not to overeat.

Adolescent Sex Differences in Body Composition

The increasing tendency for fat deposition in the teenage girl, in comparison to greater increase in lean body mass in the teenage boy, makes weight management a greater problem for the girl. Guidance from parents is needed in a supportive, accepting manner.

Dental Caries

Incidence

Over the past two decades a significant, if not surprising, decline in the dental caries rate has begun to appear. According to data from a previous National Caries Prevalence Survey involving schoolchildren ages 5 to 17, the incidence of caries has declined 32% over the past 10 years.[66] This study also registered an increase of 9% in the incidence of caries-free children compared to data of the prior decade. Observers have attributed some of this decline to increased use of fluoridated public water supplies and better dental hygiene with fluoridated toothpastes among children. However, during this same period, the use of kcaloric sweeteners in foods consumed by children has not declined. For example, although from 1963 to 1980 there was a downward trend in the consumption of refined cane and beet sugar, there was a compensating increase in corn sweeteners. The net result is that total use of sugars appears to be relatively unchanged.

Etiology

Three factors combine to produce tooth decay: the susceptible host, oral bacteria, and diet.

Susceptible Host

Inherent differences in caries susceptibility vary widely among individual children. Some of these are hereditary differences in the anatomic characteristics of the tooth, but the ultimate shape of the tooth is influenced by interrelationships among these inherited characteristics and the environment that sustains its development during its formative period. Since teeth formed are stable structures, it is evident that this positive nutritional influence has effect only during growth and development of the enamel-forming organ in the gums and the tooth bud. Certain vitamins and minerals, especially vitamins A and D, calcium, and phosphorus, play a part during this period.

Oral Bacteria

In human beings, streptococci constitute the highest number of bacteria in the dental plaque, the gelatinous coating of the teeth. These organisms seem to have a particular affinity for carbohydrates and act on them rapidly, producing acids that lower the pH of the dental plaque and erode the enamel. However, the oral flora is complex, and bacterial effects vary because of symbiosis between two or more microorganisms. It is their substrate that is mandatory for the metabolism of caries-producing organisms. This substrate is carbohydrates—starches and sugars.

Diet

As food accumulates in the mouth, it provides the necessary medium for the normal growth of acidogenic microorganisms that cause tooth decay. In sites of greatest food particle retention, around irregular tooth formations in which bits of the offending food particles may easily lodge or stick, the bacterial activity is greatest. Current studies indicate that a sticky sweet texture is not necessarily the main culprit, because a number of carbohydrate food forms and the tooth structure contribute to the problem.[67] Exposure to fluoride and comprehensive dental care provide the major means of preventing dental caries.

Dietary Implications

Although the problem of dental caries has decreased in recent years, it is by no means solved. Recent advances in the knowledge of nutrition and its relationship to caries provide helpful steps in that direction. Two guidelines seem apparent: (1) increase the intake of fresh fruits and vegetables that require more chewing and act as "natural toothbrushes" and reduce the intake and frequency of carbohydrate snacks and (2) use fluoridated public water supplies where possible, along with fluoridated toothpaste and flossing in regular tooth care.

To Sum Up

Nutritional therapy of the hospitalized infant or child should be based on the unique needs of the age group in terms of mental and physical development, dietary modifications, and foods readily accepted.

A major barrier to nutritional therapy for hospitalized children is food rejection. Children may be too ill to eat, too anxious about family separation and being in an unfamiliar environment, or too frightened by the illness itself. Relieving anxiety and fear is as important as the methods used to encourage food acceptance during the hospital stay—for example, allowing self-selection, providing a warm mealtime atmosphere via group eating and special holiday celebrations, using familiar foods, and involving family members.

Disorders seen in children include gastrointestinal problems, such as infantile colic, diarrhea, and feeding problems caused by congenital defects such as cleft lip and palate; malabsorption problems caused by celiac sprue and cystic fibrosis; other genetic diseases—disorders of amino acid metabolism such as PKU and disorders of carbohydrate metabolism such as galactosemia; food allergies, especially to cow's milk but also to eggs, wheat, and other foods; obesity; and dental caries.

QUESTIONS FOR REVIEW

1. Identify possible causes and solutions for colic, vomiting, constipation, and diarrhea in infancy or early childhood.
2. What causes cleft lip and palate? How does this defect affect the feeding process in infancy? Describe the surgical repair schedule and appropriate feeding methods during this period.
3. What is the underlying cause of celiac sprue? Describe its clinical signs and dietary management.
4. What is the underlying metabolic defect that causes cystic fibrosis? Describe its clinical symptoms and nutritional management.
5. What is the underlying metabolic defect that causes phenylketonuria (PKU)? How does this condition affect the untreated child? Describe the current program for newborn screening, nutritional management, and monitoring provided for children with PKU.
6. What is the underlying metabolic defect that causes galactosemia? How does this condition affect the untreated child? Describe the current program for newborn screening, nutritional management, and monitoring provided for children with galactosemia.
7. What is the underlying cause of food allergies? Describe symptoms of milk allergy and recommendations for therapy and family education.
8. What factors have generally contributed to the growing rate of obesity in childhood? What recommendations would you make to a new mother to help her reduce her child's risk of becoming obese?
9. Discuss four factors that influence susceptibility to dental caries and how the condition may be controlled.

REFERENCES

1. Powell GF: Nutrition in nonorganic failure to thrive, *Clin Nutr* 4(2):54, 1985.
2. Fomon SJ: *Infant nutrition,* Philadelphia, 1974, WB Saunders.

3. Cervisi J et al: Office management of the infant with colic, *J Pediatr Health Care* 5:184, 1991.
4. Clyme P, Kulczycki A: Human breast milk contains bovine IgG: relationship to infant colic? *Pediatrics* 87(4):439, 1991.
5. World Health Organization: News from WHO's diarrheal disease control programme, *WHO Chronicle* 38:212, 1984.
6. American Academy of Pediatrics, Committee on Nutrition: The use of oral fluid therapy and post-treatment feeding following enteritis in children in a developed country, *Pediatrics* 75:358, 1985.
7. Cloeson M, Merson MH: Global progress in the control of diarrheal diseases, *Pediatr Infect Dis J* 9:345, 1990.
8. Santosham M, Greenough WB: Oral rehydration therapy: a global perspective, *J Pediatr* 118(suppl 4):445, 1991.
9. Snyder JD: Use and misuse of oral therapy for diarrhea: comparison of US practices with American Academy of Pediatrics recommendations, *Pediatrics* 87(1):28, 1991.
10. Brown KH: Dietary management of acute childhood diarrhea: optimal timing of feeding and appropriate use of milks and mixed diets, *J Pediatr* 118(suppl):92, 1991.
11. Lifshitz F et al: Refeeding infants with acute diarrheal disease, *J Pediatr* 118(suppl):99, 1991.
12. Lebenthal E, Lu R-B: Glucose polymers as an alternative to glucose in oral rehydration solutions, *J Pediatr* 118(suppl):62, 1991.
13. Farnan S: Nutrition and feeding of children with cleft lip/palate, *Nutr News,* 3(2):1, 1988.
14. Brooks MD: Nutrition overview of cleft lip and palate, *Top Clin Nutr* 3(3):9, 1988.
15. Zeman FJ: *Clinical nutrition and dietetics,* ed 2, New York, 1991, Macmillan Publishing.
16. Kennedy-Caldwell C, Caldwell MD: Pediatric enteral nutrition. In Rombeau JL, Caldwell MD: *Enteral and tube feeding,* vol 1, *Clinical nutrition,* Philadelphia, 1984, WB Saunders.
17. Trier JS: Celiac sprue, *N Engl J Med* 325(24):1709, 1991.
18. Anson O et al: Celiac disease: parental knowledge and attitudes of dietary compliance, *Pediatrics* 85:98, 1990.
19. Skerritt JH, Hill AS: Self-management of dietary compliance in coeliac disease by means of ELISA "home test" to detect gluten, *Lancet* 337:379, 1991.
20. Roberts L: CF screening delayed for awhile, perhaps forever, *Science* 247:1296, 1990.
21. Rock MJ et al: Newborn screening for cystic fibrosis complicated by age-related decline in immunoreactive trypsinogen levels, *Pediatrics* 85:1001, 1990.
22. Marcus MS et al: Nutritional status of infants with cystic fibrosis associated with early diagnosis and intervention, *Am J Clin Nutr* 54:578, 1991.
23. Cystic Fibrosis Foundation: Guidelines for patient services, evaluation, and monitoring in cystic fibrosis centers, *Am J Dis Child* 144:1311, 1990.
24. Roberts L: The race for the cystic fibrosis gene, *Science* 240:141, 1988.
25. Thomas PJ et al: Cystic fibrosis transmembrane conductance regulator: nucleotide binding to a synthetic peptide, *Science* 251:553, 1991.
26. Lehrman S: Genetic testing puts society on the spot, *San Francisco Examiner,* p. E-1, 1992.
27. Roberts L: Cystic fibrosis corrected in the lab, *Science* 249:1503, 1990.
28. Verma IM: Gene therapy, *Sci Am* 263(5):68, 1990.
29. Moran A et al: Pancreatic endocrine function in cystic fibrosis, *J Pediatr* 118:715, 1991.
30. Ramsey BW et al: Nutritional assessment and management in cystic fibrosis, *Am J Clin Nutr* 55:108, 1992.
31. Brady MS et al: Effectiveness of enteric coated pancreatic enzymes given before meals in reducing steatorrhea in children with cystic fibrosis, *J Am Diet Assoc* 92(7):813, 1992.
32. Luder E et al: Efficacy of a nonrestricted diet in patients with cystic fibrosis, *Am J Dis Child* 143:458, 1989.
33. Luder E et al: Current recommendations for breast-feeding in cystic fibrosis centers, *Am J Dis Child* 144:1153, 1990.
34. Holliday KE et al: Growth of human milk-fed and formula-fed infants with cystic fibrosis, *J Pediatr* 118(1):77, 1991.
35. Wilson-Goodman V et al: Factors affecting the dietary habits of adolescents with cystic fibrosis, *J Am Diet Assoc* 90(3):429, 1990.
36. Luder E, Gildride JA: Teaching self-management skills to cystic fibrosis patients and its effect on their caloric intake, *J Am Diet Assoc* 89(3):359, 1989.
37. Wdowik MJ, Carlyle TL: Nutrition education for children with cystic fibrosis, *J Nutr Educ* 24(4):195, 1992.
38. Bowser EK: Evaluating enteral nutrition support in cystic fibrosis, *Top Clin Nutr* 5(3):55, 1990.
39. Bowser EK: Criteria to initiate and use supplemental gastrostomy feedings in patients with cystic fibrosis, *Top Clin Nutr* 5(3):62, 1990.
40. Sapienza C: Parental imprinting of genes, *Sci Am* 263(4):1990.
41. Begley S: A new genetic code, *Newsweek* CXX(8):77, 1992.
42. Schuett VE: Inborn errors of metabolism in the United States: an overview, *Top Clin Nutr* 2(3):1, 1987.
43. Clemens PC et al: Newborn screening for hyperphenylalaninemia on day 5: is 240 μmol/liter the most appropriate cut-off level? *Prev Med* 19:54, 1990.
44. McMurray MP et al: Bone mineral status in children with phenylketonuria—relationship to nutritional intake and phenylalanine control, *Am J Clin Nutr* 55:997, 1992.
45. Azen CG et al: Intellectual development in 12-year-old children treated for phenylketonuria, *Am J Dis Child* 145:35, 1991.

46. Waisbren SE, Levy HL: Effects of untreated maternal hyperphenylalaninemia on the fetus: further study of families identified by routine cord blood screening, *J Pediatr* 116(6):926, 1990.

47. Rohr FJ et al: Maternal PKU: report from the PKU Collaborative Study, *Metabol Curr* 1(1):1, 1988.

48. Elsas LJ, Acosta PB: Nutrition support of inherited metabolic disease. In Shils ME, Young VR, eds: *Modern nutrition in health and disease,* ed 7, Philadelphia, 1988, Lea & Febiger.

49. Schuett VE: *Low protein food list, low protein cookery for phenylketonuria,* ed 2, Madison, 1988, University of Wisconsin Press.

50. Jahn D: Inside, looking out: one mother's view on phenylketonuria, *Top Clin Nutr* 2(3):87, 1987.

51. Martin SB, Acosta RB: Nutrition support of phenylketonuria and maple syrup urine disease, *Top Clin Nutr* 2(3):9, 1987.

52. Wagstaff J et al: Severe folate deficiency and pancytopenia in a nutritonally deprived infant with homocystinuria caused by cystathionine beta-synthase deficiency, *J Pediatr* 118(4):569, 1991.

53. Selhub J, Miller JW: The pathogenesis of homocystinemia: interruption of the coordinate regulation by S-adenosylmethionine of the remethylation and transsulfuration of homocystine, *Am J Clin Nutr* 55:131, 1992.

54. Edstrom CS: Hereditary fructose intolerance in the vomiting infant, *Pediatrics* 85(4):600, 1990.

55. Bishop JM et al: Natural history of cow milk allergy: clinical outcome, *J Pediatr* 116:862, 1990.

56. Sampson HA et al: Safety of casein hydrolysate formula in children with cow milk allergy, *J Pediatr* 118:520, 1991.

57. Björkstén B: Dietary management of food allergy, *Semin Pediatr Gastroenterol Nutr* 3(2):13, 1992.

58. Nash JM et al: Allergies, *Time* 139(25):54, 1992.

59. Balfour IC et al: Pediatric cardiac rehabilitation, *Am J Dis Child* 145:627, 1991.

60. Ballew C et al: Comparison of three weight-for-height indices in blood pressure studies in children, *Am J Epidemiol* 131(3):532, 1990.

61. Gutin B et al: Blood pressure, fitness, and fatness in 5- and 6-year-old children, *JAMA* 264:1123, 1990.

62. Epstein LH et al: Growth in obese children treated for obesity, *Am J Dis Child* 144:1360, 1990.

63. Epstein LH et al: Ten-year follow-up of behavioral, family based treatment for obese children, *JAMA* 264(19):2519, 1990.

64. Stunkard AJ, Berkawitz RI: Treatment of obesity in children, *JAMA* 264(19):2550, 1990.

65. Agras WS et al: Influence of early feeding style on adiposity at 6 years of age, *J Pediatr* 116:805, 1990.

66. National Institutes of Health: The prevalence of dental caries in the United States children: The National Dental Caries Prevalence Survey 1979-1980, Department of Health and Human Services, Pub No 82:2245, Washington, DC, 1981, US Government Printing Office.

67. Kashket S et al: Lack of correlation between food retention on the human dentition and consumer perception of food stickiness, *J Dent Res* 70(10):1314, 1991.

FURTHER READING

Dietitians urged to educate parents about preventing diarrheal dehydration in children, *J Am Diet Assoc* 90(11):1550, 1990.

This brief notice to dietitians and other health care team professionals urges us to reach and teach parents of young children how to use simple oral rehydration therapy (ORT) to prevent serious diarrhea. Most parents do not know or understand ORT and often give children inappropriate household drinks such as colas, sweetened juices, or sports beverages, which only make the diarrhea worse. For more information, write to The National ORT Project (a coalition of child health organizations for teaching health professionals and parents about ORT), 2626 Pennsylvania Ave., N.W., Suite 301, Washington, DC 20037.

Brady MS et al: Effectiveness of enteric coated pancreatic enzymes given before meals in reducing steatorrhea in children with cystic fibrosis, *J Am Diet Assoc* 92(7):813, 1992.

Wdowik MJ, Carlyle TL: Nutrition education for children with cystic fibrosis, *J Nutr Educ* 24(4):195, 1992.

Wilson-Goodman V et al: Factors affecting the dietary habits of adolescents with cystic fibrosis, *J Am Diet Assoc* 90(3):429, 1990.

These three articles provide helpful information about current care of cystic fibrosis patients, with renewed emphasis on enzyme therapy that makes an increased aggressive diet possible and approaches to help children and adolescents learn about diet and enyzme therapy for their increased normal growth needs. Cystic fibrosis is often in the news these days, with new discoveries about the causative gene and national gene testing programs underway. For more information, write to the Cystic Fibrosis Foundation, 6931 Arlington Road, Bethesda, MD 20814.

CASE STUDY

The Child with Phenylketonuria

Anne Brown, a 4-year-old white female with phenylketonuria (PKU), came in with her mother to the special PKU clinic for her regular progress visit with the PKU team members. The pediatrician-geneticist noted that her general health was good. Her medical record indicated that she had had no illnesses, all her vaccinations were up to date, and her previous complete blood count results were all within normal limits. A review of Anne's regular blood tests monitoring her phenylalanine levels showed that for the most part her PKU was managed well by her mother's careful control of her diet. Only one test was elevated, and Mrs. Brown explained that Anne had had an ear infection at that time.

Her blood test revealed a phenylalanine level of 363 μmol/L (6 mg/dl). She was 107 cm (42 in) tall and weighed 18 kg (40 lb). She apparently was a well-nourished, alert, and happy little girl.

When Anne and her mother next saw the team nutritionist, Mrs. Brown asked about the possibility of modifying Anne's diet. Anne was still drinking Lofenalac, which was carefully prepared each day by her mother according to the nutritionist's instructions. She had been following the diet recommended for her very well, but her mother was worried about Anne's increasing interest in the foods eaten by her non-PKU brother, 2-year-old Fred. Apparently, when Mr. Brown had learned that Fred did not have PKU also and would not need a special diet, he immediately started making plans to introduce the child to his own favorites, which include steak and hamburgers. He had also been constantly urging his wife to start the younger child on solid foods early during infancy. Even now he wants meat on the table with every meal to make sure his son grows strong and healthy.

After commending Mrs. Brown's excellent care of Anne and her special diet, the metabolic nutritionist explained why Anne needed to continue her current PKU food plan. Then the nutritionist made another appointment with Mrs. Brown for the following week and asked that her husband come with her to the clinic.

Questions for Analysis

1. How is PKU diagnosed? What are the dietary implications during the neonatal period? What are the results of PKU if it is not controlled?
2. What is the acceptable range for levels of serum phenylalanine in children with PKU as compared with the normal level? Is Anne's level acceptable?
3. If you were in the position of the nutrition counselor, based on your study of phenylketonuria and its nutritional management, what advice would you offer Mrs. Brown regarding the "relaxation" of her daughter's diet now or in the near future? Explain the physiologic bases of the advice you offer.
4. What issues do you expect to arise during the follow-up appointment with both of Anne's parents? How would you counsel with them to help them resolve each nutrition-related issue?

Preventing Malnutrition in the Pediatric Ward

Medical technology has a certain irony. It keeps children alive who have historically fatal pediatric diseases only to have them suffer and sometimes die from malnutriton induced by altered metabolic and energy demands of the illness or its therapy.

Malnutition in the pediatric ward is associated with many of the same problems seen in adult wards: (1) *nonspecific effects of disease,* such as pain, nausea, fever, and gastrointestinal upset; (2) *iatrogenic starvation* induced by medical therapy; (3) *malabsorption* caused by disease of the small bowel, liver, or pancreas, as well as prematurity; (4) *increased basal metabolic rate,* raising kcalorie requirements; and (5) *altered metabolic pathways* for essential nutrients. In addition to these problems, the hospitalized child, up to a certain age, is unable or limited in ability to communicate problems or concerns. This makes it essential for pediatric health workers to be extremely observant and thorough when evaluating the nutritional status of every child.

Preventing malnutrition in this population requires a nutritional assessment, a nutritional care plan based on assessment results, and the use of appropriate feeding techniques. These processes must be designed not only to meet current nutritional requirements but also to meet the requirements for growth, which in infancy and adolescence is rapid enough to put the child at risk easily.

Nutritional assessment

Several nutritional assessment factors should be monitored to meet the metabolic requirements of the hospitalized child:

1. *Weight-height standard.* A recent and continuing weight loss indicates *acute* malnutrition, which increases the possibility of infection. This evidence of malnutrition is measured by determining the percentage of the weight-height standard each child has achieved: 90% (5th percentile) indicates *mild* malnutrition; 80%, *moderate* malnutrition; and 70%, *severe* malnutrition. These figures have also been used to evaluate adolescents. Their interpretation, however, is limited by the influence of the rate of sexual maturity on these values.
2. *Height.* Stature below normal for age may be associated with prior or chronic malnutrition. It is not considered a risk factor for infection or other nutrition-related problems.
3. *Arm anthropometry.* Midarm circumference and skinfold thickness, with calculated midarm muscle circumference, are measures used to assess protein and fat stores. Hospitalized children with values between the 5th and 15th percentiles are considered low normal; below the 5th percentile, depleted. These methods identify patients with low protein stores, even when the body weight is normal.
4. *Laboratory values.* Twenty-four hour creatinine excretion, serum proteins (especially albumin and transferrin, although prealbumin and retinol-binding protein have also been suggested because of a shorter half-life), total lymphocyte count, and intradermal skin tests are used to evaluate protein status. Although useful assessment tools, these values are strongly affected by trauma, infection, anemia, and corticosteroid therapy.

Nutritional care planning

Planning a child's diet based on body stores evaluated during the assessment must include a consideration of the nutritional effects of illness as follows:

1. *Metabolic rate.* Metabolic rate increases between 20% and 50% occur in patients with congestive heart failure, infection, and injury.
2. *Energy needs.* Energy needs double in patients with burn injury over more than 30% of their bodies. Attempts to meet elevated kcalorie requirements with too much glucose can result in hyperventilation. Thus sources of nutrients required to meet

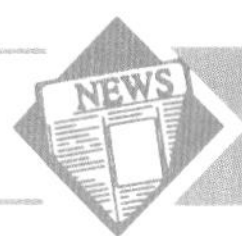

altered nutritional needs become critical in pediatric care.

Specific nutritional problems of disorders commonly associated with malnutrition in the pediatric patient are summarized in Table 5-4.

Low birth-weight, preterm infants

The feeding of premature infants during the first few weeks of life, especially their protein requirement, is still a subject of considerable controversy. Usually these small babies in the hospital's intensive care nursery are enterally fed special "preemie" commercial formulas with a relatively higher protein and energy content: 2.4 to 3.0 g/100 kcal of protein and 67 kcal/dl, as compared with regular "term" formulas: 2.2 g/100 kcal of protein and 67 kcal/dl. In a few instances, they may be fed breast milk with some form of fortification. When they achieve a body weight of 1800 to 2000 g, the formula is generally changed to a term formula in preparation for hospital discharge. These term formulas usually contain 1.5 g/dl of protein with a whey-to-casein ratio of either 60:40 or 18:82.

The American Academy of Pediatrics has recognized the indefinite state of knowledge concerning nutrition for preterm infants and stated that the basic goal is to achieve a postnatal growth that approximates the growth *in utero* of the normal fetus at the same postconception age. Yet the usual preterm and term formulas provide amounts of protein well in excess of that provided in the breast milk at comparable time periods. In fact, a recent study has demonstrated that similar growth and biochemical responses were achieved by a formula with a protein content close to that of human milk as compared with a standard infant formula, suggesting that the protein content of formulas be reduced to amounts close to those found in human milk.

Enteral and parenteral support may become necessary for infants born prematurely or for other children with inflammatory bowel disease, short-bowel syndrome, cancer, or intractable diarrhea. Diarrheal diseases especially pose a malnutrition and dehydration burden, not only in undeveloped countries but also in America. Despite modern advances in hygiene and sanitation, diarrheal illnesses remain among the most common problems requiring pediatric care. In a recent 5-year period studied, an average of 220,000 children under 5 years of age were hospitalized each year with gastroenteritis, representing 10.6% of all hospitalizations for young children of these ages. Major therapy includes (1) fluid and electrolyte replacement, (2) dietary intake, (3) symptomatic therapy with antidiarrheal compounds, and (4) specific therapy with antimicrobial agents. Specific nutritional problems of disorders commonly associated with malnutrition in the pediatric patient are summarized in Table 5-4.

Malnutrition is avoided by carefully evaluating each hospitalized child for inadequate nutrient levels in the blood and diet, altered metabolic rate or nutrient absorption, status of the gastrointestinal tract, and growth. By incorporating appropriate nutritional therapies into the health care plan for seriously ill patients, the pediatric health care team can avoid making the cure worse than the disease.

REFERENCES

American Academy of Pediatrics, Committee of Nutrition: Nutritional needs of preterm infants. In *Pediatrics nutrition handbook*, ed 2, Elk Grove Village, Ill, 1985, The Academy Press.

Bhatia J, Rassin DK: Feeding the premature infant after hospital discharge: growth and biochemical responses, *J Pediatr* 118:515, 1991.

Brown KH: Dietary management of acute childhood diarrhea: optimal timing of feeding and appropriate use of milks and mixed diets, *J Pediatr* 118(suppl):92, 1991.

Glass RI et al: Estimates of morbidity and mortality rates for diarrheal diseases in American children, *J Pediatr* 118(suppl):27, 1991.

Merritt RJ, Hack S: Infant feeding and enteral nutrition, *Nutr Clin Prac* 3(2):47, 1988.

Michielutte R et al: The relationship between weight-height indices and the triceps skinfold measure among young children ages 5 to 12, *Am J Public Health* 74:604, 1984.

Chapter 6

Gastrointestinal Diseases

CHAPTER OUTLINE

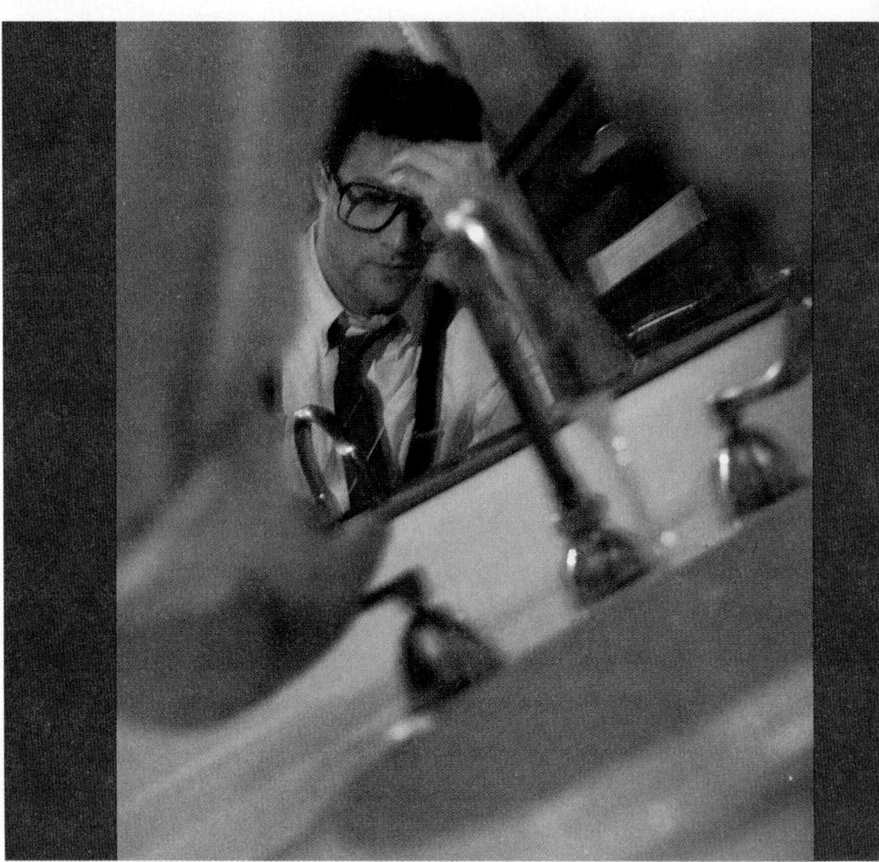

This chapter considers diseases that affect the various parts of the gastrointestinal tract. This basic body system receives our food, processes it, extracts its nutrients, and eliminates its wastes. To the extent that disease or malfunction at any point along the way interferes with this finely meshed process, nutritional therapy must modify food intake accordingly and at the same time maintain the body's optimal nutritional status and the individual's personal needs.

Surrounding every stomach is a person. The gastrointestinal tract is a sensitive mirror of the individual human condition, its physiologic function reflecting physical and psychologic conditioning. In adapting nutritional therapy for patients with gastrointestinal disorders, we deal not only with specific food items per se but also, and perhaps more so, with the state of the body that receives them.

The digestion and absorption of the food a person eats are accomplished in the gastrointestinal tract through a series of intimately related secretory and neuromuscular mechanisms. This network of functions forms the basis for general nutritional therapy in various gastrointestinal diseases that hinder the normal operation of these mechanisms. In this chapter we relate these basic functions and the healing process to the nutritional therapy indicated.

Nutritional Management

When food is taken into the mouth, the act of eating stimulates the gastrointestinal tract into accelerated action. Throughout the digestive process, highly coordinated systems and interactive functions respond. Secretory functions provide the necessary environment and agents for chemical digestion. Neuromuscular functions provide the necessary motility for mechanical digestion and move the food mass along the gastrointestinal tract. Absorptive functions enable the nutrients to enter the body's circulation and nourish the cells. Psychologic factors influence the overall individual response pattern. This highly individual and interrelated functional network forms the basis for nutritional therapy in disease or malfunction.

After food is taken into the mouth, masticated, and swallowed, the esophagus conducts the food mass to the stomach by peristalsis and gravity. The *gastroesophageal sphincter muscle* at the entry to the stomach forms a controlling valve. It relaxes to receive the food, then closes to hold each bolus for digestive action of enzymes in the gastric acid mix. Then a number of small intestine conditions may interfere with normal food passage and create malabsorption problems. These overall conditions vary widely from brief periods of functional discomfort to serious disease and complete obstruction. Nutritional therapy in any case is adapted to the degree of dysfunction in choice of food and feeding mode.

Oral Problems

The oral cavity, involving the mouth and pharynx, receives the food as it is eaten and passes it into the gastrointestinal tract for processing. Oral problems such as tissue inflammation and dental disease, as well as problems with salivation and swallowing, interfere with the normal actions of the oral cavity and affect the body's nutritional status.

Tissue Inflammation and Dental Disease

Tissue Inflammation

The tissues of the mouth often reflect a person's basic nutritional status. In malnutrition they deteriorate, becoming inflamed and more vulnerable to local infection or injury, causing pain and difficulty with eating. These conditions in the oral cavity include (1) *gingivitis*, inflammation of the gums, involving the mucous membrane with its supporting fibrous tissue encircling the base of the teeth; (2) *stomatitis*, inflammation of the oral mucosa lining the mouth; (3) *glossitis*, inflammation of the tongue; and *cheilosis*, a cracking and dry scaling process at the corners of the mouth affecting the lips and corner angles, making opening the mouth to receive food difficult.

These oral tissue problems may also be nonspecific and unrelated to nutritional factors. In some instances, gingivitis and stomatitis occur in many persons in mild form in relation to another disease or to stress. Occasionally, a severe form of *acute necrotizing ulcerative gingivitis* occurs, commonly called "trench mouth" (from its prevalence among soldiers in the World War I trenches). It is caused by a specific infectious bacterium *Fusobacterium nucleatum*, often in conjunction with a spirochete *Treponema vincentii*, and is also known as Vincent's disease, from the Paris physician Henri Vincent (1862-1950), who first identified the disease process. Hormonal changes, abnormal diet, or emotional stress may be contributing factors. The gums around the bases of the teeth become puffy, shiny, and tender, overlapping the teeth margins. Affected gums often bleed, especially during toothbrushing. This is a serious condition that destroys gum tissue and the supporting tissues of the teeth, and requires a course of antibiotic treatment.

Food intake in these conditions often decreases because of the pain and creates a major problem in maintaining adequate nutrition. Generally, patients are given high-protein, high-kcalorie liquids and then soft foods, usually nonacidic and without strong spices to avoid irritation. Temperature extremes may also be avoided if they cause pain. The diet is gradually advanced to unrestricted foods according to individual toleration and is often supplemented with vitamins. In severe disease, the use before meals of a mouthwash containing a mild topical local anesthetic helps relieve the pain of eating.

Dental Problems

The incidence of *dental caries* has recently been reduced in children and young adults (see Chapter 5).

However, it is still present in many older adults, especially those unable to afford regular dental care, and causes tooth loss and chewing problems. In older adults, some 65 million in the United States alone, *periodontal disease* is a major cause of tooth loss.[1] Especially if dental caries is untreated, or if dental hygiene is poor, gum tissue at the base of the teeth becomes damaged and pockets form between the gums and the teeth. Dental *plaque* forms from a sticky deposit of mucus, food particles, and bacteria, and it hardens into *calculus*, a mineralized coating developed from the plaque and saliva. These hardened calculuses then collect in the pocket openings at the base of the teeth, where the bacteria attack the periodontal tissue. The result is inflammation and bacterial erosion of bone tissue surrounding affected teeth and subsequent tooth loss. Preventive care, of course, through daily dental care with fluoridated toothpaste, careful flossing, and periodic plaque removal by the dentist and dental hygienist is the best approach. Extensive tooth loss leads to the need for replacement by *dentures*, which in many elderly people become ill-fitting and hinder adequate chewing. All of these dental problems need to be reviewed in any patient's nutritional history so that food textures and forms can be adjusted according to individual needs.

Salivary Glands and Salivation

Three pairs of glands secrete saliva via ducts into the mouth. The largest pair are the *parotid glands*, which lie over the angle of the jaw, just below and in front of the ear. The parotid ducts run forward and inward, opening inside the cheeks. The pair of *sublingual glands* lie under the tongue in the floor of the front of the mouth, one on each side of the *frenulum*, the central band of tissue that attaches the underside of the tongue to the floor of the mouth. They form a low ridge on each side of the frenulum. This ridge has a row of small openings through which the saliva flows. The third pair are the *submandibular glands*, which lie toward the back of the mouth close to the sides of the jaw. Their ducts run forward and open under the tongue, one on each side of the frenulum.

Disorders of the salivary glands affect eating, because saliva carries an amylase that begins starch breakdown and is vital in moistening the food to facilitate chewing and swallowing. Problems may arise from infection, such as the *mumps* virus that attacks the parotid glands or *calculuses* that may form in the ducts, damming the saliva flow and requiring surgical removal. Other problems come from *excessive salivation*, which occurs in numerous disorders affecting the nervous system such as *Parkinson's disease* and from local disorders such as mouth infections or injury. Excessive salivation may arise from any disease or drug that causes overactivity of the parasympathetic division of the autonomic nervous sytem, which controls the salivary glands.

Conversely, *lack of salivation*, which causes *dry mouth*, may be a temporary condition caused by fear, salivary gland infection, or action of *anticholinergic drugs* that hinder the normal action of neurotransmitters. Permanent dry mouth is rare but does occur in *Sjögren's syndrome* (Henrik Samuel Conrad Sjögren, Swedish ophthalmologist, born 1899), a symptom complex of unknown etiology that is thought to be an abnormal immune response. Sjögren's syndrome usually occurs in middle-aged or older women and is marked by conjunctival keratosis, *xerostomia* (dry mouth), and enlargement of the parotid glands and often is associated with rheumatoid arthritis. It may also result from radiation therapy. There is difficulty in swallowing and speaking, interference with taste, and tooth decay. The extreme mouth dryness may be partially relieved by spraying the inside of the mouth with an artificial saliva solution.

Swallowing Disorders

The process of swallowing involves highly integrated actions of the mouth, pharynx, and esophagus (Fig. 6-1). After food is chewed in the mouth and mixed well with saliva, the tongue pushes it to the back of the mouth and the voluntary muscles in the palate

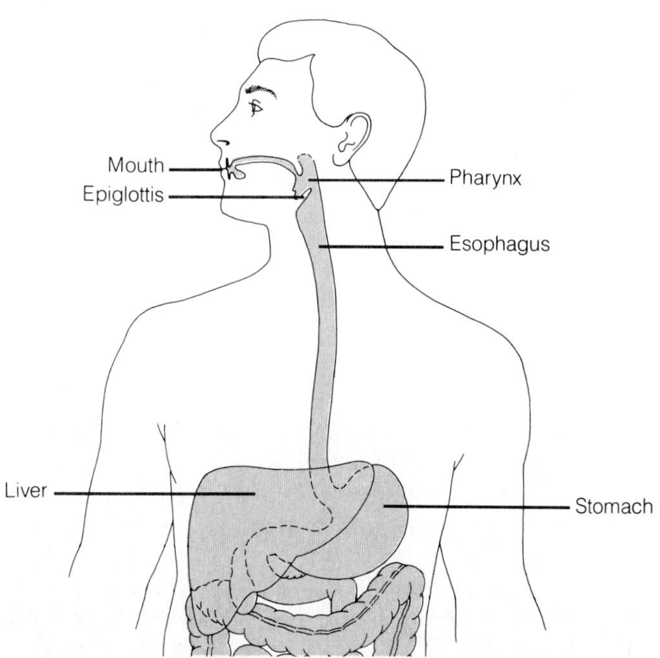

FIG. 6-1 Parts of mouth, pharynx, and esophagus involved in the swallowing process.

push the food into the *pharynx* (throat). The rest of the swallowing act is involuntary and automatic as food is propelled by a series of reflexes that are rapid, powerful, and almost impossible to stop. Entry of the food into the pharynx causes the *glottis* (the vocal cords of the larynx) and the *epiglottis* (the lidlike cartilage structure overhanging the entrance to the larynx) to seal off the trachea. The circular sphincter muscle at the top of the esophagus relaxes, and the muscles of the pharynx seize the food and squeeze it in the form of a *bolus* (rounded lump) into the open esophageal sphincter, which closes behind it. Powerful peristaltic contractions propel the food bolus toward the stomach. Finally, circular sphincter muscles at the end of the esophagus relax and allow the bolus of food to enter the stomach, then constrict to close the passage again.

Swallowing difficulty, known medically as *dysphagia,* is a fairly common problem with a wide variety of causes. It may be only temporary, as a piece of food lodged in the back of the throat, for which the **Heimlich maneuver** is appropriate first aid, or it may be involved with the insufficient production of saliva and xerostomia. Dysphagia may be more serious if it is caused by a nervous system disorder such as *myasthenia gravis* (see Chapter 14), by a stroke (see Chapter 8), or by other neuromuscular or structural impairments of the upper digestive tract.[2] Such dysfunctional swallowing often causes children and adults alike to aspirate food particles, in turn causing coughing and choking episodes that must be evaluated carefully by the interdisciplinary team providing care.[3,4] The team includes the physician, nurse, clinical dietitian, physical therapist, and especially the occupational therapist, who has had special training in swallowing problems.[2] Thin liquids are the most difficult food forms for patients with dysfunctional swallowing. In the oral phase of swallowing, liquids require greater oral coordination and finer motor control than do solids, and patients have a greater risk of aspiration, decreased fluid intake, and inadequate hydration.[5,6] To test various food and commercial agents for thickening liquids for individuals with swallowing disorders, Stanek et al.[6] recently compared several levels of viscosity in different thickening agents to help individuals with dysphagia. They tested a number of agents with three base liquids—water, apple juice, and milk—and three levels of viscosity: (1) a low level equal to that of infant formula, (2) a medium level equal to that of apricot nectar, and (3) a high level equal to that of yogurt. At all levels they found baby rice cereal to be the most effective food agent, with the least amount required to achieve the desired thickening and being the least costly. The charted results, including energy-nutrient values, provide excellent references for practitioners.

Esophageal Problems

General Problems along the Esophagus

The esophagus is a long, muscular tube lined with mucous membranes that extends from the pharynx, or throat, to the stomach (Fig. 6-1). It is bounded on both ends by circular muscles, or sphincters, that act as valves to control food passage. The upper sphincter remains closed except during swallowing, thus preventing airflow into the esophagus and stomach. Disorders along the tube that may disrupt normal swallowing and food passage include *esophageal spasm,* uncoordinated contractions of the esophagus; *esophageal stricture,* a narrowing caused by a scar from previous inflammation or ingestion of caustic chemicals or by a tumor; and *esophagitis,* an inflammation. These problems hinder eating and require medical attention through *dilation,* stretching procedures or surgery to widen the tube, and drug therapy.

Lower Esophageal Sphincter Problems

Defects in the operation of the lower esophageal sphincter (LES) muscles may come from changes in the smooth muscle itself or from neuroendocrine problems associated with its nerve-muscle stimuli or its hormonal control. For example, gastrin increases LES pressure, whereas secretin, cholecystokinin, and glucagon decrease it. In general, these LES problems arise from spasm, stricture, or incompetence.

Achalasia

Spasms occur when the LES muscles maintain an excessively high muscle tone, even while resting, and thus fail to open normally when the person swallows. This condition is called **achalasia,** from its unrelaxed

Heimlich maneuver • A first-aid maneuver to relieve a person who is choking from blockage of the breathing passageway by a swallowed foreign object or food particle. Stand behind the victim and clasp the hands around the victim's waist, placing one fist just under the sternum (breastbone) and grasping the fist with the other hand. Then make a quick, hard, thrusting movement inward and upward.

achalasia • Failure of the smooth muscle fibers of the gastrointestinal tract to relax at any point of juncture of its parts; especially failure of the esophagogastric sphincter to relax when swallowing because of degeneration of ganglion cells in the wall of the organ. The lower esophagus also loses its normal peristaltic activity. Also called cardiospasm.

TABLE 6-1

Dietary Principles for Care of Achalasia

Principles	Foods included
Energy nutrients	Moderate protein and carbohydrates and increased fat to help reduce LES pressure and gastric secretion
Texture	Liquid or semisolid food as tolerated Moderate to low fiber if it aids swallowing
Temperature	No very hot or very cold foods
Irritants	No citrus juices to injure mucosa if retained No highly spiced foods to irritate if retained
Meal pattern	Frequent, small meals as tolerated
Eating pace	Eat slowly in small bites and swallows

Adapted from Zeman FJ, Ney DM: *Applications of clinical nutrition,* Englewood Cliffs, NJ, 1988, Prentice Hall.

muscle state, and is also known as *cardiospasm,* from the proximity to the heart, although it has no relation at all to heart action. Patients apparently have fewer ganglion cells than normal in the myenteric plexus and vagus nerves of the enteric nervous system. There may also be a physiologic association with surrounding inflammatory cells and a viral agent. Because of the muscle tone and peristalsis of the disorder, the esophagus becomes misshapen, enlarged in the upper portions and constricted in the lower part and appearing on x-ray (after administration of an oral barium solution) as a full bag or a funnel. Patient symptoms include swallowing problems, frequent vomiting, a feeling of fullness in the chest, weight loss from eating difficulty, serious malnutrition, and pulmonary complications and infection caused by aspiration of food particles, especially during sleep hours.

Surgical treatment involves dilating the LES or slitting the muscle, an *esophagomyotomy,* which improves the stricture but does not correct the decreased peristalsis.[1] The patient's postoperative course usually involves oral fluids beginning on day 1, with a regular diet within about 5 days, according to toleration. Possible side effects of the surgery, however, include gastric reflux and subsequent esophagitis. Nutritional care must follow individual tolerations carefully. Some general guidelines for nutritional management of achalasia are given in Table 6-1.

Diffuse Esophageal Spasm and Stricture

Backup of gastric contents into the lower esophagus and disordered peristalsis result in diffuse esophageal spasm, an early stage of achalasia.[7] Strictures from the irregular muscle actions, a tumor, or burns and scars from ingestion of caustic household chemicals such as lye narrow the lumen and interfere with food intake, causing the same symptoms that occur with achalasia. Thus the nutritional management is the same as that for achalasia.

Gastroesophageal Reflux Disease

Chronic *gastroesophageal reflux disease (GERD)* results from ongoing lower esophageal sphincter problems. Clinicians are beginning to view "acid setting up shop in the esophagus" as serious and as difficult for the patient and the physician as the formation of peptic ulcers in the stomach or duodenum.[8] The true incidence of GERD is difficult to establish because many cases go undetected, and it is estimated that only the "tip of the iceberg" of chronic sufferers are seen clinically.[9] Regurgitation of the acid gastric contents into the lower part of the esophagus creates continuing tissue irritation. The hydrochloric acid and pepsin cause tissue erosion with symptoms of substernal burning, cramping, pressure sensation, or severe pain. These symptoms are aggravated by lying down or by any increase of abdominal pressure, such as that caused by tight clothing. This condition is related to (1) an *incompetent* (lacking strength and ability, nonfunctioning) gastroesophageal sphincter, (2) frequency and duration of the acid reflux, and (3) the inability of the esophagus to produce normal secondary peristaltic waves to prevent prolonged contact of the esophageal mucosa with the acid pepsin. A hiatal hernia may or may not be present.

Clinical Symptoms

The most common symptom is **pyrosis**—heartburn. It is frequently severe, occurring 30 to 60 minutes after eating. Surveys in the United States have reported that this common symptom occurs in 33% of persons with GERD at least once a month and in 7% daily.[9] Sometimes substernal pain radiates into the neck and jaw or down the arms. In addition to a hiatal hernia, the acid reflux may be caused by pregnancy, obesity, pernicious vomiting, or nasogastric tubes. Other symptoms include iron deficiency anemia with chronic tissue bleeding or aspiration, which may cause cough, dyspnea, or pneumonitis.

Complications

The most common complications are **stenosis** and esophageal ulcer. Also, significant **gastritis** in the herniated portion of the stomach may cause **occult bleeding** and anemia.

Treatment

Obesity is often an associated or precipitating factor. Thus weight reduction is essential. The patient needs to avoid lying down immediately after meals and to sleep with the head of the bed elevated. Frequent use of antacids helps to control the symptoms. From 85% to 90% of persons with esophagitis respond to weight

TABLE 6–2

Dietary Care of Gastroesophageal Reflux

Outcome	Action
Decrease esophageal irritation	Avoid common irritants such as coffee, carbonated beverages, tomato and citrus juices, and spicy foods
	Avoid any foods such as rich disserts that may cause heartburn
Increase lower esophageal sphincter pressure	Increase protein foods
	Decrease fat to about 45 g/day or less; use nonfat milk
	Avoid strong tea, coffee, and chocolate if poorly tolerated
	Avoid peppermint and spearmint
Decrease reflux frequency and volume	Eat small, frequent meals
	Sip only a small amount of liquid with meal; drink mostly between meals
	Avoid constipation; straining increases abdominal pressure reflux
Clear food materials from the esophagus	Sit upright at the table or elevate the head of bed
	Do not recline for 2 hours or more after eating

Adapted from Zeman FJ, Ney DM: *Applications of clinical nutrition,* Englewood Cliffs, NJ, 1988, Prentice Hall.

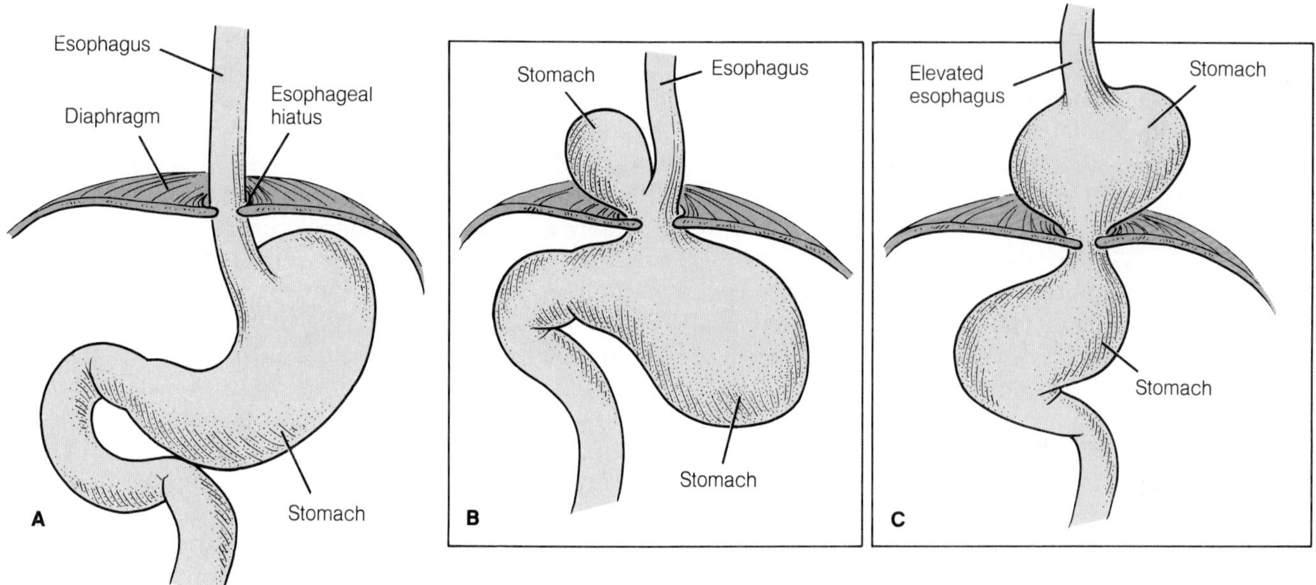

FIG. 6-2 Hiatal hernia compared with normal stomach placement. **A,** Normal stomach. **B,** Paraesophageal hernia (esophagus in normal position). **C,** Esophageal hiatal hernia (elevated esophagus).

reduction and conservative measures. Table 6-2 summarizes these management principles.

Hiatal Hernia

Normally the lower end of the esophagus enters the chest cavity at the *hiatus,* an opening in the diaphragmatic membrane, and immediately joins the upper portion of the stomach. A hiatal hernia occurs when a portion of the upper part of the stomach at this entry point of the esophagus protrudes through the hiatus alongside the lower portion of the esophagus (Fig. 6-2).

pyrosis • Heartburn.

stenosis • Narrowing or stricture of a body duct or canal.

gastritis • Inflammation of the stomach.

occult bleeding • Obscure, difficult to detect bleeding concealed from observation; such a small blood loss that it can be detected only by a microscope or chemical test.

Clinical Symptoms

The hiatal hernia is associated with reflux of acid gastric contents and causes symptoms similar to those already described.

Complications

Food may easily be captured in the herniated area of the stomach and, mixed with acid and pepsin, may be regurgitated into the lower portion of the esophagus. As indicated, gastritis may occur in the herniated portion of the stomach and cause bleeding and anemia.

Treatment

Since obesity is also frequently associated with hiatal hernias, weight reduction is a primary consideration. Avoiding abdominal pressure caused by tight clothing helps to relieve discomfort. Patients need to avoid leaning over or lying down immediately after meals and to sleep with the head of the bed elevated. The last meal of the day should be eaten early enough so that no food mass is left in the herniated area or stomach on retiring. Antacids help to relieve the burning sensation. Large hiatal hernias or smaller sliding hernias may require surgical repair.

Stomach Problems

Gastrointestinal problems arising in the stomach include generalized nausea and vomiting commonly experienced by many persons and the major clinical problem of peptic ulcer disease.

Nausea and Vomiting

The problems of nausea and vomiting, the involuntary forcible expulsion of the stomach contents through the mouth, are more of a symptom than a disease. They are commonly associated with overindulgence in food or alcohol or with toxic reactions to contaminated food and allergic responses to specific foods. They are also common adverse side effects of many drugs. Vomiting may also result from inflammation, irritation, or distention of the stomach. Many other situations provoke vomiting, including high levels of certain substances in the blood, pressure within the skull, severe headaches, or balance disturbances. Persistent vomiting requires investigation by a physician.

In any case the vomiting center in the brainstem is activated and causes nerve messages to pass toward the abdomen. These messages cause the diaphragm to press down on the stomach and the muscles in the abdominal wall to contract. As a result the sphincter muscle between the stomach and the esophagus relaxes and the stomach contents are propelled upward through the esophagus toward the mouth. The epiglottis closes over the larynx to prevent the vomited material from entering the trachea. The underlying cause is usually simple, such as stomach irritation by infection or overindulgence in food or alcohol. However, it may be related to medications or may be a sign of a more serious disorder and should always be fully explored in the nutritional history.

Peptic Ulcer Disease

Incidence

In the previous century peptic ulcer disease was an uncommon disorder. However, during the early part of the 1900s, the disease began to increase greatly. In the 1940s at least 10% to 15% of men were reported to have duodenal ulcers, with unreported cases in women and children adding to those figures.[10] This increase seems to have peaked about the mid-1950s, and over the past 15 to 20 years, knowledge of the disease process and its medical management has progressed rapidly. Awareness of the possible genetic implications has increased, considering that about 40% of adult patients and 50% of children with the disease have family histories of peptic ulcer disease.[11] Yet in spite of remarkable changes in occurrence, the peptic ulcer is one of the most prevalent gastrointestinal disorders and still is a common, chronic, and recurring disease.[10] Now with an aging population, an increased number of older adult patients, men and women, have the disease. It may occur together with other diseases such as rheumatoid arthritis and cirrhosis or in other stressful illnesses or injuries such as burns. The physiologic stress of illness and the added psychologic stress contribute to stress erosive gastritis and stress ulceration.[12-14] Major complications of peptic ulcer disease are bleeding, perforation, and obstruction, but less than 2% of the patients under treatment experience such a complication in any given year.[10]

Etiology

Peptic ulcer is the general term given to an eroded mucosal lesion in the central portion of the gastrointestinal tract. The areas affected include the lower portion of the esophagus, the stomach, and the first portion of the duodenum, the duodenal bulb. Esophageal and gastric ulcers are less common. Most ulcers occur in the duodenal bulb, where gastric contents emptying into the duodenum through the pyloric valve are most concentrated. Gastric ulcers usually occur along the lesser curvature of the stomach. Peptic ulcer itself is a **benign** disease. Gastric ulcers, however, are more prone to develop into **malignant** disease.

Clinicians agree that in the past few years we have seen a revolution in our understanding of the pathophysiology of peptic ulcer disease.[15,16] Three basic causative factors seem to prevail[17]:

- *Gastric acid and pepsin.* There is hypersecretion of gastric hydrochloric acid and pepsinogen, the inactive gastric proenzyme that the acid quickly converts to the active protein enzyme pepsin. The amount of acid varies: (1) a normal to small increase with most gastric ulcers, except those situated in the lower inner curvature of the antrum near the pyloric valve, which is often associated with decreased mucosal tissue defense; (2) a larger increase with duodenal ulcers, which occurs just across the pyloric valve in the duodenal bulb, where concentrated acid flows from the stomach; and (3) massive secretions in special cases of the **Zollinger-Ellison syndrome.** Nonetheless, the classic medical dictum—"no acid, no ulcer"—still holds.
- *Nonsteroidal antiinflammatory drugs (NSAIDs).* Widely used NSAIDs, as well as the common analgesic aspirin (acetylsalicylic acid—ASA), irritate the gastric mucosal tissue and cause bleeding, erosion, and ulceration, especially with prolonged or excessive use. Recent study shows that the underlying physiologic cause of these NSAID effects relates to the protective functions of *prostaglandins,* local hormonelike compounds in the mucosal tissue (see Chapter 2). These important protective compounds regulate mucus production, bicarbonate secretion, and mucosal blood flow and acid secretion by the oxyntic (parietal) cells. NSAIDs inhibit these protective prostaglandin actions leading to acute mucosal injury. The NSAID group of drugs are so named to distinguish them from the corticosteroids, synthetic variants of the natural adrenal hormones, which have extensive side effects involving glucose and sodium metabolism. The NSAIDs include a dozen antiinflammatory drugs such as ibuprofen (Advil, Motrin), perhaps more well known because it requires no prescription, and ketoprofen (Orudis), fenoprofen (Nalfon), and others.
- *Helicobacter pylori infection. H. pylori* are common spiraling, rod-shaped bacteria inhabiting the gastrointestinal area around the pyloric valve, the lower gastric antrum, and the upper duodenal bulb. Infection by this organism, from host or bacterial factors such as a toxin, is a major determinant of chronic active gastritis. Mounting evidence supports the role of *H. pylori* as a necessary ingredient, along with acid and pepsin, in the ulcerative process. Ongoing work indicates that the organism secretes a chemical substance that controls leukocyte concentrations as part of the inflammatory process.[18] However, the reason the majority of infected persons never develop peptic ulcer disease, whether from host susceptibility or bacterial virulence, is still unclear. Studies thus far suggest that impairment of the host mucosal defenses is probably more important.[17]

Clinical Symptoms

Increased gastric tone and painful hunger contractions when the stomach is empty are basic symptoms of peptic ulcer. The amount and concentration of hydrochloric acid is increased in the duodenal ulcer but may be normal in the gastric ulcer. The complication of bleeding and risk of perforation occur when the mucosal erosion extends to involve blood vessels serving the tissue area. Nutritional deficiencies are evident in low plasma protein levels, anemia, and loss of weight. Hemorrhage may be the first sign of the ulcer in some patients. Confirmation of the diagnosis comes from clinical findings, x-ray tests, and visualization by fiberoptic gastroscopy.

Medical Management

In treating patients with peptic ulcer disease, the physician has four basic goals: (1) to alleviate the symptoms, (2) to promote healing, (3) to prevent recurrences, and (4) to prevent complications. In addition to general traditional measures, the rapidly expanding knowledge base provided by recent research and the development of a number of new drugs have increased the physician's available management tools.[10,15,16]

General therapeutic measures. Adequate rest, relaxation, and sleep have long been a foundation for general care of peptic ulcer disease to enhance the body's natural healing process. Positive stress coping and relaxation skills, which help patients deal with personal psychosocial stressors, can be learned and practiced. Simple encouragement to talk about anxieties, anger, and frustrations helps to make patients feel better, and as soon as they are able, appropriate physical activity helps work out tensions. Habits that

benign • Not malignant or recurrent; favorable for recovery.

malignant • An abnormal condition such as a tumor that tends to become progressively worse and results in death.

Zollinger-Ellison syndrome • An intractable, sometimes fulminating, atypical peptic ulcer disease, characterized by extreme gastric hyperacidity.

contribute to ulcer development, such as smoking and alcohol use, should be eliminated. Common drugs such as aspirin and other NSAIDS should be avoided.

Drug therapy. Current medical management of peptic ulcer disease has been greatly facilitated by a wider choice of drugs to control underlying physiologic causes and clinical symptoms and to support healing. Some of these major drugs are listed in the following discussion. In various ways, they suppress gastric acid and pepsin secretion, protect mucosal tissue, buffer acid, and eliminate infection.

HISTAMINE H_2-RECEPTOR ANTAGONISTS. These agents, commonly called *H_2-blockers,* are popular drugs for controlling gastric acid secretion. Histamine, a metabolic product of the amino acid histidine, occurs in all body tissues and controls widespread functions associated mainly with muscle action and secretions. Normally, histamine attaches to its specific cellular **receptors** (type H_2) on the oxyntic (parietal) acid-producing cells of the gastric mucosa and mediates their secretion of hydrochloric acid. These drugs competitively block the cell entry and function of histamine. This action makes the cells far less responsive, not only directly to the histamine but also indirectly to stimulation of acetylcholine and gastrin, thus effectively controlling acid and pepsin.[15,16] Currently four of these drugs are in use:

- *Cimetidine* (Tagamet)
- *Ranitidine* (Zantac)
- *Famotidine* (Pepcid)
- *Nizatidine* (Axid)

PROTON PUMP INHIBITORS. This is a new class of drugs, more potent than the H_2-blockers, that also suppress gastric acid, but by a different action. Without competition, they irreversibly prevent operation of the *H^+,K^+-ATPase* enzyme located in the oxyntic cell membrane that actively secretes a hydrogen (H^+) ion in exchange for a potassium (K^+) ion.[15,16] Thus without available H^+ ions, the hydrochloric acid (HCl) cannot be made. Then without the acid, ulcers heal rapidly: 50% by 2 weeks, 90% by 4 weeks, and all by 6 to 8 weeks. Thus far, the first of these drugs approved for use with ulcers resistant to conventional therapy is *omeprazole.*

MUCOSAL PROTECTORS. Drugs of this type act as *cytoprotective* agents by helping the stomach heal itself. They guard the mucosal tissue from further injury or enhance tissue-nourishing blood supply, thus allowing the tissue to heal. Both drugs in this class are relatively new and serve as examples. The first, *sucralfate,* is a complex salt of sucrose sulfate and aluminum hydroxide that provides a surface barrier over the ulcer, effectively preventing gastric acid or pepsin from reaching it to cause further erosion.[19] When the tablets or a liquid suspension are taken in the presence of the stomach acid and mucins, they form a viscous gel-like suspension that binds to the ulcer base and covers it from harm while it heals. This gel-like substance binds strongly to the defective ulcer area and to the normal mucosa. It also forms complexes with pepsin that inactivate the pepsin.[15,16] The second protective drug, *misoprostol,* is a synthetic class E_1 prostaglandin analogue. This new drug enhances mucosal defenses by increasing blood flow and mucus production and has been shown to be effective in reducing the incidence of gastric ulcers in patients taking NSAIDs, as in older persons with chronic arthritis.[15,16,20] The FDA has approved this particular prophylactic use. At this time, it is the only commercially available prostaglandin agent. Thus two cytoprotective drugs, *sucralfate* (Carafate) and *misoprostol,* are being used in peptic ulcer therapy.

ANTACIDS. Substances that counteract or neutralize acidity have long been a standard part of treatment for peptic ulcer disease. Common antacids vary in terms of their acid-neutralizing capacity, composition, and sodium content. Of the topical antacids in which sodium content is relatively low, those with a base of magnesium-aluminum or aluminum are preferred over those with a calcium base, which are thought to stimulate acid secretion as well as cause hypercalcemia.[15,16] Usually, magnesium-aluminum compounds, such as Mylanta II or Maalox TC (therapeutic choice) are the antacids of choice.[12] These drugs are effective and relatively safe when used properly.[21] Examples of the two main types include *magnesium-aluminum hydroxide* (Maalox TC, Mylanta II) and *aluminum hydroxide* (Basaljel, Amphojel).

ANTIBIOTICS. Since the discovery of the association of *Helicobacter pylori* infection with peptic ulcer disease, various antibiotics for its control are being studied. Although the organism is easily suppressed, it seems to be more difficult to eradicate.[15,16] However, combinations being used by investigators include each of the following bactericidal or suppressant agents:

- *Bismuth* (Pepto-Bismol), bismuth subsalicylate; or colloid bismuth subcitrate
- *Metronidazole* (Flagyl, Protostat), a bacterial and protozoan killer
- *Amoxicillin* (Amoxil, Polymox), a penicillin derivative; or *tetracycline* (Achromycin-V, Panmycin), a frequently used wide spectrum antibiotic

Other drugs for general needs include substitution of the mild, nonirritating analgesic drug *acetaminophen* (Tylenol) for commonly used aspirin and other NSAIDs. Also, if mild sedation is needed, the physician may briefly use a tricyclic antidepressant such as *amitriptyline* (Elavil) to aid the initial need for relaxation and sleep.

TABLE 6-3

Recurrent Peptic Ulcer Risk Factors

Chance of recurrence	Risk factors
Possible	Positive family history
	Emotional stress
	Continued use of concentrated alcohol
Good	History of recurrences and complications
	Continued use of aspirin and other NSAIDs
	Increased *Helicobacter pylori* infection
Strong	Poor compliance with maintenance diet-drug plan
	Continued smoking (10 or more cigarettes/day)
	Gastric acid hypersecretion

Adapted from Earnest DL: Maintenance therapy in peptic ulcer disease, *Med Clin North Am* 75(4):1013, 1991.

Overall, effective medical management in general has made major advances in correcting factors that promote peptic ulcer formation or failure to heal and in decreasing its incidence. The main challenge now is to develop a maintenance therapy that prevents its recurrence.[22] Currently the best approach seems to include continuous low-dose drug therapy, intermittent full-dose treatment, or symptomatic self-care with the same agents used to heal the ulcer. Success rates hinge on the relative strength of risk factors that influence recurrence (Table 6-3).

Nutritional Management

Over the past 15 to 20 years the revolutionary advances in scientific knowledge of peptic ulcer disease and development of many new effective drugs have also brought welcome reevaluation of the role of nutrition in its basic care. Most gastroenterologists, both academic and clinical, now see little or no role for diet in the traditional sense and certainly ascribe no therapeutic value to the old restrictive milk-based "ulcer diets," which in some ways, such as acid stimulation and animal fat, may even be harmful.[15,16,23] In its earlier position paper, the American Dietetic Association has long since stated the ineffectiveness and potential harm of the past generation of bland diet routines.[24] Nutrition specialists, in their teaching and clinical practice, have fully agreed.[25,26]

Current positive nutritional approach. Instead of former highly restrictive "special" diets for peptic ulcer disease, which were often nutritionally inadequate, the current nutritional practice is that of the basic health maintenance or preventive approach in overall health care today.[27] As with any disease process involving tissue injury, the prime nutritional requirement is sufficient energy-nutrient intake supplied by a regular well-balanced diet to support the primary medical management of (1) tissue healing and (2) tissue maintenance of its structural and functional integrity. Initial and periodic nutritional assessment is needed to determine energy-nutrient status and any areas of individual need.

Dietary principles. The basic nutritional principles of a well-balanced diet are found in the regular guidelines of the RDA energy-nutrient standards and the U.S. Dietary Guidelines for health promotion (see Chapter 1). In addition to the major goal of optimal nutritional support, a second dietary goal is to avoid stimulating excess acid secretion and directly irritating the gastric mucosa. Only a few related food factors or habits have been shown to cause excess acid secretion and irritation[25,26]:

- *Meal pattern.* Eat three regular meals a day without frequent snacks, especially at bedtime. Any food intake stimulates more acid output.
- *Food quantity.* Avoid stomach distention with large quantities of food at a meal.
- *Milk intake.* Avoid drinking milk frequently. It stimulates significant gastric acid secretion, has only a transient buffering effect, and its animal fat content is undesirable. Also, the milk sugar lactose creates problems of abdominal cramping, gas, and diarrhea for many persons with lactose intolerance caused by a deficiency of the enzyme lactase.
- *Seasonings.* Individual tolerance is the rule. However, several agents have caused variable results and may need to be watched: hot chili peppers, black pepper, chili powder.
- *Dietary fiber.* There is no evidence for restricting dietary fiber. Some fibers, especially soluble forms, are beneficial (see *To Probe Further,* p. 106).
- *Coffee.* Avoid regular and decaffeinated coffee. Coffee stimulates acid secretion and may cause dyspepsia. The comparative effect of regular tea and colas may be milder with some persons, but these beverages also stimulate acid secretion.
- *Citric acid juices.* These juices may induce gastric reflux and discomfort in some persons.

receptor • Any one of various specific protein molecules in surface membranes of cells and cell organelles to which complementary molecules, such as hormones, neurotransmitters, drugs, viruses, or other antigens or antibodies may become bound.

Dietary Fiber and Peptic Ulcer Disease

TO PROBE FURTHER

With the current liberalization to a regular diet for persons with peptic ulcer disease, the question previously raised about dietary fiber in this treatment program is of particular interest. A group of European clinicians have studied this question.

The investigators randomly selected 73 patients for their study from a large group of recently healed peptic ulcer patients. Over 6 months the control group of 35 patients were fed the old traditional low-fiber or bland diet. The study group of 38 patients were fed a moderately high-fiber diet, with emphasis on whole grain breads and cereals, including wheat or mixtures of wheat with barley, rye, and oat, as well as liberal use of fibrous vegetables and fruits.

At the end of the test period, 28 patients (80%) in the control group fed the low-fiber diet experienced recurrence of their ulcer disease. In the study group fed the high-fiber diet, however, only 17 patients (45%) had a recurrence of their disease. The investigators concluded from their study that, contrary to popular opinion and practice, more attention to dietary fiber in nutritional therapy for duodenal ulcer may indeed be beneficial. They noted, however, that the most frequent recurrence of disease in both groups was among smokers as compared with nonsmokers. In a subsequent study by this same group of investigators, the addition of low-dose antacids to the fiber diet enhanced the healing effect.

Current medical management of peptic ulcer disease vindicates these earlier test results in effect by the use of regular diets for all ulcer patients. Now aided by the development of new effective drugs, practical care no longer involves the old bland low-fiber diets, much to the positive nutritional support benefit for the patient.

REFERENCES

Marotta RB, Floch MH: Diet and nutrition in ulcer disease, *Med Clin North Am* 75(4):967, 1991.

Rubin W: Medical treatment of peptic ulcer disease, *Med Clin North Am* 75(4):981, 1991.

Rydning A et al: Prophylactic effect of dietary fiber in duodenal ulcer disease, *Lancet* 2:736, 1982.

Rydning A et al: Healing of benign gastric ulcer with low-dose antacids and fiber diet, *Gastroenterology* 91:56, 1986.

- *Alcohol.* Avoid alcohol in concentrated forms, such as 40% (80 proof) alcohol. Other less concentrated forms of wine, taken with food in moderate amounts, are tolerated well by some patients. Avoid beer; it has been shown to be a potent stimulant of gastric acid. For patients who find it particularly difficult to avoid alcohol and coffee completely, some physicians have suggested they may try a small serving of wine with the dinner meal occasionally or a small cup *(demitasse)* of coffee at the close of the meal to minimize the acid secretion.
- *Smoking.* The habit of smoking is often associated with food intake. It is best eliminated completely at any time. It not only affects gastric acid secretion but also influences the effectiveness of drug therapy.

The following list is a summary of the principles of nutrition and diet for support of medical management of peptic ulcer disease.

Eat a regular diet with optimal energy-nutrient balances to meet individual health needs.

Respect individual responses or tolerances to specific foods experienced at any time, remembering that the same food may evoke different responses at different times depending on the stress factor.

Eat three regular meals a day and avoid between-meal snacks, remembering that every time food is taken into the stomach, it causes acid secretion.

Eat slowly and savor the food in a calm environment.

Avoid common irritants with foods such as hot chili peppers or black pepper.

Avoid frequently drinking milk and regular and decaffeinated coffee, tea, and colas.

Avoid alcohol, especially high-proof beverages and beer.

Avoid aspirin and nonsteroidal antiinflammatory drugs (NSAIDs).

Eliminate smoking—this not only helps the ulcer, but it also helps food taste better.

Personal focus. Sound nutritional management plays an important supportive role in the total medical care of peptic ulcer disease. The individual must be the focus of treatment. The patient is not "an ulcer," but a *person* with an ulcer. The course of the disease is conditioned by the patient's unique makeup and life situation, and its presence in turn affects the patient's life. Therefore two basic principles guide this personal approach:

1. *The patient must be treated as an individual.* A careful initial history gives information about daily living situations, attitudes, food reactions, and tolerances. On the basis of such a history, a reasonable and adequate nutritional support program may be worked out with the patient.
2. *The activity of the patient's ulcer influences dietary management.* During acute periods of active ulceration, a more moderate food plan may be needed to control acidity and initiate healing, based on nutritional needs and individual tolerances. However, when pain disappears, regular meals may be planned using a variety of foods. Sound nutrition and improved emotional outlook, and thus recovery, are more likely to be supported by such a program. During quiet periods and for long-term prophylaxis when the patient is asymptomatic, judicious choices from a wide range of foods and regular, unhurried eating habits provide the best course of action.

Small Intestine Diseases

Conditions of Malabsorption and Diarrhea

Malabsorption

There are multiple causes of a malabsorption condition.[28] It may result from maldigestion problems, for example, pancreatic disorders, biliary disease, bacterial overgrowth, or ileal disease. It may also result from intestinal stasis, mucosal alterations, intestinal resection, or lymphatic obstruction. Malabsorption may reflect an underlying genetic disease such as cystic fibrosis and its complication of pancreatic insufficiency, which in turn creates a lack of the pancreatic enzymes amylase, trypsin, and lipase (see Chapter 24). It may be induced by a deficiency of intestinal enzymes such as disaccharidases, as in lactose intolerance caused by lactase deficiency. It may result from neoplastic disease such as cancer and its treatment by radiation and chemotherapy, which may affect the absorbing surface mucosa. And malabsorption may reflect biochemical defects such as in pernicious anemia or gluten-induced enteropathy.

Diarrhea

General diarrhea may result from basic dietary excesses, with fermentation of sugars involved or excess fiber stimulation of intestinal muscle function.[29] In other cases it may result from a specific foodborne infectious organism or from acute food poisoning with bacterial toxin. In the case of lactose intolerance, the accumulated concentration of lactose in the intestine creates increased osmotic pressure, effectively drawing water into the gut and stimulating *hypermotility,* abdominal cramping and diarrhea (see Chapter 6). Milk treated with lactase enzyme is tolerated by these persons without the intestinal difficulty encountered with regular milk. Secretory, osmotic, and inflammatory processes in the intestine result in increased losses of fluid and electrolytes from diarrhea (see *Issues and Answers,* p. 117).[30]

Celiac Sprue

Celiac sprue is an intestinal malabsorption disease that affects children and adults. Sensitive persons have a defect in mucosal cells that causes an inability to metabolize *gluten,* a plant protein in grains such as wheat and rye (see Chapter 6). The offending agent in gluten is the *gliadin* fraction. As little as 3 g/day of gliadin in a sensitive person's diet produces diarrhea and steatorrhea. In adults with this disease, the mucosal tissue breakdown may diffusely involve the entire intestinal mucosa, with more severe effects on the upper small intestine. As a result, absorption of all nutrients is greatly impaired, especially fat, although absorption of sugar, protein, vitamins, and minerals is also hindered. Clinical symptoms and nutritional management with a special *gluten-free diet* are discussed in detail in Chapter 5.

Inflammatory Bowel Disease

The general term *inflammatory bowel disease (IBD)* is now used to apply to two conditions having similar symptoms but different underlying clinical problems—*Crohn's disease* and *ulcerative colitis.* Both of these conditions produce extended mucosal tissue lesions. However, although they differ in extent and nature of these lesions, they have been classed medically in a single group because they are similar in their clinical symptoms and management.[31,32]

Incidence

The incidence of these diseases, especially Crohn's disease, has increased worldwide. A recent epidemiologic study in Denmark, for example, indicated a sixfold increase in Crohn's disease, present in all age groups and both sexes, over the 25-year period from 1962 to 1987.[31] In the United States incidence rates of 4 to 6 per 100,000 adults per year and prevalence rates of 40 to 100 per 100,000 have been reported.[33] Crohn's disease and ulcerative colitis have similar clinical and pathologic features despite differences in their incidence in ethnic populations, climates, dietary habits, and customs. Crohn's disease is particularly prevalent in industrialized areas of the world. It also appears among otherwise low-risk persons who move from rural to urban centers. These factors suggest a role for pathogenic agents in the environment. The demographic characteristics of patients are the same

CLINICAL APPLICATION

Drug Therapy Effects on Nutritional Status of Patients with Inflammatory Bowel Disease

Those involved in the care of patients with inflammatory bowel disease must consider the effect of drug therapy on their nutritional status in addition to the effects of malabsorption caused by the disease itself. Commonly used medications with significant effects on patient nutrition include prednisone, sulfasalazine, azathioprine or mercaptopurine, and cholestyramine.

Prednisone is a corticosteroid and thus triggers gluconeogenesis. As a result it stimulates appetite, protein catabolism, and fluid retention. Prednisone has an antagonistic effect on vitamin D, resulting in reduced calcium transport and ultimately the bone disease osteomalacia. The drug also inhibits collagen synthesis, a function of ascorbic acid, and the complete breakdown of tryptophan, a function of vitamin B_6, thereby increasing the patient's need for these nutrients as well.

Although *sulfasalazine* (sulfa drug) is an effective treatment for inflammatory bowel disease, it affects nutritional status by inducing nausea, vomiting, and anorexia. These effects may be lessened by taking the drug with food. In addition, plenty of water (about 1.5 qt/day) is needed during the day to facilitate renal elimination. Folate deficiency is associated with this drug, either because of the mild hemolysis or decreased absorption induced in many patients. Iron needs are also sometimes increased as a result of the hemolysis.

Azathioprine (Imuran) and its active derivative *mercaptopurine* (Purinethol), immunosuppressants also used in cancer chemotherapy, carry side effects of nausea and vomiting, sore mouth, and loss of appetite. These effects cause loss of nutrients, risk malnutrition, and require the nutritional support efforts described in the following discussion.

Cholestyramine (Questran) is an anion exchange resin used to treat diarrhea. It is associated with malabsorption of fat and fat-soluble vitamins. Iron and vitamin B_{12} requirements are sometimes increased as well because of reduced absorption.

To correct specific nutrient deficiencies during drug therapy, first identify the specific deficiency, and then plan to correct it by foods, oral supplementation, or formula. Although several elemental and chemically defined formulas are available for tube feeding, the oral route is preferred. Most patients can consume a nutritious diet as long as levels of fat and lactose, both poorly absorbed in inflammatory bowel disease, are carefully monitored. In addition, conference with the physician about the possibility of reducing the medication dosage to enhance the patient's recovery from damage caused by malabsorption or nutrient antagonist effects of the drug may be desired. ◆

REFERENCES

Christie PM, Hill GL: Effect of intravenous nutrition on nutrition and function in acute attacks of inflammatory bowel disease, *Gastroenterology* 99:730, 1990.

Peppercorn MA: Advances in drug therapy for inflammatory bowel disease, *Ann Intern Med* 112:50, 1990.

Podolsky DK: Inflammatory bowel disease, Part II, *N Engl J Med* 325(14):1008, 1991.

Polk DB et al: Improved growth and disease activity after intermittent administration of a defined formula in children with Crohn's disease, *JPEN* 16(6):499, 1992.

for both diseases. Incidence is highest among teenagers, with a secondary peak at ages 55 to 60.

Etiology

Although epidemiologic and clinical studies continue to increase knowledge of the disease processes involved, the causes of these two inflammatory bowel diseases remain unknown. A number of observations indicate that genetic factors may predispose persons to the development of IBD, in particular (1) its increased incidence among children whose parents have IBD; (2) its incidence in certain close-knit population groups; and (3) the high rate of IBD among identical (monozygotic) twins compared with fraternal (dizygotic) twins.[34,35]

Ulcerative colitis and Crohn's disease have severe, often devastating tissue effects and nutritional consequences, but they are distinguished by two main differences: (1) *anatomic distribution* of the inflammatory process and (2) the nature of *tissue changes* involved. First, Crohn's disease occurs in any part of the gastrointestinal tract. About 40% of the patients have colon and small intestine disease, about 30% have disease in the small intestine, and the remaining 30% have only colorectal disease. In contrast, ulcerative colitis is confined to the colon and rectum. Second, in Crohn's disease, the inflammatory tissue changes become a chronic recurring illness, the lesions of which penetrate any part of the intestinal wall (that is, a **transmural** pattern occurs), which may penetrate the entire wall. Often this extensive tissue involvement leads to stricture, with partial or complete obstruction, and to **fistula** formation.[32] In contrast, inflammatory tissue changes in ulcerative colitis are usually acute, lasting for a brief period and limited to the mucosal and submucosal tissue layers of the intestine.

Clinical Symptoms

The common clinical symptom is a chronic bloody diarrhea that occurs at night as well as during the day. Ulceration of the mucous membrane of the intestine leads to various associated nutritional problems such as anorexia, nutritional edema, anemia, avitaminosis, protein losses, negative nitrogen balance, dehydration, and electrolyte disturbances. Clinicians have observed evidence of specific deficiencies of zinc and vitamin E, with improvement occurring when supplements of the particular nutrient involved are taken. There is general weight loss, often general malnutrition, fever, skin lesions, and arthritic joint involvement. In Crohn's disease, the overall malnutrition resembles kwashiorkor and is an important cause of abnormal immunologic function.[36]

Medical Management

The medical management of IBD centers on drug therapy to control the inflammatory process and promote tissue healing. In addition to the mainstays for medical therapy that have remained unchanged for decades, the ongoing development of new agents, better analogues of older agents, and improved modes of drug delivery hold even greater promise for future therapy.[32,37] Currently, the physician has available three types of drugs to use in developing individual therapy for IBD: (1) a corticosteroid—*prednisone*; (2) an antiinflammatory agent—*sulfasalazine,* which is a combination of sulfapyridine and 5-aminosalicylic acid; and (3) an immunosuppressant agent especially for Crohn's disease—*mercaptopurine.*[32,38] Effects of these drugs become important aspects of planning supportive nutritional care (see the *Clinical Application*, p. 108).

Nutritional Management

Nutritional therapy centers on supporting the healing process and avoiding nutritional deficiency states. Therapy in serious conditions includes elemental diets—absorbable isotonic preparations of amino acids, glucose, fat, minerals, and vitamins. In patients who tolerate these supplements, gastrointestinal protein losses diminish and nutrition improves, accompanied by clinical remission. In cases where the small bowel has been shortened or the disease process is extensive, as in Crohn's disease, parenteral intravenous hyperalimentation (TPN) is most effective (see Chapter 4).[15] Such vigorous nutritional therapy is helpful in childhood Crohn's disease to prevent severe growth retardation. Nutritional repletion is accompanied by improvement in symptoms. There is diminished gastrointestinal secretion and motility, decreased disease activity, relief of partial intestinal obstruction, occasional closure of enteric fistulas, and renewed immunocompetence. Nutrient supplements are usually necessary to avoid deficiencies in agents such as zinc, copper, chromium, selenium, and other nutrients.

General Continuing Nutritional Management

Continuing dietary therapy for ulcerative colitis and Crohn's disease is based on restoring optimal nutrient intake, removing deficits, preventing local trauma to the inflamed areas, and controlling less easily absorbed materials such as fats. To help secure additional kcalories, medium-chain triglycerides (MCT), as in the commercial preparations Portagen or MCT oil, may be used instead of regular fats. The focus of the diet centers on protein and energy, minerals and vitamins, and texture, with supplemental feedings as needed.

High protein. There are large losses of protein from the intestinal mucosal tissue by exudation and bleeding, as well as losses associated with impaired intestinal absorption. Healing occurs only if adequate protein is provided. The total diet needs to supply adequate protein, about 100 g/day in highly malnourished patients, for necessary tissue synthesis and healing. Tasteful ways of including protein foods of high biologic value (eggs, meat, and cheese) can be devised to tempt poor appetites. If milk causes some difficulty, it may be omitted at first, then added as tolerated individually.

High energy. About 2500 to 3000 kcal/day may be needed to restore nutritional deficits from daily losses in the stools and the consequent weight loss. Also, the negative nitrogen balance is overcome only if sufficient kcalories are present to support and protect the main anabolic function of protein.

Increased minerals and vitamins. When anemia is present, iron supplements may be used. Extra vitamins associated with the healing process and with the metabolism of the increased kcalories and protein are especially needed. These are the B vitamins, including thiamin, riboflavin, and niacin, and ascorbic acid. Trace minerals such as zinc, which participates in tissue synthesis, along with vitamin E, which contributes to tissue integrity, are also essential. Usually supplements of these vitamins and minerals are routine. Potassium therapy may be indicated if undue losses from diarrhea and tissue destruction occur, causing hypokalemia.

Dietary fiber control. Over the past years, on the belief that dietary fiber or residue would irritate the mucosal lining, a diet low in dietary fiber or residue has sometimes been used until healing is well-estab-

transmural • Through the wall of an organ; extending through or affecting the entire thickness of the wall of an organ or cavity.

lished. However, the old bland, low-residue diets, most of which restricted milk, are based on old literature, tradition, and studies on laboratory animals, factors which some investigators even then seemed to suggest.[39,40] These unappetizing and often less than nourishing diets seem to have been based more on past anecdotal accounts and beliefs rather than on human scientific study.[41] A more recent 5-year trial has shown that Crohn's disease patients on regular diets, including normal use of whole grain foods, fruits, and vegetables, required 20% less hospitalization than the control group fed traditional bland, low-residue diets and were subjected to fewer operations. These results suggest that routine low-fiber, low-residue diets for inflammatory bowel disease should go the way of these diets for use with diverticular disease. Rather, as is the current therapy in peptic ulcer disease, a regular highly nourishing diet, respecting individual tolerances and disease status, seems more appropriate. Certainly, as some clinicians indicate in the case of Crohn's disease, it warrants further research attention.[42] The primary concern is supplying the necessary nutrition in as appetizing a manner as possible.

Perhaps no other condition better illustrates the need for a close working relationship between the physician, clinical dietitian, nurse, and patient than does inflammatory bowel disease. The appetite is poor, but adequate nutritional intake is imperative. In many creative ways, individually explored and implemented, the fundamental therapeutic needs must be met. This is done through vigorous nutritional care using a range of feeding modes, including enteral or parenteral nutrition support as needed, always with personal supportive warmth and encouragement.[43-45]

Short-Bowel Syndrome

Etiology

Short-bowel syndrome (SBS) is a pattern of varying metabolic and physiologic consequences that occur with extensive dysfunction of the small or large intestine.[46] It results from intrinsic disease such as Crohn's disease or radiation enteritis, surgical bypass, or massive surgical resection of parts of the intestine. These resections may be required for massive abdominal injury and trauma, vascular problems such as blood clots leading to death of the tissue involved, Crohn's disease with complications such as extensive fistulas, radiation injury, congenital abnormalities, or malignancy.

Clinical Symptoms

Clearly, the severity of the clinical problem remaining and its clinical symptoms vary with factors such as length and location of the remaining intestine, presence or absence of the ileocecal valve, any disease of the colon, and mucosal integrity and function of the remaining gut. Consider the complex nature and functions of the small intestine, for example. Its estimated length is between 12 and 20 ft (about 365 to 600 cm) and it receives about 7 to 9 L/day of nutrient-filled fluid. So efficiently does it do its specialized jobs along the way that only 100 to 200 cc of feces remains to be excreted. Now think of the metabolic impact if 80% or more of the ileum, which has a functional length of about 400 cm, is surgically removed. Among numerous other results, hepatic synthesis cannot maintain a sufficient circulating bile pool to sustain normal fat digestion, and steatorrhea and a chain of metabolic events follow.[46] Also, without the normal enterohepatic circulation that occurs in the distal part of the ileum, the liver's usually efficient regulation of cholesterol is affected.[47]

Nutritional Management

Because degrees of surgical resection create different problems, the nutritional management of each SBS patient must be tailored to meet individual needs and residual functional capacity. Early feeding usually supplies nutritional support needs through enteral oral supplements or enteral tube-feeding, if possible, or by TPN if indicated (see Chapters 3 and 4).[46] Frequent monitoring of nutritional responses, especially fluid and electrolyte balances and malnutrition signs, is essential. Later weaning to an oral diet with vitamin and mineral supplementation follows as tolerated, with continued nutritional assessment. Vitamin D (cholecalciferol) deficiency is one of the common nutritional deficits but can be more easily met with its intermediate metabolic product, oral 25-hydroxycholecalciferol.[48] As adaptation occurs, some moderate liberalization of early fat restriction may add needed kcalories in the form of more easily absorbed medium-chain triglycerides (MCT oil) in foods.

Large Intestine Diseases

Diverticular Disease

Etiology

At points of weakened musculature in the bowel wall, along the track of blood vessels entering the bowel from without, small tubular sacs may form that protrude from the intestinal lumen of the colon. The direct cause is a progressive increase in intraluminal pressures from segmental circular muscle contractions that normally move the remaining food mass along and form the feces for elimination. When pressures become sufficiently high in one of these segments, and dietary fiber is insufficient to maintain the necessary intraluminal bulk for preventing development of high intracolonic pressures, a small protrusion of the muscle layer, a *diverticulum,* forms at that point. The formation and presence of these small diverticula in the colon, not uncommon in elderly persons, is called *diverticulosis.* This condition does not present any problem unless these small sacs become infected and inflamed from fecal irritation and colon bacteria, a state called **diverticulitis.** The commonly used collective term covering diverticulosis and diverticulitis is *diverticular disease.*

Clinical Symptoms

As the inflammatory process grows, increased hypermotility and intraluminal pressures from luminal segmentation cause pain. The pain and tenderness are usually localized in the lower left side of the abdomen and are accompanied by nausea, vomiting, distention, intestinal spasm, and fever. If the process continues, intestinal obstruction or perforation may necessitate surgical intervention.

Nutritional Management

Diverticular disease is a common gastrointestinal disorder among middle-aged and elderly persons and may often be accompanied by malnutrition. Thus assessment of nutritional status of these patients, including sensitive laboratory tests, is important so that aggressive nutritional therapy hastens recovery from an attack and shortens the hospital stay.[49] Generally, the most reliable laboratory test indicators are the serum proteins with short half-lives, prealbumin (2 days) and transferrin (8 to 10 days), as compared with the longer half-life of albumin (20 days) (see Chapter 7). Current studies and clinical practice have demonstrated better management of chronic diverticular disease with an increased amount of dietary fiber than with old practices of restricting fiber. In acute episodes of the active disease, the amount of dietary fiber may need to be moderately reduced. The relationship of dietary fiber and diverticular disease has been further reinforced by studies of populations, such as those in Japan since the current westernizing of its culture.

Irritable Bowel Syndrome

Incidence

Data from the second National Health and Nutrition Examination Survey (NHANES II, 1976-1980) indicated that almost 5 million Americans, about 3% of the population, self-reported problems consistent with the condition now called irritable bowel syndrome (IBS). The rates reported for women were 3.2 times those for men, 5.3 times higher for whites than for blacks, and highest among those ages 45 to 64 years.[50,51] Follow-up national surveys in the mid-1980s documented between 2.4 and 3.5 yearly visits to physicians for IBS and more than 2.2 million medications prescribed.[51] Currently, gastroenterologists estimate that 15% to 20% of the general U.S. population have symptoms of IBS, about 5% of whom seek medical help and become patients.[52]

Etiology

Although the IBS is one of the most common of all gastrointestinal disorders, its precise nature and cause continue to puzzle practitioners. It has aptly been called by some gastroenterologists "a dilemma within a dilemma surrounded by dilemmas."[53]

Clinical Symptoms

A recent international working team report has more clearly defined IBS for medical diagnostic guidance as a functional, nonorganic disorder and has outlined its characteristic symptoms for general care.[54] The three major types of symptoms of IBS have been classified as follows: (1) *pain,* chronic and recurrent, occurring in any area of the abdominal region; (2) *bowel dysfunction,* small volume, varying from constipation or diarrhea to an intermittent combination of both; and (3) *flatulence,* excess gas formation with increased distention and bloating, accompanied by rumbling abdominal sounds *(borborygmi),* belching, and passing of gas. Patients appear tense and anxious, and stress is a major triggering factor. Studies indicate that these patients with IBS have high scores on a variety of scales measuring depression, anxiety, interpersonal sensitivity, and *somatization*—the transference of anxiety to body symptoms, but with no pattern of psychologic symptoms. Somatization is unique to patients with this diagnosis.[55]

Medical Management

Over the years management of IBS has frustrated many physicians, as well as their patients. After comprehensive tests and examinations to rule out organic disease, drug therapy consists largely of (1) moderate use of *antidepressant agents* for transient reactions to situational stress factors seen in the larger patient group in general medical care, with referrals as needed to counseling or psychiatric services, and

diverticulitis • Inflammation of "pockets" of tissue (diverticula) in the lining of the mucous membrane of the colon.

(2) frequent use of *anticholinergic agents* for reducing the impact of neurotransmitters of the enteric nervous system on smooth muscles of the intestine causing spastic contractions.[53,56] Other drugs used include stool bulk formers and antidiarrheal agents.

Nutritional Management

Because the nature of IBS varies among individual patients, a highly individual and personal approach to nutritional care is essential. The initial nutritional assessment must include a detailed dietary history. This history should include much more data than the food habits and practices in a regular diet history (see Chapter 1). It must compile specific symptom-related information, including date of the IBS onset and reaction-associated foods such as wheat, corn, dairy products, coffee, tea, or citrus fruits that may suggest food intolerance or an IBS subset of food allergy.[57,58] The dietary history must include a sensitive and supportive personal history of the role of stress-related triggering of attacks and current living situation, personal concerns, and experiences associated with symptoms. In addition to this detailed history, baseline measures of nutritional status should include the usual anthropometry with calculations for body mass index and midarm muscle circumference, as well as biochemical markers of short-life serum proteins such as prealbumin or transferrin, with the longer-life turnover of albumin for comparison (see Chapter 1).

With this careful history as a base, a reasonable and appropriate food plan may be developed with the patient, followed by periodic food records and related symptoms for continued counseling and adjustments. In general, the food plan gives attention to the following basic principles:

- *Increase dietary fiber.* Increased dietary fiber aids functions of the large intestine mainly by (1) increasing and softening the fecal output, (2) regulating transit time of the final food mass through the colon, and (3) lowering segmental pressures in the final section of the colon, especially the sigmoid area. A regular diet with optimal energy-nutrient composition and dietary fiber food sources—such as whole grains, fruits, and vegetables—should provide the basic therapy. Then moderate supplemental dietary fiber may be used if needed, with controlled additions of bran, often better tolerated in cooked forms, or more soluble forms of bulking agents such as psyllium seed products (Metamucil).
- *Recognize gas formers.* Some foods are recognized gas formers for many people because of the presence of known constituents such as certain oligosaccharides as in the case of legumes. Others provide gaseous discomfort on an individual basis, such as the cruciferous family of vegetables including cabbage, brussels sprouts, broccoli, turnips, and radishes. A new product containing an agent to assist the intestinal digestion of oligosaccharides in beans and other legumes, appropriately called "beanase" enzyme by the manufacturer (Lactaid), is being marketed under the trade name Beano. The use of a few drops of the agent mixed with mashed beans has been shown to reduce breath hydrogen, and its clinical value is undergoing continued testing.[56]
- *Respect food intolerances.* Lactose intolerance, caused by a deficiency of the digestive enzyme lactase, is a well-known disorder resulting in intestinal cramping, bloating, and diarrhea after drinking milk or eating dairy products. However, preparations of lactase enzyme such as Lactaid allow lactose-intolerant persons to use dairy products. In other cases similar intestinal problems for some persons result from either a sorbitol or fructose intolerance. Sorbitol is a sugar alcohol used in many dietetic foods and drugs as an artificial sweetener. Only 10 g of sorbitol solution produces abdominal pain, bloating, and diarrhea in such intolerant adults.[59] Significant amounts of sorbitol are found in common foods such cherries, pears, peaches, and plums; as a sweetener in sugarless gum and chocolate; and in dietetic jams and jellies. Fructose is simple sugar found in fruits and is a digestive product of sucrose. Symptoms relate to the fermentation effect of colonic bacteria on malabsorbed sugars.[57]
- *Reduce total fat intake.* Excess fat delays gastric emptying and contributes to malabsorption problems in the intestines and diarrhea. For healthier diets in general, moderation in total dietary fat also helps reduce risks of fatty buildup in major blood vessels that leads to heart disease problems.
- *Avoid large meals.* Large amounts of food in one meal create discomfort from gastric distention and gas generated in the stomach, especially meals of high kcaloric content. Smaller, more frequent meals may reduce these symptoms.
- *Decrease air-swallowing habits.* Certain habits of eating contribute to gas swallowed or generated in the stomach. These include eating rapidly, in addition to eating large amounts, and excessive fluid intake, especially carbonated beverages. Habits of chewing gum and smoking also contribute.

For any member of the health care team helping a patient to manage IBS, success is often elusive. However, experienced practitioners have learned that an honest and creative relationship with the patient is basic.[60] Two such approachs include avoiding dogma and helping the patient to cope. Life-style and diet are highly personal and individual. Thus wise nutritional management involves both in realistic counseling toward a healthier life.

Constipation

A common disorder, usually of short duration, constipation is characterized by retention of feces in the colon beyond the normal emptying time. It is a problem for which Americans spend more than $200 million each year for over-the-counter laxatives and untold millions more for prescription drugs and other medical services. The regularity of elimination is highly individual, and it is not necessary for good health to have a bowel movement every day. Extended constipation is usually the result of nervous tension and worry and changes in social settings. Such situations include vacations and travel, thus alterations in usual routines. It may also be caused by prolonged use of laxatives and cathartics, low-fiber diets, or lack of exercise, which cause decreased intestinal muscle tone. General measures such as improved dietary and bowel habits, life-style changes with emphasis on a regular well-balanced diet with increased dietary fiber, and increased exercise and relaxation periods are usually sufficient to remedy the situation. The diet should include whole grains, vegetables, fruits, especially naturally laxative fruits such as dried prunes and figs; and increased fluid intake. If chronic constipation persists, however, supplemental agents that increase stool bulk may be necessary; these include bran or more soluble fiber forms. Taking laxatives or enemas on a regular basis is to be avoided. The problem of constipation occurs in all age groups, but is almost epidemic in elderly persons. In all cases a personalized approach to management of constipation is fundamental.[61]

To Sum Up

The nutritional management of gastrointestinal disease is based on careful consideration of four major factors: (1) *secretory functions,* providing the chemical agents and environment necessary for digestion to occur; (2) *neuromuscular functions,* required for motility and mechanical digestion; (3) *absorptive functions,* enhancing the entry of nutrients into the circulatory system; and (4) *psychologic factors,* reflected by changes in gastrointestinal function.

Esophageal problems vary widely from simple *dysphagia* to serious disease or obstruction. Nutritional therapy and mode of intake vary according to the degree of dysfunction.

Peptic ulcer disease is a common gastrointestinal problem affecting millions of Americans. It is an erosion of the mucosal lining, mainly the duodenal bulb and less commonly the lower antrum portion of the stomach. It results in increased gastric tone and painful hunger contractions on an empty stomach, as well as nutritional problems such as low plasma protein levels, anemia, and weight loss. Current medical management consists of acid and infection control with a coordinated system of new drugs, rest, and a regular diet with a few food and drink considerations to supply the essential nutritional support for tissue healing.

Intestinal diseases are classified as (1) *anatomic changes,* such as the development of small tubular sacs branching off the main alimentary canal in *diverticular disease;* (2) *malabsorption,* from multiple maldigestive and malabsorptive conditions; and (3) *inflammatory bowel disease,* the result of mucosal changes and infectious processes, as seen in *ulcerative colitis* or *Crohn's disease* or in *short-bowel syndrome* resulting from surgical resection of parts of the intestine. Nutritional therapy usually involves fluid and electrolyte replacement, modification in the diet's protein and energy content and food texture, and increased vitamins and minerals, with continuous adjustment of the diet according to changes in toleration for specific foods. In some cases intravenous therapy, or TPN, is required. However, oral intake of fluids, supplements, formula, or food is generally preferred.

QUESTIONS FOR REVIEW

1. What is the basic principle of diet planning for patients with esophageal problems? Outline a general nutritional care plan for a patient with gastroesophageal reflux disease complicated by a hiatal hernia.
2. In current practice, what are the basic principles of diet planning for patients with peptic ulcer disease? How do these principles differ from former traditional therapy?
3. Outline a course of nutritional management for a person with peptic ulcer disease based on the current approaches to medical management. How would you plan nutritional education for continuing self-care and avoidance of recurrence?
4. Describe the etiology, clinical signs, and treatment of the following intestinal diseases: malabsorption and diarrhea, inflammatory bowel disease, diverticular disease, irritable bowel syndrome, and constipation.

REFERENCES

1. Zeman FJ: *Clinical nutrition and dietetics,* ed 2, New York, 1991, Macmillan Publishing.
2. Yankelson S et al: Dysphagia: a unique interdisciplinary treatment approach, *Top Clin Nutr* 4:43, 1989.
3. Loughlin GM: Respiratory consequences of dysfunctional swallowing and aspiration, *Dysphagia* 3:126, 1989.

4. Tuchman DN: Cough, choke, sputter: the evaluation of the child with dysfunctional swallowing, *Dysphagia* 3:111, 1989.
5. Dantas RD et al: Effects of swallowed bolus variables on oral and pharyngeal phases of swallowing, *Am J Physiol* 258:G675, 1990.
6. Stanek K et al: Factors affecting use of food and commercial agents to thicken liquids for individuals with swallowing disorders, *J Am Diet Assoc* 92(4):488, 1992.
7. Zeman FJ, Ney DM: *Applications of clinical nutrition,* Englewood Cliffs, NJ, 1988, Prentice Hall.
8. Gelfand MD: Gastroesophageal reflux disease, *Med Clin North Am* 75(4):923, 1991.
9. Kitchin LI, Castell DO: Rationale and efficiency of conservative therapy for gastroesophageal reflux disease, *Arch Intern Med* 151:448, 1991.
10. Katz J: The course of peptic ulcer disease, *Med Clin North Am* 75(4):1013, 1991.
11. Gryboski JD: Peptic ulcer disease in children, *Med Clin North Am* 75(4):889, 1991.
12. Miller TA et al: Stress erosive gastritis, *Curr Probl Surg* 28:458, 1991.
13. Pilchman J et al: Cytoprotection and stress ulceration, *Med Clin North Am* 75(4):853, 1991.
14. Schindler BA, Ramchandani D: Psychologic factors associated with peptic ulcer disease, *Med Clin North Am* 75(4):865, 1991.
15. Rubin W: Medical treatment of peptic ulcer disease, *Med Clin North Am* 75(4):981, 1991.
16. Isenberg JI et al: Acid-peptic disorders. In Yamada T, ed: *Textbook of gastroenterology,* Philadelphia, 1991, JB Lippincott.
17. Mertz HR, Walsh JH: Peptic ulcer pathophysiology, *Med Clin North Am* 75(4):799, 1991.
18. Craig P et al: *Helicobacter pylori* secretes a chemotactic factor for monocytes and neutrophils, *Gastroenterology* 98:33, 1990.
19. McCarthy DM: Sucralfate, *N Engl J Med* 325(14):1017, 1991.
20. Graham D: Prevention of gastroduodenal injury induced by chronic nonsteroidal anti-inflammatory drug therapy, *Gastroenterology* 96:675, 1989.
21. Bauerfeind P et al: Fate of antacid gel in the stomach, site of action and interaction with food, *Dig Dis Sci* 35(5):553, 1990.
22. Earnest DL: Maintenance therapy in peptic ulcer disease, *Med Clin North Am* 75(4):1013, 1991.
23. Farrar GE: Remember the Sippy regimen for peptic ulcer? *Clin Ther* 11:278, 1989.
24. American Dietetic Association: Position paper on bland diet in the treatment of chronic ulcer disease, *J Am Diet Assoc* 59:244, 1971.
25. Marotta RB, Floch MH: Diet and nutrition in ulcer disease, *Med Clin North Am* 75(4):967, 1991.
26. Montgomery KL: Peptic ulcer disease. In Pemberton C et al, eds: *Mayo Clinic diet manual,* ed 6, St Louis, 1989, Mosby.
27. Food and Nutrition Board Committee on Diet and Health, National Academy of Sciences—National Research Council: *Diet and health: implications for reducing chronic disease risk,* Washington, DC, 1989, National Academy Press.
28. Caspary WF: Physiology and pathophysiology of intestinal absorption, *Am J Clin Nutr* 55(suppl):299S, 1992.
29. Kruis W et al: Effects of diets high and low in refined sugars on gut transit, bile acid metabolism, and bacterial fermentation, *Gut* 32:367, 1991.
30. Banwell JG: Pathophysiology of diarrheal disorders, *Rev Infect Dis* 12(suppl 1):530, 1990.
31. Podolsky DK: Inflammatory bowel disease, Part I, *N Engl J Med* 325(13):928, 1991.
32. Podolsky DK: Inflammatory bowel disease, Part II, *N Engl J Med* 325(13):1008, 1991.
33. Farthing MJG: Gastrointestinal dysfunction in inflammatory bowel disease, *Clin Nutr* 2(suppl 4):5, 1983.
34. Bennett RA et al: Frequency of inflammatory bowel disease in offspring of couples both presenting with IBD, *Gastroenterology* 100:1638, 1991.
35. Tysk C et al: Ulcerative colitis and Crohn's disease in unselected population of monozygotic and dizygotic twins: a study of heritability and the influence of smoking, *Gut* 29:990, 1988.
36. Ainley C et al: The influence of zinc status and malnutrition on immunological function in Crohn's disease, *Gastroenterology* 100:1616, 1991.
37. Peppercorn MA: Advances in drug therapy for inflammatory bowel disease, *Ann Intern Med* 112:50, 1990.
38. O'Brien JJ et al: Use of azathioprine or 6-mercaptopurine in the treatment of Crohn's disease, *Gastroenterology* 101:39, 1991.
39. Donaldson RM: The muddle of diets for gastrointestinal disorders, *JAMA* 225:1243, 1973.
40. Bingham S: Low residue diets: a reappraisal of their meaning and content, *J Hum Nutr* 33:5, 1979.
41. Christian GM et al: Milk and milk products in low-residue diets: current hospital practices do not match dietitians' beliefs, *J Am Diet Assoc* 91(3):341, 1991.
42. Rosenburg IH, Jenkins DJA: Nutrition and diet in management of diseases of the gastrointestinal tract: small intestine and colon. In Shils ME, Young VR, eds: *Modern nutrition in health and disease,* ed 7, Philadelphia, 1988, Lea & Febiger.
43. Polk DB et al: Improved growth and disease activity after intermittent administration of a defined formula diet in children with Crohn's disease, *J Parenter Enteral Nutr* 16(6):499, 1992.
44. Teahon K et al: Ten years' experience with an elemental diet in the management of Crohn's disease, *Gut* 31:1133, 1990.
45. Christie PM, Hill GL: Effect of intravenous nutrition on nutrition and function in acute attacks of inflammatory bowel disease, *Gastroenterology* 99:730, 1990.

46. Purdum PP, Kirby DF: Short-bowel syndrome: a review of the role of nutrition support, *J Parenter Enteral Nutr* 15(1):93, 1991.
47. Åkerlund J-E et al: Hepatic metabolism of cholesterol in Crohn's disease: effect of partial resection of ileum, *Gastroenterology* 100:1046, 1991.
48. Leichtmann GA et al: Intestinal absorption of cholecalciferol and 25-hydroxycholecalciferol in patients with both Crohn's disease and intestinal resection, *Am J Clin Nutr* 54:548, 1991.
49. Wunderlich SM, Tobias A: Relationship between nutritional status indicators and length of hospital stay for patients with diverticular disease, *J Am Diet Assoc* 92(4):430, 1992.
50. Sandler RS: Epidemiology of irritable bowel syndrome in the United States, *Gastroenterology* 99:409, 1990.
51. Schuster MM: Diagnostic evaluation of the irritable bowel syndrome, *Gastroenterol Clin North Am* 20(2):269, 1991.
52. Thompson WC: Symptomatic presentations of the irritable bowel syndrome, *Gastroenterol Clin North Am* 20(2):235, 1991.
53. Subrameni K, Janowitz HD: The irritable bowel syndrome, a continuing dilemma, *Gastroenterol Clin North Am* 20(2):363, 1991.
54. Drossman DA et al: Identification of the subgroups of functional gastrointestinal disorders, *Gastroenterol Int* 3:159, 1990.
55. Whitehead WE, Crowell MD: Psychologic considerations in the irritable bowel syndrome, *Gastroenterol Clin North Am* 20(2):249, 1991.
56. Friedman G: Treatment of the irritable bowel syndrome, *Gastroenterol Clin North Am* 20(2):325, 1991.
57. Friedman G: Diet and the irritable bowel syndrome, *Gastroenterol Clin North Am* 20(2):313, 1991.
58. Mullin GE: Food allergy and irritable bowel syndrome, *JAMA* 265(13):1736, 1991.
59. Jain NK et al: Sorbitol intolerance in adults, *Am J Gastroenterol* 8:678, 1985.
60. Wingate DL: The irritable bowel syndrome, *Gastroenterol Clin North Am* 20(2):351, 1991.
61. Donatelle EP: Constipation: pathophysiology and treatment, *Am Fam Physician* 42(5):1335, 1990.

FURTHER READING

Christian GM et al: Milk and milk products in low-residue diets: current hospital practices do not match dietitians' beliefs, *J Am Diet Assoc* 91(3):341, 1991.

This group of dietitians present results of their survey showing a diminishing use of the low-residue diet in the treatment of intestinal disorders.

Donatelle EP: Constipation: pathophysiology and treatment, *Am Fam Physician* 42(5):1335, 1990.

This family physician provides an excellent review of this common problem, especially among elderly hospitalized patients, and includes a full-page table of laxative products with evaluations and comments.

Marotta RB, Floch MH: Diet and nutrition in ulcer disease, *Med Clin North Am* 75(4):967, 1991.

This clinical dietitian-physician team reviews the new directions for treatment of peptic ulcer disease and the use of regular diets for nutritional support rather than the various old bland diet therapies.

Stanek K et al: Factors affecting use of food and commercial agents to thicken liquids for individuals with swallowing disorders, *J Am Diet Assoc* 92(4):488, 1992.

Three clinical dietitians provide helpful material from their testing of various thickening agents for liquids to make them more easily swallowed by persons with swallowing problems and include a full-page table of the agents used and their test results.

Thompson WG: *Gut reactions,* New York, 1989, Plenum Press.

This book, written by a well-known gastroenterologist especially for persons with irritable bowel syndrome, provides much helpful information for patients with this difficult chronic disorder.

Wunderlich SM, Tobias A: Relationship between nutritional status indicators and length of hospital stay for patients with diverticular disease, *J Am Diet Assoc* 92(4):429, 1992.

These two clinical dietitians apply nutritional assessment laboratory tests for short-life serum protein markers such as prealbumin and transferrin for early detection of malnutrition commonly seen in chronic diverticular disease patients, so that immediate nutritional support shortens their hospital stay and its economic costs.

CASE STUDY

The Patient with Peptic Ulcer Disease

Lowell Randolph is a 40-year-old businessman who was admitted to the city hospital 3 weeks ago after an incidence of vomiting bright-red blood. A medical history revealed that a dull, gnawing pain in the upper abdomen began several months ago and has increased in severity during that time. It became more severe after his most recent out-of-state trip to one of his stores. Because the pain was usually accompanied by headaches, he took aspirin to help relieve it.

Initial hospital treatment consisted of blood transfusions, intravenous fluids and electrolytes, and vitamin C. Mr. Randolph continued to feel nauseated and weak but stopped vomiting. However, he passed several large, tarry stools during the first 24 hours. His initial nutritional assessment results included the following: weight, 68 kg (150 lb); height, 179 cm (70 in); albumin, 2.8 g/dl; prealbumin, 14 mg/dl; transferrin, 18% saturation value; hemoglobin, 11 g/dl; and hematocrit, 35%. His medications included cimetidine, sucralfate, magnesium-aluminum hydroxide, and triple antibiotic therapy.

The patient began slowly to tolerate sips of clear liquids, then advanced to a regular diet as tolerated, showing continued improvement. Before he was discharged at the end of the second week, the nutritionist and the nurse discussed general nutritional needs with Mr. Randolph and his wife. They advised him to eat his meals regularly in as relaxed a setting and manner as possible, eliminate his frequent between-meal snacks, and take his multivitamin supplement daily with his meals. Also, they reviewed his general guidelines sheet, listing a few food-related items or habits to avoid. They also advised him to stop smoking and to rest as much as possible before returning to work. His physician had also advised him to reduce his work load and scheduled a follow-up appointment in 1 week.

Mrs. Randolph accompanied her husband to the next appointment and reported that she was pleased with his ability to put aside business duties and take more time to enjoy his family. Mr. Randolph stated that his two teenaged sons had been surprisingly supportive in assisting him in following the prescribed regimen and that he plans to make it his general habit.

Questions for Analysis

1. The x-ray diagnosis of Mr. Randolph's illness was a gastric ulcer in the antrum lesser curvature. What does this mean? Where do most ulcers occur? Why?
2. What factors contributed to Mr. Randolph's ulcer? What effect did each of them have?
3. Evaluate the results of Mr. Randolph's initial nutritional assessment data. How would you use this information in nutritional counseling?
4. Identify Mr. Randolph's basic nutritional needs. Outline a teaching plan based on these needs that you would use to help him with his new diet plan. How would you include his wife in formulating and implementing his nutritional care plan?
5. What role does vitamin C play in Mr. Randolph's therapy? What other vitamins and minerals play a significant role in his care? Describe each role.
6. Why should Mr. Randolph give up coffee, cigarettes, and alcohol? What problems do you think he may encounter in trying to change these habits?

Nutritional Aspects of Diarrhea

Gastrointestinal disease so often presents barriers to efficient nutrient absorption that nutritional deficiencies are planned for automatically. Ironically these conditions also lead frequently to diarrhea, all of which result in loss of fluids and electrolytes. As expected, their replacement is the initial and primary concern of therapy. However, different types of diarrhea also present other differences; the control of type-specific problems requires different modes of treatment coordinated with the treatment of the disease it accompanies. Before looking into possible treatment modes, examine first three of the most common types of diarrhea: watery, fatty, and small volume.

Watery diarrhea occurs when the amount of water and electrolytes moving into the intestinal mucosa exceeds the amount absorbed into the bloodstream. This movement of water and electrolytes into the mucosa may be secretive or osmotic.

If this movement of water and electrolytes into the mucosa is *secretive,* it may be active or passive. *Active movement* occurs with excessive gastric hydrochloric acid secretion or enterotoxin-induced infections such as cholera. *Passive movement* occurs with a rise in hydrostatic pressure that accompanies infectious diseases such as salmonellosis or tuberculosis, nonbacterial infections, fungal infections, renal failure, irradiation enteritis, and inflammatory bowel disease. Other conditions associated with watery diarrhea include hyperthyroidism, thyroid carcinoma, and hypermotility of the gastrointestinal tract.

If this movement of water and electrolytes into the mucosa is osmotic, it occurs when these nutrients are not absorbed because of intolerable levels of nonabsorbable particles present in the intestinal chyme. Such particles include lactose (milk sugar) in lactase-deficient individuals or gluten (grain protein) in persons with a reduced gastrointestinal transit time caused by the removal of part of the intestinal tract.

Fatty diarrhea, or steatorrhea, occurs with maldigestion or malabsorption. *Maldigestion* involves a lack of enzymatic activity required to completely digest food, such as reduced pancreatic exocrine activity (release of intestinal enzymes from the pancreas) caused by pancreatic insufficiency. *Malabsorption* means that digested materials do not make it across the intestinal mucosa to enter the bloodstream. This failure occurs in conditions in which the intestinal villi are destroyed, such as celiac disease.

Small-volume diarrhea occurs mainly when the rectosigmoid area of the colon is irritated, such as in inflammatory bowel disease (Crohn's disease or ulcerative colitis). It also occurs when inflammatory conditions affect areas adjacent to the colon, as in pelvic inflammatory disease, diverticulitis, appendicitis, and hemorrhagic ovarian cysts.

The metabolic consequences of each type of diarrhea are similar. Uncontrolled, they result in *syncope, hypokalemia, acid-base imbalances,* and *hypovolemia,* with resulting *renal failure.* They may also be accompanied by low levels of fat-soluble vitamins, B_{12}, or folic acid or eventually lead to protein-energy malnutrition. In addition to these conditions, each type of diarrhea also manifests problems associated with the disorder it accompanies. Workers with the Memorial Sloan-Kettering Cancer Center in New York and the Department of Medicine at Brooke Army Medical Center in Texas have developed recommendations for treating gastrointestinal diseases associated with each type of diarrhea. These are summarized here in the following discussion, with the focus on the diarrheal aspects of disease.

Watery diarrhea often accompanies inflammatory bowel conditions, such as Crohn's disease, for which diet therapy involves (1) increased protein and kcalories, (2) low fats and lactose, and (3) avoidance of foods that stimulate peristalsis. Thus secretive diarrhea is reduced by eliminating foods that may stimulate gastric acid secretion, and all types of watery diarrhea are avoided by reducing the motility of the gastrointestinal tract. In other conditions in which osmotic diarrhea occurs, such as *dumping syndrome,* this problem is avoided by giving fluids *between* meals to avoid any extreme difference in osmotic pressures on either side of the intestinal wall. Small, frequent meals also help prevent this problem, as well as painful distention.

Fatty diarrhea frequently accompanies conditions associated with maldigestion, such as chronic pancreatitis. The dietary management of this disease involves (1) frequent meals, high in protein and carbohydrates and low in fat; (2) use of medium chain triglycerides, which are more easily absorbed under adverse conditions; and (3) avoiding gastric stimulants, especially caffeine and alcohol. Fatty diarrhea also accompanies conditions of malabsorption, such as gluten-sensitive enteropathy. In addition to diet management strategies listed, treating this type of diarrhea also requires the removal of products that damage the mucosal villi, including lactose and gluten, which are found in wheat, rye, barley, and oats, and food products and fillers such as hydrolyzed vegetable protein products. It sometimes requires restricting fat as well. In both cases the primary concern is to monitor fats that would otherwise appear in the feces. As the therapy progresses, the fat content of the meal can be increased as tolerated to normal levels to improve palatability.

Small-volume diarrhea may accompany diverticulosis of the colon. A high-residue diet is recommended to increase fecal bulk, thereby preventing diarrhea. To prevent flatulence and distention, however, the fiber—such as wheat bran, fruits, and vegetables—should be added to the diet gradually.

All types of diarrhea result in malnutrition, primarily

Continued.

because of electrolyte and fluid losses. It is important to identify the *type* of diarrhea occurring with each patient. Only then can an effective nutritional management strategy be designed to replace those losses, as well as to eliminate or prevent other nutrition-related problems that are possible for each case.

REFERENCES

1. Banwell JG: Pathophysiology of diarrheal disorders, *Rev Infect Dis* 12(suppl 1):30, 1990.
2. Barrett KE, Dharmsathaphorn K: Secretion and absorption: small intestine and colon. In Yamada T, ed: *Textbook of gastroenterology,* Philadelphia, 1991, JB Lippincott.

CHAPTER 7

Diseases of the Liver, Gallbladder, and Pancreas

CHAPTER OUTLINE

Diseases of the Liver
Diseases of the Gallbladder
Diseases of the Pancreas

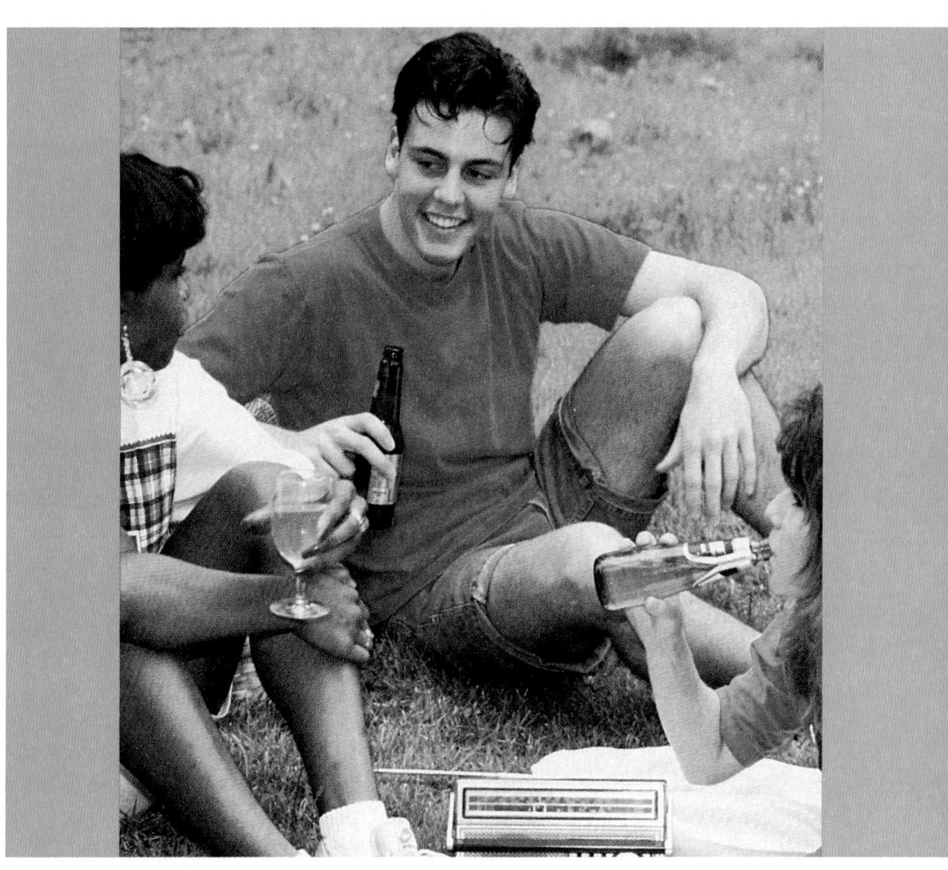

This chapter is a companion to the preceding one and focuses on the accessory organs of the gastrointestinal system. Three organs—the liver, gallbladder, and pancreas—serve the needs of the gastrointestinal tract, but their actions also have far reaching effects throughout the body.

Through its vast network of biochemical reactions, the liver controls a major portion of the body's internal environment. When the liver is diseased and its usual cellular activities do not proceed normally, repercussions of this diminished capacity are reflected in numerous metabolic difficulties.

The much smaller, adjacent gallbladder receives the watery bile of the liver and concentrates, stores, and releases it as needed. The pancreas also affects the entire body through its controlling enzymes and hormones.

In this chapter, we examine these three vital accessory organs and see their roles in health diminished by various diseases. Our nutritional care must be developed from this relationship of normal metabolic function and disease interference and its impact on the quality of individual lives and life itself.

Diseases of the Liver

Structures and Functions of the Liver

The liver has rightly been called the "metabolic capital" of the body. It is a highly active, vital organ. A clear understanding of the normal structures and functions of the liver in relation to its vital metabolic tasks is an essential first step in establishing a valid rationale for nutrient modifications in liver disease. These metabolic functions have been studied in previous chapters of this text. At this point, we briefly review the "big picture" of the liver's main anatomy and physiology as a framework for its major metabolic functions, thus gaining a better understanding of its clinical problems in disease as a basis for nutritional therapy.

Hepatic Structures and Vascular System

The liver is the largest of the body's internal organs, weighing in adulthood about 1.1 to 1.5 kg (2.5 to 3.3 lb). It is a somewhat cone-shaped, red-brown organ consisting of two major lobes enclosed within an overall connective tissue capsule lying immediately below the diaphragm and occupying the upper right portion of the abdominal cavity. Its vast specialized network of cells and circulating channels within each of its thousands of microscopic functional units is uniquely designed to accomplish its multiple metabolic tasks.

Lobules and vascular network. The basic functional unit of the liver is the *liver lobule,* a small cylindric structure several millimeters in length and about 0.8 to 2.0 mm in diameter. The human liver contains some 50,000 to 100,000 of these powerful individual lobules. Each lobule contains organized groups of the functional cells, the *hepatocytes,* and is surrounded by branches of the interrelated vascular system serving its functional metabolic needs. The following are vessels of the hepatic vascular system[1]:

- *Hepatic artery* branches bring large amounts of freshly oxygenated blood from the heart to perfuse the liver tissue lobules and their cells. This amount totals about 25% of the entire output of the heart.
- *Portal vein* branches bring blood from two sources, the small intestine and the spleen. The mesenteric vein brings the larger amount (80%) of the portal circulation, nutrient-rich blood absorbed directly from the small intestine and ready to be metabolized or stored. The splenic vein brings the remaining 20%, blood drained from the spleen and the stomach. These venous circulations perfuse each lobule to enhance the metabolic work of the hepatocytes and drain into the central hepatic vein to carry carbon dioxide and metabolic products via the vena cava back to the heart for circulation to body cells.
- *Bile ducts* drain the bile secreted by the liver through a branching series of channels and canals that form the *biliary tree.* The bile collects into the main hepatic duct, which carries it on to the gallbladder.
- *Lymphatic vessels* drain the liver lobules of large quantities of lymph. About half of all the lymph formed in the body under resting conditions is from the liver.

Structural scheme of the lobules. Thus the unique structural design of these basic functional units of the liver enable this vital organ to do its life-sustaining work. Each liver lobule is constructed around a central vein that empties into the hepatic veins and flows on into the vena cava. From this central vein many *hepatic cellular plates* radiate outward like spokes in a wheel (Fig. 7-1). Each hepatic plate of functional liver cells is one or two cells thick, which are separated by small bile *canaliculi* and *portal venules* from which blood flows into flat, branching *hepatic sinusoids* between the plates and into the central vein. In this pattern, these liver cells are continuously exposed to portal venous blood. Also, special large *Kupffer cells* line these branching channels around the cellular plates. These are tissue macrophages capable of engulfing bacteria and any other foreign matter in the blood and disposing of them. An average of 1450 ml of blood per minute flows through this combined portal and arterial liver circulation, which amounts to about 29% of the resting cardiac output.

Metabolic Functions

The liver has many metabolic functions related to the three energy-yielding macronutrients (carbohydrates,

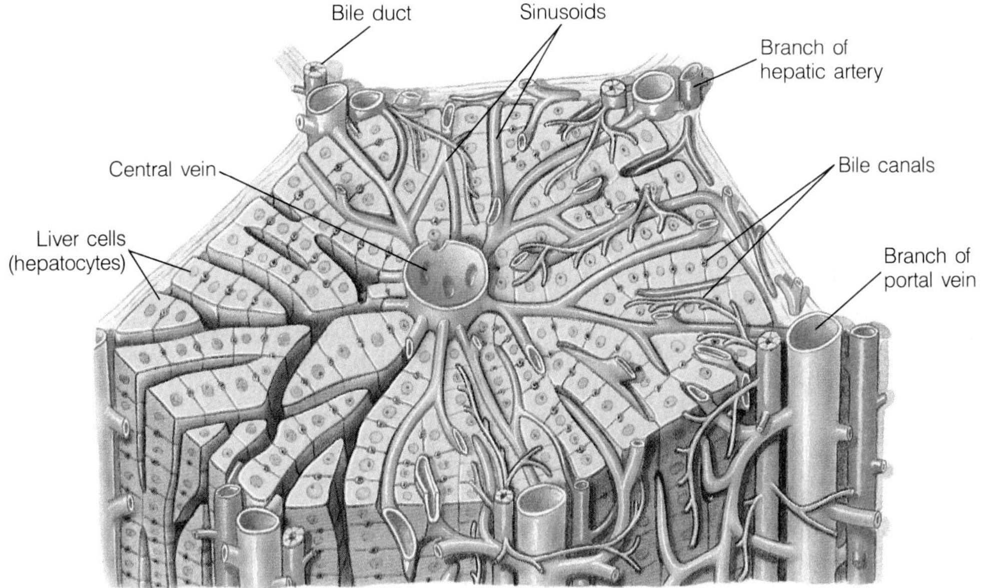

FIG. 7-1 Liver structure showing hepatic lobule and hepatic cell.

fat, and protein), the micronutrients (vitamins and minerals), and fluid-electrolyte-plasma protein balances. Some of the key metabolic activities of the liver are outlined for review:

Carbohydrate metabolism

- Formation and storage of glycogen in glycogenesis
- Conversion of galactose and fructose to glucose
- Conversion of amino acid residues to glucose in gluconeogenesis
- Formation of many important chemical compounds from carbohydrate intermediates

Fat metabolism

- Fat conversion to transport form with formation of lipoproteins
- Oxidation of fatty acids to acetoacetic acid and then to acetylcoenzyme A (acetyl-CoA) for use in the citric acid cycle to yield energy
- Formation of cholesterol and phospholipids
- Formation of bile salts
- Conversion of carbohydrate and protein intermediates to fat through lipogenesis

Protein metabolism

- Deamination of amino acids
- Provision of lipotropic factor for fat conversion to lipoproteins
- Formation of plasma proteins
- Urea formation for removal of ammonia from body fluids
- Many amino acid interconversions; transamination and amination; and synthesis of nonessential amino acids (purines and pyrimidines), creatine, phosphate, and others

Other related functions

- Formation of *25-hydroxycholecalciferol,* the intermediate product in the synthesis of active vitamin D hormone, *1-alpha-25-dihydroxycholecalciferol*
- Formation of the blood coagulation factors fibrinogen, prothrombin, accelerator globulin, and factors VII, IX, and X; all except fibrinogen and accelerator globulin require vitamin K
- Storage of iron as ferritin
- Storage of large amounts of vitamins A, D, and B_{12} and of smaller amounts of other B-complex vitamins and vitamin K
- Conjugation and biliary excretion of steroid hormones and thyroxin
- Detoxification of many different drugs and their excretion in bile
- Conjugation and biliary excretion of bilirubin, the greenish yellow pigment released from the heme of hemoglobin in the breakdown of red blood cells

Circulatory Functions

Blood storage. In effect, the liver is a large, expandable venous organ. It stores large quantities of blood in its network of blood vessels. Normally, the blood volume of the hepatic veins and sinuses is about 450 to 650 ml, some 10% of the body's total blood volume.[1,2] However, the liver expands or contracts as needed to alter its blood volume. For example, when the pressure is high in the right atrium of the heart,

CLINICAL APPLICATION — Jaundice: When to Expect It and What to Do About It

Since jaundice is not usually a life-threatening condition, it is easy for the health care professional to take it lightly. The resulting yellow-to-orange skin color seems harmless, only reflecting an accumulation of excessive bile pigments in the blood that results from a rise in *bilirubin,* a product of heme released when red blood cells are destroyed. Certainly the underlying condition resulting in hemolysis is the major issue.

This may be true in a biologic sense. However, in a psychologic sense it can be devastating. The embarrassment of an altered body image, with accompanying depression and withdrawal, can affect the appetite and willingness to comply with the therapy that is recommended for the illness. To promote a healthy recovery, health workers must treat jaundice as seriously as these effects dictate. Several actions would be helpful:

1. Explain to the patient the reason for jaundice.
   - *Prehepatic jaundice.* Prehepatic jaundice most often is caused by a massive breakdown in red blood cells. It is seen most often in Rh factor sensitization, hemolytic anemias, sickle cell anemia, massive lung infarctions, transfusion reactions, and septicemia. The result is an excessive amount of bilirubin in a form that cannot be excreted, that is, fat-soluble. The body's bilirubin transport system, based on albumin, then deposits the excess in the patient's skin and in a few other tissues.
   - *Hepatic jaundice.* In hepatic jaundice the liver cannot convert fat-soluble bilirubin into the water-soluble form required for its removal from the blood. This condition is seen in hepatitis, cirrhosis, metastatic cancer, and prolonged drug use, especially of drugs broken down by the liver.
   - *Posthepatic jaundice.* Posthepatic jaundice occurs when the flow of bile into the duodenum is blocked. Since bile carries water-soluble excretable bilirubin, this blockage backs up the bile, resulting in a backlog of bilirubin in the blood. Blockage often occurs with inflammation, scar tissue, stones, or tumors in the liver, bile, or pancreatic systems.
2. Explain to the patient assessment procedures and tests. A careful and comprehensive assessment process involving members of the health care team provides vital information for medical, nutritional, and nursing care plans.
   - *Include a careful history and anthropometry.* A full personal, family, psychosocial, medical, and nutritional history will help detect any possible hepatic virus sources and current nutritional status and needs.
   - *Check anthropometric data.* Routine body measures including skinfold thicknesses help determine nutritional status.
   - *Evaluate results of routine biochemical tests.* Relate these tests to medical diagnosis and nutritional status and needs.
   - *Explain each procedure.* A clear explanation of each procedure will help the patient participate more meaningfully in diagnostic and care-planning processes and will allay anxieties about the jaundice.
3. Identify nutrition-related problems. Jaundice is often associated with anorexia, indigestion, nausea, and vomiting.
   - *Help resolve nutrition-related problems.* To overcome indigestion or anorexia, recommend small meals that offer some of the patient's favorite foods. To overcome nausea or vomiting, simple foods may be necessary. Also, foods rich in fat and caffeine should be avoided.
   - *Encourage the patient to discuss personal feelings and concerns.* Such information is essential for the nurse and nutritionist to develop a treatment plan. Also, this counseling may help the patient feel psychologically stronger and ready to contribute to the health care process.
   - *Discuss pertinent needs with the patient's family and friends.* Often other significant persons avoid the patient out of embarrassment or lack of understanding. A discussion of the patient's need for support may help other persons accept the patient socially and support any other efforts made to resolve the underlying health problem.
   - *Make appropriate referrals as needed.* If jaundice was caused by alcohol or drug abuse, the patient and possibly the patient's family may require special counseling. Referral to community programs after hospital discharge may help provide needed follow-up therapy. ◆

REFERENCE

Sherlock S: *Diseases of the liver and biliary system,* ed 8, Cambridge, Massachusetts, 1989, Blackwell Scientific Publications.

which receives blood via the vena cava from the liver, back pressure develops in the liver. The liver then expands to hold as much as an extra 0.5 to 1 L of blood temporarily in the hepatic veins and sinuses. This occurs particularly in cardiac failure with peripheral congestion. Thus this valuable blood volume capacity enables the liver to act as a reservoir at times of excess blood volume and to supply extra blood at times of diminished blood volume.

Lymph flow. The large pores of the hepatic sinusoids are permeable to fluid and proteins, allowing these to flow in the lymph channels, called Disse's spaces, surrounding each cellular plate in the liver lobule. The liver lymph has a protein concentration about that of plasma. Because of this great permeability and the collecting spaces of the liver sinusoids, large quantities of lymph, about half of all the lymph formed in the resting body, is from the liver.[1] When hepatic venous pressure rises at the point where the liver veins empty into the vena cava, excessive fluids begin to leak through the outer surface of the liver directly into the abdominal cavity. This abdominal fluid is almost pure plasma, carrying 80% to 90% as much protein as normal plasma and represents considerable nutrient loss.[1] This accumulation of nutrient-rich free fluid in the abdominal cavity is called **ascites.**

Diagnostic Liver Function Tests

Based on these multiple liver functions, a number of liver function tests have been developed to aid the physician in determining the nature of the liver disease and in initiating appropriate treatment. Some of these tests are not specific to liver disease, are influenced by factors outside the liver, and are complicated by the liver's large reserve and ability to regenerate tissue. Thus they vary in usefulness. Nonetheless, selected tests are valuable parts of nutritional assessment. Several types of tests commonly used are described in the following discussion. In each case, a particular aspect of liver function or response is measured.

Dye tests. The *BSP* test measures the ability of the liver to retain the dye *sulfobromophthalein* (Bromsulphalein) and then concentrate and secrete it. Thus it tests the general function of the liver. After parenteral injection, the dye is bound to serum albumin, taken up by the liver, conjugated, and excreted in bile. Increased retention of the dye indicates disease in the liver or biliary ducts but does not distinguish the location. Because of some recent reactions to the BSP injections, another less toxic dye, *indocyanine green (ICG),* is being used in some cases in clinical practice.[3]

Van den Bergh's test. This test measures the relative amounts of conjugated bilirubin and total bilirubin. The amount of unconjugated bilirubin is then obtained by subtraction. An increased unconjugated bilirubin value indicates the presence of diseased, nonfunctioning hepatocytes unable to conjugate the bilirubin normally. In liver disease, up to 85% of total serum bilirubin is the unconjugated form.[1,3] An increased conjugated bilirubin value indicates functioning hepatocytes but some biliary obstruction hindering normal excretion.

Serum bilirubin concentration. About 200 mg of bilirubin is formed daily by the liver, mostly from heme being released from hemoglobin breakdown as old red blood cells die after an average life span of 120 days. First, the bilirubin is bound with albumin for transport in the blood circulation; then within hours it is taken up by the liver, released from the albumin and conjugated, mostly with glucuronic acid, and excreted in the bile. An increased serum bilirubin value indicates the inability of the liver to conjugate and excrete it.

Prothrombin time. This test measures blood clotting time, although it is not specific to liver disease. Nonetheless, liver disease is a frequent cause of impaired coagulation.[3] A lack of liver synthesis of blood clotting factors contributes to a prolonged clotting time.

Albumin concentration. Quantitatively, albumin is the most important of a number of plasma proteins formed in the liver, so testing for it helps determine the quality of liver synthesis functions. However, because of its relatively long half-life of 20 days, albumin is a better index of chronic liver disease. Also, nutritional factors such as the availability of amino acids are critical determinants of the rate of albumin synthesis. The shorter half-life (2 days) of prealbumin, a glycoprotein synthesized by the liver, makes it a more sensitive indicator in tests for acute liver injury or for day-to-day monitoring.[3]

Aminotransferases (transaminases). Two tests for blood levels of key cell enzymes that catalyze the process of transamination in the metabolism of specific amino acids are used: (1) aspartate aminotransferase (AST), also called serum glutamic-oxaloacetic transaminase (SGOT); and (2) alanine aminotransferase (ALT), also called serum glutamic-pyruvic transaminase (SGPT). Both are important markers of functional liver cell injury. AST is also found in other tissues such as the heart, muscles, kidney, and brain, but ALT is limited primarily to the liver. A rise in the level of these transaminases, especially ALT, indicates damaged liver cells that cannot maintain normal concentrations of cell enzymes required for specific reactions in the metabolism of nutrients.

A number of other tests for serum levels or tissue reserves of nutrient metabolites of the liver may reflect liver cell damage. Such tests include, for example, tests for glucose tolerance, glycogen reserves, triglycerides, phospholipids, cholesterol and cholesterol esters, ketones, urea nitrogen, ammonia, and various plasma proteins.

Viral Hepatitis

Etiology

Viral hepatitis, inflammation of the liver, is a major public health problem throughout the world affecting hundreds of millions of people. It is a cause of considerable illness and death in human populations from the acute infection or its effects, which may include chronic active hepatitis, cirrhosis, and primary liver cancer. During the past few years, knowledge of the viruses causing different types of hepatitis has grown rapidly. Currently, five totally unrelated and often highly unusual human hepatitis viruses have now been discovered and described[4]:

- *Hepatitis A virus (HAV).* HAV, the infectious agent of hepatitis type A, formerly called infectious hepatitis, was discovered as early as 1973 in the feces of infected patients and is transmitted by the oral-fecal route. It is still ranked by the World Health Organization (WHO) as a prevalent infection worldwide. This virus is spread by common contaminated water and food, especially where there is overcrowding and poor hygiene and sanitation. Such a high-risk environment was shown by a recent major outbreak in mainland China in 1988 involving 1 to 2 million persons. As was observed in this outbreak, the infection is often minor in children and young adults, but mortality increases with age.[5] Although HAV infection does not lead to chronic hepatitis and cirrhosis, it is a serious illness. A new HAV vaccine has recently been developed that is far more effective than the former large and painful injection of gamma globulins, antibodies isolated from blood.[6] This new vaccine protects travelers to developing countries, where the virus is **endemic** and may contaminate water and food.
- *Hepatitis B virus (HBV).* HBV, the infectious agent of hepatitis type B, formerly called serum hepatitis, is mainly spread sexually and by needle-sharing drug abusers. It has now been implicated worldwide as the major etiologic factor in chronic liver disease and associated liver cancer. Current studies indicate that the HBV infection is closely related to the body's immune system. The current estimate of carriers is 300 million worldwide, 75% of whom are Asians. The WHO indicates that about 40% of these infected persons will eventually die of chronic active hepatitis or liver cancer.[7] An improved vaccine was developed in 1986 and is now being used with high-risk groups such as health care personnel and babies of antibody-carrier mothers in most developed countries. In some endemic areas, all newborn babies are routinely vaccinated.
- *Hepatitis C virus (HCV).* After definitive isolation of HBV in the 1960s and HAV in the 1970s, there remained patients with clinical viral hepatitis without identification of either the A or B virus. Thus the term non-A, non-B hepatitis (NANB) was coined to describe these cases. Recent identification of the major non-A, non-B virus, now termed hepatitis C virus (HCV), has resulted from major advances in molecular biology and cloning techniques.[8] HCV is associated with various high-risk populations with autoimmune chronic active hepatitis, liver cirrhosis, and liver cancer and with hemophiliacs receiving blood transfusions, intravenous drug users, and hemodialysis patients. The only antiviral treatment of proven value in studies thus far is **interferon-alpha.**[9,10] This protein substance, normally made by cells as a defense against viral infection, is now produced in quantity by laboratory recombinant gene techniques.
- *Hepatitis D virus (HDV).* In 1977, a new viral **antigen** was found in patients with chronic HBV infection. Follow-up studies proved that this antigen was related to a new virus, originally called *delta* virus, the Greek letter δ for D, but now in the alphabetic naming system termed hepatitis virus D or HDV. HDV is endemic in Italy, the Middle East, and parts of Africa and South America, but is relatively rare in Western Europe, North America, and Asia. It may occur as a superinfection with HBV antigen carriers, causing a severe, sometimes **fulminant,** form of acute hepatitis. In other cases, it may occur as a coinfection with HBV that is usually self-limiting as acute HBV, but the degree of attending illness may be greater. In any case, HDV appears to be directly toxic to functional liver cells. Interferon-alpha has been shown to have only a transient effect on HDV. Control of HDV infection is by HBV vaccination.[4]
- *Hepatitis E virus (HEV).* Scientific detective work spanning almost three decades has finally unraveled the puzzle of the newest of the known viral liver disease agents, hepatitis E virus. This interesting history began in 1955, after a massive outbreak of hepatitis occurred in Delhi, India, affecting nearly 30,000 persons when drinking water was contaminated by the overflow of an open sewer. Study of this outbreak and nine subsequent Indian epidemics over the intervening years indicated two unique characteristics of its pattern: (1) a benign self-limiting course followed for the majority of the population with no chronic problems, but 10% of the women affected in their third trimester of pregnancy died of fulminant liver failure; and (2) the source of the infection was the oral-fecal route of contamination, entirely different from the blood-borne non-A, non-B hepatitis (type C). Finally, in 1983, advanced technology led to identification of this new viral hepatitis

agent, an enteric non-A, non-B type that severely affects pregnant women and is now classed as HEV. Sporadic imported cases from epidemics in various countries of Asia, Africa, and Central and South America have been reported in the United States.[4]

Clinical Symptoms

The viral agents of hepatitis produce diffuse injury to liver cells, especially the **parenchymal cells.** In milder cases the liver injury is largely reversible, but with increasing severity more extensive **necrosis** occurs. In some cases, massive necrosis may lead to liver failure and death. A cardinal symptom of hepatitis is *anorexia,* contributing to the risk of malnutrition. Varying clinical symptoms appear depending on the degree of liver injury. The most obvious sign is **jaundice,** which gives the person a yellow appearance. It serves as a rough index of the severity of the disease. However, jaundice is frequently not seen, although it may be present in many persons. In an outbreak of hepatitis, for example, many infected persons may be **nonicteric** and thus go undiagnosed and untreated. Malnutrition and impaired **immunocompetence** contribute to the development of spontaneous infections and continuing liver disease. General symptoms, in addition to the main sign of anorexia, include malaise, weakness, nausea and vomiting, diarrhea, headache, fever, enlarged and tender liver, and enlarged spleen. When jaundice develops, it usually follows a **preicteric** period of 5 to 10 days, deepens for 1 to 2 weeks, and then levels off and decreases. At this crisis point, sufficient recovery of injured cells has taken place to begin the convalescent period. Convalescence requires from 3 weeks to 3 months, and optimal care during this time is essential to avoid relapse.

Treatment

The importance of bed rest in the treatment of acute hepatitis has been clearly demonstrated. Physical exercise increases the severity and duration of the disease. A daily intake of about 3000 ml of fluid guards against dehydration and gives a general sense of well-being and improved appetite. Optimal nutrition provides the foundation for recovery of the injured liver cells and overall return of strength; it is a major aspect of basic care.[11] The principles of diet therapy relate to the liver's function in the metabolism of each nutrient.

Nutritional Therapy

Initial assessment includes an extensive history to evaluate possible infection sources, food and alcohol habits, and nutrient-energy computations; anthropometric data to determine any degree of malnutrition; review of laboratory test results to indicate liver function and nutritional status; and clinical observations for any evidence of nutritional deficiencies or signs of jaundice. On the basis of this analysis of personal nutritional needs and therapeutic requirements for liver tissue healing, the nutritional therapy focuses on the following guidelines:

1. *Adequate protein.* Protein catabolism is accentuated by liver disease and may be prolonged by inappropriate protein restriction. Adequate protein must be provided not only to promote liver tissue repair but also to maintain all of the body's essential functions. Protein also provides lipotropic agents such as methionine and choline for the conversion of fats to lipoproteins for removal from the liver, thus preventing fatty infiltration. The daily diet should supply high-quality protein in the amount of 1.5 to 2.0 g/kg actual body weight, or about 100 to 150 g. This amount is usually sufficient to achieve a positive nitrogen balance.
2. *High carbohydrate.* Sufficient available glucose must be provided to restore protective glycogen reserves and to meet the energy demands of the disease process. Also, an adequate amount of glucose ensures the use of protein for vital tissue regeneration, the so-called protein-sparing ac-

endemic • A disease of low morbidity that remains constantly in a human community but is clinically recognizable in only a few.

interferon-alpha • One of a class of small soluble proteins produced and released by cells invaded by a virus, which induces in noninfected cells the formation of an antiviral protein that interferes with viral multiplication.

fulminant • Sudden, severe; occurring suddenly with great intensity.

parenchymal cells • Functional cells of an organ as distinguished from the cells comprising its structure or framework.

necrosis • Cell death caused by progressive enzyme breakdown.

jaundice • A syndrome characterized by hyperbilirubinemia and deposits of bile pigment in the skin, mucous membranes, and sclera, giving a yellow appearance to the patient.

icterus • An alternate term for jaundice. Nonicteric indicates absence of jaundice. Preicteric indicates a state before development of icterus, or jaundice.

immunocompetence • The ability or capacity to develop an immune response, that is, antibody production or cell-mediated immunity, following exposure to an antigen.

tion of carbohydrates. The diet should supply about 50% to 55% of the total kcalories as carbohydrates, or about 300 to 400 g of carbohydrates daily.

3. *Moderate fat.* An adequate but not excessive amount of fat in the diet makes the food more palatable, and therefore the anorectic patient is more encouraged to eat. If steatorrhea is present, a more easily absorbed medium-chain triglyceride product such as MCT oil may be used for a brief time, and then regular vegetable oil products and small amounts of butterfat may be resumed to ensure adequate amounts of essential linoleic acid. The diet should supply about 30% to 35% of the total kcalories as fat, or about 80 to 100 g/day.
4. *Increased energy.* For hospitalized patients, the resting energy requirements, or basal energy expenditure (BEE), is estimated by the classic Harris-Benedict equations (see p. 55). For total energy needs, malnourished patients should receive 150% of these calculated BEE values. Ambulatory patients require more energy intake to cover added, though limited, physical activity, or a total of about 2500 to 3000 kcal/day. This increased energy intake is needed to meet energy demands of the tissue regeneration process, to compensate for losses resulting from fever and general debilitation, and to renew strength and recuperative powers.
5. *Micronutrients.* Fat-soluble vitamins in water-soluble form should be provided in amounts twice the normal recommended dietary allowance (RDA) levels. Other water-soluble vitamins also require supplementation.
6. *Meals and feedings.* The problem of supplying a diet adequate to meet the increased nutritive demands for a patient whose illness makes food almost repellent is delicate and calls for creativity and supportive encouragement. The food may need to be in liquid form at first, using concentrated formulas such as the one in Table 7-1 for frequent feedings, with the fat content modified as needed according to toleration. As the patient better tolerates solid food, prepare and serve appetizing and attractive food. Cater to the patient's food preferences to support increased intake. Since nutritional therapy is the key to recovery, a major nutritional and nursing responsibility is devising ways to encourage this essential optimal food intake. A suggested total food intake for the day (Table 7-2) can also be modified in fat as needed. The clinical dietitian and the nurse work together closely to achieve this overall nutritional goal. All staff attendants follow appropriate precautions in handling the patient's tray to prevent spread of the infection.

TABLE 7-1

High-Protein, High-Kilocalorie Formula for Patient with Hepatitis

Ingredients	Amount	Approximate food value	
Milk	1 cup	Protein	40 g
Egg substitute	Equivalent of 2 eggs	Fat	30 g
Skimmed milk powder or Casec	6 to 8 tbsp 2 tbsp	Carbohydrates	70 g
Sugar	2 tbsp	Kilocalories	710
Ice cream	2.5 cm (1 in) slice or 1 scoop		
Cocoa or other flavoring	2 tbsp		
Vanilla	Few drops, as desired		

TABLE 7-2

High-Protein, High-Carbohydrate, Moderate-Fat Daily Diet

Food	Amount
Milk	1 L (1 qt)
Egg substitute	Equal to 1-2 eggs
Lean meat, fish, or poultry	224 g (8 oz)
Vegetables (4 servings)	
Potato or substitute	2 servings
Green leafy or yellow	1 serving
Other vegetables (including 1 raw)	1-2 servings
Fruit (3-4 servings, includes juices often)	
Citrus (or other good source of ascorbic acid)	1-2
Other fruit	2 servings
Bread and cereal (whole grain or enriched)	6-8 servings
Cereal	1 serving
Sliced bread or crackers	5-6
Butter or fortified margarine	2-4 tbsp
Jam, jelly, honey, and other carbohydrates	As patient desires and is able to eat them
Sweetened fruit juices	To increase carbohydrates and fluids

Cirrhosis

Cirrhosis is the general term used for advanced stages of liver disease, whatever the initial cause of the disease may be. Among all digestive diseases, cirrhosis of the liver is the leading nonmalignant cause of death

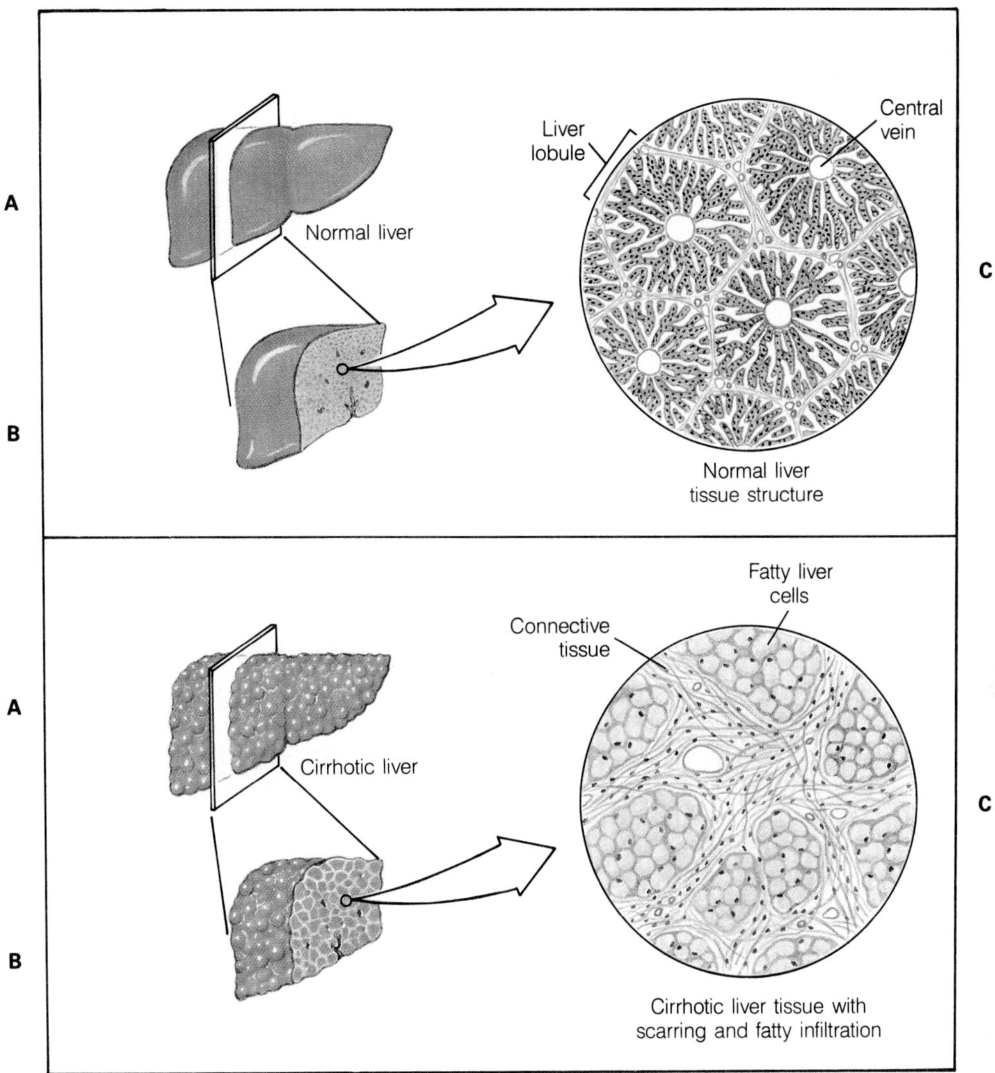

FIG. 7-2 Comparison of normal liver and liver with cirrhotic tissue changes. **A,** Anterior view of organ; **B,** cross-section; **C,** tissue structure.

in the United States and most of the developed world.[12] These deaths occur largely among young and middle-aged adults. In 1989, for example, three fifths of the 26,694 deaths caused by chronic liver disease and cirrhosis occurred among persons between the ages of 25 and 64 years.[13] The French physician René Laënnec (1781-1826) first used the term *cirrhosis* (from the Greek word *kirrhos,* meaning "orange yellow") to describe the diseased liver's abnormal color and rough surface. The cirrhotic liver is a firm, fibrous, dull yellowish mass with orange nodules projecting from its surface (Fig. 7-2).

Etiology

Some forms of cirrhosis result from biliary obstruction, with a blockage in the biliary ducts causing *cholestasis,* accumulation of bile in the liver. The focal lesions in primary biliary cirrhosis affect the *cholangioles,* the small biliary vessels, causing destructive cholangitis.[14] Other cases may result from liver necrosis of undetermined causes (idiopathic postnecrotic cirrhosis) or in some cases from previous viral hepatitis. A common problem, however, is fatty cirrhosis, *steatosis,* associated with the complicating factor of malnutrition. This continuing malnutrition, together with

> **cirrhosis** • Chronic liver disease characterized by loss of functional cells, with fibrous and nodular regeneration.

the impaired immunocompetence of *chronic active hepatitis,* accounts for the frequent occurrence of infectious relapse.[15] An increasingly poor food intake with advancing disease leads to multiple nutritional deficiencies. Damage to the liver cells occurs as fatty infiltration causes cellular destruction and fibrotic tissue changes. Ironically, such liver tissue damage and cirrhosis has also resulted from the toxic effects of prolonged chronic use of self-prescribed "therapeutic" doses of vitamin A for general health purposes. In one recent study of 41 liver disease patients with vitamin A hepatotoxicity, the smallest continuous daily dose leading to cirrhosis was 25,000 IU during 6 years, and the highest was greater than 100,000 IU taken during 2.5 years.[16]

Clinical Symptoms

Early signs of cirrhosis include gastrointestinal disturbances such as nausea, vomiting, anorexia, distention, and epigastric pain. In time, jaundice may appear, with increasing weakness, edema, ascites, gastrointestinal bleeding tendencies, and iron deficiency or hemorrhagic anemia. A folic acid deficiency, **macrocytic anemia,** may also be observed. Steatorrhea is a common symptom.

The nutritional deficiency produces multiple problems:

1. Low plasma protein levels from reduced synthesis by the failing liver and reduced dietary protein intake lead to failure of the capillary fluid shift mechanism, and the decreased colloidal osmotic pressure contributes to *ascites,* a lost accumulation of nutrient-rich fluid in the peritoneal cavity that accelerates protein-energy malnutrition.[17] Increased tubular resorption of sodium also adds to the ascites.
2. Lipotropic agents are not supplied to effect fat conversion to lipoprotein, and damaging fat accumulates in the liver tissue.
3. Blood clotting mechanisms are impaired, since factors such as prothrombin and fibrinogen are not adequately produced.
4. General tissue catabolism and negative nitrogen balance continue the overall degenerative process.

As the disease progresses, the increasing fibrous scar tissue impairs blood circulation through the liver, and portal hypertension develops.[18] Contributing further to the problem is the continuing ascites. The impaired portal circulation with increasing venous pressure may lead to esophageal **varices,** with danger of rupture and fatal massive hemorrhage. A major means of medical management of esophageal varices is by *injection sclerotherapy.* In this procedure, using a conventional fiber endoscope with local anesthesia and sedation, the physician injects a sclerosing (hardening) solution such as 5% ethanolamine or 5% morrhuate sodium just above the gastroesophageal junction.[19] The involved vein area becomes thrombosed or hardened to prevent bleeding. The surface area is then covered with a mucosal protective agent such as sucralfate (see p. 104).[18,19]

Treatment

General treatment of cirrhosis is usually aimed at correcting fluid and electrolyte problems and providing nutritional support to encourage hepatic repair as much as possible.

Nutritional Therapy

The following are guidelines for nutritional support of patients with cirrhosis of the liver:

1. *Protein according to tolerance.* In the absence of impending hepatic encephalopathy (see the following discussion), the protein intake should be continued at the level indicated for hepatitis, about 1.5 to 2.0 g/kg actual body weight, or about 100 to 150 g daily, to correct the malnutrition, regenerate functional liver tissue, and replenish plasma proteins. However, if signs of hepatic encephalopathy appear, the protein is decreased to individual tolerance.
2. *Low sodium.* Sodium is usually restricted to about 1000 mg daily to help reduce the fluid retention. Outlines of these low-sodium diet plans are given in Chapter 8.
3. *Texture.* If esophageal varices develop, it may be necessary to give soft foods that are smooth in texture to prevent the danger of rupture.
4. *Optimal general nutrition.* The remaining overall diet principles outlined for hepatitis are continued for cirrhosis for the same reasons. Kcalories, carbohydrates, and vitamins, especially B-complex vitamins plus folic acid, are supplied according to individual need and deficiency. Moderate fat is used. Alcohol is strictly forbidden.

Hepatic Encephalopathy

The term **encephalopathy** refers to any disease or disorder that affects the brain, especially chronic degenerative conditions. The brain effect in hepatic encephalopathy is a major serious complication of end-stage liver disease brought on by an accumulation of toxic substances in blood as a result of liver failure and characterized by impaired consciousness, memory loss, personality change, tremors, seizures, stupor, and coma.

Etiology

The precise cause of hepatic encephalopathy cannot always be attributed to a single agent or mechanism. However, approaches are based on the general concept that the failing liver no longer inactivates or detoxifies certain substances or metabolizes others. A key component involved is an elevated blood level of ammonia, though it is by no means the sole agent. On the basis of duration of disease and its causes, hepatic encephalopathy has been classed as chronic or acute.

The majority of cases develop from advanced cirrhosis and portal hypertension and are classed as *chronic hepatic encephalopathy*, or more specifically *portal-systemic encephalopathy (PSE)*.[18,20] PSE results when the failing cirrhotic liver diverts the incoming portal circulation carrying potentially toxic substances such as ammonia into the collateral systemic circulation by which they flow on to the brain. The resulting encephalopathy may range from trivial disorientation to full-blown coma depending on the degree of disease. Causes of chronic hepatic encephalopathy include the following[20]:

- *Excessive dietary protein and azotemia.* Increased amounts of nitrogen-containing compounds brought to the failing liver add to the metabolic problem of **azotemia.**
- *Sedatives and tranquilizers.* Excessive central nervous system depressant drugs contribute to toxicity.
- *Gastrointestinal hemorrhage.* Bleeding from esophageal varices, for example, puts still more nitrogen-containing plasma proteins into the portal circulation.
- *Acid-base disturbances.* Metabolic alkalosis or acidosis occurs as compensating control of the acid-base balance system cannot function.
- *Serum electrolyte abnormalities.* Hypokalemia and hypomagnesemia contribute to central nervous system problems.

Much more rare is *acute hepatic encephalopathy* occurring within 8 weeks after the onset of acute liver failure without previous chronic liver disease. This acute form has a high mortality of up to 80%. Its causes include the following[20,21]:

- *Fulminant viral hepatitis.* Fulminant hepatitis B virus is the most prevalent cause, with coinfection of hepatitis D virus increasing the severity of acute hepatic encephalopathy. Other cases may be caused by an increased antibody response to hepatitis viruses A and C. The prognosis in any case is grave.
- *Drug toxicity.* Examples of the three forms of drug toxicity are (1) overdosage (acetaminophen), (2) direct hepatotoxicity (carbon tetrachloride), and (3) hypersensitivity (halothane gas anesthesia).

Thus in various ways two basic factors are involved in the development of hepatic encephalopathy:

- *Ammonia formation.* The excess formation of ammonia and its increased level in the blood, *hyperammonemia,* is generally toxic in nature and is associated in varying degrees with a failing liver. It is based on the cirrhotic changes in the liver that diminish portal blood circulation and develop collateral systemic circulation, bypassing the liver and its urea cycle, which removes ammonia from the blood and converts it to urea for excretion. Instead, the toxic ammonia is shunted into the systemic blood circulation, carrying its toxic effects to the brain.
- *Amino acids and neurotransmitters.* The failing liver induces an amino acid imbalance, with an accumulation of more aromatic amino acids (phenylalanine, tyrosine, and tryptophan), as well as methionine and histidine, in the central nervous system. These amino acids are all neurotransmitter precursors, and the imbalance of their products may lead to encephalopathy.

In the diseased liver, its normal metabolic and detoxification functions cannot take place. The resulting hepatic encephalopathy brings changes in consciousness, behavior, and neurologic status. Ammonia is formed predominantly in the gastrointestinal tract as the result of the enzymatic action of dietary protein. Gastrointestinal bleeding adds still another source, and intestinal bacteria produce still more ammonia.

Clinical Symptoms

The patient's typical response involves disorders of consciousness and alterations in motor function. There is apathy, confusion, inappropriate behavior, and drowsiness progressing to coma. Facial expressions are described as an absent stare. The speech may be slurred and monotonous. A typical motor system change is the coarse, flapping tremor known as **asterixis,** observed in the outstretched hands (Fig. 7-3). It occurs as a result of a sustained contraction in a group of muscles. The breath may have a fecal odor, **fetor hepaticus.**

macrocytic anemia • An anemia (deficiency of normal red blood cells) characterized by abnormally large red blood cells.

varices • Varicose veins; enlarged and tortuous veins, full of twists, turns, curves, or windings.

encephalopathy • Any degenerative disease of the brain.

azotemia • A term meaning nitrogen, the essential life element; referring to an excess of urea and other nitrogenous substances in the blood.

asterixis • Neuromotor disturbance marked by an inability to hold outstretched hands in a steady position, resulting in an intermittent flapping of the hands, characteristic of hepatic coma.

fetor hepaticus • The peculiar odor of the breath that is characteristic of advanced liver disease.

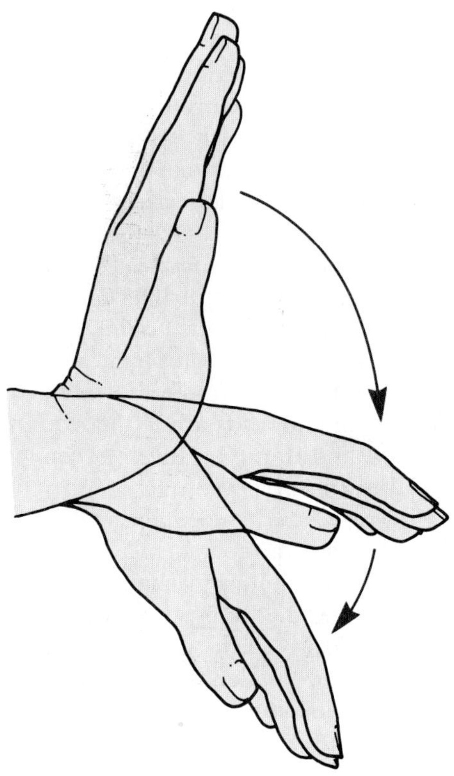

FIG. 7-3 Asterixis, the "flapping" effect of the outstretched palms-down hand seen in hepatic encephalopathy.

Treatment

A fundamental principle of therapy is the removal of the sources of excess ammonia. A Sengstaken-Blakemore tube, as well as the procedure of injection sclerosing (see p. 128), may be used to depress varices and stop bleeding. Parenteral fluid and electrolytes are used to restore normal balances. The nonabsorbable synthetic disaccharide *lactulose* is used to reduce intestinal ammonia. Lactulose reduces absorption of intestinal ammonia by creating an acidic pH of about 5.5, decreasing intestinal transit time (cathartic effect), and may stimulate secretion of nitrogenous compounds from the mucosa into the intestinal lumen.[22] Intestinal sterilization may also be attempted with an antibiotic such as neomycin to reduce the urea-splitting organisms within the bowel. It acts by trapping nitrogen in the stools, thus decreasing ammonia production.

Nutritional Therapy

The following are guidelines for nutritional support of patients with hepatic encephalopathy:

1. *Low protein.* General dietary protein intake is reduced individually as necessary to restrict the exogenous source of nitrogen in amino acids. The amount of restriction varies with the circumstances, but the usual amounts range from 30 to 50 g/day, depending on whether symptoms are severe or mild. A simple method for controlling dietary protein uses a base meal pattern containing approximately 15 g of protein and then adds small items of protein foods according to the level of total protein desired (Table 7-3).
2. *Branched-chain amino acids.* The three branched-chain amino acids (BCAAs)—*leucine, isoleucine,* and *valine*—are not catabolized by the liver but are taken up preferentially by extrahepatic tissues. Thus their metabolism proceeds without dependence on healthy liver tissue, as is the case with the other amino acids. They provide a useful energy source, as well as a better tolerated source of needed protein that may be utilized directly by the muscles, heart, liver and brain.[23] Successful treatment of hepatic encephalopathy using oral BCAA formula has been reported, with the patients becoming neurologically normal.[24] Thus several special nutritional support products have been developed with a higher ratio of BCAAs to aromatic amino acids (AAAs)—phenylalanine, tyrosine, and tryptophan—for use in enteral or parenteral nutrition support therapy, depending on the condition of the patient. The clinical use of BCAA supplementation in enteral and parenteral nutrition support formulations is an important part of standard forms of therapy in liver failure and may improve chance of survival.[25]
3. *Kilocalories and vitamins.* Adequate energy intake is crucial to the patient's recovery, especially through the impact of caloric intake on liver glycogen reserves and the protective role of these reserves in the healing process. The amounts of kcalories and vitamins are prescribed according to individual need. About 2000 kcal is sufficient to prevent catabolism, with sufficient carbohydrates as the primary essential energy source and some fat as tolerated. Vitamin K is usually given parenterally, along with other vitamins that may be deficient. Close attention is also given to possible mineral deficiencies. In addition to common vitamin and mineral deficiencies seen in malnutrition, zinc deficiency specifically has been found to induce episodes of hepatic encephalopathy in patients with chronic liver disease.[26]
4. *Fluid intake.* Fluid intake is carefully controlled in relation to output.

Liver Transplantation

Indications

The development of liver transplantation as an acceptable therapy for end-stage liver disease has been

TABLE 7–3

Low-Protein Diets (15 g, 30 g, 40 g, and 50 g Protein)

General description

- The following diets are used when dietary protein is to be restricted.
- The patterns limit foods containing a large percentage of protein, such as milk, eggs, cheese, meat, fish, fowl, and legumes.
- Avoid meat extractives, soups, broth, bouillon, gravies, and gelatin desserts.

Basic meal patterns (contains approximately 15 g of protein)

Breakfast	Lunch	Dinner
½ cup fruit or fruit juice	1 small potato	1 small potato
½ cup cereal	½ cup vegetable	½ cup vegetable
1 slice toast	Salad (vegetable or fruit)	Salad (vegetable or fruit)
Butter	1 slice bread	1 slice bread
Jelly	Butter	Butter
Sugar	1 serving fruit	1 serving fruit
2 tbsp cream	Sugar	Sugar
Coffee	Coffee or tea	Coffee or tea

For 30 g protein	Examples of meat portions
Add: 1 cup milk 28 g (1 oz) meat, 1 egg, or equivalent	28 g (1 oz) meat = 1 thin slice roast, 4 × 5 cm (1½ × 2 in) 1 rounded tbsp cottage cheese 1 slice American cheese
For 40 g protein	
Add: 1 cup milk 70 g (2½ oz) meat, or 1 egg and 42 g (1½ oz) meat	70 g (2½ oz) meat = Ground beef patty (5 can be made from 448 g [1 lb]) 1 slice roast
For 50 g protein	
Add: 1 cup milk 112 g (4 oz) meat, or 2 eggs and 56 g (2 oz) meat	112 g (4 oz) meat = 2 lamb chops 1 average steak

an important recent medical advance. In a single recent year, 1989, approximately 2200 liver transplants were performed in the United States, and the average 1-year survival was 72%.[27] Candidates for transplant include patients with end-stage chronic liver disease or acute fulminant liver failure with hepatic encephalopathy, progressive liver diseases for which conventional treatment has failed and the prognosis of which indicates a survival of less than 10%. In such cases, **orthotopic** (normal placement) liver transplantation remains the best chance of prolonged survival. Less suitable cases include problems such as alcoholic cirrhosis and malignant tumors, and contraindicated cases are those complicated by sepsis or advanced lung and kidney disease. Basic consideration of individual cases involves three aspects—the prognosis without transplantation, the complications present, and the quality of life reported by the patient.[28] A number of post-transplant women, after return of fertility with the new healthy liver, have been able to conceive and maintain the high-risk pregnancy to a successful outcome with closely monitored medical management, although preeclampsia is a common complication.[29] Clinicians suggest that contraception be considered immediately following transplantation and advise waiting 9 to 12 months before conceiving. They recommended a barrier method because birth control pills may interfere with accurate **cyclosporine** dosing for maintaining the transplant.

orthotopic • Occurring at the normal place in the body; placement of a transplanted organ in the position formerly occupied by tissue of the same kind.

cyclosporine • An immunosuppressant drug widely used following organ transplants to control the immune system and prevent rejection of the new tissue.

Nutritional Therapy

As with all major surgery, aggressive nutritional support reduces risks. Careful pretransplant nutritional assessment and support helps prepare the patient for major surgery and may require enteral or parenteral nutrition support for optimal postoperative nutritional status. Practical food handling precautions have also been recommended for use before and after surgery to minimize bacterial development[2]:

- Avoid fermented dairy products such as cheese, yogurt, and buttermilk.
- Avoid raw vegetables and unpeeled fruit.
- Avoid foods kept warm or at room temperature for long periods.
- Use refrigerator or microwave for defrosting frozen foods.
- Serve and eat prepared foods immediately.
- Cover and freeze leftovers immediately.
- Use refrigerated foods within 2 days.
- Maintain clean technique and an immaculate preparation area.

Alcoholic Liver Disease

Problem of Alcohol Dependence

About two thirds of all American adults drink alcohol at least occasionally, and it is estimated that about 18 million currently experience problems from alcohol use. About 7% of these persons develop moderate to serious levels of alcohol dependence symptoms.[30] Current U.S. national health promotion and disease objectives for the year 2000 include a goal to reduce alcohol (and other drug) abuse and the health problems it brings to Americans of all ages, from the birth defects of fetal alcohol syndrome and the alcoholic dependence of one in four American adolescents to the early deaths of young and middle-aged adults from chronic alcoholic liver disease.[31,32] The economic cost of problems associated with alcohol abuse was estimated in 1990 to be $70 billion.[33]

Alcohol Intake and Metabolism

Beverage alcohol—either ethyl alcohol or *ethanol* (CH_3CH_2OH)—is widely enjoyed socially. But its abuse creates major problems of alcoholism or alcohol dependency and serious social, economic, physiologic, and disease effects. The liver must metabolize this excessive intake, so it often bears the main burden of tissue damage and serious progressive alcoholic liver disease.

Alcohol intake. Alcohol is a drug. Thus as with any drug, its effects depend on the dose amount, which depends on the type of drink a person consumes, how much, and how often. Alcoholic drinks come in many forms and contain different amounts of pure alcohol. Decreasing the volume of beverages with higher alcohol content gives servings containing approximately equal amounts of pure alcohol. On the average, most beers are about 3.8% alcohol; unfortified table wines, about 12%; and fortified wines (made by adding brandy) such as sherry or port, about 20%. Distilled liquors such as whiskey, rum, gin, or brandy vary with *proof degrees,* which differ in different countries. One U.S. proof equals 0.5% alcohol, so 80-proof whiskey contains 40% alcohol. The grams of alcohol in common size servings of alcoholic beverages may be calculated by the following equation, considering 1 oz is approximately equal to 30 ml:

$$\text{Volume of drink (ml)} \times \text{percent alcohol} = \text{amount of alcohol (g)}$$

For example, calculate the amount of alcohol in an average 5-oz serving of table wine (12% alcohol):

$$150 \text{ ml wine } (5 \times 30) \times 0.12 = 18 \text{ g alcohol}$$

A sweet variation of fortified wine, made by stopping the fermentation of the sugar base with the addition of concentrated alcohol, making a drink high in sugar and alcohol, is favored by "street" alcoholics and often substituted for food. Such intake provides some energy but no protein and practically no vitamins and minerals, which contributes to serious malnutrition.

Alcohol metabolism. Alcohol is largely metabolized by two body systems: (1) the *alcohol dehydrogenase (ADH) system* and (2) the *microsomal ethanol oxidizing system (MEOS).*[34] A general diagram of the interaction of these two systems and the flow of metabolic effects is shown in Fig. 7-4. The major route of alcohol oxidation by initial conversion to *acetaldehyde* is controlled by the cell enzyme *alcohol dehydrogenase.* This reaction takes place in the cell cytoplasm. Acetaldehyde in mitochondria and cytoplasm is toxic, causing membrane damage and cell necrosis.[19] The acetaldehyde is converted to acetyl-CoA with *acetaldehyde dehydrogenase (ALDH)* acting as a coenzyme. The acetyl-CoA is normally a pivotal product of cell metabolism, being broken down to acetate, which is oxidized to carbon dioxide and water or enters the citric acid cycle for energy production. In this alcoholic environment, however, these normal pathways are depressed. The cell enzyme *nicotinamide adenine dinucleotide (NAD)* is a cofactor and hydrogen acceptor when alcohol is converted to acetaldehyde and then to acetyl-CoA.[19] The *NADH* generated moves into the mitochondria and changes the oxidation-reduction

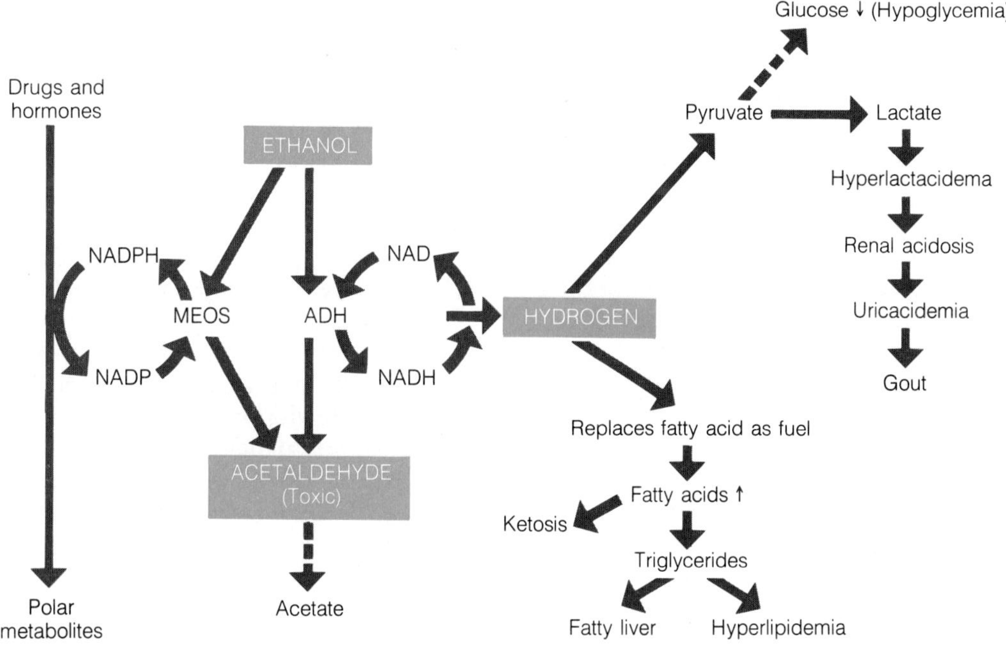

FIG. 7-4 Diagram of alcohol (ethanol) metabolism in liver cells through the alcohol dehydrogenase *(ADH)* system and the alternate microsomal ethanol oxidizing system *(MEOS)*. Broken lines indicate depressed metabolic pathways. *NAD,* Nicotinamide adenine dinucleotide; *NADP,* nicotinamide adenine dinucleotide phosphate. *(Adapted from Sherlock S:* Diseases of the liver and biliary system, *ed 8, Cambridge, Mass, 1989, Blackwell Scientific Publications.)*

(redox) balance of the liver. The hydrogen replaces fatty acid as a fuel, followed by triglyceride accumulation, a fatty liver, and hyperlipidemia. The changed redox state of the liver inhibits protein synthesis and increases lipid peroxidation, with subsequent damage to lipid cell wall structures. The citric acid cycle is reduced, adding to the decrease in fatty acid oxidation. Continuing metabolic ripple effects lead to hypoglycemia, increased lactic acid, renal acidosis, increased uric acid, and gout. To a much smaller degree, some of the excessive alcohol is metabolized by the alternate system MEOS. This system is induced by alcohol and is involved in general drug detoxification functions of the liver.[19]

Progression of hepatic injury sometimes continues after cessation of alcohol intake. The tissue changes resemble those of chronic active hepatitis and have been attributed to additional *immunologic mechanisms* triggered by the alcohol effect on liver cells.[15] Alcoholic liver disease may well be in part the result of an "immune attack" on the hepatocytes.[34]

Nutritional Concerns and Care

Numerous nutritional problems occur in the alcoholic patient with major liver disease and malnutrition. Clinical malnutrition is often a complex of many factors and has been defined by experienced clinicians as a pathologic state in which the person (1) fails to ingest sufficient kcalories, protein, and micronutrients to meet nutritional needs; (2) experiences a series of functional changes that bring on body composition changes; and (3) eventually develops abnormalities in clinical, biochemical, and nutritional status.[35] Thus our major concerns focus on these three aspects—food intake, digestion and absorption, and nutrient metabolism.

Alcohol dependency and food intake. The amount and form of alcohol ingested largely determine the appetite and degree of hunger that drive food intake. Chronic alcoholics with liver disease tend to have anorexia and altered taste sensation, with episodes of nausea and vomiting associated with alcohol-related gastritis and pancreatitis.[35] Cultural and social factors, as well as personal psychologic state and economic means, influence food consumed. The small amount of food that may be eaten is often inadequate in protein and specific nutrients such as zinc and B-complex vitamins. Also, those with limited funds are often driven to feed their addiction with more alcohol rather than to nourish their bodies with needed food.

Alcohol effects on digestion and absorption. Even if food is consumed, alcoholism and chronic alcoholic liver disease cause a secondary malnutrition from maldigestion and malabsorption.[36] Chronic heavy drinking has a damaging toxic effect over time, not only on liver cells but also on gastrointestinal mucosal tissue and secretory cells and on cells of the pancreas. The highly synchronized structures and functions of these organs that control normal digestion and absorption become disordered and dysfunctional, with multiple effects on secretions and nutrients.

Alcohol effects on nutrient metabolism. Chronic alcoholism is the major cause of cirrhosis. This form of progressive liver disease has been named *Laënnec's cirrhosis,* for the French physician who first described it from the diseased liver's orange nodular appearance (p. 127). Alcohol abuse so injures liver tissues by its direct toxic effect and its indirect cell metabolic effect that normal function is increasingly depressed. Widespread cellular injury occurs as alcohol alters the biochemical activation and degradation of many key nutrients.[36] This altered body chemistry interferes in turn with the normal functioning of the body's organ systems, and the prognosis is grave. Excessive consumption of alcohol correlates with deaths from cirrhosis in most countries, and in the United States, cirrhosis largely caused by heavy alcohol consumption is the ninth leading cause of death in adults.[19,31]

Nutritional therapy. For the most part, nutritional management of alcoholic liver disease relates to the stage and nature of the disease process, such as hepatitis, cirrhosis, and complications of hepatic encephalopathy. A major effort is made to combat the high malnutrition rate. Malnutrition is virtually 100% in patients with alcoholic hepatitis and cirrhosis caused by anorexia, nausea and vomiting, poor diet (quality and quantity), malabsorption, the energy cost of alcohol metabolism, and the hypermetabolic and hypercatabolic state.[35] Nutritional care is generally based on the following guidelines, adjusted according to individual patient status:

- *Energy.* Increased energy intake, about 2500 to 3000 kcal mainly from carbohydrate sources and fat as tolerated, is required to meet hypermetabolic needs and counteract increased catabolism.
- *Protein.* To maintain nitrogen balance, the protein need is about 60 to 80 g/day. With the complication of hepatic encephalopathy, standard drug therapy with *lactulose* allows the patient to consume 60 g of protein daily from a regular diet. If regular diet protein in this amount is not tolerated, half of the need, 30 to 40 g/day, may be supplied by the regular diet and the remaining half by BCAA supplementation with a special formula such as Hepatic Aid (McGaw).[35,37]
- *Micronutrients.* Vitamin and mineral supplementation to about twice the adult RDA standard is needed to meet the increased metabolic needs and to restore tissue needs from the malnourished deficiency levels.
- *Nutritional support therapy.* Aggressive nutritional support, enteral or parenteral as needed, improves nutritional status and liver function in malnourished patients. Various forms have been used, including high-kcalorie enteral feedings, oral BCAA supplementation, standard total parenteral nutrition (TPN) solutions, and TPN solutions high in BCAA (see Chapters 3 and 4).[35]

For intensive care to succeed, vigorous encouragement of oral intake is essential. Supportive nursing and nutritional attention often increases the patient's appetite and food intake. Studies of vigorous nutritional support show significant improvement in liver function and nutritional status.[35]

Diseases of the Gallbladder

Metabolic Functions

The gallbladder is a small, pear-shaped organ that usually lies in a depression known as the "gallbladder bed" on the lower surface of the liver at the boundary between the right and left lobes. The interior mucosal surface epithelium is quite similar to that of the small intestine, having mucosal folds with numerous surface villi and microvilli to increase its absorbing surface area.[38] The structure of the gallbladder is well suited to its physiologic function of concentrating the bile, which flows from the liver through the common hepatic duct and the cystic duct to enter the neck of the gallbladder.

Bile produced by the hepatic cells is efficiently concentrated and stored in the gallbladder. Liver bile consists largely of bile salts, with additional amounts of bilirubin (a major end product of hemoglobin decomposition), cholesterol, fatty acids, and the usual plasma electrolytes—sodium, potassium, calcium, chloride, and bicarbonate. When bile is concentrated in the gallbladder, water and most of the electrolytes are resorbed by the gallbladder mucosa, leaving the remaining ingredients, especially the bile salts, in a highly concentrated form in the gallbladder bile. The liver secretes about 600 to 800 ml of bile daily, which the gallbladder normally concentrates fivefold to tenfold. Thus this constant concentrating power enables the gallbladder to accommodate the daily bile in its small capacity of 40 to 70 ml. Through the cholecystokinin (CCK) mechanism, the presence of fat in the duodenum stimulates contraction of the gallbladder and the consequent release of bile into the common duct and then into the small intestine. Bile serves two important roles related to the digestion and absorption of fats in the small intestine: (1) emulsifying agent preparing fat for enzymatic digestion and (2) micelle formation for transporting fat into the small intestine wall during the initial stage of absorption. These tasks completed, the bile returns to the small intestine, where it rejoins the constantly cycling enterohepatic circulation of bile salts between the liver, gallbladder, and small intestine, to repeat these essential tasks.

Cholecystitis and Cholelithiasis

The prefix *chole-* of the two terms *cholecystitis* and *cholelithiasis* comes from the Greek word *cholē,* which means "bile." Thus *cholecystitis* is an inflammation of the gallbladder, and *cholelithiasis* is the formation of gallstones.

Cholecystitis

Inflammation of the gallbladder may occur alone or with gallstones. Acute cholecystitis without stones occurs frequently in patients who are critically ill with conditions such as sepsis, shock, burns, or cancer. The reason is not entirely clear, but investigators indicate that impaired gallbladder emptying and bile stasis from the physiologic stress may be important factors.[39] However, in 90% to 95% of patients, acute cholecystitis is associated with gallstones and is due to the obstruction of the cystic duct by stones, resulting in acute inflammation of the organ.[40]

Cholelithiasis

Gallstones have an ancient history. They have been found in autopsy studies of 35-centuries-old Egyptian and Chinese mummies and remain today the most prevalent disease affecting the biliary system.[40] Gallstones can be classified into two main groups: cholesterol and pigment stones.

Cholesterol stones. In the United States and most Western countries, more than 75% of gallstones are cholesterol stones. They usually result from a low-grade chronic infection. The infectious process produces changes in the gallbladder mucosa, which affect its absorptive powers. Normally the cholesterol in bile, which is insoluble in water, is kept in solution by the hydrotropic action of the other bile ingredients, especially the bile acids. However, when mucosal changes occur in cholecystitis, the absorptive powers of the gallbladder may be altered, affecting the solubility ratios of the bile ingredients. Excess water or excess bile acid may be absorbed. Under these abnormal absorptive conditions cholesterol may precipitate, causing gallstones of almost pure cholesterol to form. Also, a high dietary fat intake over a long period of time predisposes persons to gallstone formation because of the constant stimulus to produce more cholesterol as a necessary bile ingredient to metabolize the fat.

Pigment stones. Both black and brown pigment gallstones, though they differ in chemical composition and clinical features, are colored by the presence of *bilirubin,* the pigment in red blood cells. They are associated with chronic hemolysis in conditions such as sickle cell disease, thalassemia, cirrhosis, long-term TPN, and advancing age.[40] Pigment stones are often found in the bile ducts and may be related to a bacterial infection with *Escherichia coli.*

Clinical Symptoms

When inflammation, stones, or both are present in the gallbladder, contraction from the *cholecystokinin-pancreozymin (CCK-PZ) mechanism* causes pain. Sometimes the pain is severe. There is fullness and distention after eating and particular difficulty with fatty foods.

Treatment

Surgical removal of the gallbladder, a cholecystectomy, has been the usual treatment for cholecystitis and cholelithiasis (see Chapter 11). It is usually simple, safe, and curative, and still the choice for many patients. More than 500,000 cholecystectomies are performed in the United States each year. However, several new nonsurgical treatments for removing the stones have been developed, though they are still in experimental stages (see *To Probe Further,* p. 136).[40] These methods are based on principles of chemical stone dissolution *(litholysis)* and mechanical stone fragmentation *(lithotripsy).* Chemical dissolution procedures include (1) oral doses of two naturally occurring bile acids, chenodeoxycholic acid (CDCA) and ursodeoxycholic acid (UDCA), and (2) direct instillation of liquid contact solvents. Mechanical fragmentation procedures include (1) extracorporeal shock wave lithotripsy (ESWL) using ultrasonographic targeting of electromagnetic waves and (2) laser beams.[41-44]

If the patient is obese, as many persons with gallbladder disease are, some gradual weight loss before surgery is advisable. Among obese persons predisposed to cholesterol gallstones, rapid weight loss with very low-kcaloric dieting has been shown to lead to the formation of gallstones.[45,46]

Dissolution and Fragmentation: Alternate Solutions to the Problem of Gallstones

TO PROBE FURTHER

The 25 million Americans with gallstones may be able to have relief without surgery. Chemical dissolution by use of a drug, alone or combined with mechanical fragmentation by ultrasound waves, offers possible alternatives.

Chenodiol (chenodeoxycholic acid) and its companion *ursodiol* (ursodeoxycholic acid) are two natural bile acids that reduce the concentration of cholesterol in bile and dissolve cholesterol stones harmlessly, thus sparing many persons the discomfort, risk, and cost of major surgery. Their biologic activity prevents excessive cholesterol from separating out of bile to form the most common type of gallstone. Other stones consisting of combinations of calcium carbonate, bilirubin, and other compounds make up only 15% to 20% of all gallstones.

These two naturally occurring bile acids, CDCA and UDCA, have been studied for a number of years and are now used to treat gallstones in more than 40 countries. Clinically, they appear to be effective at dissolving "floating" gallstones less than 1.25 cm (½ in) in diameter with few side effects (such as diarrhea) and only temporary reversible changes in some liver enzymes. This makes it potentially beneficial to patients who are surgical risks because of other medical problems.

Other nonsurgical methods of removing gallstones are also now in experimental stages of development and may expand these alternatives still further. An additional chemical dissolution method is the instillation of liquid solvents such as methyl tert-butyl ether directly into the gallbladder or the common bile duct. Additional mechanical fragmentation by pulsed lasers is being studied.

These alternate means may help patients avoid gallbladder surgery, but they do not eliminate the need for a diet emphasizing carbohydrates and fiber and controlling fat with an eye to weight management. Further, most of these alternatives work mainly on small stones rather than on larger clumps of cholesterol. Also, they are not recommended for everyone. Chronic liver disease or a bile duct obstruction may rule them out, as does pregnancy. For many persons however, these alternatives may provide long sought, successful treatments. Those who suffer from gallstones may be able to say good-bye to pain, indigestion, nausea, and jaundice without fear of surgery.

REFERENCES

Albert MB, Fromm H: Nonsurgical alternatives in the management of gallstones, *Intensive Care Med* 4(1):3, 1989.

Editorial: Bile acid therapy in the 1990s, *Lancet* 340:1260, 1992.

Hochberger J et al: Lithotripsy of gallstones by means of a quality-switched giant-pulse neodymium: yttrium-aluminum-garnet laser, *Gastroenterology* 101(5):1391, 1991.

Nutritional Therapy

The following are guidelines for nutritional support of patients with cholecystitis or cholelithiasis:

1. *Fat.* Because fat is the principal cause of contraction of the diseased organ and the consequent pain, it may be poorly tolerated. Kcalories for energy needs should come principally from carbohydrate foods, especially during acute phases. The diet may be limited in fat to 20 to 30 g daily. Later the patient may tolerate 50 to 60 g, so that the diet may be made more palatable. A diet plan for a low-fat regimen is given in Table 7-4. Control of fat also contributes to weight control, a primary goal since obesity and excess food intake have been repeatly associated with the development of gallstones.
2. *Kcalories.* If weight loss is indicated, kcalories should be reduced according to patient need. Usually a low-kcalorie reduction diet has a low fat ratio and meets the needs of the patient with gallbladder disease for fat control.
3. *Cholesterol and "gas formers."* For healthy eating in general, dietary fat and cholesterol should be reduced from America's usual high-fat fare. The body synthesizes sufficient cholesterol daily to meet its needs. As for use of so-called gas formers such as legumes or cabbage or fiber, these foods affect individuals differently, so the person with gallbladder disease may eat these or not according to individual comfort and desire. Blanket restriction seems unwarranted, since food tolerances are highly individual (see Chapter 6). Repeated surveys of hospitalized patients fail to show differences in food tolerances attributable to specific gastrointestinal disorders. Patients with gallbladder disease have no more incidence of specific food intolerances than do patients without gastrointestinal disease.

Diseases of the Pancreas

Metabolic Functions

The pancreas is a soft, flattened, elongated gland, 12 to 20 cm long in the adult and weighing 85 to 95 g.[47]

TABLE 7–4

Low-Fat and Fat-Free Diets

Low-fat diet

General description

- This diet contains foods that are low in fat.
- Foods are prepared without the addition of fat.
- Fatty meats, gravies, oils, cream, lard, avocados, desserts containing eggs, butter, cream, and nuts are avoided.
- Foods should be used in amounts specified and only as tolerated.
- The sample pattern contains approximately 85 g protein, 50 g fat, 220 g carbohydrates, and 1670 kcal.

	Allowed	Not allowed
Beverages	Skimmed milk, coffee, tea, carbonated beverages, fruit juices	Whole milk, cream, evaporated and condensed milk
Bread and cereals	All kinds	Rich rolls or breads, waffles, pancakes
Desserts	Jell-O, sherbet, water ices, fruit whips made without cream, angel food cake, rice and tapioca puddings made with skimmed milk	Pastries, pies, rich cakes and cookies, ice cream
Fruits	All fruits, as tolerated	Avocados
Eggs	3 allowed per week, cooked any way except fried	Fried eggs
Fats	3 tsp butter or margarine daily	Salad and cooking oils, mayonnaise
Meats and fish	Lean meat such as beef, veal, lamb, liver, lean fish and fowl, baked, broiled, or roasted without added fat	Fried meats, bacon, ham, pork, goose, duck, fatty fish, fish canned in oil, cold cuts
Cheese	Dry or fat-free cottage cheese	All other cheeses
Potato or substitute	Potatoes, rice, macaroni, noodles, spaghetti, all prepared without added fat	Fried potatoes, potato chips
Soups	Bouillon or broth, without fat; soups made with skimmed milk	Cream soups
Sweets	Jam, jelly, sugar, sugar candies without nuts or chocolate	Chocolate, nuts, peanut butter
Vegetables	All kinds as tolerated	The following should be omitted if they cause distress: broccoli, cauliflower, corn, cucumber, green pepper, radishes, turnips, onions, dried peas, and beans
Miscellaneous	Salt in moderation	Pepper, spices, highly spiced food, olives, pickles, cream sauces, gravies

Suggested menu pattern

Breakfast
- Fruit
- Cereal
- Toast, jelly
- 1 tsp butter or margarine
- Egg 3 times per week
- Skimmed milk, 1 cup
- Coffee, sugar

Lunch and dinner
- Meat, broiled or baked
- Potato
- Vegetable
- Salad with fat-free dressing
- Bread, jelly
- 1 tsp butter or margarine
- Fruit or dessert, as allowed
- Skimmed milk, 1 cup
- Coffee, sugar

Fat-free diet

General description

The following additional restrictions are made to the low-fat diet to make it relatively fat free.

1. Meat, eggs, and butter or margarine are omitted.
2. A substitute for meat at the noon and evening meal is 84 g (3 oz) of fat-free cottage cheese.

It lies to the rear of the other abdominal organs, its head to the right below the liver, nested in the curves of the duodenum, with its tapering tail slanting upward to the left under the stomach. The main pancreatic duct extends from the tail of the pancreas through the elongated center of the gland, collecting its vital secretions of enzymes for digesting all three major types of food—proteins, carbohydrates, and fats—and eventually connecting with the common bile duct before opening into the duodenum.

The pancreas is largely an *exocrine* gland, secreting its enzymes and electrolytes outward into a system of ducts that carry them into the gastrointestinal tract to digest foods. At the same time, about 2% of its tissue makes up an *endocrine* gland, as its scattered clusters or islets of endocrine tissue secrete their hormones inward directly into their own capillary network for transport to body cells. This endocrine portion consists of about 1 million islets of Langerhans, mostly concentrated in the pancreas tail, where about 80% of the cells produce insulin, 15% make glucagon, and the remaining 5% contain somatostatin (see Chapter 27.[47]

Acute Pancreatitis

Collectively, biliary tract stone disease and alcohol abuse account for about 80% of all cases of acute pancreatitis.[48] Gallstones and *biliary sludge,* a viscous sediment that sometimes accumulates in the gallbladder and is composed of calcium-bilirubin granules and cholesterol crystals embedded within a mucous gel, impede normal flow of secretions.[48,49] These biliary substances may block normal outflow of pancreatic enzymes, causing the backup of powerful activated proteolytic enzymes, beginning with trypsin, to digest tissues of the organ itself.

Alcohol abuse stimulates release of the intestinal hormone secretin, which in turn increases secretion of pancreatic enzymes. When the pancreas becomes severely damaged or when the ducts become blocked, large quantities of pancreatic secretions pool in the damaged areas. In these conditions, the effect of trypsin inhibitor may be overwhelmed, and if it is unchecked, the rapidly activated enzymes literally digest the pancreas in a few hours.[1] This acute critical course and its accompanying shock may be lethal or, if the rapid course is stemmed, may lead to chronic pancreatic insufficiency.

Less commonly, acute pancreatitis results from a viral infection such as mumps; injury such as through biliary tract surgery or a blow to the abdomen; certain drugs, for example, tetracycline, thiazide diuretics, and sulfonamides; or induction of hypercalcemia by pharmacologic doses of calcium.[48,50] Genetic disease such as cystic fibrosis also leads to pancreatic insufficiency (see Chapter 5).

Chronic Pancreatitis

Alcohol in Western societies (70% to 80%) and malnutrition worldwide are the major causes of chronic pancreatitis.[51] Chronic excessive alcohol consumption produces pancreatitis by interfering with the intracellular transport and discharge of digestive enzymes, causing their activation and the autodigestion of the pancreas. Rarely is chronic pancreatitis hereditary. In some cases, it is preceded by severe acute pancreatitis. It may also result from *hemochromatosis,* or excess iron in the blood.

Chronic pancreatitis usually produces the same symptoms as the acute form, although the pain may last longer and attacks may increase as the disease progresses. There is frequent nausea and vomiting. A principal sign of progressive chronic pancreatitis is malabsorption caused by a deficiency of pancreatic enzymes and subsequent steatorrhea. Weight loss and general malnutrition follow. Diabetes mellitus may develop because of insufficient insulin produced by the pancreatic islets of Langerhans.

Nutritional Concerns and Care

Acute Pancreatitis

Every effort is made to avoid stimulating pancreatic secretions and adding to the severe pain. Thus nothing is given by mouth and needed fluids and electrolytes are supplied intravenously. Clear fat-free liquids or a chemically defined formula may be tolerated as the patient's condition improves, progressing with continued improvement to frequent small meals of high-protein, high-carbohydrate, low-fat foods. Alcohol is strictly forbidden. If the disease state does not improve and the patient is unable to consume sufficient food, or if there are complications such as abscesses or fistulas, parenteral nutrition support may be required to sustain recovery (see Chapter 4). Studies have shown that patients with severe acute pancreatitis who were started on TPN within 72 hours of the disease had fewer complications and recovered more rapidly, indicating that in such cases TPN is safe, effective, and well tolerated.[52]

Chronic Pancreatitis

Nutritional concerns focus on preventing malnutrition and treating the malabsorption caused by the pancreatic insufficiency and subsequent lack of digestive enzymes. In general, basic nutritional therapy follows the principles detailed in Chapter 5 for managing the chronic pancreatic insufficiency of cystic fibrosis:

- *Food plan.* Normal food pattern, increased in energy-nutrient values to about 150% of the RDAs, depending on the energy-nutrient loss from malabsorption. Considering individual condition and toleration, the goal is sufficient energy intake to maintain an ideal weight-height ratio. Generally, the total increased kcalories are divided about 20% as protein, 40% as carbohydrates, and 40% as fat, a ratio also suitable for diabetes. The fat allowance is fairly moderate and need not be lower with enzyme replacements.

- *Enzyme replacement.* New capsule-encased enteric coated microspheres of pancreatic enzymes to replace normal enzyme loss caused by pancreatic insufficiency. Current products such as Pancrease (McNeil Pharmaceutical), in large enough doses to reduce the nutrient loss of steatorrhea and to correct maldigestion, help support energy-nutrient needs. The pH-sensitive enteric coating protects the enzymes from acid breakdown in the stomach (pH 2). The coating dissolves only at an alkaline pH of 6 or greater, which is the normal pH of the upper small intestine. Pancrease and the similar products Cotazyme and Viokase are all substances made from hog pancreas and contain the pancreatic enzymes peptidase, lipase, and amylase.
- *Vitamin and mineral supplementation.* Supplements of vitamins A and E particularly, with vitamins D and K as needed. Fat-soluble vitamins are best absorbed when taken in the morning with fat-containing meals and pancreatic enzymes. B-complex vitamins also replace losses.
- *Nutritional support.* Enteral support by nasoenteric or enterostomy tube-feeding or parenteral support by peripheral vein or TPN as needed.

Abstinence from alcohol should also be a goal, but with patients whose pancreatic disease is largely the result of alcohol dependency, that is difficult to achieve. Extended group support programs may be helpful.

To Sum Up

The liver performs three primary functions: (1) *metabolic,* influencing the fate of all nutrients, some drugs, and steroid hormones; (2) *secretory,* producing bile for the gastrointestinal tract; and (3) *vascular,* filtering and storing blood. The gallbladder concentrates, stores, and releases bile as required to help digest and absorb fats.

Common liver disorders include *hepatitis,* usually caused by viral infection, and *cirrhosis,* advanced stages of chronic liver disease and tissue necrosis. Uncontrolled cirrhosis leads to a major complication of end-stage hepatic disease, *hepatic encephalopathy.* Although nutrient and kcalorie levels required vary with each condition, the nutritionist and the nurse are faced with the problem of overcoming anorexia in the patient. Providing concentrated liquid formulas is one solution. However, solid food served with an appetizing and attractive appearance is also used to provide optimal nutrient levels. In some extreme cases, TPN may be required.

Diseases of the gallbladder include *cholecystitis,* an inflammation that interferes with the absorption of water or bile acids, and *cholelithiasis,* or gallstone formation. Cholecystitis may lead to gallstones by creating an environment that causes excess cholesterol to precipitate out of solution in the bile. For this reason, 80% of gallstones are made up of cholesterol. Treatment involves surgical removal of the gallbladder or dissolution of the stones by procedures using the drug chenodeoxycholic acid or ultrasound. In either case the patient must follow a low-fat diet to avoid distention and pain after surgery and to reduce the possibility of gallstone formation in the future.

Pancreatitis may occur in acute and chronic forms. In both forms, alcohol abuse is a primary cause. Other causes include biliary disease, malnutrition, drug reactions, abdominal injury, and genetic predisposition. In acute pancreatitis, pain is severe because of autodigestion of pancreatic tissue by pooled activated enzymes. Initially, nothing is allowed by mouth to avoid stimulating more enzyme action and feeding is by vein, with a gradual return to small, frequent meals as the attack subsides. In chronic pancreatitis the nutritional problems are malnutrition and maldigestion from lack of enzymes because of pancreatic insufficiency. Nutritional care focuses on a nourishing diet with enzyme replacement and vitamin-mineral supplementation.

QUESTIONS FOR REVIEW

1. How are the major metabolic functions of the liver affected in liver disease? Give some examples.
2. What is the rationale for treatment in the spectrum of liver disease—hepatitis, cirrhosis, and hepatic encephalopathy?
3. Develop a 1-day food plan for a 45-year-old male, 183 cm (6 ft 1 in) tall, weighing 90 kg (200 lb), with infectious hepatitis; another plan for a similar patient with cirrhosis of the liver; and another for a patient with hepatic encephalopathy. What principles of diet therapy apply for each?
4. What are the principles of nutritional therapy in treating gallbladder disease? Write a 1-day meal plan for a 30-year-old woman, 165 cm (5 ft 6 in) tall, weighing 81 kg (180 lb), who has an inflamed gallbladder with stones and is awaiting a cholecystectomy.
5. Compare acute and chronic forms of pancreatitis in terms of etiology, symptoms, and nutritional therapy. What role does special enteral or parenteral nutrition support play in this therapy?

REFERENCES

1. Guyton AC: *Textbook of medical physiology,* ed 8, Philadelphia, 1991, WB Saunders.
2. Zeman FJ: *Clinical nutrition and dietetics,* ed 2, New York, 1991, Macmillan Publishing.
3. Moseley RH: Approach to the patient with abnormal liver chemistries. In Yamada T, ed: *Textbook of gastroenterology,* vol 2, New York, 1991, JB Lippincott.
4. Lau JYN et al: Viral hepatitis, *Gut* 32(suppl 9):47, 1991.
5. Yang NY et al: Inapparent infection of hepatitis A virus, *Am J Epidemiol* 127:599, 1988.
6. Hoffman M: Hepatitis A vaccine shows promise, *Science* 254:1581, 1991.
7. *Bull World Health Organ* 66:443, 1988.
8. Choo QL et al: Isolation of a cDNA clone derived from a blood-borne non-A, non-B viral hepatitis genome, *Science* 244:359, 1989.
9. Bisceglie AM et al: Recombinant interferon alpha therapy for chronic hepatitis C—a randomized double-blind, placebo-controlled trial, *N Engl J Med* 321:1506, 1989.
10. Marcellin P et al: Recombinant human α-interferon in patients with chronic non-A, non-B hepatitis: a multicenter randomized trial from France, *Hepatology,* 13:393, 1991.
11. Silk DBA et al: Nutritional support in liver disease, *Gut* 32(suppl 9):29, 1991.
12. Everhart JE, Hoofnagle JH: Hepatitis B-related end-stage liver disease, *Gastroenterology* 103(5):1692, 1992.
13. National Center for Health Statistics: Advance report of the final mortality statistics, 1989, *Monthly Vital Statistics Report* 40(suppl 8):1, Hyattsville, Md, 1992, Public Health Service.
14. Neuberger J et al: Primary biliary cirrhosis, *Gut* 32(suppl 9):573, 1991.
15. Johnson PJ, McFarland IG: Chronic active hepatitis, *Gut* 32(suppl 9):63, 1991.
16. Geubel AP et al: Liver damage caused by therapeutic vitamin A administration: estimate of dose-related toxicity in 41 cases, *Gastroenterology* 100:1701, 1991.
17. Dolz C et al: Ascites increases the resting energy expenditure in liver cirrhosis, *Gastroenterology* 100:738, 1991.
18. MacDougall BRD et al: Portal hypertension—25 years of progress, *Gut* (suppl 9):18, 1991.
19. Sherlock S: *Diseases of the liver and biliary system,* ed 8, London, 1989, Blackwell Scientific.
20. Conn HO: The hepatic encephalopathies. In Conn HO, Bircher J, eds: *Hepatic encephalopathy: management with lactulose and related carbohydrates,* East Lansing, Mich, 1989, Medi-Ed Press.
21. Highes RD et al: Acute liver failure, *Gut* 32(suppl):586, 1991.
22. Bircher J, Ullrich D: Clinical pharmacology of lactulose. In Conn HO, Bircher J, ed: *Hepatic encephalopathy: management with lactulose and related carbohydrates,* East Lansing, Mich, 1989, Medi-Ed Press.
23. Fischer JE: Branched-chain-enriched amino acid solutions in patients with liver failure: an early example of nutritional pharmacology, *J Parenter Enteral Nutr* 14(suppl 5):29, 1990.
24. Marchesini G et al: Long-term oral branched-chain amino acid treatment in chronic hepatic encephalopathy: a randomized double-blind casein-controlled trial, *J Hepatol* 11:92, 1990.
25. Hiyama DT, Fischer JE: Nutritional support in hepatic failure: the current role of disease-specific therapy. In Fischer, ed: *Total parenteral nutrition,* ed 2, Boston, 1991, Little, Brown.
26. Van der Rijt CCD et al: Overt hepatic encephalopathy precipitated by zinc deficiency, *Gastroenterology* 100:1114, 1991.
27. *Annual report of the US Scientific Registry for Organ Transplantation Network 1990,* Richmond, Va, UNOS, and Bethesda, Md, Division of Organ Transplantation, Health Resources and Scientific Administration.
28. O'Grady JG, Portman B: Liver transplantation, *Gut* 32(suppl 9):79, 1991.
29. Laifer SA et al: Pregnancy in liver transplant patients—and vice versa, *Gastroenterology* 10(5):1443, 1991.
30. National Institute on Alcohol Abuse and Alcoholism, US Department of Health and Human Services: *Seventh special report to the US Congress on alcohol and health,* Washington, DC, 1988, US Government Printing Office.
31. US Department of Health and Human Services, Public Health Services: *Healthy people 2000: national health promotion and disease prevention objectives,* Pub No 91-50212, Washington, DC, 1990, US Government Printing Office.
32. Dryfoos JG: *Working paper on youth at risk: one in four in jeopardy,* Hastings-on-Hudson, 1987, The Carnegie Corporation.
33. Rice DP et al: *The economic costs of alcohol and drug abuse and mental illness,* San Francisco, 1990, Institute for Health and Aging, University of California—San Francisco.
34. Thomson AD et al: Alcoholic liver disease, *Gut* 32(suppl 9):97, 1991.
35. Marsano L, McClain CJ: Nutrition and alcoholic liver disease, *J Parenter Enteral Nutr* 15(3):337, 1991.
36. Leiber CS: Alcohol, liver, and nutrition, *J Am Coll Nutr* 10(12):602, 1991.
37. Weber FL et al: Effects of branched-chain amino acids on nitrogen metabolism in patients with cirrhosis, *Hepatology* 11:942, 1990.
38. Pellegrini CA, Duh Q-Y: Gallbladder and biliary tree: anatomy and structural anomalies. In Yamada T, ed: *Textbook of gastroenterology,* vol 2, New York, 1991, JB Lippincott.
39. Adam A, Roddi ME: Acute cholecystitis: radiological management, *Baillieres Clin Gastroenterol* 5(4):787, 1991.
40. Lee SP, Sekijima J: Gallstones. In Yamada T, ed: *Textbook of gastroenterology,* vol 2, New York, 1991, JB Lippincott.
41. Albert MB, Fromm H: Nonsurgical alternatives in the management of gallstones, *Intensive Care Med* 4:3, 1989.

42. Jones SN et al: Non-operative management of gallstones—a preliminary review. *Clin Radiol* 40:591, 1989.
43. Hochberger J et al: Lithotripsy of gallstones by means of quality-switched giant-pulse neodymium: yttrium-aluminum-garnet laser, *Gastroenterology* 101(5):1391, 1991.
44. Fromm H, Albert MB: Mechanical and chemical management of gallstones. In Yamada T, ed: *Textbook of gastroenterology,* vol 2, New York, 1991, JB Lippincott.
45. Liddle RA et al: Gallstone formation during weight reduction dieting, *Arch Intern Med* 149:1750, 1989.
46. Marks JW et al: The sequence of biliary events preceding the formation of gallstones in humans, *Gastroenterology* 103:566, 1992.
47. Moossa AR, Mulholland MW: Pancreas: anatomy and structural anomilies. In Yamada T, ed: *Textbook of gastroenterology,* vol 2, New York, 1991, JB Lippincott.
48. Steer ML: Acute pancreatitis. In Yamada T ed: *Textbook of gastroenterology,* vol 2, New York, 1991, JB Lippincott.
49. Editorial: Biliary sludge: more than a curiosity, *Lancet* 339:1087, 1992.
50. Reber HA: Acute pancreatitis—another piece of the puzzle? *N Engl J Med* 325(6):423, 1991.
51. Owyang C, Levitt M: Chronic pancreatitis. In Yamada T, ed: *Textbook of gastroenterology,* vol 2, New York, 1991, JB Lippincott.
52. Kalfarentzos FL et al: Total parenteral nutrition in severe acute pancreatitis, *J Am Coll Nutr* 10(2):156, 1991.

FURTHER READING

Albert MB, Fromm H: Nonsurgical alternatives in the management of gallstones, *Intensive Care Med* 4(1):1989.

Editorial: Bile acid therapy in the 1990s, *Lancet* 340:1260, 1992.

A good review and current comments on the status of nonsurgical procedures for removing gallstones and the new alternate laparoscopic version of cholecystectomy for the 1990s.

Fischer JE: Branched-chain-enriched amino acid solutions in patients with liver failure: an early example of nutritional pharmacology, *J Parenter Enteral Nutr* 14(suppl 5):24, 1990.

Marsano L, McClain J: Nutrition and alcoholic liver disease, *J Parenter Enteral Nutr* 15(3):337, 1991.

These clinicians provide a clear understanding of the metabolic action of branched-chain amino acids as a nutritional and pharmacologic therapy in liver failure, and they provide a review of the vital role of nutrition in alcoholic liver disease as demonstrated in the recent Veterans Administration Cooperative Study on Alcoholic Hepatitis.

Hoffman M: Hepatitis A vaccine shows promise, *Science* 254:1581, 1991.

This brief news comment reports interesting background information on the long-awaited recent development of the new hepatitis A vaccine, a boon to world travelers.

CASE STUDY

The Patient with Infectious Hepatitis

James Coleman is a 44-year-old male hospital administrator, 177 cm (5 ft 11 in) tall, 74 kg (165 lb), who was seen initially in Memorial Hospital 6 weeks ago complaining of a lack of energy, poor appetite, and severe headaches that began 3 weeks before, following his return from a trip to Paris. Since then, he has experienced nausea and diarrhea on eating. His wife, a clinical dietitian, noticed signs of jaundice in her husband beginning the day before he was admitted.

Mr. Coleman's physician ordered laboratory tests for serum albumin, bromosulfophthalein (BSP), hippuric acid, galactose tolerance, serum bilirubin, prothrombin time and response to vitamin K, cephalin cholesterol flocculation, thymol turbidity, cholesterol/cholesterol ester ratio, lactate dehydrogenase (LDH), and serum glutamic-pyruvic and serum glutamic-oxaloacetic transaminases. Results indicated impaired liver function. A physical examination revealed an enlarged tender liver and an enlarged spleen, with a diagnosis of infectious hepatitis.

The physician ordered a diet high in protein, carbohydrates, kcalories, and vitamins and moderately low in fats. During the first 4 days, the patient experienced anorexia. Attempts at eating resulted in nausea. On the request of his wife, the physician changed the diet to full liquid. With daily encouragement, Mr. Coleman's appetite gradually improved. He advanced to solid food and 3 days later consumed 75% to 90% of his meals. On discharge shortly afterward he was advised to rest as much as possible.

Mrs. Coleman called several times during his first week home for advice on encouraging her husband to stop working. A follow-up visit was arranged a few days later to evaluate the prescribed treatment, especially the need to rest. A number of relaxation techniques were discussed. As of 2 weeks ago, Mrs. Coleman reported that her husband had reduced his work load significantly and was adapting well to the diet.

Questions for Analysis

1. What is the relationship between normal liver functions and the effects or symptoms seen in infectious hepatitis?
2. For each laboratory test ordered, discuss its physiologic basis and significance in diagnosing hepatitis. Give normal values for each.
3. What problems can you identify in Mr. Coleman's nutritional care? What is the basis for each? How would you resolve them?
4. Explain the rationale for the hospital diet ordered for Mr. Coleman. Which vitamins and minerals would be the most essential for his progress?

Nutritional Management of the Alcoholic Patient

You have just picked up the chart of a newly admitted patient. The term *alcoholic* appears on the history form. Before reading any further, you assume the diagnosis is cirrhosis. What would you also assume about his diet? Is it (a) low in protein? (b) high in kcalories, half of which are provided by ethanol? (c) low in vitamins, especially in the B family? or (d) all of the above?

Many professionals would select (d) because research on nutrition and alcoholism has, since the 1940s, focused on skid-row alcoholics who squander most of their income on the bottle, leaving little with which to guard their nutritional status via nutritious foods or to maintain living quarters with facilities for cooking them properly. Conversely, a few professionals may have selected (b) as an answer, assuming that the wealthy can afford "plenty of food," as well as 12-year-old Scotch and expensive liqueurs.

These two disparate images of people suffering from alcoholism, the skid-row street person and affluent obese drinker, have been so firmly implanted in our minds that it sometimes leads the health professional to look for the following symptoms that are not always there.

Cirrhosis

Only half of all American alcoholics develop cirrhosis of the liver.

Nineteenth century malnutrition

Beriberi and pellagra, signs of thiamin and niacin deficiency, respectively, have occurred in persons with alcoholism and sometimes still do. However, studies of alcoholic patients reveal that thiamin and niacin intakes meet or exceed RDAs in the diets of most subjects.

Inadequate protein intake

Dietary studies usually indicate that patients frequently have protein intakes at RDA levels or above, certainly far from inadequate.

Excessive kilocalorie intake

Reports of kcalorie intake of patients without liver disease show levels even somewhat *lower* than that recommended, and most patients are at or below the 25th percentile of weight for height.

However, such reports do not indicate that the health professional may be wasting time looking for the effects of skid-row poverty everywhere in the heterogenous population of 10 million alcoholics in the United States. Alcoholism crosses all economic, sexual, age, and racial barriers. So it should not be surprising to learn that studies of veterans have indicated *no* statistical difference in the prevalence of malnutrition, infection, anemia, or even death rates between alcoholic and nonalcoholic populations.

The widespread incidence of alcoholism indicates that the *individual* with this problem must be evaluated as such. This is not to discount that the individual may present the following *expected findings:*

- *Cirrhosis,* or inflammation of the liver caused by the toxic effects of ethanol or by malnutrition resulting from the replacement of essential nutrients with ethanol
- *Anorexia,* accompanying ethanol-induced gastritis or pancreatitis
- *Infection,* caused by low immune response resulting from low serum protein levels
- *Hypovitaminosis A,* especially in patients with cirrhosis, since inadequate liver function reduces levels of vitamin A carrier proteins such as prealbumin
- *Fragile bones,* caused by malabsorption of calcium, phosphate, and vitamin D in postmenopausal women with liver disease caused by alcoholism

However, the patient may also present the *unexpected*—a well-nourished body.

This does not mean that the well-nourished individual with alcoholism is a healthy individual. The alcoholism itself is a disease, a separate entity that must be addressed whether any other health problems exist. The thorough health care professional develops a care plan not only for the patient's obvious health problems but also for the problems of alcoholism. These sensitive professionals keep abreast of alcohol programs available in the patient's community and learn how to identify and assess an alcohol problem by asking the right questions. Such questions include the following:

- Do you drink alcohol?
- What do you like to drink?
- How much do you drink? (How much liquor do you put in your glass? How much ice and mixer do you usually use in your glass?)
- How often do you drink?
- How much do you usually drink in a 24-hour period? How much *can* you drink in 24 hours?
- When was the last time you had a drink? What did you drink? How much did you drink?

By encouraging the patient to identify drinking habits and informing him or her that these habits could pose as great a physiologic problem as an obvious injury or disease, you may be helping the patient to take the first step on the road to recovery.

REFERENCES

Marsano L, McClain CJ: Nutrition and alcoholic liver disease, *J Parenter Enterol Nutr* 15(3):337, 1991.

Owyang C, Levitt M: Chronic pancreatitis. In Yamada T, ed: *Textbook of gastroenterology,* vol 2, New York, 1991, JB Lippincott.

Thomson AD et al: Alcoholic liver disease, *Gut* 32(suppl 9):97, 1991.

CHAPTER 8

Diseases of the Heart, Blood Vessels, and Lungs

CHAPTER OUTLINE

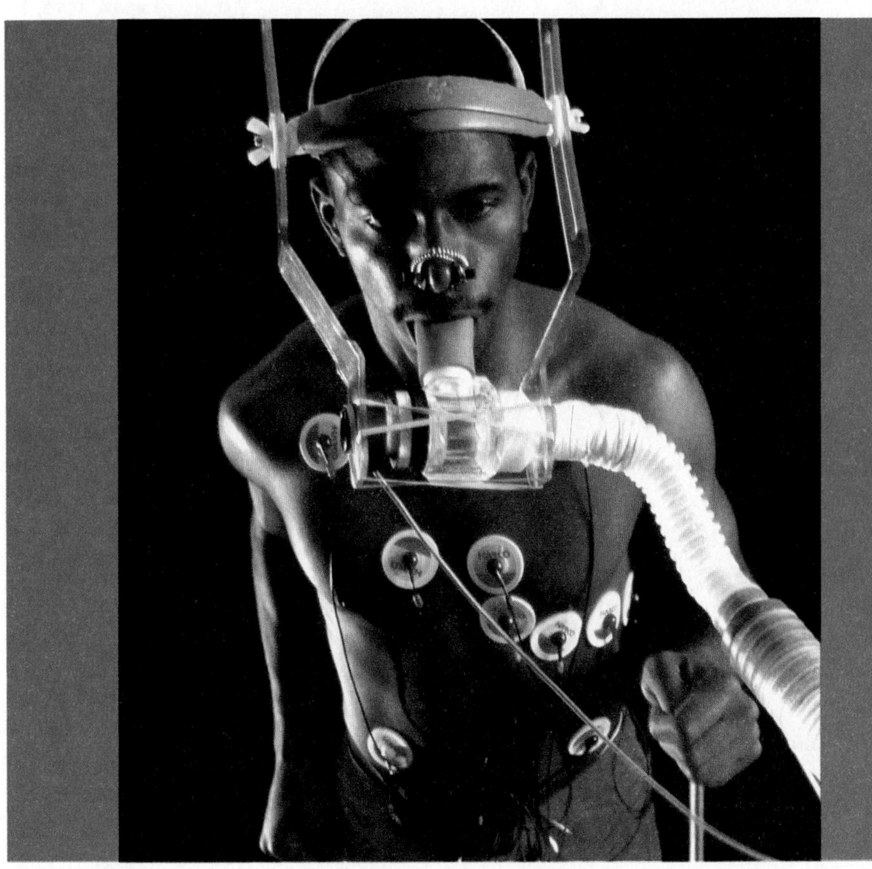

This chapter deals with the interrelated diseases of the circulatory system—the heart, blood vessels, and lungs. In recent decades these diseases of modern civilization have become the major causes of death in the United States and most other Western societies. The magnitude of this health care problem is enormous.

Coronary heart disease, and its underlying blood vessel disease arteriosclerosis, *is a leading cause of death in the United States. More than two Americans each minute suffer heart attacks and about half that number suffer cerebrovascular accidents (strokes). Targets of modern medical research and practice center on elevated blood levels of fat and cholesterol and hence on nutritional efforts to reduce dietary sources of these offenders.*

Elevated blood pressure continues to contribute a major risk factor in the development of heart disease and other blood vessel problems. Also, rising problems with pulmonary circulation have now made chronic obstructive pulmonary disease the fifth major cause of death in the United States.

In this chapter we examine the health problems that relate to the blood circulation and the vital organs that maintain it and in turn how nutritional therapy relates to modification of key nutrients involved.

Interactions of the Circulatory System

For normal operation of the body's life-sustaining blood circulation to service cell metabolism, efficient interaction of three major organ systems is essential. First, a healthy heart muscle must provide a never-ceasing pump to keep the lifeblood constantly flowing. Second, a vast network of healthy blood vessels, from large arteries to minute capillaries, must transport multiple metabolites and nutrients to nourish every single body cell. Third, healthy lungs must provide the necessary oxygen–carbon dioxide gas exchange to sustain continuing metabolic life.

Heart: The Central Pump

The heart lies in the center of the chest with its right margin directly underneath the right side of the *sternum* (breastbone) and its remaining body leaning to the left. Its lowest point, the apex, lies directly underneath the left nipple. This muscular pump beats rhythmically and continuously throughout life to send blood to the lungs and the rest of the body, contracting more than 2.5 billion times during an average lifetime.

Structure and Function

The wall of the heart is composed of three layers: (1) the *endocardium,* a smooth membrane lining the interior surface; (2) the *myocardium,* the thick interconnecting network of muscle fibers comprising the heart muscle; and (3) the *epicardium,* a tough protective outer membrane. In brilliant functional design the heart is actually two separate pumps: a *right heart* that pumps the blood through the lungs and a *left heart* that pumps the blood through the peripheral organs.[1] A thick central muscular wall, the *septum,* divides the

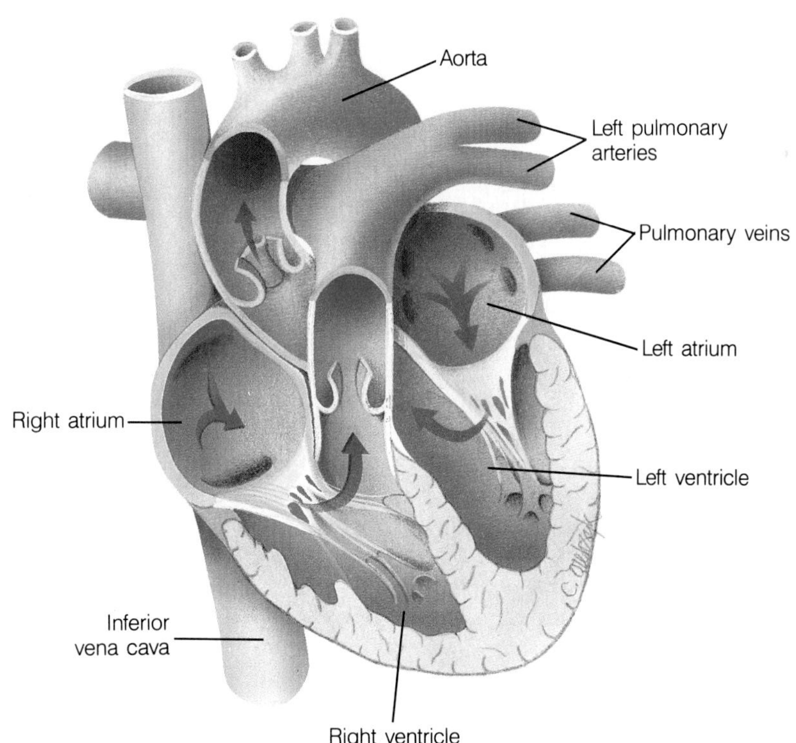

FIG. 8-1 The normal human heart. Anterior internal view showing cardiac circulation. *(From Seeley RR, Stephens TD, Tate P:* Anatomy and physiology, *ed 2, St. Louis, 1992, Mosby.)*

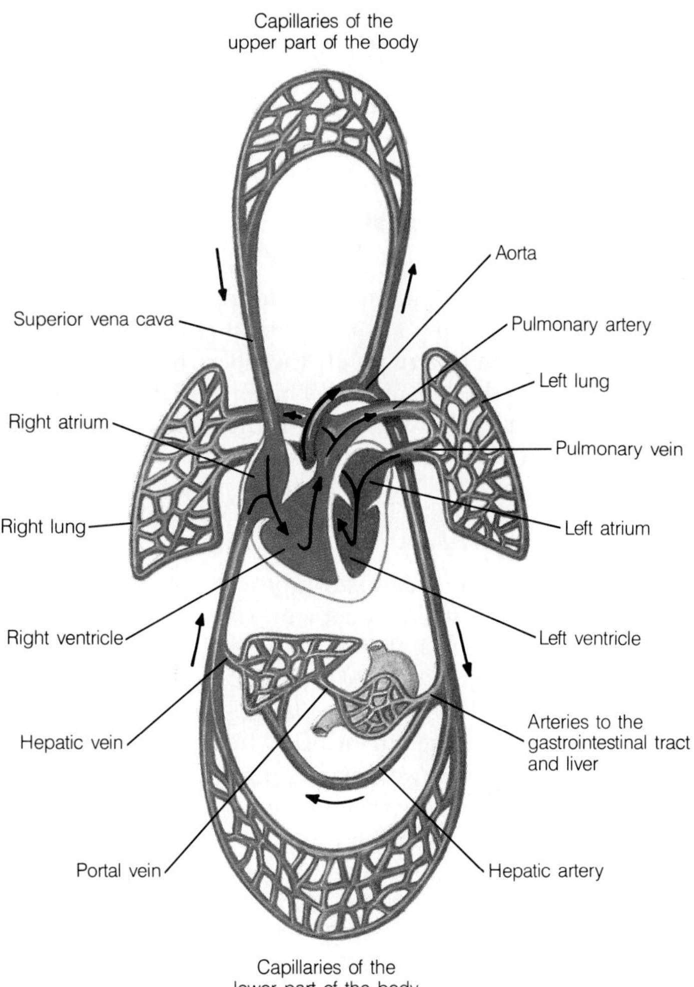

FIG. 8-2 General scheme of the human overall circulatory system showing relative arrangement of heart, blood vessels, and lungs.

interior cavity into right and left halves, each with a small upper chamber, the **atrium,** and a lower, somewhat larger one, the **ventricle,** joined by special one-way valves to prevent backflow. In both of the separate pumps, the atrium functions mainly as a blood reservoir and a primer pump and the ventricle supplies the major force that propels the blood forward into circulation.

The route of blood through the heart may be traced in Fig. 8-1. The right side of the heart receives deoxygenated blood from the entire body into its atrium by two large veins, the superior and inferior *vena cava,* and transfers it into the right ventricle, from which it is pumped via the *pulmonary artery* to the lungs to receive fresh oxygen in exchange for its carbon dioxide load. The left side of the heart then receives this oxygenated blood from the pulmonary veins into the left atrium and transfers it into the left ventricle, from which it is forcefully pumped via the body's major midline artery, the *aorta,* into branching systemic circulation throughout all the body tissues. The broad overall scheme of the body's blood circulation and the central control position of the heart is outlined in Fig. 8-2.

Cardiac Cycle

The period of time from the beginning of one heart beat to the beginning of the next is called the *cardiac cycle.* The pumping action of the heart muscle in one beat has three phases regulated by electric waves that spread from the heart's own pacemaker, the *sinoatrial node.* The three phases of the cardiac cycle are called *diastole, atrial systole,* and *ventricular systole* and are clearly seen in an *electrocardiogram* tracing (Fig. 8-3).[1]

Diastole. In diastole, the resting phase, the heart fills with blood as deoxygenated blood flows into the right side and at the same time oxygenated blood flows into the left side. The heart muscle is at rest, and the electric impulse begins to spread from the sinoatrial node (Fig. 8-3, *diastole*).

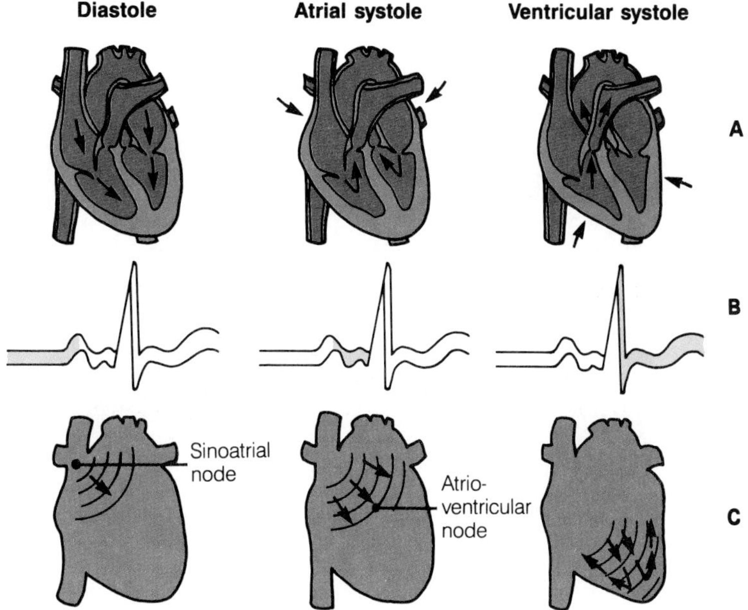

FIG. 8-3 Three phases of one heart beat that comprise the cardiac cycle. **A,** Heart action and blood flow at each phase as incoming blood is received and efficiently pumped out with heart muscle contraction. **B,** Electrocardiogram tracing of each phase. **C,** Action of the heart's own pacemaker, the sinoatrial node, sending electric waves that are picked up by the atrioventricular node and passed on to both ventricles, the major strong muscular pumps, signaling strong contractions that empty the heart.

Atrial systole. In the second phase, atrial systole, both atriums (upper heart chambers) contract simultaneously and squeeze more blood into the ventricles (lower heart chambers), completely filling them. The electric impulse reaches the atrioventricular node (Fig. 8-3, *atrial systole*).

Ventricular systole. In the final phase, ventricular systole, both ventricles contract, pumping deoxygenated blood from the right ventricle into the pulmonary artery and oxygenated blood from the left ventricle into the aorta, emptying both lower chambers. Waves of electric activity cover the ventricles and stimulate this forceful emptying, and then the cycle begins again (Fig. 8-3, *ventricular systole*).

Blood Vessels: Transport and Regulatory Systems

General Structure and Function

Blood vessels are uniquely structured to meet their functional needs. Basically the arteries and veins are pliable tubes with relatively thick walls composed of three layers: (1) a smooth inner lining, (2) a muscular elastic middle layer, and (3) a fibrous outer layer (Fig. 8-4). The thicker muscle layer in arteries controls pulsing pressures from the heart beat and the thinner walls of veins distend to provide blood reservoirs as needed.

Arterial pressure controls. The walls of arteries are far stronger than those of veins to accommodate the greater pressure pulsations from the heart beat. The artery walls are also capable of distending somewhat to help receive each new surge of blood and thus reduce resistance to flow. Fortunately, this capacity gradually reduces the pressure pulsations through the large arteries and the smaller branching venules, so that by the time the blood reaches the outer capillaries the pressure pulsations are almost zero, effectively providing a tissue blood flow hardly affected by the pulsating nature of heart pumping and allowing the blood to efficiently nourish the cells.[1]

atrium • An anatomic chamber; usually used alone to designate one of the pair of smaller upper chambers of the heart with thin muscular walls that receives blood from the body's inflowing circulation via the superior and inferior vena cavas and delivers it to the thicker-walled ventricles.

ventricle • A small cavity; one of a pair of lower chambers of the heart with thick muscular walls that make up the bulk of the heart and force blood out into body circulation to the lungs for oxygenation and then into systemic body circulation to service the cells.

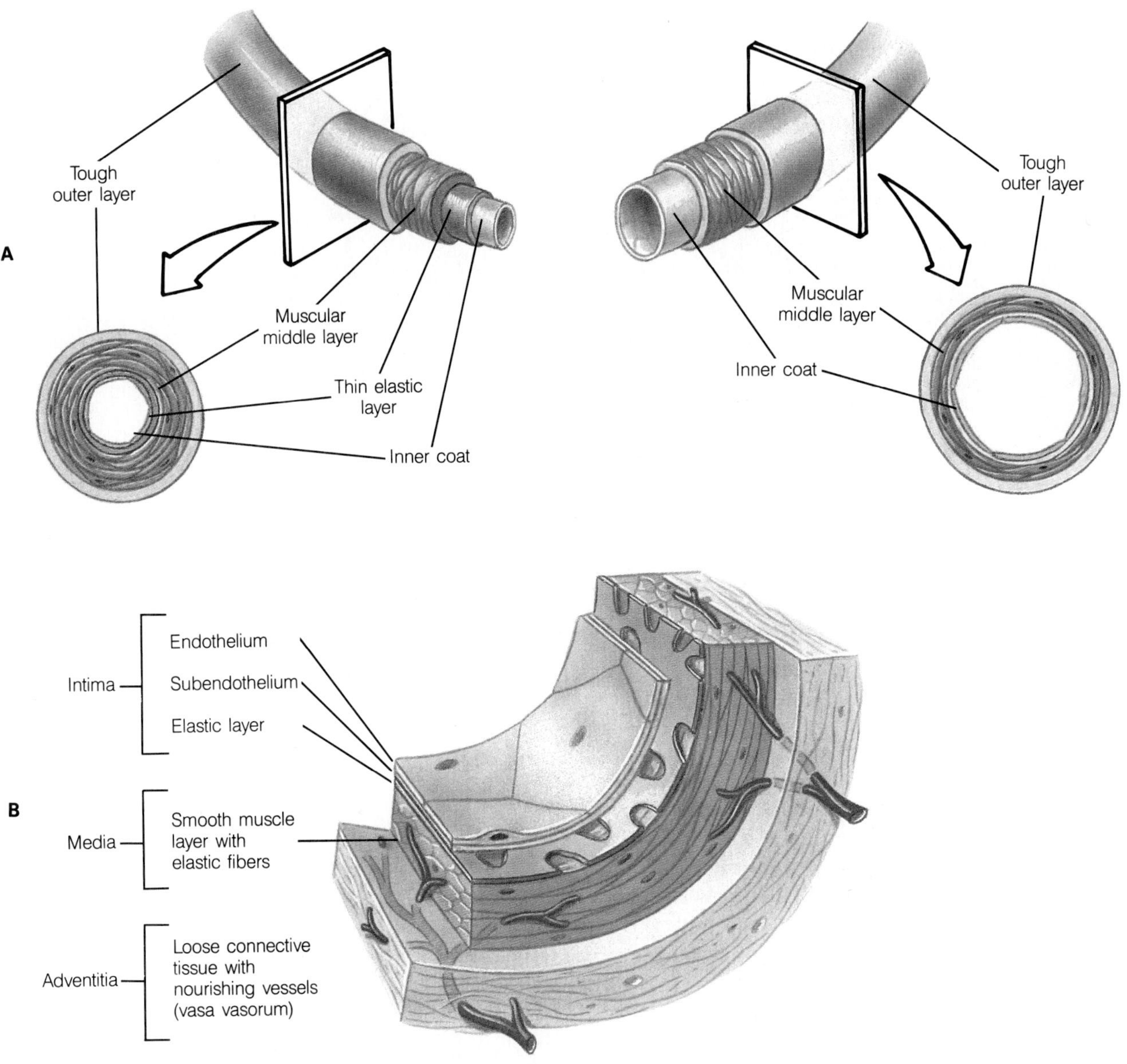

FIG. 8-4 Blood vessel structure. **A,** Comparative wall thicknesses and inner lumen size of arteries (left) and veins (right). **B,** Cutout of vessel wall showing three basic layers of tissue involved: intima, media, and adventitia.

Venous pump. Veins have thinner walls and are far more able to distend than arteries, allowing them to serve as blood reservoirs as needed. Most veins, especially those in the legs, contain small valves that squeeze blood through every time a person moves or tightens a muscle. This system of valves and muscles, called the "venous pump," is so arranged that the only direction blood flows is toward the heart in surface and deep tissue veins (Fig. 8-5).[1] When veins become overstretched by excess venous pressure lasting weeks or months, as in pregnancy, or when a person stands most of the time, the veins accumulate more blood and the valves are pulled apart, causing the venous pump to fail. The result is *varicose veins,* protrusions of the veins beneath the skin of the legs. Surrounding venous and capillary pressures cause leakage of fluid, and edema forms in the lower leg and ankle. The edema in turn prevents sufficient diffusion of nutrients from the capillaries serving the muscle and skin cells, resulting in painful and weak muscles and possible skin ulcers. Obvious treatment is elevation of the legs and tight leg binders. Varicose vein surgery may be indicated.

Special Endothelial Regulation

An important single-cell layer of *endothelial cells* lines the interior surface of the blood vessels, as well as the interior surface of intersecting lymph vessels. These

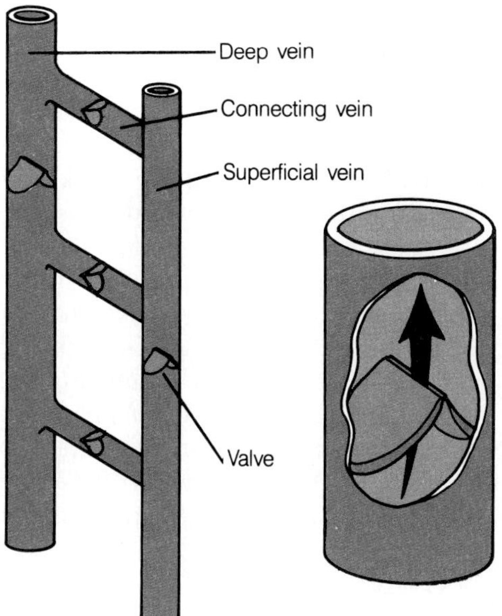

FIG. 8-5 Venous "pump" involving vein valves and adjacent muscles to ensure constant blood flow toward the heart with no backflow. Every time the legs are moved, leg muscles tighten and compress nearby veins, overcoming hydrostatic pressure and gravity and "pumping" blood through the vessel's system of valves to the heart. *(Adapted from Guyton AC:* Textbook of medical physiology, *ed 8, Philadelphia, 1991, WB Saunders.)*

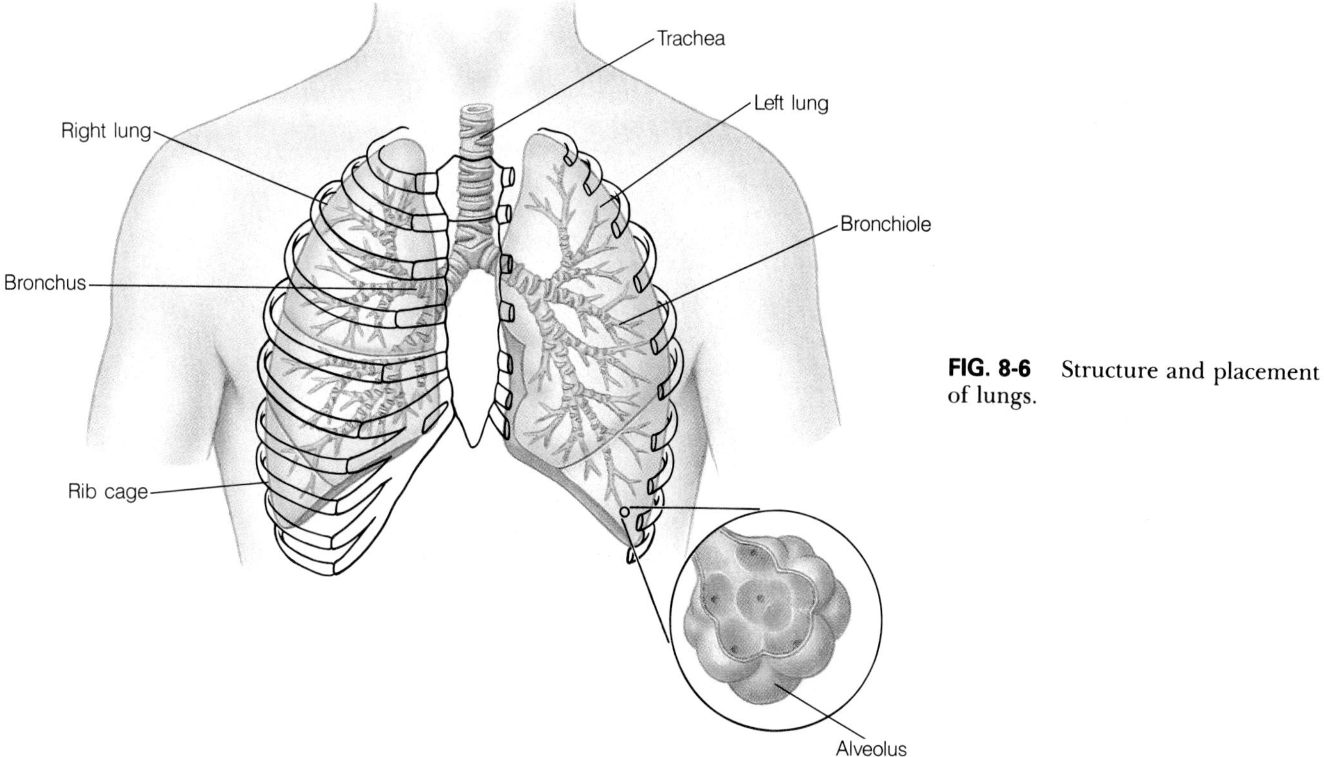

FIG. 8-6 Structure and placement of lungs.

cells are *squamous* in shape—thin, elongated, and flat—providing a smooth surface that aids the flow of blood and lymph and helps to prevent *thrombus,* or blood clot, formation. Blood vessels have been viewed traditionally as mere "plumbing," that is, as conduits to carry this vital body fluid to the tissues to service the cells, as the term circulation implies. However, researchers are now discovering that blood vessels play a far more dynamic role in regulating blood pressure and blood clotting as well as their own growth.[2] The key to these regulatory functions, according to these researchers and their growing body of new findings, lies in the endothelial cells, which form an essential protective interface between the blood and the vessel walls of arteries, arterioles, veins, and venules. The smallest vessel wall, the capillary membrane, is composed of only this single-cell layer of flat, thin endothelial cells. Together in all of these blood vessels, these thin, flat, elongated endothelial cells constitute a major line of defense for the cardiovascular system. Endothelial injury is now recognized as a major underlying link to cardiovascular disease and hypertension.[2,3] A functionally intact **endothelium** and the release of its key substance, initially named *endothelium-derived relaxing factor (EDRF),* affects vascular tone and hence relates to hypertension and arteriosclerosis. EDRF is now known to be *nitric oxide (NO),* synthesized specifically from the amino acid arginine.[3] Scientists are just beginning to discover some of the extraordinarily beneficial roles that NO has in human physiology and health. Helping to maintain blood pressure by dilating blood vessels is only one but has given strong support to its current "Molecule of the Year" award.[4,5]

Lungs: Oxygen Station

Structure and Function

The lungs lie in the chest within the rib cage behind the heart immediately connected with a network of blood vessels that comprise the pulmonary circulation (Fig. 8-6) and provide a constant supply of oxygen through the *respiratory system.* Oxygen-laden air inhaled through the nose or mouth travels down a central tube, the *trachea* (windpipe), and branches in the chest into two main *bronchi* (air passages), which supply the right and left lungs. Each of the two main air passages in turn forms a bronchial tree, branching out into smaller bronchi and then into still smaller *bronchioles,* which open out into tiny grapelike clusters of air sacs, the *alveoli.* Through the thin walls of the tiny alveoli the gases oxygen and carbon dioxide diffuse

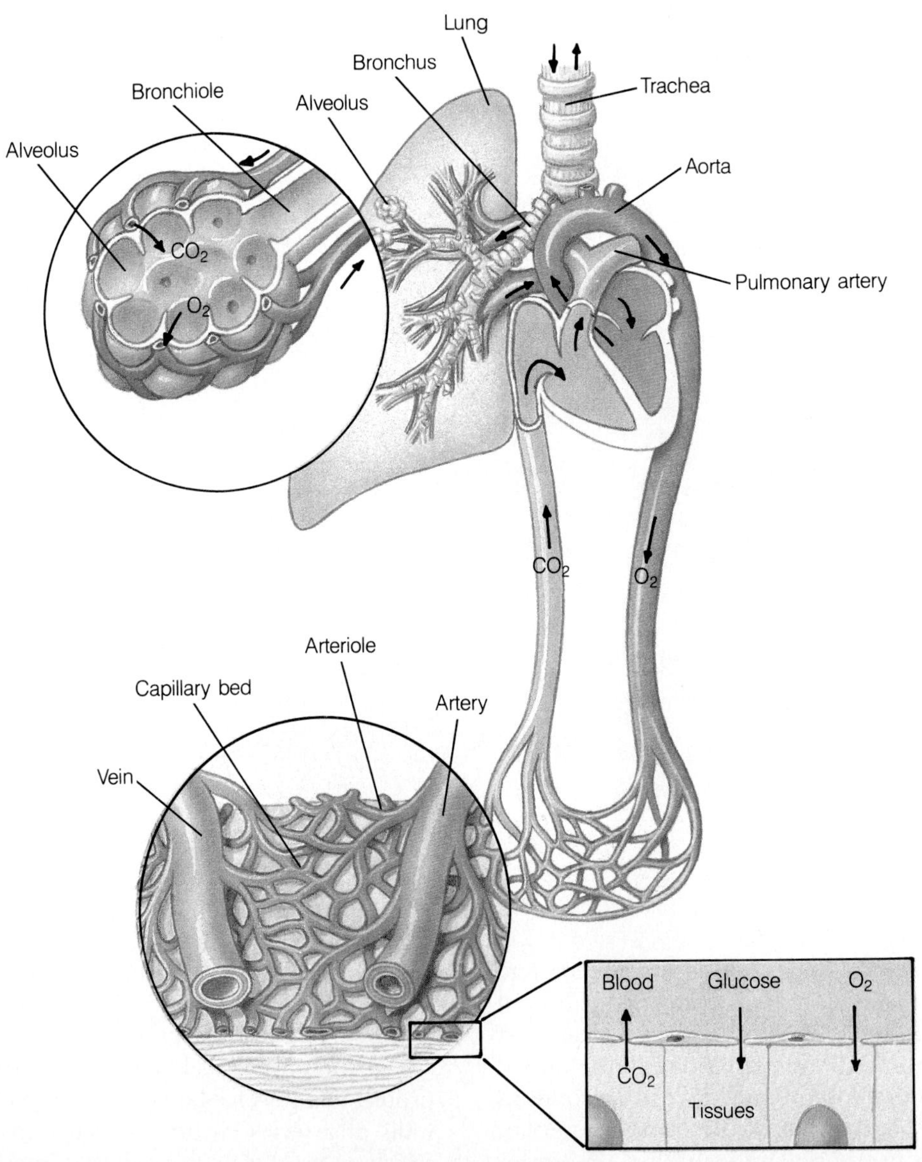

FIG. 8-7 Interacting pulmonary and systemic circulatory systems, showing oxygenation of blood in the lungs and metabolic transfers in body tissues.

into and out of the blood. An extensive capillary network fans out through each lung, surrounding each twig of alveoli, where oxygen is absorbed and carbon dioxide is released and exhaled into the air (Fig. 8-7). To facilitate the task of respiration, each lung is covered with a double membrane called the *pleura,* which allows the lungs to slide freely as they expand and contract during breathing.

Oxygen Uptake

When oxygen has diffused from the alveoli into the pulmonary blood, it combines with hemoglobin, forming oxyhemoglobin as a carrier. The hemoglobin in red blood cells allows blood to transport 30 to 100 times as much oxygen as could be transported simply in the form of dissolved oxygen in the water of the blood.[1] The oxygenated blood returns through the pulmonary circulation to the heart to be pumped through the body network of main arteries and arterioles and finally is transported to a feathery network of tissue capillaries where the oxygen is released to the cells for use in cell metabolism of the nutrients. These metabolic cell actions form large quantities of carbon dioxide, which in turn enters the tissue capillaries and is transported back to the lungs for expiration and exchange for more oxygen.

Diseases in any of these vital organs that form the body's circulatory system—heart, blood vessels, and lungs—have devastating effects. We turn now to consider such disorders in each of the organ systems involved.

Coronary Heart Disease

The Problem of Atherosclerosis

Atherosclerosis, the major **arteriosclerosis** disease and the underlying pathologic process in coronary heart disease, is paramount in ongoing study in modern medicine. The characteristic lesions involved, as they have been observed at autopsy, are raised fibrous **plaques** (Fig. 8-8). They appear on the interior surface, the **intima,** of the blood vessel as discrete lumps elevated above the unaffected surrounding regions of the tissue and ranging in color from pearly gray to yellowish gray. The main cellular component of the plaque is a smooth muscle cell similar to the major cell of the normal artery wall. The plaque usually contains fatty material such as lipoproteins, the carriers of cholesterol in the blood, which are found inside and outside the cells. Deep in the lesions is debris from dead and dying cells, as well as various amounts of lipids. Crystals of cholesterol are visible with the unaided eye in the softened cheesy debris of advanced lesions.

It is this fatty debris that suggested the original name **atherosclerosis,** from the Greek words *athera* (gruel) and *sclerosis* (hardening). This fatty degeneration and thickening narrows the vessel lumen; develops a blood clot, a *thrombus,* from its irritating presence, which may thicken into a circulating *embolus;* and eventually may cut off the blood flow in the involved artery (Fig. 8-8). If the artery involved is a major coronary vessel, a heart attack occurs. The tissue area serviced by the involved artery is deprived of its vital oxygen and nutrient supply (**ischemia**), and the cells die. The localized area of dying or dead tissue is called an **infarct.** Because the artery involved supplies the cardiac muscle, the *myocardium,* the result is called an acute *myocardial infarction (MI).* The two major *coronary arteries* with their many branches, are so named because they lie across the brow of the heart muscle and resemble a crown (Fig. 8-8).

Thus the focus of the problem in coronary heart disease is the development of these characteristic fatty plaques called **atheromas.** Injury to the important inner endothelial lining of the blood vessel wall may lead to a thickening thrombosis and lipid deposits, with the development of atherosclerosis. Analysis of the fatty plaques involved has shown considerable content of lipid materials, especially cholesterol crystals. A growing mass of evidence from large clinical trials relates these lipids and other life-style risk factors to incidence of the disease process in numerous population groups (Table 8-1).

endothelium • The layer of epithelial cells originating from the mesoderm that lines the cavities of the heart, the blood and lymph vessels, and the serous cavities of the body.

arteriosclerosis • A blood vessel disease characterized by thickening and hardening of artery walls with loss of functional elasticity, mainly affecting the intima (inner lining) of the arteries.

plaque • Thickened deposits of fatty material, largely cholesterol, within the arterial wall that eventually may fill the lumen and cut off blood supply to the tissue served by the damaged vessel.

intima • A general term indicating an innermost part of a structure or vessel; inner layer of the blood vessel wall.

atherosclerosis • A common form of arteriosclerosis in which cheesy yellow plaques of cholesterol and fatty material form within the artery wall.

ischemia • The deficiency of blood to a particular tissue caused by functional blood vessel constriction or actual obstruction.

infarct • An area of tissue necrosis caused by local ischemia resulting from obstruction of blood circulation.

atheroma • A mass of fatty plaque formed in inner arterial walls in atherosclerosis.

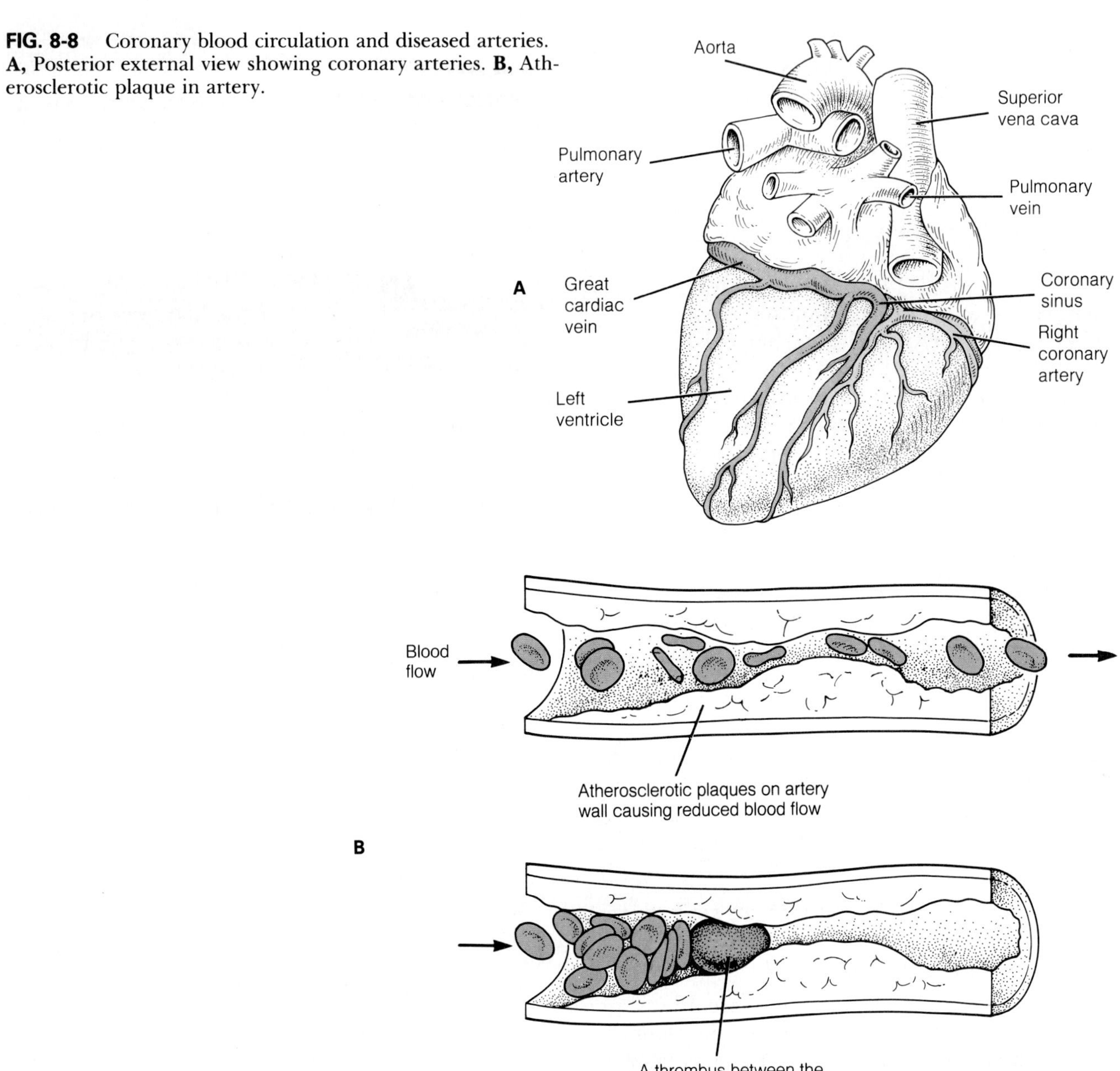

FIG. 8-8 Coronary blood circulation and diseased arteries. **A,** Posterior external view showing coronary arteries. **B,** Atherosclerotic plaque in artery.

TABLE 8–1

Multiple Risk Factors in Cardiovascular Disease

Personal characteristics (no control)	Learned behaviors (intervene and change)	Background conditions (screen and treat)
Sex	Stress and coping	Hypertension
Age	Smoking cigarettes	Diabetes mellitus
Family history	Sedentary life-style	Hyperlipidemia (especially hypercholesterolemia)
	Obesity	
	Food habits	
	Excess fat	
	Excess sugar	
	Excess salt	

Etiology: Relationship to General Lipid Metabolism

Over the past few years, large-scale studies have demonstrated repeatedly a definite association between types of dietary fat and elevated blood lipid levels, especially cholesterol.[6] Dietary substitution of foods high in polyunsaturated fatty acids for foods high in saturated fatty acids, as well as total dietary fat reduction, has produced a lowering of blood cholesterol. The work of many investigators has brought forth an increasing understanding about the mechanisms for synthesis, transport, and catabolism of cholesterol, thus control of blood cholesterol levels, and has paved

Role of Nonfat Factors in Atherosclerosis

TO PROBE FURTHER

Nutrients other than fat play an important role in preventing or promoting atherosclerosis by changing blood levels of cholesterol, high density lipoprotein-cholesterol (HDL-C), and triglycerides.

Calcium. Large amounts of calcium have been shown to lower our cholesterol and triglyceride levels. Most Americans, including American women, fail to take in the 800 mg/day recommended daily allowance (RDA).

Carbohydrates. The body tends to manufacture triglycerides when sucrose is consumed in large amounts. Although the evidence is not conclusive, this and other research data tend to suggest that a diet rich in simple carbohydrates may well increase the risk in susceptible individuals of forming atherosclerotic plaque.

Chromium. Cholesterol levels drop while HDL-C levels rise when the diet is supplemented with chromium. Thus chromium may have a protective role against plaque formation. The American diet may be marginal in this trace element.

Fiber. Cardiovascular disease is less common in populations that have high-fiber diets than it is in populations in developed countries in which a more refined lower-fiber diet is consumed. Soluble dietary fiber—hemicellulose, gums, and pectin—has lowered cholesterol levels in human beings during controlled studies, although at different rates. Research continues to determine the most effective types and amounts of dietary fiber to use in reducing the risk of cardiovascular disease.

Iron. Severe deficiency of iron (anemia) increases blood lipids, but moderate anemia may actually lower cholesterol levels. This is an important nutrient to watch, since iron deficiency anemia strikes most often during early infancy and childhood, when protective measures should begin.

Zinc. In experiments a zinc deficiency lowers blood cholesterol levels. High intake apparently reduces HDL-C levels. Although conclusive evidence is not yet available, these preliminary findings suggest that large amounts of zinc may increase the risk of disease.

This information suggests that the entire diet, not just the fat component, must be examined to help control or prevent atherosclerosis.

REFERENCES

Anderson JW et al: Lipid responses of hypercholesterolemic men to oat-bran and wheat-bran intake, *Am J Clin Nutr* 54:678, 1991.

Mertz W: Trace minerals and atherosclerosis, *FASEB J* 41:2807, 1982.

Story JA: Dietary carbohydrates and atherosclerosis, *FASEB J* 41:2797, 1982.

the way for present practice and future directions.[7,8] The following are some findings from current research:

1. *Low density lipoprotein-cholesterol cell receptors.* The discovery by Goldstein and Brown of cell-surface receptors for low density lipoprotein-cholesterol (LDL-C), the basis of their 1985 Nobel prize in medicine, is fundamental for understanding how plasma cholesterol levels are controlled.[9]
2. *Drug development.* The Lipid Research Clinics Coronary Primary Prevention Trial reported as early as 1984 that lowering the plasma cholesterol level by *bile acid binding* in the gut reduces the incidence of coronary heart disease, including myocardial infarction.[10] Such binding agents include the earlier cholestyramine (Questran) and colestipol (Colestid). A more recent class of cholesterol-lowering drugs, *cholesterol-synthesis inhibitors,* compete with the rate-limiting enzyme in cholesterol synthesis, 3-hydroxy-3-methylglutaryl coenzyme A reductase (HMG CoA). The first of these agents approved is lovastatin (Mevacor). Others are in stages of development and testing.
3. *Knowledge of advanced lesion development.* Ongoing clinical and experimental work has expanded knowledge of the cholesterol-interactive mechanisms involved in the development of atherosclerotic lesions. The trail leads from high plasma LDL-C through the early precursor fatty streak, to endothelial injury and its effect on the artery wall, the resulting platelet aggregation and release of platelet-derived growth factor (PDGF), and on to cell proliferation and advanced lesion as shown in Fig. 8-9.[11,12] Further angiographic studies, using magnetic resonance imaging and ultrafast computed tomography to indicate results of diet (cholesterol-fat control) and drug therapy (colestipol/niacin) have shown that atherosclerosis can be stabilized and reversed and that new lesion formation can be reduced.[13,14]

Scientists continue to refine their knowledge about coronary heart disease, the underlying pathologic process atherosclerosis, and how lowered blood choles-

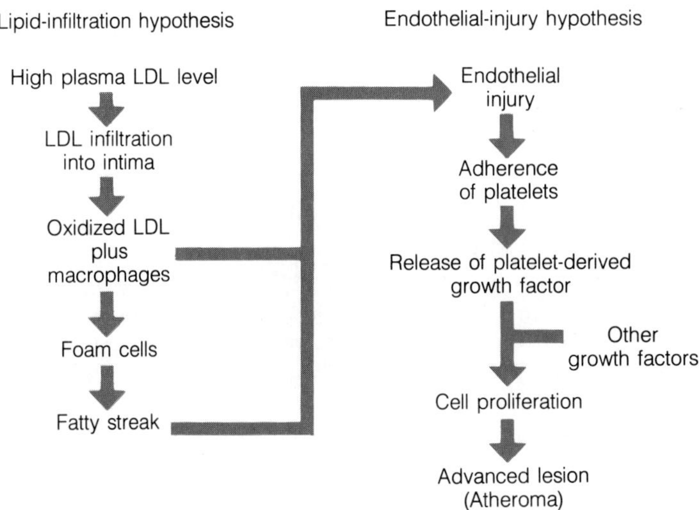

FIG. 8-9 Possible linkages of the lipid-filtration and endothelial-injury routes to development of atherosclerotic lesions in arteries. *LDL,* Low density lipoprotein; *PDGF,* platelet-derived growth factor. *(Modified from Steinberg D, Witztum JL: Lipoproteins and atherogenesis: current concepts,* JAMA *264(23):3047, 1990.)*

terol levels help control the disease process. A broad international consensus has emerged, which the cholesterol-lowering guidelines of the U.S. Consensus Conference (NIH, 1985) and the follow-up National Cholesterol Education Program reflect.[15-17] A concerted effort has been made to control cholesterol levels as a major means of controlling heart disease. Advancing research knowledge indicates two things about atherosclerosis: (1) elevated serum cholesterol level is a major contributor to the disease process and (2) dietary fat intake, especially saturated fat, affects serum cholesterol levels. These major strides, incorporated in the National Research Council's recent review, *Diet and health: implications for reducing chronic disease risks,* have given impetus to our nutrition intervention efforts.[18]

Hyperlipoproteinemia

As indicated by many studies, increased blood concentrations of certain cholesterol-carrying lipoproteins, the LDLs and the beta–very-low density lipoproteins (beta-VLDL), which are derived either from chylomicrons or from VLDLs by the action of lipoprotein lipase, are without question atherogenic.[12] Lipoproteins are the major transport forms of lipids, especially cholesterol, in the blood. An increase in one or more of these plasma lipoproteins creates the condition called **hyperlipoproteinemia.** A more general term referring to elevation of one or more of the broad plasma lipid classes is *hyperlipidemia.*

Classes of Lipoproteins

The lipoproteins in the blood are produced mainly in two places: (1) in the intestinal wall after initial ingestion, digestion, and absorption of exogenous fat from a meal, and (2) in the liver, from endogenous fat sources. The major intestinal wall lipoproteins formed from exogenous fat sources are called *chylomicrons.* They have the highest lipid content of all the lipoproteins, mostly *triglycerides* from the meal just consumed, with a small amount of protein as a carrier substance; thus they have the lowest density of the lipoproteins. The other four major lipoproteins are produced mainly in the liver, with some synthesized in the serum and in the intestinal wall. They carry fat and cholesterol to the tissues for use in energy production and for interchange with other products of cell metabolism. These lipoprotein groups are classified according to their fat content and thus their density, with those having the highest fat content possessing the lowest density:

- *Chylomicron.* Chylomicrons have the highest lipid content, lowest density, and are composed mostly of exogenous triglycerides (TGs), with a small amount of carrier protein. They accumulate in portal blood following a meal and are efficiently cleared from the blood by the specific enzyme *lipoprotein lipase.*
- *Very-low density lipoprotein.* VLDL still carries a large lipid (TG) content but includes about 10% to 15% cholesterol, and it is formed in the liver from endogenous fat sources.

TABLE 8–2

Characteristics of the Classes of Lipoproteins

Characteristic	Chylomicrons	Very low density (VLDL)	Intermediate density (IDL)	Low density (LDL)	High density (HDL)
Composition					
Triglycerides (TGs)	80%-95%; diet, exogenous	60%-80%; endogenous	40%; endogenous	10%-13%; endogenous	5%-10%; endogenous
Cholesterol	2%-7%	10%-15%	30%	45%-50%	20%
Phospholipid	3%-6%	15%-20%	20%	15%-22%	25%-30%
Protein	1%-2%	5%-10%	10%	20%-25%	45%-50%
Function	Transport dietary TGs to plasma and tissues, cells	Transport endogenous TGs to cells	Continue transport of endogenous TGs to cells	Transport cholesterol to peripheral cells	Transport free cholesterol from membranes to liver for catabolism
Place of synthesis	Intestinal wall	Liver	Liver	Liver	Liver
Size, density					
Description	Largest, lightest	Next largest, next lightest	Intermediate size, lighter	Smaller, heavier	Smallest, densest, heaviest
Density	0.095	0.095-1.006	1.00-1.03	1.019-1.063	1.063-1.210
Size in nanometers (nm)	75-100	30-80	25-40	10-20	7.5-10

- *Intermediate density lipoprotein.* IDL continues the delivery of endogenous TGs to cells and carries about 30% cholesterol.
- *Low density lipoprotein.* LDL carries in addition to other lipids about two thirds or more of the total plasma cholesterol. LDL is formed in the serum from catabolism of VLDL. Because LDL carries cholesterol to the cells for deposit in the tissues, it is considered the main agent in elevated serum cholesterol levels.
- *High density lipoprotein.* HDL carries less total lipid and more protein. It is formed in the liver from endogenous fat sources. Because HDL carries cholesterol from the tissues to the liver for catabolism and excretion, higher serum levels of HDL are considered protective against cardiovascular disease. The "normal" (statistical) range for HDL-C is 30 to 80 mg/dl. Thus a value below 30 mg/dl implies significant risk, and a value of 75 mg/dl or above contributes to protection and decreased risk.

The characteristics of these classes of lipoproteins are summarized in Table 8-2. Note the comparative functions of LDL and HDL. Because LDL carries cholesterol to the peripheral cells, for example, it contributes the "cholesterol of concern" in familial hypercholesterolemia and is a more valid measure of risk status than is the total cholesterol value.[19,20] The LDL value may be calculated by the following formula:

LDL = Total cholesterol - (20% TG + HDL)

Functional Classification of Lipid Disorders

Current clinical practice is based on a useful functional classification that reveals two important factors: (1) recognition of the genetic factors involved and (2) focus on the role of *apoproteins* in the course of lipoprotein formation, transport, or destruction. Both of these factors will be encountered in readings and in clinical work with patients. Thus the outline provided in this discussion and the later summary in Table 8-4 of this current functional approach are useful in understanding the clinical problems involved in dealing with atherosclerosis and in counseling patients and clients. We first identify the apoproteins; then we briefly outline the current functional classification of lipid disorders.

Apoproteins

The term **apoprotein** refers to a major protein part of a combined metabolic product, in this case a specific protein part of a combined lipid and protein molecule (Fig. 8-10). These apoproteins are increasingly rec-

hyperlipoproteinemia • An elevated level of lipoproteins in the blood.

apoprotein • A separate protein compound that attaches to its specific receptor site on a particular lipoprotein and activates certain functions such as synthesis of a related enzyme; for example, lipoprotein lipase (apoprotein C-II).

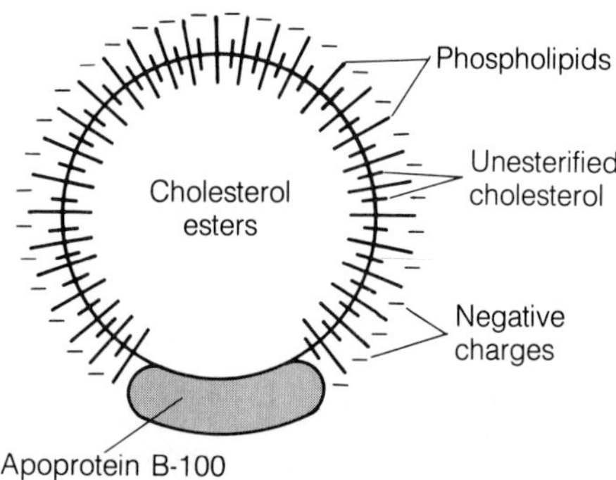

FIG. 8-10 Composition and structure of low density lipoprotein (LDL), primary transporter of cholesterol in human plasma. Apoprotein B-100 binds to LDL and provides recognition site for transport into cells. *(Modified from Guyton AC:* Textbook of medical physiology, *ed 8, Philadelphia, 1991, WB Saunders.)*

ognized as important parts of the lipoprotein molecule as more of them are identified, analyzed, and classified by letter and number. For example, apoprotein B is a common attachment to LDLs that serves two basic functions: (1) it aids in transport of lipids in a water medium, the blood, and (2) it transports lipids into the cells for metabolic uses. When apoprotein B-100, a single large protein molecule with a molecular weight of 400,000, attaches to one pole of the LDL, it provides a recognition site for the LDL receptors on the cell, causing the entire LDL to be transported by pinocytosis to the inside of the cell where it is digested and the LDL components are used for the cell.[1] The smaller apoprotein B-48, so named because it appears to be about 48% the size of apoprotein B-100, is necessary for assembly of chylomicrons.[21]

Various types of lipoproteins have specific receptor sites for particular apoproteins to which the apoprotein is attracted and which in large measure determine function.

Function

When lipoproteins are synthesized in the intestinal wall, liver, and serum, the protein component is made up of varying kinds of apoprotein parts. These genetically determined components influence the structure, receptor binding, and metabolism of lipoproteins. It is this apoprotein component that helps to form the special spherical droplets of lipid material for transport in the bloodstream. Apoprotein determination is currently a useful laboratory tool for identifying persons at high risk for coronary heart disease.[12,21] A particularly interesting and rapidly developing area of apoprotein B research is the structure and functional significance of lipoprotein(a), a remarkable apoprotein B-100–containing lipoprotein synthesized in the intestine that transports cholesterol, binds to blood clots, and raises the risk of a heart attack.[22] It apparently is the cause for much of the previously unaccountable risk for coronary heart disease.

Classes

A number of apoproteins and their corresponding apolipoproteins have been identified. The class designations in common use are apoprotein A, B, C, and E. In turn a class may consist of several different proteins; for example, A-I, A-II, A-III, and A-IV and C-I, C-II, C-III. All of these classes of apoproteins are made by the liver, and the intestinal mucosa makes A and B apoproteins. Table 8-3 lists the various classes of apoproteins associated with specific classes of lipoproteins.

The current functional approach classifies lipid disorders in four major groups based on the underlying functional problem: (1) defects in apolipoprotein synthesis, (2) enzyme deficiencies, (3) LDL-receptor deficiency, and (4) other inherited hyperlipidemias.

Defects in Synthesis of Apolipoproteins

Apolipoprotein A Deficiency

In the absence of apoprotein A, plasma HDL cannot be formed properly, and the cholesterol esters accumulate in the tissues. These lipid deposits are frequently yellow to red in color from lipid-soluble pigments such as carotenes. The blood triglyceride level is high and the cholesterol is low. This familial *alpha-lipoprotein* (HDL) deficiency is also called Tangier disease.

Apolipoprotein B Deficiency

This form of lipid disorder, from a lack of apoprotein B with an absence of LDL, is fortunately a rare inherited disease, because the consequences are serious. Triglyceride and cholesterol metabolism generally fail. The afflicted child is unable to transport ingested fat through the intestinal mucosa and into the circulation. Consequently, the cells become stuffed with multiple fat droplets, and the excess appears in foul-smelling stools. Without the necessary apoprotein B, no chylomicrons or VLDLs and thus no LDLs can be formed. General degeneration of nerve and muscle tissues occurs, probably caused by the deficiency of essential fatty acids, various lipid-soluble nutrients, and the lipid imbalance in general.

Apolipoprotein C Deficiency

In the absence of apolipoprotein C-II, lipoprotein lipase (LPL) cannot be activated. This important enzyme efficiently catalyzes the hydrolysis of triglycerides, present in heavy loads in circulating chylomicrons after meals and in VLDLs, to monoglycerides,

TABLE 8–3

Apoproteins in the Structure of Human Plasma Lipoproteins

Apoprotein	Related lipoprotein*	Tissue origin	Function†
A-I	CM, VLDL, HDL	Intestine, liver	Activates LCAT
A-II	CM, VLDL, HDL	Intestine, liver	Unclear
A-III	Subfraction of HDL		Catalyzes transfer of cholesterol esters among lipoproteins
A-IV	CM, VLDL, HDL, free in plasma	Intestine, liver	?Activates LCAT
B-48	CM	Intestine	Secretes CM, transports cholesterol and TGs
B-100	VLDL, IDL, LDL	Liver	Secretes VLDL, recognizes LDL receptor
C-I	CM, VLDL, HDL	Liver	Inhibits hepatic uptake of lipoproteins
C-II	CM, VLDL, HDL	Liver	Activates lipoprotein lipase
C-III	CM, VLDL, HDL	Liver	Inhibits lipoprotein lipase and premature remnant clearance
D	HDL	Spleen, liver, intestine, and adrenal glands	Functions in cholesterol ester transfer complex
E	CM, VLDL, IDL, trace amounts in LDL and HDL	Liver, macrophages, and body tissues except the intestine	Recognizes remnant and LDL receptor, acts as regulator in immune system, modulates cell growth

***CM,* Chylomicron; *HDL,* high density lipoprotein; *IDL,* intermediate density lipoprotein; *LDL,* low density lipoprotein; *VLDL,* very-low density lipoprotein.
†*LCAT,* lecithin-cholesterol acyltransferase; *TG,* triglyceride.

diglycerides, and free fatty acids. Apolipoprotein C-II is a 79-amino acid protein present in chylomicrons, VLDLs, and HDLs, serving as a cofactor for LPL, and hence is essential for normal triglyceride hydrolysis. The absence of apoprotein C-II, thus the presence of only inactive LPL, causes chylomicron triglycerides to accumulate in the blood, and the lipid disorder *familial hyperchylomicronemia syndrome* develops.[23] Even after a 12-hour fast, chylomicrons, which are normally cleared rapidly from circulation, are still present and give the blood a milky appearance. Major associated illness is pancreatitis, which may lead to pancreatic insufficiency and in some cases premature cardiovascular disease. Prominent fatty **xanthomas,** or lipid deposits, develop on the skin but recede with treatment, which consists of a low-fat diet restricting fat to about 15% of the total kcal/day, or 20 g, with medium-chain triglyceride oil to supplement kcalories.

Apolipoprotein E Deficiency

This familial lipid disorder occurs with a lack of apolipoprotein E and is characterized by a low concentration, 10% to 50% of normal, of LDL. However, chylomicron formation does not take place. These cholesterol ester-rich chylomicron remnants are not bound to the apoprotein E receptors in the liver, since these receptor proteins are deficient. Thus they accumulate in the blood, which causes the appearance of xanthomas. These small fatty plaques are usually yellow to orange in color from their content of lipid-soluble pigments. They may be unsightly but are not dangerous like the xanthomas that characterize atherosclerosis. Continuing apolipoprotein E deficiency results in premature atherosclerotic disease.

Enzyme Deficiencies

Familial Lipoprotein Lipase Deficiency

The lipid disorder resulting from LPL deficiency produces symptoms similar to those described in the previous discussion that result from a deficiency of apoprotein C-II, which normally activates the serum fat-clearing factor LPL, but the underlying metabolic problem is different. In this genetic disease the necessary enzyme is absent. As a result the food fat cannot be cleared, and the chylomicrons, with their triglyceride load, accumulate in the portal blood system. In children with this disease the main symptom is also abdominal pain caused by acute inflammation of the pancreas from the heavy fat load. The condition may be treated by a diet low in fats, a limit of 15% of total kcal/day, or 20 g.

Familial Lecithin Cholesterol Acyltransferase Deficiency

The plasma enzyme **lecithin cholesterol acyltransferase (LCAT)** is necessary for the normal transport of cholesterol as cholesterol esters. Without this

xanthoma • A plaque of yellow lipid deposits in the skin that appears as fatty streaks or nodules.

LCAT (lecithin-cholesterol acyltransferase) • Plasma enzyme necessary for normal transport of cholesterol as cholesterol esters; its deficiency is a result of a rare genetic defect and causes a lipid disorder characterized by high serum levels of free unesterified cholesterol.

enzyme the immature ("newborn") HDLs cannot develop into mature HDL-C carriers. All the other circulating lipoproteins are abnormal, containing low amounts of cholesterol esters and high concentrations of free cholesterol and lecithin. Large LDL particles, rich in unesterified (free) cholesterol, accumulate. In childhood opaque densities appear in the cornea; later, anemia and kidney damage develop.

LDL-Receptor Deficiency

In familial hypercholesterolemia the LDL receptors are defective, thus blocking the removal of LDL-C from the blood.[20] It is characterized by increased LDL and therefore increased total cholesterol levels. Also, the tendency is for the LDL precursor, VLDL, to be elevated. This lipid disorder is associated with an increased frequency of atherosclerosis and is one of the most commonly occurring forms of elevated lipid patterns. The nutritional therapy consists of a reduction of dietary cholesterol levels to 300 mg or less and use of unsaturated fats in limited amounts. If needed, additional drug therapy is used with agents such as colestipol, an oral ion-exchange resin that acts to bind bile acids in the gut, and sometimes nicotinic acid, a form of niacin that inhibits mobilization of fatty acids from adipose tissue.[19] In addition, the drug lovastatin, which inhibits the cell enzyme necessary for liver cholesterol synthesis, may be indicated.

Other Inherited Hyperlipidemias

Familial Hypertriglyceridemia

This condition is characterized by high levels of endogenously produced VLDLs carrying triglycerides through the bloodstream. Cholesterol levels may also rise, and glucose intolerance is frequently present. This lipid pattern is also commonly associated with non-insulin-dependent diabetes mellitus, obesity, coronary heart disease, and many other conditions, including alcoholism and progestational hormone therapy. The nutritional management consists of weight reduction and a decrease of dietary sugars, fats, and cholesterol.

Familial Multiple Hyperlipoproteinemia

This is another relatively common condition in which either the VLDL or the LDL blood levels may be elevated. Since these lipoproteins transport cholesterol in the bloodstream, the nutritional therapy is a low-cholesterol diet that provides approximately 300 mg/day.

Familial Hyperlipoproteinemia

This lipid pattern is complex, involving elevation of chylomicrons and VLDLs. Thus serum levels of triglycerides and cholesterol are elevated. Glucose intolerance also occurs, as does a frequent association with obesity and diabetes. Although the condition is familial, its precise genetic associations are not clear. The nutritional treatment consists of weight reduction followed by a maintenance diet of controlled carbohydrate and fat intake.

The summary of these lipid disorders in Table 8-4 provides a review of the basic related conditions and nutritional therapies. The concepts of fatty acids, saturation and unsaturation, essential fatty acids, and related fat substances such as cholesterol and lipoproteins need to be clearly understood in theory and in terms of foods. Patients and clients need brief, concise explanations of their various diet recommendations and the rationale behind each. Each individual food plan also needs to be related to family food patterns and to family support. Often misunderstandings obtained from lay articles or public advertising of various food products need to be clarified or corrected.

TABLE 8-4

Functional Classification of Lipid Disorders

Type of defect or lipid disorder	Abnormal lipid pattern	Clinical characteristics	Nutritional therapy
Defective synthesis of apolipoproteins			
Apolipoprotein A deficiency	Decreased HDL Increased tissue cholesterol Decreased serum cholesterol Increased serum TG	Rare Genetic Tangier disease	Low cholesterol Low fat
Apolipoprotein B deficiency	High mucosal tissue fat No lipoprotein synthesis possible	Rare Genetic Serious prognosis for child Malabsorption Steatorrhea	Very low fat

TABLE 8–4

Functional Classification of Lipid Disorders—cont'd

Type of defect or lipid disorder	Abnormal lipid pattern	Clinical characteristics	Nutritional therapy
Defective synthesis of apolipoproteins—cont'd			
Apolipoprotein C deficiency	Increased TG Increased chylomicrons	Rare Genetic Early childhood Abdominal pain (pancreatitis) Lipemia, retinalis Xanthomas Hepatosplenomegly	Very low fat (20 g) High carbohydrate Medium-chain triglycerides (MCTs)
Apolipoprotein E deficiency	Increased chylomicron remnants Decreased serum LDL Increased cholesterol Increased TG	Relatively uncommon Genetic Xanthomas Premature atherosclerosis	Low cholesterol (<300 mg) Low saturated fat Increased substitution of polyunsaturated fat Weight reduction
Enzyme deficiency			
Lipoprotein lipase deficiency	Increased chylomicrons	Rare Genetic Early childhood Abdominal pain (pancreatitis) Lipemia, retinalis Xanthomas Hepatosplenomegaly	Very low fat (20 g) High carbohydrate MCTs
Lecithin-cholesterol acyltransferase deficiency	Overall abnormal lipid pattern: all lipoproteins have low amounts of cholesterol esters and high concentrations of free cholesterol and lecithin Accumulation of large LDL particles rich in unesterified cholesterol	Rare Genetic Abnormal cornea Anemia Kidney damage	Low cholesterol Low fat
LDL-receptor deficiency			
Familial hypercholesterolemia	Increased LDL Increased total cholesterol Increased VLDL	Common Genetic Increased atherosclerosis All ages Xanthomas	Low cholesterol (<300 mg) Low saturated fat Substitution of polyunsaturated fat
Other inherited hyperlipidemias			
Familial hypertriglyceridemia	Increased VLDL Increased TG Increased cholesterol Sometimes increased blood sugar	Common Genetic Glucose intolerance Possible type II (non-insulin dependent) diabetes mellitus Obesity Accelerated atherosclerosis	Weight reduction Low, simple carbohydrates Low saturated fat Low cholesterol
Familial multiple hyperlipoproteinemia	Increased VLDL Increased LDL	Fairly common Genetic Adult Xanthomas; vascular disease	Low cholesterol (<300 mg) Low saturated fat Substitution of polyunsaturated fat Weight reduction
Familial type V hyperlipoproteinemia	Increased chylomicrons Increased VLDL Increased cholesterol Increased TG	Rare Glucose intolerance Obesity Abdominal pain (pancreatitis) Hepatosplenomegaly	Weight reduction Controlled carbohydrate and fat intake High protein

TABLE 8-5

The Prudent Diet as Compared with the Usual American Diet

	Prudent diet	Usual American diet
Total kcalories	Sufficient to maintain ideal body weight	Often excessive for need
Cholesterol	300 mg	600-800 mg
Total fats (% of kcalories)	30%-35%	40%-45%
Saturated	10% or less	15%-20%
Monounsaturated	15%	15%-20%
Polyunsaturated	10%	5%-6%
P/S ratio (polyunsaturated/saturated fat in the diet)	1-1.5 : 1	0.3 : 1
Carbohydrates (% of kcalories)	50%-55%	40%-45%
Starch (complex CHO)	30%-35%	20%-25%
Simple sugars	10%	15%-20%
Proteins (% of total kcalories)	12%-20%	12%-15%
Sodium	130 mEq	200-250 mEq

TABLE 8-6

American Heart Association Revised Prudent Diet Guidelines for Lowering Elevated Blood Lipid Levels

	Step 1 % total kcalories	Step 2 % total kcalories
Total fat	<30	<30
Saturated	<10	<7
Monounsaturated	10-15	10-15
Polyunsaturated	10	10
Carbohydrates	50-60	50-60
Protein	15-20	15-20
Cholesterol	<300 mg/day	<200 mg/day

TABLE 8-7

Step 1 and Step 2 Diets for Treating High Plasma Cholesterol in Adults (NCEP)*

Nutrient	Step 1 % total kcalories	Step 2 % total kcalories
Total fat	30	30
Saturated	10	7
Monounsaturated	10-15	10-15
Polyunsaturated	10	10
Carbohydrates	50-60	50-60
Protein	10-20	10-20
Cholesterol	300	200
Total kcalories	Sufficient to achieve and maintain desirable weight	Sufficient to achieve and maintain desirable weight

*National Cholesterol Education Program, adult treatment panel guidelines.

General Principles of Nutritional Therapy: Fat-Modified Diets

The two major lipid factors of concern are (1) the total amount of fat in the diet and (2) the kind of fat used in terms of cholesterol and saturated fats. These two principles were first applied in the generally used approach of the "prudent" food pattern originally proposed a decade ago by the American Heart Association (AHA) and compared with the usual American diet still followed by too many persons (Table 8-5).[24] The initial AHA prudent diet has been revised to meet current lipid-lowering recommendations (Table 8-6). The reports of the Expert Panel on Detection, Evaluation, and Treatment of High Blood Cholesterol in Adults issued in 1988 and the expert Panel of Population Strategies issued in 1990 further refined these dietary principles with specific guidelines for practitioners.[16,17] These current dietary recommendations for adults are shown in Table 8-7, and the related food guide for adults is given in Table 8-8. The related National Cholesterol Education Program treatment criteria for adults is shown in Table 8-9 and illustrated in Fig. 8-11. This stepwise approach calls first for a vigorous dietary effort to lower the elevated serum cholesterol level before drugs are added.

Recent recommendations for children and adolescents, especially for those in high-risk families, have focused on similar guidelines for helping children and adolescents develop early food habits on a healthy, less rich and excessive basis.These recommendations have been made for public health (population) needs, especially for children from high-risk families, and for individual needs of children and adolescents with identified high serum levels of total cholesterol and LDL-C (Tables 8-10 through 8-12).[25] A general population (Step 1) food guide for children and adolescents is provided in Table 8-13.

Amount of Fat

Almost half of the kcalories of the average American's diet is contributed by fat. It is recommended currently that this be moderated to at most 30% of the total kcalories or lowered further to 20% for higher levels of serum cholesterol. Limiting the total amount of fat, as well as increasing physical exercise, is especially indicated when weight management is needed.

Kind of Fat

About two thirds of the total fat in the American diet has been of animal origin and therefore is mainly saturated fat. The remaining one third has come from vegetable sources and is mainly unsaturated fat. How-

TABLE 8–8

Step 1 Diet Guide: Modifications to Lower Plasma Cholesterol in Adults (NCEP)*

Food groups	Choose	Decrease
Fish, chicken, turkey, and lean meats (3-oz cooked portions)	Fish; poultry without skin; lean cuts of beef, lamb, pork, or veal; shellfish	Fatty cuts of beef, lamb, or pork, spare ribs, organ meats, regular cold cuts, sausages, hot dogs, bacon, sardines, roe
Skimmed and low-fat milk, cheese, yogurt, and dairy substitutes	Skimmed or 1%-fat milk (liquid, powdered, evaporated), buttermilk	Whole milk: (4% fat) regular, evaporated, condensed; cream, half & half, 2% milk, imitation milk products, most nondairy creamers, whipped toppings
	Nonfat (0% fat) or low-fat yogurt	Whole milk yogurt
	Low-fat cottage cheese (1% or 2% fat)	Whole milk cottage cheese (4% fat)
	Low-fat cheeses, farmer or pot cheeses (all of these should be labeled no more than 2 to 6 g fat per oz)	All natural cheeses (e.g., blue, Roquefort, Camembert, cheddar, Swiss)
		Low-fat or "light" cream cheese, low-fat or "light" sour cream
		Cream cheeses, sour cream
	Sherbet, sorbet	Ice cream
Eggs	Egg whites (2 whites = 1 whole egg in recipes), cholesterol-free egg substitutes	Egg yolks
Fruits and vegetables	Fresh, frozen, canned, or dried fruits and vegetables	Vegetables prepared in butter, cream, or other sauces
Breads and cereals	Homemade baked goods using unsaturated oils sparingly, angel food cake, low-fat crackers, low-fat cookies	Commercially baked goods: pies, cakes, doughnuts, croissants, pastries, muffins, biscuits, high-fat crackers, high-fat cookies
	Rice, pasta	Egg noodles
	Whole grain breads and cereals (e.g., oatmeal, whole wheat, rye, bran, multigrain)	Breads in which eggs are major ingredient
Fats and oils	Baking cocoa	Chocolate
	Unsaturated vegetable oils: corn, olive, rapeseed, safflower, sesame, soybean, sunflower	Butter, coconut oil, palm oil, palm kernel oil, lard, bacon fat
	Margarine or shortenings made from one of the unsaturated oils listed above	
	Diet margarine	
	Mayonnaise, salad dressings made with unsaturated oils listed above	Dressings made with egg yolk
	Low-fat dressings	
	Seeds and nuts	Coconut

*National Cholesterol Education Program.

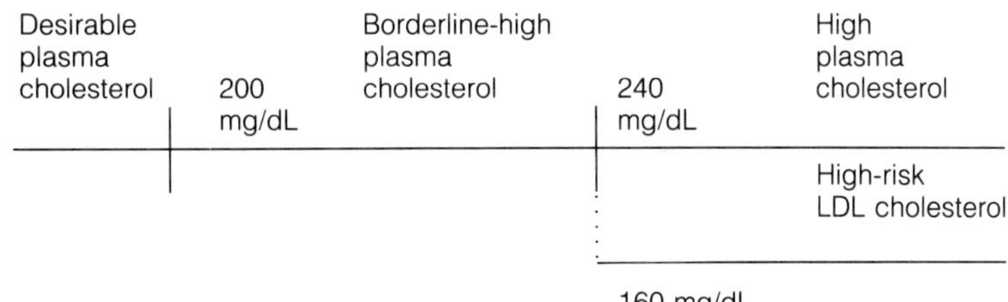

FIG. 8-11 Classification spectrum by total and low density lipoprotein (LDL) cholesterol levels. Initial classification by plasma total cholesterol followed by LDL cholesterol evaluation for persons with high levels. *(National Cholesterol Education Program, adult treatment panel guidelines.)*

TABLE 8–9

Evaluation Criteria for Screening and Monitoring Adults for Treatment of Elevated Blood Cholesterol (NCEP)*

Type of test	Blood level classifications (mg/dl)
Total plasma cholesterol	
Desirable level	<200
Borderline high level	200-239
High level	≥240
LDL cholesterol	
Borderline high risk	130-159
High risk	≥160

*National Cholesterol Education Program, adult treatment panel guidelines.

TABLE 8–10

Current Versus Recommended Nutrient Intake in Children and Adolescents

	Current	Recommended
Saturated fatty acids (% of kcalories)	14	<10
Total fat (% of kcalories)	35-36	Average no more than 30
Polyunsaturated	6	Up to 10
Monounsaturated	13-14	10-15
Cholesterol (mg/day)	193-296	<300

From preliminary data from USDA's 1987-1988 Nationwide Food Consumption Survey and National Cholesterol Education Program: *Recommendations for Children and Adolescents,* USDHHS (PHS), NIH Pub No 91-2732.

TABLE 8–11

Cutpoints of Total and LDL-Cholesterol for Dietary Intervention in Children and Adolescents with a Family History of Hypercholesterolemia or Premature Cardiovascular Disease

Category	Total cholesterol (mg/dl)	LDL-C (mg/dl)	Dietary intervention
Acceptable	<170	<110	Recommended population eating pattern
Borderline	170-199	110-129	Step 1 Diet prescribed, other risk factor intervention
High	≥200	≥130	Step 1 Diet prescribed, then Step 2 Diet if necessary

From National Cholesterol Education Program, *Report of the expert panel on blood cholesterol levels in children and adolescents,* USDHHS (PHS), National Institutes of Health, Washington, D.C., 1991, US Government Printing Office.

TABLE 8–12

Characteristics of Step 1 and Step 2 Diets for Lowering Blood Cholesterol in Children and Adolescents

	Recommended intake	
Nutrient	**Step 1 diet**	**Step 2 diet**
Total fat	Average of no more than 30% of total kcalories	Same
Saturated fatty acids	Less than 10% of total kcalories	Less than 7% of total kcalories
Polyunsaturated fatty acids	Up to 10% of total kcalories	Same
Monounsaturated fatty acids	Remaining total fat kcalories	Same
Cholesterol	Less than 300 mg/day	Less than 200 mg/day
Carbohydrates	About 55% of total kcalories	Same
Protein	About 15%-20% of total kcalories	Same
Kcalories	To promote normal growth and development and to reach or maintain desirable body weight	Same

Modified from National Cholesterol Education Program, *Report of the expert panel on blood cholesterol levels in children and adolescents,* USDHHS (PHS), NIH Pub NO 91-2732 National Institutes of Health, Washington, D.C., 1991, US Government Printing Office.

TABLE 8–13

Foods to Choose and Decrease for the Step 1* and Step 2 Diets for Children and Adolescents

Food group	Choose	Decrease
Meat, poultry, fish	Beef, pork, lamb; lean cuts trimmed well before cooking	Beef, pork, lamb; regular ground beef, fatty cuts, spare ribs, organ meats, sausage, regular luncheon meats, wieners, bacon
	Poultry without skin	Poultry with skin, fried chicken
	Fish, shellfish	Fried fish, fried shellfish
	Processed meat prepared from lean meat (e.g., turkey ham, tuna wieners)	Regular luncheon meat (e.g., bologna, salami, sausage, wieners)
Eggs	Egg whites (2 whites = 1 whole egg in recipes), cholesterol-free egg substitute	Egg yolks (if more than 4 per week on Step 1 or if more than 2 per week on Step 2; includes egg used in cooking
Dairy products	Milk: skim or 1% fat (fluid, powdered, evaporated), buttermilk	Whole milk (fluid, evaporated, condensed), 2% low-fat milk, imitation milk
	Yogurt: nonfat or low-fat yogurt or yogurt beverages	Whole milk yogurt, whole milk yogurt beverages
	Cheese: low-fat natural or processed cheese (part-skim mozzarella, ricotta) with no more than 6 g fat per oz on Step 1, or 2 g fat per oz on Step 2	Regular cheeses (American, blue, Brie, cheddar, Colby, Edam, Monterey Jack, whole milk mozzarella, Parmesan, Swiss), cream cheese, Neufchâtel cheese
	Cottage cheese: low-fat, nonfat, or dry curd (0 to 2% fat)	Cottage cheese (4% fat)
	Frozen dairy dessert: ice milk, frozen yogurt (low-fat or nonfat)	Ice cream
		Cream, half & half, whipping cream, nondairy creamer, whipped topping, sour cream
Fats and oils	Unsaturated oils: safflower, sunflower, corn, soybean, cottonseed, canola, olive, peanut	Coconut oil, palm kernel oil, palm oil
	Margarine made from unsaturated oils listed above, light or diet margarine	Butter, lard, shortening, bacon fat
	Salad dressings made with unsaturated oils listed above, low-fat or oil-free	Dressings made with egg yolk, cheese, sour cream, whole milk
	Seeds and nuts: peanut butter, other nut butters	Coconut
	Cocoa powder	Chocolate
Breads and cereals	Breads: whole grain bread, hamburger and hot dog bun, corn tortilla	Bread in which eggs are a major ingredient, croissants
	Cereals: oat, wheat, corn, multigrain	Granola made with coconut
	Pasta	Egg noodles and pasta containing egg yolk
	Rice	
	Dry beans and peas	
	Crackers, low-fat: animal-type, graham, saltine-type	High-fat crackers
	Homemade baked goods using unsaturated oil, skim or 1% milk, and egg substitute: quick breads, biscuits, cornbread muffins, bran muffins, pancakes, waffles	Commercial baked pastries, muffins, biscuits
	Soup: chicken or beef noodle, minestrone, tomato, vegetarian, potato	Soup containing whole milk, cream, meat fat, poultry fat, or poultry skin
Vegetables	Fresh, frozen, or canned	Vegetables prepared with butter, cheese, or cream sauce
Fruits	Fruit: fresh, frozen, canned, or dried	Fried fruit or fruit served with butter or cream sauce
	Fruit juice: fresh, frozen, or canned	
Sweets and modified fat desserts	Beverages: fruit-flavored drinks, lemonade, fruit punch	
	Sweets: sugar, syrup, honey, jam, preserves, candy made without fat (candy corn, gumdrops, hard candy), fruit-flavored gelatin	Candy made with chocolate, coconut oil, palm kernel oil, palm oil
	Frozen desserts: sherbet, sorbet, fruit ice, popsicles	Ice cream and frozen treats made with ice cream
	Cookies, cake, pie, pudding prepared with egg whites, egg substitute, skim milk or 1% milk, and unsaturated oil or margarine; gingersnaps; fig bar cookies; angel food cake	Commercial baked pies, cakes, doughnuts, high-fat cookies, cream pies

*The Step 1 Diet has the same nutrient recommendations as the eating pattern recommended for the general population.

Modified from the National Cholesterol Education Program, *Report of the expert panel on blood cholesterol levels in children and adolescents,* USDHHS (PHS), National Institutes of Health, Washington, D.C., 1991, US Government Printing Office.

ever, this ratio has gradually been changing over the past few years with the use of less animal and more plant fat. This has been the general goal of the prudent diet (Table 8-6), illustrated by its breakdown of total fat according to degree of saturation with emphasis on unsaturated fats reflected in the **polyunsaturated/saturated (P/S) ratio.** The current stepwise guidelines place greater emphasis on control of cholesterol and total fat and its degrees of saturation according to serum levels of LDL-C, patient or family history of coronary heart disease, and other risk factors (Table 8-7). The serum cholesterol values used in the program as guidelines for testing and monitoring are shown in Table 8-9 and Fig. 8-11.

Additional Dietary Factors

In addition to the primary focus on lipid factors (cholesterol and relative amounts of fat according to degree of saturation), the added factors of dietary fiber, omega-3 long-chain fatty acids, and sodium also need consideration.

Dietary fiber. Studies indicate that water-soluble types of dietary fiber have a significant cholesterol-lowering effect.[26-29] Soluble fiber includes gums, pectin, certain hemicelluloses, and storage polysaccharides. Foods rich in soluble fiber are oat bran and dried beans, with barley and fruits having lesser amounts. Oat bran, for example, contains a primary water-soluble gum, beta-glucan, which is a lipid-lowering agent.[26] Soluble fiber increases intestinal transit time, delays gastric emptying, and slows glucose absorption. In the colon it is almost completely fermented into short-chain fatty acids, which may inhibit liver cholesterol synthesis and help clear LDL-C. Insoluble fiber—cellulose, lignin, and many hemicelluloses—found in vegetables, wheat, and most other grains do not have lipid-lowering effects. Thus an increased use of soluble fiber food sources, especially oat bran and legumes, has beneficial effects.

Omega-3 fatty acids. Studies have indicated that the omega-3 fatty acids *eicosapentaenoic acid (EPA)* and *docosahexaenoic acid (DHA)*, which are found mostly in seafood and marine oils, (1) change the distribution of fatty acids in plasma and in phospholipids to alter platelet activity and reduce platelet aggregation that increases blood clotting, thus reducing the rate of coronary thrombosis; (2) decrease the synthesis of VLDLs; and (3) have antiinflammatory effects.[30,31] Food value tables on the content of omega-3 fatty acids and other fat components of selected foods have been developed.[32]

Sodium. Reduction of dietary sodium to a moderate intake between 1.5 to 3.0 g/day is recommended to help control any potential cardiac edema in coronary disease or reduce the added risk factor of hypertension.[33,34]

Acute Cardiovascular Disease: Myocardial Infarction

Medical Therapy

Initial medical treatment of myocardial infarction, or heart attack, usually includes strong analgesics for the severe unremitting pain, oxygen therapy, and intravenous fluids for shock. The antiarrhythmic drug lidocaine may also be given by intravenous injection to reduce the risk of *ventricular fibrillation* (irregular heartbeat). In addition, diuretic drugs may be given for heart failure to avoid accumulation of fluid in the lungs, and beta-blockers that occupy the beta-receptors and prevent the stimuli of norepinephrine to the muscles may be used in some cases to reduce the force and speed of the heartbeat and risk of further heart muscle damage. In some hospitals patients who arrive shortly after the heart attack are now treated with a thrombolytic drug, *streptokinase,* to dissolve blood clots, especially those in the arteries of the heart and lung. Streptokinase is an enzyme produced by streptococcus bacteria that dissolves the fibrin of blood clots. It is fast-acting, always given only in hospitals by the physician, and most effective on newly formed clots. The physician releases the enzyme at the site of the clot via a catheter inserted into an artery. Used in the early stages after the attack, it reduces heart muscle damage. Following the clot-dissolving drug therapy, *angioplasty* may be used to widen the narrowed coronary arteries. In this procedure, done under local anesthesia and guided by x-ray imaging, a sausage-shaped balloon at the tip of a catheter is inserted into the artery and positioned at the narrowed point in the artery. The balloon is inflated and deflated a few times to widen the blood vessel and then it is withdrawn.

Nutritional Therapy

In the initial acute phase of cardiovascular disease, a myocardial infarction requires close attention to dietary modifications. The basic clinical objective is cardiac rest. Thus all care is directed toward ensuring that this requirement for restoring the damaged heart to normal functioning is followed. The diet is therefore modified in energy value and texture, as well as in fat and sodium.

Kcalories. A brief period of undernutrition during the first few days after the attack is advisable. The metabolic demands for digestion, absorption, and metabolism of food require a generous cardiac output volume. Small intakes of food at a time spread over the day decrease the level of metabolic activity to one that the weakened heart can accommodate. The patient progresses to more food as healing occurs. During the initial recovery stages the diet may be limited to about 1200 to 1500 kcal to continue cardiac rest from metabolic work loads. If the patient is obese, as is frequently the case, this kcalorie level may be continued for a longer period to help the patient begin gradually to lose some of the excess weight.

Texture. Early feedings generally include foods soft in texture or easily digested to avoid excess effort in eating. Smaller meals served more frequently may give needed nutrition without undue strain or pressure. Avoid temperature extremes in solid and liquid foods.

Lipids. The general prudent diet (Table 8-6) controls the amount and kind of fat for most needs. If the patient has a diagnosed lipid disorder, additional specific modifications of lipid components may be added according to individual needs.

Sodium. A moderately reduced sodium content in the foods selected is also emphasized. This helps control any tendency for fluid to accumulate in the body tissues. Added tissue fluid causes more work for the heart to maintain an increased blood volume circulation.

Additional Risk Factors

Heavy coffee drinking has an effect on blood cholesterol levels and also disrupts heart rhythms. An abnormal heart rhythm is seen after only one or two cups of coffee in patients with a history of irregular heart rate. The best practice is to avoid caffeine, or limit regular coffee to 2 cups/day.[35] Heavy use of alcohol also increases triglycerides and atherosclerotic risk. If alcohol is used, the amount should be moderate. Some data indicate that small amounts of alcohol play a protective role by contributing to an increased level of serum HDL, but there is no basis for recommending either that patients increase their intake or that they start its use if they do not already drink.[36]

Chronic Coronary Heart Disease: Congestive Heart Failure

In chronic coronary heart disease a condition of congestive heart failure may develop over time. The key event is loss of a critical quantity of functioning myocardial calls after an injury to the heart, which may be an acute myocardial infarction, toxins (alcohol or cytotoxic drugs), viral or bacterial infection, or prolonged cardiovascular stress (hypertension or valvular disease). To compensate for the myocardial cell loss, hemodynamic and neurohormonal mechanisms are activated to enhance the contracting force of the heart muscle and preserve cardiac function. However, the progressively weakened heart muscle, the myocardium, is unable to maintain an adequate cardiac output to sustain normal blood circulation. The resulting fluid imbalances cause edema, especially **pulmonary edema,** to develop. This brings problems in breathing called respiratory distress or *dyspnea,* which places added stress on the laboring heart. Thus heart failure is now considered a disorder of circulation, not merely a disease of the heart.[37]

Etiology: Relationship to Sodium and Water Metabolism

Imbalance in capillary fluid shift mechanism. As the heart fails to pump out the returning blood fast enough, the venous return is retarded, and a disproportionate amount of blood accumulates in the vascular system working with the right side of the heart. As venous pressure rises in a "backup" pressure effort, the balance of filtration pressures necessary to maintain the normal *capillary fluid shift mechanism* is overcome. Fluid that normally flows between the interstitial spaces and the blood vessels is held in the tissue spaces rather than being returned to circulation.

Hormonal mechanisms. Two hormonal mechanisms are involved in fluid balance in the normal circulation; both contribute to cardiac edema.

RENIN-ANGIOTENSIN-ALDOSTERONE MECHANISM. In its usual operation this basic fluid balance mechanism ensures normal fluid balances. In this case, however, it only compounds the edema problem. As the heart fails to propel the blood circulation forward, the deficient cardiac output effectively reduces the renal blood flow. The decreased renal blood pressure triggers the renin-angiotensin system. Renin is an enzyme from the renal cortex that combines in the blood with its substrate, angiotensinogen, which is produced in the liver, to produce in turn angiotensin I and II. Angiotensin II acts as a stimulant to the adrenal

polyunsaturated/saturated (P/S) ratio • Ratio of polyunsaturated to saturated fats in the diet.

pulmonary edema • The accumulation of fluid in tissues of the lung.

CLINICAL APPLICATION

The Spice of Life: Breaking Up the Salt Monopoly

If you counsel persons about sodium-restricted diets, you probably spend a lot of time answering the question, "Is there life without salt?" The standard reply is something like, "Of course there is. You'll just have to get used to the natural flavor of foods." This answer usually falls flat.

We learn to like the taste of salt; it's a taste that "accumulates" over the years. That's why it's unreasonable, for example, to expect a middle-aged man who has just discovered he has hypertension to suddenly give up his lifetime seasoning habits. It's overly optimistic to expect anyone raised on hot dogs, potato chips, and TV dinners to fall in love with the flavor of fresh broccoli overnight if it has never been a favorite food.

There is hope, however. Subjects in one study developed a lower tolerance for salty foods after following a low-sodium diet for 5 months. So if you can convince clients to reduce their salt intake for a significant period, you might get them to fall out of love with the taste of salt.

There's still the problem of getting clients to use less salt to begin with. The solution is to introduce them to the world of salt-free seasonings. Some persons are already familiar with a variety of alternate seasonings and only need some recipes that show how to use them creatively. Those who think that gourmet cooking means just using pepper instead of salt need a little extra help in selecting and using salt-free seasonings successfully. The following are some suggestions for guidelines:

- Stop adding salt at the table; it's pure habit. Get rid of the shaker—throw it away, hide it, or get it out of sight—anything to remove the reminder.
- If foods taste too bland without added salt, sprinkle them with fresh lemon juice, not salt.
- When cooking, cut the amount of salt in the recipe in half and avoid other sodium rich seasonings (see Appendix I).
- If you're already a good cook, or even if you're not, refer to guides for hints on spicing up old favorites without salt (see Appendix J).
- If you're not the world's greatest chef, enroll in a basic cooking class at a local adult education center or community college and use these guidelines when preparing meals at home. You may also want to check the foods section of your local newspaper for listings of special low-sodium cooking classes offered by local health organizations.
- Relax for a moment while dinner is simmering on the stove and enjoy the wonderful new aromas filling your kitchen. Sodium reduction introduces you to a flavorful new adventure with food. ◆

REFERENCES

Bertino M et al: Long-term reduction in dietary sodium alters the taste of salt, *Am J Clin Nutr* 36:1134, 1982.

Wylie-Rossett J: Spices to the rescue, *Prof Nutr* 14:4, Spring 1982.

glands, causing them to produce aldosterone, the hormone that in turn effects a resorption of sodium in an ion exchange with potassium in the distal tubules of the nephrons, and water resorption follows.[38] Ordinarily this is a lifesaving mechanism to protect the body's vital water supply. In congestive heart failure, however, it only adds to the edema problem. The mechanism reacts as if the body's total fluid volume is reduced, when in truth the fluid is excessive. It simply is not in normal circulation but is being retained in the body's tissues.

ANTIDIURETIC HORMONE MECHANISM. The normally functioning antidiuretic hormone (ADH) mechanism also adds to the edema problem. The cardiac stress and reduced renal flow cause the release of vasopressin, the ADH from the pituitary gland. This hormone stimulates still more water resorption in the distal tubules in the nephrons, further increasing the problem of edema.

Increased cellular free potassium. As the reduced blood circulation depresses cellular metabolism, protein catabolism releases protein-bound potassium in the cell, increasing intracellular osmotic pressure from free potassium. Sodium ions in the surrounding extracellular fluid increase to prevent hypotonic dehydration. The increased extracellular sodium in time adds still further to the tissue water retention.

Nutritional Therapy

The basis for all care of the person with congestive heart disease is reduction of the work load of the heart. Medical management involves oxygen therapy, decreased physical activity, and drug therapy with (1) diuretic agents to control the fluid congestion in the lungs and (2) digitalis drugs to strengthen contractions of the heart muscle. Nutritional management involves the following:

- *Low sodium.* Sodium restrictions of 500-1000 mg/day (see the *Clinical Application* above) with individual fluid restriction as needed to help reduce fluid retention, with amounts depending on the severity of the heart failure and tissue fluid accumulation.

- *Food texture and meal pattern.* Food with relatively soft texture requiring little physical effort to eat and divided into small feedings eaten slowly.
- *Kcalories.* Decreased to reduce any obesity as well as to decrease the work of the heart to meet circulatory demands for digestion and absorption.
- *Vitamins and minerals.* Full allowance of vitamins and minerals, with special attention to any drug-nutrient interactions causing losses. For example, potassium replacement is needed when potassium-losing diuretics are used, and added vitamin B_6 may be needed when the vasodilator *hydralazine* is used for hypertension control. This drug binds vitamin B_6 and increases its excretion.

Cardiac Cachexia

Etiology

Sometimes with prolonged myocardial insufficiency and heart failure an extreme clinical condition of *cardiac cachexia* develops.[39,40] This is a progressive and profound state of malnutrition. The oxygen supply by fluid-congested lungs is insufficient to meet the demands of red blood cell formation by the bone marrow or the energy needs for basic breathing. The enlarged laboring heart is unable to maintain a sufficient blood supply to the body tissues, all the while confronting an increased metabolic rate and energy demand in its struggle to do so. As a result, nutrient delivery to cells is impaired by the insufficient circulatory system. In addition, *iatrogenic* nutrient losses occur from removal of body fluids to reduce edema and from diuretic drug-induced loss of fluid and electrolytes. A protein-losing enteropathy also develops, hindering nutrient absorption. The overall anorexia is deepened by the edema, unpalatable sodium-restricted diets, drug reactions, and postoperative complications of cardiac surgery that reduce food intake. It should be no surprise that the incidence of *nosocomial* (hospital-induced) cardiac cachexia is not an uncommon occurrence.

Nutritional Therapy

Nutritional therapy for the congestive heart failure patient with cardiac cachexia requires continuous individual assessment and management according to status and treatment response. The goal is to help restore heart-lung function as much as possible and provide support for rebuilding body tissue. Team care involving the physician, nutritionist, nurse, patient, and family is essential (see Chapter 1). Nutritional support requires attention to energy, nutrients, feeding plan, and supplementation:

- *Energy.* General maintenance needs include sufficient kcalories to cover basal energy expenditures (BEE) and resting energy expenditures (REE), plus energy for minimal activity, the hypermetabolism of severe congestive heart failure, and more if major surgery is planned.[39,40] Depending on the extent of malnutrition indicated by the nutritional assessment, an increase of 30% to 50% of BEE needs may be indicated.
- *Fluids.* Fluid intake should be sufficient but not excessive, at a rate of about 0.5 ml/kcal/day or 1000 to 1500 ml/day.
- *Protein.* Approximately 0.8 to 1.0 g of protein per kilogram of body weight is needed to replace tissue losses and cover malabsorption.
- *Fat.* Using a medium-chain triglyceride (MCT) oil for part of the fat allowance modifies losses from malabsorption.
- *Sodium.* Sodium restriction varies with individual status, usually in a range of 500 to 2000 mg/day.
- *Mineral and vitamin supplementation.* To meet needs for tissue rebuilding, malabsorption losses, and hypermetabolic state, general supplementation at 1.5 to 2.0 times the RDAs, with follow-up monitoring of blood concentrations, is usually provided.
- *Feeding plan.* Small, frequent feedings are better tolerated. Large meals add to the risk of carbon dioxide accumulation and respiratory failure.
- *Enteral and parenteral nutrition support.* If regular dietary intake is less than 1500 kcal, the diet may be supplemented with enteral feeding of a high caloric density formula (see Chapter 3). If regular intake falls to less than 500 kcal/day, the patient requires carefully monitored parenteral nutrition support feedings (see Chapter 4).

Essential Hypertension and Vascular Disease

The Problem of Hypertension

Incidence

High blood pressure is one of the most prevalent vascular diseases worldwide.[41] It presents a problem in the lives of some 62 million Americans and is a major factor in the half million strokes and 1.25 million heart attacks that occur each year.[42,43] The major portion of persons with hypertension, at least 95%, have **essential hypertension,** meaning that its cause is unknown. It has become the fourth largest public health problem

> **essential hypertension** • An inherent form of hypertension with no specific discoverable cause; considered to be familial; also called primary hypertension.

in America and has earned an inevitable reputation as the "silent killer," because it carries no overt signs. This indicates its potentially serious implications if it is not treated and controlled. However, it has been demonstrated that control can be accomplished with use of the current antihypertensive drugs as needed, but other sociocultural factors such as access to medical care, health education, and life-style also play roles.[41,44,45] It appears from current analysis that such sociocultural factors influence mass *population* hypertension and stroke risk in the "high normal blood pressure and mild hypertensive" groups that benefit least from the medical detection-and-medication approach.[45]

Public Awareness

Fundamental work of the National Heart, Lung, and Blood Pressure Institute of the National Institutes of Health during the past decade has initiated a public education campaign about the serious problem of hypertension and has followed through with a successful clinical trial to demonstrate the value of a planned stepwise care program. As a result, public awareness of the successful treatment of hypertension with a variety of drugs, singly and in combinations, and of the potential preventive care for persons with high-normal and mildly hypertensive blood pressures through nondrug programs, has grown widely.[46-48]

Nondrug Approaches

A significant result of these ensuing years of clinical experience, within the broader current preventive move in health care, has been a renewed focus on nonpharmacologic approaches to the control of hypertension. This approach has shown that these nondrug therapies, such as diet, exercise, and behavior modification, are effective in treating mild hypertension and are an important adjunct in more severe cases. The goal of all therapy is to reduce as much as possible the quantity of drugs required. Subsequent studies have continued to show the effectiveness of nondrug nutritional therapy.[48,49] These therapies have included weight reduction, regular physical exercise, reduction of salt intake, reduction of dietary fat and cholesterol, and relaxation and stress management. Thus nutritional therapy has proved to have a fundamental role in the care of persons with hypertension and needs to be pursued aggressively to avoid, where possible, some unwanted biochemical effects and considerable cost of lifetime drug treatment.[50,51]

Blood Pressure Controls

Arterial Blood Pressure

Blood pressure, as commonly measured, is an indication of the pressure in the arteries of the upper arm, as measured by an instrument for determining the force of the pulse, a *sphygmomanometer.* The upper figure recorded is the systolic pressure from the contraction of the heart muscle. The lower figure recorded is the diastolic pressure, produced during the relaxation phase of the cardiac cycle (see p. 146). Thus the upper limit of normal adult blood pressure is recorded as 150/89. Several factors contribute to maintaining the fluid dynamics of normal blood pressures: (1) increased pressure on the forward blood flow, (2) increased resistance from the containing blood vessels, and (3) increased viscosity of the blood itself, making movement through the vessels more difficult. Of these factors, increased blood viscosity is a rare event. Thus in discussing high blood pressure in general terms, we are dealing with the first two factors, the pumping pressure of the heart muscle propelling the blood forward and the resistance to its forward flow presented by the vessel walls.

Muscle Tone of Blood Vessel Walls

In hypertension the body's normally finely tuned mechanisms that maintain fluid dynamics are not operating effectively. These systems include several that act to dilate or constrict the blood vessels to meet whatever need is present at a given time. In a hypertensive person, however, these systems cannot achieve their goals. If not effectively treated, uncontrolled elevated blood pressure results. Three main systems operate to maintain normal blood pressure:

1. *Neuroendocrine adrenergic system.* The nervous impulses that control muscle function throughout the body are generally stimulated in a variety of brain centers. They are instantaneously relayed through the nervous system to blood vessel wall muscles and the heart muscle. These nerve impulses are mediated by neuroendocrine chemical transmitter substances, the most common being *norepinephrine.* Adrenergic nerve fibers of the sympathetic nervous system release these neurotransmitters at nerve fiber junctions (*synapses*). The hormone norepinephrine is also secreted by the adrenal medulla, the central zone of the adrenal gland, especially in response to stress. This explains the more forceful heart muscle contraction observed early in the development of essential hypertension and the increased heart rate as the disease is manifested.
2. *Renin-angiotensin-aldosterone system.* This system operates essentially to conserve sodium and body fluids, but it also exerts a *vasopressor* effect.
3. *Kallikrein-kinin system.* Another important system that helps control blood pressure is the kallikrein-kinin system, which operates in a fashion similar to the renin-angiotensin system. **Kallikrein** is an enzyme that operates on its specific

substrate, the *kininogens* and their activated **kinin** substances, the most significant one of which is **bradykinin.** This is a small peptide of only nine amino acids that dilates the blood vessels and increases their permeability, thus reducing blood pressure. It also acts as a smooth muscle constrictor as needed. The kinins work with a second group of substances, the *prostaglandins*. Together they achieve an important down-regulating effect on arterial pressure.

Step-Care Treatment Approach

Based on the national studies indicated and widespread community screening programs, medical treatment has centered on an improved "step-care" method of identifying types of blood pressure levels and matching standard treatment programs to these diagnosed types. Increased emphasis is being given to nondrug therapies, limited use of drugs, and "step-down" weaning from drugs as life-style habits improve.[50,51] Identification of patients with hypertension according to degree of severity generally improves basic care, but as with any care each person's total needs must be considered. These steps of care are termed mild, moderate, or severe.

Mild Hypertension

Diastolic pressure is 90 to 104 mm Hg in the mild form. Initial consideration is given to other risk factors such as weight or stress. Individual treatment is initiated using nondrug approaches and centers on nutritional therapies of weight management, sodium and fat and cholesterol restriction, and behavioral techniques including smoking cessation, regular physical exercise, and stress reduction.

Moderate Hypertension

With moderate hypertension the diastolic pressure is 105 to 119 mm Hg. Prompt evaluation and treatment are indicated. A combination of drugs may be used: (1) a diuretic agent to decrease the blood volume and (2) a blocking agent to decrease muscle constriction of blood vessel walls. The basic nutritional therapy already outlined serves as support, with the goal of reducing the quantity of medication required.

Severe Hypertension

In severe hypertension the diastolic pressure is 120 to 130 mm Hg and above. Immediate evaluation and vigorous drug therapy are needed. Diuretic and beta-blocker agents are continued, and a third drug may be added, a peripheral vasodilator, to assist in reducing arterial resistance to blood flow. In all cases the implications for diet therapy revolve around potassium replacement in the use of diuretics and nutritional guidance for weight management and sodium restriction (p. 172). In addition to the supportive nutritional therapy, additional nondrug therapies include physical exercise, not smoking, and stress-reduction activities.

Cerebrovascular Accident

Incidence

Atherosclerotic vascular injury and hypertension may also affect blood vessels in the brain. Depending on the size of the blood vessel involved and the extent of tissue it serves, the result varies from small, passing *transient ischemic attacks (TIAs)* to larger vessel involvement serving more tissue and a *cerebrovascular accident (CVA)* or disabling stroke to major artery involvement causing massive hemorrhage and a fatal stroke. Over the past two decades, with the declining U.S. early death rate from heart disease, stroke stands in fourth place, following cancer, heart disease, and injuries, in the leading causes of death of adults ages 25 to 65.[52] Of the nearly 150,000 Americans who die annually of stroke, approximately 13% are ages 25 to 65, but the larger majority are older, ages 55 to 65. Among all U.S. population groups, black men have the highest rate of stroke, with a resulting death rate about twice that of white men and substantially higher than for black women.[53,54]

Treatment

Treatment of recurrent TIAs includes cessation of smoking, drug therapy for hypertension, and moderate dietary control of sodium, sometimes with fat and cholesterol modification as needed. Because the proportion of elderly persons in the population has been progressively increasing and age appears to be the most important risk factor for stroke, the number of elderly stroke patients is gradually increasing, and their evaluation and management needs particular attention.[55] In the case of a CVA, a permanent disability may result that requires rehabilitation care. Such disabling conditions are discussed in more detail in Chapter 14.

kallikrein • Any of a group of proteolytic enzymes in the blood and various glands that release kinins (for example, bradykinin) from various globulins.

kinin • Any of a group of endogenous peptides that cause vasodilation, increase vascular permeability, cause hypotension, and induce contraction of smooth muscle.

bradykinin • A nine-amino acid peptide chain formed from kallidin II by the action of kallikrein; a powerful vasodilator that causes increased capillary permeability and also constricts smooth muscle.

Peripheral Vascular Disease

Etiology

Peripheral vascular disease (PVD) is characterized by narrowing of blood vessels in the legs and sometimes in the arms, restricting blood flow and causing pain in the affected area. The most common cause of PVD is *atherosclerosis,* in which typical fatty plaques form on the inner walls of arteries. Contributory risk factors include hypertension and inadequately controlled diabetes mellitus. However, the greatest risk factor is cigarette smoking, which constricts blood vessels. More than 90% of patients with PVD are or were moderate to heavy smokers. Two less common causes of PVD are (1) *Buerger's disease,* in which the arteries, veins, and nerves in the legs, and occasionally in the arms, become severely inflamed and narrowed, blocking off the blood supply to toes and fingers and creating severe sensitivity to cold, and (2) *Raynaud's disease,* in which exposure to cold causes small arteries in the fingers and toes to contract suddenly and cut off the blood supply. In all of these PVD conditions, cigarette smoking is a strong risk factor and must be stopped.

Symptoms and Complications

As narrowing of the arteries develops gradually because of atherosclerosis (the most common cause), an aching, tired feeling occurs in the leg muscles when walking. Resting the leg for a few minutes relieves the pain, but it recurs shortly when walking is resumed. For this reason the symptom is called **intermittent claudication.** Sometimes, sudden arterial blockage occurs when a blood clot develops on top of a plaque of atherosclerosis or a clot formed in the heart is carried to and obstructs a peripheral artery. The blockage causes sudden severe pain in the affected area, which becomes cold and either pale and blue and has no pulse. Movement and sensation are lost.

Treatment

By far the most important treatment for the patient is to stop smoking. As with coronary vessels, surgery on the diseased vessels is sometimes required: (1) *arterial reconstructive surgery* to bypass them, (2) *endarterectomy* to remove the obstructing fatty deposits on the inner linings, or (3) *balloon angioplasty* to widen them. Drug therapy may include **antiplatelet** or anticoagulant agents to prevent blood clotting. Nutritional therapy consists of the regular fat and cholesterol modifications described for coronary heart disease. Exercise is also important. The person should walk every day, gradually increasing to about an hour, stopping whenever intermittent pain occurs and resuming when it stops. Regular inspection of the feet, daily washing and stocking change, good-fitting shoes to avoid pressure, and scrupulous foot care (ideally by a *podiatrist*) is essential to prevent infection. In severe cases in which *gangrene* (tissue death) has developed, amputation may be necessary, with the fitting of an artificial limb.

Chronic Obstructive Pulmonary Disease

Clinical Characteristics

Progressive congestive heart failure, as well as other respiratory problems, contributes to lung disease and the risk of respiratory failure. Malnutrition is common with the debilitating condition of *chronic obstructive pulmonary disease (COPD).* This term describes a group of disorders, including chronic bronchitis and emphysema, in which air flow to the lungs is limited and respiratory failure develops. Malnutrition usually accompanies COPD, and its presence increases the morbidity and mortality associated with the disease process. Anorexia and significant weight loss reflect a growing inability to maintain adequate nutritional status, which in turn severely compromises pulmonary function.[56] Progression of the disease with its increasing shortness of breath prevents the person affected from living a normal life. Eventually, in progressive respiratory failure the person becomes dependent on a mechanical respirator.

Nutritional Therapy

Ratio of Fuel Macronutrients

Respiratory failure is actually a failure of the pulmonary exchange of oxygen and carbon dioxide. Thus its common manifestations are **hypoxemia,** deficient oxygenation of the blood, and **hypercapnia,** excess carbon dioxide in the blood. Nutritional therapy is guided by the *respiratory quotient (RQ),* the ratio of carbon dioxide produced and oxygen consumed, per unit of time, by each of the fuel nutrients. This becomes apparent in the following special diet nutrient ratios used[57]:

- *Fat.* Contrary to generally recommended diets, fat is the favored fuel source in COPD because of its lower oxidative RQ value of 0.7, compared with 1.0 for carbohydrates. Further, fat is a concentrated source of needed kcalories and is lower in osmolality than carbohydrates and does not contribute to the hyperglycemia often seen in critically ill patients fed formulas largely composed of dextrose and amino acids. Fat should provide about 30% to 50% of the nonprotein kcalories in the diet.
- *Carbohydrates.* Conversely, a lower than usual amount of carbohydrates is recommended because of the less favorable RQ value. The metabolic effect of larger amounts of carbohydrates is to increase oxygen consumption and carbon dioxide production and retention, which is a critical imbalance for a patient with failing respiratory function. Carbohydrates should provide approx-

imately 50% of the nonprotein kcalories in the diet.

- *Protein.* The need for protein in ill persons' diets to counteract the catabolic effect of metabolic stress on the body tissue protein is well understood. The recommended dietary protein amount for this purpose ranges from 1.0 to 2.5 g/kg body weight/day, adjusted according to the degree of malnutrition and stress. However, in respiratory failure more is not better, and protein allowances need to be judiciously prescribed. Thus in a prudent diet for failing pulmonary function, protein should provide about 15% of the total kcalories.

Energy Needs

Adequate energy intake is based on extent of protein-energy malnutrition and loss of lean body mass. However, as with protein, kcalorie increases are approached with caution to avoid the dangers of hypercaloric feeding in a patient with limited respiratory reserve.[58] For general purposes BEE and REE needs are estimated by the classic Harris-Benedict equations (p. 55), although these calculations may underestimate REE somewhat in patients with COPD, because of the disease-related REE increase from metabolically active tissue in COPD.[59] A metabolic activity factor (MAF) may be added according to the degree of stress involved (see Chapter 11). For the respiratory patient an MAF of 1.0-1.2 times BEE is adequate for maintenance, and 1.4-1.6 times BEE is needed for restoring lean body mass. An alternate method of estimating energy needs, based on body weight, is allowing 25 to 35 kcal/kg body weight/day for maintenance and 45 kcal/kg body weight/day for rebuilding lean tissue mass.[56,60]

Special Enteral Feeding

Enteral feeding is the preferred mode of feeding, orally for dietary supplementation if possible or by nasoenteric tube if needed (see Chapter 3). Appropriate formulas based on the recommended nutrient ratios discussed, such as Pulmocare (Ross), are available.

General guidelines for dietary modifications in chronic pulmonary disease for professional use based on these nutritional support principles are available.[61] Suggestions for use in counseling COPD clinical patients in menu planning and food preparation are included.

Education and Prevention

General Background and Practical Guidance: "Why" and "How"

Personal life-style habits, especially rich food and limited exercise patterns, play large roles in creating risks for heart disease and hypertension problems. Thus a large part of the health team's work is to help individuals change longstanding habits rooted in the larger society's way of life, both in treating present disease and in preventing disease development. This is not an easy task, but it is our primary task. Persons want to know *why* such personal habit change is important, which requires a sound knowledge base as a motivational factor, and they want to know *how* to achieve these desired changes in practical ways in their life situation. All the while, they need to feel a sense of being in control of their own lives and their own decision making. So a partnership with patients that empowers each one to achieve that degree of self-care with constant support in that development is a basic part of the healing process. It is the primary goal of our therapy.

We turn now in this final section to look at this important area of patient education and disease prevention in relation to our major health problems of cardiovascular disease and hypertension. The major nutrient management, for the most part, focuses on fat, cholesterol, and sodium. The larger background and guidelines for fat and cholesterol control have been detailed in the previous sections of the chapter. In this final section we provide basic general guides for sodium-restricted diets and practical approaches to planning nutritional intervention and disease prevention.

Sodium in General Diets

The taste for salt is an acquired one, not a physiologic necessity. Sufficient sodium for the body's need is provided as a natural mineral in foods consumed. Some persons salt foods heavily and thus habituate their taste to high salt levels. Others acquire lighter tastes and use smaller amounts. Common daily adult intakes of sodium range widely from about 2 to 4 g with lighter tastes to as high as 10 to 12 g with heavier use.

intermittent claudication • A symptomatic pattern of peripheral vascular disease characterized by absence of pain or discomfort in a limb, usually the legs, when at rest and followed by pain and weakness when walking, intensifying until walking becomes impossible and then disappearing again after a rest period; seen in occlusive arterial disease.

antiplatelet • Anticoagulation effect. A platelet is a blood factor, a small disk-shaped structure found in clusters in the blood, chiefly known for its role in blood coagulation. It lacks a nucleus and DNA but contains active enzymes and mitochondria.

hypoxemia • Deficient oxygenation of the blood, resulting in *hypoxia,* reduced oxygen supply to tissue.

hypercapnia • Excess carbon dioxide in the blood.

Salt (sodium chloride, NaCl) intakes are about twice these amounts, since sodium (Na) makes up 40% of the NaCl molecule. The large amount of salt in the American diet, estimated to be about 6 to 15 g sodium/day (260 to 656 mEq), is largely due to the increased use of many processed food products.

Sodium-Restricted Diets

The main source of dietary sodium is sodium chloride, or common table salt. Many other less used sodium compounds, such as baking powder and baking soda, contribute small amounts; otherwise the remaining dietary source is sodium occurring in foods as a natural mineral. In general, three levels of dietary sodium restriction are used, as initially outlined by the American Heart Association, and can be achieved by a regular diet with the following basic food guides for deletion of higher salt/sodium foods:

- *Mild sodium restriction: 2 to 3 g sodium (70 to 130 mEq).* Salt may be used *lightly* in cooking, but none may be *added* at the table. Salty processed foods are avoided, for example, pickles, olives, bacon, ham, chips, and many others.
- *Moderate sodium restriction: 1 g sodium (43.5 mEq).* No salt is added in cooking, no salt is added to the food, and no salty foods are used. Beginning with this level, is some control of natural sodium foods. Higher sodium vegetables are somewhat limited in use, salt-free canned vegetables are substituted for regular canned ones, salt-free baked products are used, and meat and milk are used in moderate portions.
- *Strict sodium restriction: 0.5 g sodium (22 mEq).* This strict level is used occasionally in more severe individual cases. In addition to the deletions thus far, foods with higher natural sodium content—meat, milk, and eggs—are allowed only in small portions, and higher sodium vegetables (artichokes, beet greens, beets, carrots, celery, kale, mustard greens, spinach, Swiss chard, and turnips) are generally avoided.

Management of Hypertension

There is no question that nutritional therapy including sodium restriction plays a large role in the treatment of hypertension. Widespread studies conducted throughout the world in a variety of communities indicate that most hypertensive persons respond to some degree of sodium restriction.[62,63] Adequate potassium also relates to blood pressure control mainly through its electrolyte balance with sodium and its replacement need when potassium-losing diuretics are used.[64,65] Studies of the influence of calcium on hypertension have shown variable results, and it is difficult at this time to identify the amount of calcium that may be adequate to prevent hypertension, and the mechanism involved in a calcium effect on blood pressure remains unclear (see *Issues and Answers,* p. 177). In general the current focus of nutritional therapy is on (1) sodium restriction, (2) weight management with general nutrient balance following the Dietary Guidelines for Healthy Americans and the fat and cholesterol modifications of the National Cholesterol Education Program (NCEP), and (3) an individualized food plan.

A moderately reduced daily sodium intake of about 2 to 3 g (90 to 120 mEq) is a reasonable goal. Persons in a high-risk category for the development of hypertension should certainly reduce their sodium intake as a preventive measure.

Low-Sodium Food Plan

Food Preparation

Numerous popular guides in cookbooks and magazines for preparation of primary foods with alternative seasonings to salt and fat are increasingly available as more public awareness of healthy diets is creating a new market for them. Four references are included in the Appendix related to sodium values of foods and a salt-free seasoning guide. Use of a variety of condiments, avoiding high-sodium ones, and broad use of herbs and spices—seasoning vegetables and fruits such as onion, garlic, whole fruit and juices, especially lemon and lime juice—helps train the taste for less salt (see the *Clinical Application,* p. 166).

Food Products

Close attention to the new food product labeling system is important in the effort to control sodium. The new label regulations and format are designed to provide additional information about product ingredients so that consumers can make wise choices for controlled use, eliminating more salt, fat, and cholesterol, or other food additives. The food industry is responding to current consumer and Food and Drug Administration concerns about specific contents of food products and are providing more needed information.

Special Needs

Individual adaptation of nutritional therapy principles is fundamental to all nutritional counseling. In this case special attention needs to be given to those types of ethnic diets, such as the Chinese, that are traditionally high in sodium. Some reduced-sodium products, such as soy sauce, are now being developed and marketed. Detailed guidelines have also been prepared to assist in counseling such clients.[66]

Planning Nutrition Intervention and Education

Because coronary heart disease and hypertension and their related vascular problems assume more or less a chronic nature, an important responsibility of the health care team is educating the patient and family concerning continuing self-care needs for maintaining health.

Start Early for the Hospitalized Patient (Phase I)

The current brief hospital stay after a heart attack, as well as coronary artery bypass graft or coronary angioplasty, has limited the opportunity for preparing patients and families, especially the spouse, for convalescence and recovery at home.[67] During this period of hospitalization, or Phase I, the main concern of the patient and family is survival, and information retention is limited. The main counseling and educational goal in this initial encounter is to build a supportive bridge to immediate continuing communication and follow-up work during Phase II, the rehabilitation period to follow. Do not begin with involved so-called discharge instructions during the anxious preparation for departure. Instead, provide a firm connection for continuing personal support; supply telephone numbers for communication; briefly describe individual or group resources and programs; plan for initial follow-up contact at home, office, or clinic to provide counseling and educational services; and respond to any immediate needs expressed.

Use a Variety of Resources (Phase II)

Many excellent resources for planning and conducting individual and family patient education during Phase II rehabilitation are available for individual and group learning activities. Practical discussions need to center on aspects such as self-management development, spouse involvement, life-style risk factor changes, and food buying and preparation to make diets palatable and enjoyable.[68-71] Many helpful suggestions are included in the American Heart Association booklets and cookbook (one of our family favorites is Apricot Chicken) and in an increasing number of popular cookbooks. A survey of local markets helps identify commercial products and label information.

For those patients who are overweight, weight reduction food plans may be helpful in general weight management counseling. These plans may be further modified as needed to meet an individual patient's need for controlling sodium or a particular lipid component.

Build Family Health Habits

In the final analysis the wisest approach to the control of coronary heart disease and hypertension is that of prevention and positive health promotion and maintenance. Real contributions begin in childhood, especially in families with strong histories of heart disease and hypertension. In these developmental years, families can build sound health habits with a general focus on good nutrition, including attention to food behaviors related to fat, sugar, and salt, and a physically active life.

Target High-Risk Groups

Effective education for preventing heart and blood pressure problems also starts early and focuses on high-risk groups.

Children. Although the concept has been debated among pediatricians, preventing hypercholesterolemia and hypertension in children of high-risk families has received increased consideration. With close attention to meeting general growth needs, some preventive measures related to weight control and avoiding developing high-fat and high-salt food habits should be included.[72,73] Prevention in childhood, when food habits are developing, is easier than trying to change strong adult habits.

High-risk groups. Hypertension, for example, has been closely associated with certain high-risk groups, including black Americans, persons with a family history of hypertension, and those who are obese. Education concerning the risks of hypertension should be made available particularly to these persons. A strong family history of heart disease also should bring focus to this group.

Use Community Resources and Materials

A number of community agencies, programs, and materials provide resources on hypertension.

Community health agencies. In addition to local chapters of the American Heart Association, hypertension councils have been formed in many areas. A number of materials may be obtained, and active educational programs are sponsored in many communities.

Nutrition resources. A number of resource persons and programs may be found in most communities to assist hypertensive persons in planning self-care. These include various weight-management programs, nutritionists or registered dietitians in private practice or in local health care centers who provide nutritional counseling, or public health nutritionists and nurses in city and county public health departments. Other outreach programs of the Cooperative Extension Service, such as the highly successful course "Eating Today for a Healthier Tomorrow," reach rural and urban communities through county-city networks.[74] A number of special community cooking classes are creatively designed to develop fat- and sodium-controlled cuisines.

Educational materials. Cooking guides and informational material for diets low in fat, cholesterol, and salt may also be obtained in public bookstores and libraries.Community screening programs sponsored by industry are other sources for additional educational guidance. Through community health agencies, persons with coronary heart disease and hypertension and their families may learn to make decisions to change food habits to reduce health risks and assume even more control in managing their own health needs.

To Sum Up

Because of improved treatment programs and increased public awareness, coronary heart disease (CHD) has declined somewhat among the leading causes of death in the United States for ages 25-64, but still precedes the other major causes—cancer, injuries, and stroke—for all population deaths in this age group. The underlying pathologic process of CHD is *atherosclerosis,* which involves the formation of plaque, a fatty substance that builds up along the interior surfaces (intima) of blood vessels, interfering with blood flow and damaging blood vessels. This buildup, which may include blood clot formation, may be so severe that it cuts off supplies of oxygen and nutrients to tissue cells, which in turn begin to die. When this occurs in a coronary artery, the result is a *myocardial infarction,* or heart attack. When it occurs in a brain vessel, the result is a *cerebrovascular accident,* or stroke.

The risk for atherosclerosis increases with the amount and type of blood lipids (lipoproteins) available. Five types of lipoproteins are classified according to their content and density. Those with the lowest density are most strongly associated with atherosclerotic plaque formation. The *apoprotein* portion of lipoproteins is an important factor in the transport of lipids in blood circulation and across cell membranes. *Serum cholesterol* is also a risk factor in atherosclerotic development. The evidence is now overwhelming that elevated serum cholesterol is a causative agent in coronary heart disease, as well as extended *peripheral vascular disease* in the legs. This effect is dramatic in the presence of low density lipoproteins, major carriers of cholesterol to cells for deposit in tissues.

Dietary recommendations for acute *cardiovascular disease,* a heart attack, include caloric restriction, soft-texture foods, and small, frequent meals to reduce the metabolic demands of digestion, absorption, and metabolism and to achieve ideal body weight; restricted fat, saturated fat, and cholesterol intake; and sodium restriction. Chronic *coronary heart disease,* bringing *congestive heart failure,* possible *cardiac cachexia,* and the major risk factor in heart disease of *hypertension,* benefit from sodium restriction to overcome edema caused by inadequate cardiac output and to help control the elevated blood pressure. Restrictions usually range from mild (2 to 3 g), which may only require abstinence from the most obvious sources of sodium (table salt and preserved foods), to strict (500 mg), which requires additional control of natural sodium sources in foods.

Current dietary recommendations to prevent coronary heart disease involve reducing weight, limiting fats to 30% or less of all kcalories, maintaining an optimal ratio between polyunsaturated and monounsaturated fats and saturated fats, limiting sodium intake to 2 to 3 g per day, reducing simple carbohydrates, and increasing physical activity.

Essential hypertension, or high blood pressure of unknown cause, accounts for 95% of all hypertension. It is a major risk factor in cardiovascular disease and is controlled in its milder forms by weight management, sodium restriction, regular physical exercise, and stress-reducing activities.

QUESTIONS FOR REVIEW

1. Which types of hyperlipoproteinemia occur most often? Identify the lipids that are elevated in each case, as well as predisposing factors. Describe the types of diets recommended for each.
2. Identify four dietary recommendations made for the patient with acute cardiovascular disease. Describe how each recommendation is beneficial to recovery.
3. Discuss the three main levels of sodium restriction, describing general food choices and preparation methods.
4. What dietary changes could the average American make to reduce saturated fats and to substitute polyunsaturated fat?
5. What does the term *essential hypertension* mean? Why would weight management and sodium restriction contribute to its control?
6. Outline the nutritional therapy for cardiac cachexia, and discuss the rationale for each aspect of the feeding plan.
7. Discuss the cause and treatment of peripheral vascular disease.

REFERENCES

1. Guyton AC: *Textbook of medical physiology,* ed 8, Philadelphia, 1991, WB Saunders.
2. Marx J: Holding the line against heart disease, *Science* 248:1491, June 22, 1990.
3. Rau L: Hypertension, endothelium, and cardiovascular risk factors, *Am J Med* 90(suppl 2 A):13S, Feb 21, 1991.
4. Culotta E, Koshland DE: NO news is good news, *Science* 258:1862, Dec 18, 1992.
5. Koshland DE: The molecule of the year, *Science* 258:1861, Dec 18, 1992.

6. Gotto AM et al: The cholesterol facts: a joint statement by the American Heart Association and the National Heart, Lung, and Blood Institute, *Circulation* 81(5): 1721, 1990.
7. Grundy SM: Cholesterol and coronary heart disease: a new era, *JAMA* 256:2849, 1986.
8. Grundy SM: Cholesterol and coronary heart disease: future directions, *JAMA* 264(23):305, 1990.
9. Brown MS, Goldstein JL: A receptor-mediated pathway for cholesterol homeostasis, *Science* 232:34, 1986.
10. Lipid Research Clinics Program: The Lipid Clinics Coronary Primary Prevention Trial results: reduction in incidence of coronary heart disease, *JAMA* 251:351, 1984.
11. Ross R: The pathogenesis of atherosclerosis—an update, *N Engl J Med* 314:488, 1986.
12. Steinberg D, Witztum JL: Lipoproteins and atherogenesis: current concepts, *JAMA* 264(23):3047, 1990.
13. Blankenhorn DH et al: The influence of diet on the appearance of new lesions in human coronary arteries, *JAMA* 263:1646, 1990.
14. Blankenhorn DH: Regression of atherosclerosis: what does it mean? *Am J Med* 90(suppl 2A):42s, 1991.
15. Lowering blood cholesterol to prevent heart disease, Consensus Conference, *JAMA* 253:2080, 1985.
16. National Cholesterol Education Program: *Report of the Expert Panel on Detection, Evaluation, and Treatment of High Blood Cholesterol in Adults,* USDHHS (PHS), National Institutes of Health, National Heart, Lung, and Blood Institute, Pub No 88-2925, Washington, DC, 1988, US Government Printing Office.
17. National Cholesterol Education Program: *Report of the Expert Panel on Population Strategies for Blood Cholesterol Reduction,* USDHHS (PHS), National Institutes of Health, National Heart, Lung, and Blood Institute, Pub No 90-3046, Washington, DC, 1990, US Government Printing Office.
18. Food and Nutrition Board, Committee on Diet and Health, National Academy of Sciences—National Research Council: *Diet and health: implications for reducing chronic disease risk,* Washington, DC, 1989, National Academy Press.
19. Kane JP et al: Regression of coronary atherosclerosis during treatment of familial hypercholesterolemia with combined drug regimens, *JAMA* 264(23):3007, 1990.
20. Friday KE et al: Effects of n-3 and n-6 fatty acid-enriched diets on plasma lipoproteins and apolipoproteins in heterozygous familial hypercholesterolemia, *Arterioscler Thromb* 11(1):47, 1991.
21. Young SG: Recent progress in understanding apolipoprotein B, *Circulation* 82(5):1574, 1990.
22. Lawn RM: Lipoprotein(a) in heart disease, *Sci Am* 266(6):54, 1992.
23. Santamarina-Fojo S, Brewer HB: The familial hyperchylomicronemia syndrome, *JAMA* 265(7):904, 1991.
24. American Heart Association Nutrition Committee: Rationale of the diet-heart statement of the AHA, *Arterioscler Thromb* 4:177, 1982.
25. National Cholesterol Education Program: *Report of the Expert Panel on Blood Cholesterol Levels in Children and Adolescents,* USDHHS (PHS), National Institutes of Health, National Heart, Lung, and Blood Institute, Pub No 91-2732, Washington, DC, 1991, US Government Printing Office.
26. Davidson MH et al: The hypocholesterolemic effects of β-glucan in oatmeal and oat bran, *JAMA* 265(14):1833, 1991.
27. Anderson JW et al: Lipid responses of hypercholesterolemic men to oat-bran and wheat-bran intake, *Am J Clin Nutr* 54:678, 1991.
28. Whyte JL et al: Oat bran lowers plasma cholesterol levels in mildly hypercholesterolemic men, *JAMA* 92(4):446, 1992.
29. Demark-Wahnefried W et al: Reduced serum cholesterol with dietary change using fat-modified and oat-bran supplemented diets, *J Am Diet Assoc* 90(2):223, 1990.
30. Leaf A: Cardiovascular effects of fish oils: beyond the platelet, *Circulation* 82(2):624, 1990.
31. Li X, Steiner M: Dose response of dietary fish oil supplementations on platelet adhesion, *Arterioscler Thromb* 11(1):39, 1991.
32. Hepburn FN et al: Provisional tables on the content of omega-3 fatty acids and other fat components of selected foods, *J Am Diet Assoc* 86(6):788, 1986.
33. Reisin E: Sodium and obesity in the pathogenesis of hypertension, *Am J Hypertens* 3:164, 1990.
34. Reddy KA, Marth EH: Reducing the sodium content of foods: a review, *J Food Protection* 54(2):138, 1991.
35. Chelsky LB et al: Caffeine and ventricular arrhythmias, *JAMA* 265(17):2236, 1990.
36. Steinberg D et al: Alcohol and atherosclerosis, *Ann Intern Med* 114(11):967, 1991.
37. Packer M: Pathophysiology of chronic heart failure, *Lancet* 340:88, July 11, 1992.
38. Dargie HJ: Interrelation of electrolytes and renin-angiotensin system in congestive heart failure, *Am J Cardiol* 65:28E, March 6, 1990.
39. Heymfield S et al: Nutritional support in cardiac cachexia, *Surg Clin North Am* 61:635, 1981.
40. Ney DM: The cardiovascular system. In Zeman FJ: *Clinical nutrition and diet therapy,* ed 2, New York, 1991, Macmillan.
41. Kannel WB, Wolf PA: Inferences from secular trend analysis of hypertension control, *Am J Public Health* 82(12):1593, 1992.
42. National Center for Health Statistics: *Health, United States, 1990,* USDHHS (PHS) Pub No 91-1232, Washington, DC, 1990, US Government Printing Office.
43. National Institutes of Health, National Heart, Lung, and Blood Institute: *Morbidity and mortality chartbook on cardiovascular, lung, and blood diseases—1990,* Washington, DC, 1990, US Government Printing Office.
44. Casper M et al: Antihypertensive treatment and US trends in stroke mortality, 1962 to 1980, *Am J Public Health* 82:1600, 1992.

45. Jacobs DR et al: The US decline in stroke mortality: what does ecological analysis tell us? *Am J Public Health* 82:1596, 1992.
46. Dustin HP et al: The 1984 report of the Joint National Committee on Detection, Evaluation, and Treatment of High Blood Pressure, *Arch Intern Med* 144:1045, 1984.
47. National Institutes of Health, National Heart, Lung, and Blood Institute: *Nonpharmacological approaches to the control of high blood pressure,* final report of the Subcommittee on Nonpharmacological Therapy of the 1984 Joint National Committee on Detection, Evaluation, and Treatment of High Blood Pressure, USDHHS Pub No 1986-491-292:41147, Washington, DC, 1986, US Government Printing Office.
48. Fodor JG, Chockalingam A: The Canadian Consensus Report on Non-pharmacological Approaches to the Management of High Blood Pressure, *Clin Exp Hypertens [A],* 12(5):729, 1990.
49. Scherrer U et al: Effect of weight reduction in moderately overweight patients on recorded ambulatory blood pressure and free systolic platelet calcium, *Circulation* 83(2):552, 1991.
50. MRFIT Research Group: Mortality after 10½ years for hypertensive participants in the Multiple Risk Factor Intervention Trial, *Circulation* 82(5):1616, 1990.
51. Schieder RE et al: Antihypertensive therapy: to stop or not to stop? *JAMA* 265(12):1566, 1991.
52. US Department of Health and Human Services, Public Health Service: *Healthy people 2000: national health promotion and disease prevention objectives,* Pub No 91-50212, Washington, DC, 1990, US Government Printing Office.
53. National Center for Health Statistics: *United States, 1989, and preventive profile,* USDHHS (PHS) Pub No 90-1232, Washington, DC, 1990, US Government Printing Office.
54. Saunders E: Hypertension in Blacks, *Prim Care* 18(3):607, 1991.
55. Shuaib A, Hachinski VC: Mechanisms and management of stroke in the elderly, *Can Med Assoc J* 145(5):433, 1991.
56. Armstrong JN: Nutrition and the respiratory patient, *Nutr Support Serv* 6(3):8, 1986.
57. Miller MA: A practical approach to eating and breathing in respiratory failure, *Top Clin Nutr* 1(4):61, 1986.
58. DeMeo MT et al: The hazards of hypercaloric nutritional support in respiratory disease, *Nutr Rev* 49(4):112, 1991.
59. Schols A et al: Resting energy expenditure in patients with chronic obstructive pulmonary disease, *Am J Clin Nutr* 54:983, 1991.
60. Pingleton SK, Harmon GS: Nutritional management in acute respiratory failure, *JAMA* 257:3094, June 12, 1987.
61. Monograph: *Dietary modification in chronic pulmonary disease,* Columbus, Ohio, 1986, Ross Laboratories.
62. Kaplan NM: New evidence on the role of sodium in hypertension: the Intersalt Study, *Am J Hypertens* 3:168, 1990.
63. Law MR et al: By how much does dietary salt reduction lower blood pressure? *BMJ* 302:811, 1991.
64. Whelton PK, Klag MJ: Potassium in the homeostasis and reduction of blood pressure, *Clin Nutr* 6(2):76, 1987.
65. Russell RP: Potassium supplementation, potassium-retaining diuretics, and hazards of hyperkalemia, *Clin Nutr* 6(2):70, 1987.
66. Chew T: Sodium values of Chinese condiments and their use in sodium-restricted diets, *J Am Diet Assoc* 82(4):397, 1983.
67. Montgomery DA, Amos RJ: Nutrition information needs during cardiac rehabilitation: perceptions of the cardiac patient and spouse, *J Am Diet Assoc* 91(9):1078, 1991.
68. Barnes MS, Terry RD: Adherence to the cardiac diet: attitudes of patients after myocardial infarction, *J Am Diet Assoc* 91(11):1435, 1991.
69. McCann BS et al: Promoting adherence to low-fat, low-cholesterol diets: review and recommendations, *J Am Diet Assoc* 90(10):1408, 1990.
70. Sharlin J et al: Nutrition and behavioral characteristics and determinants of plasma cholesterol levels in men and women, *J Am Diet Assoc* 92(4):434, 1992.
71. Shenberger DM et al: Intense dietary counseling lowers LDL cholesterol in the recruitment phase of a clinical trial of men who had coronary artery bypass graft, *J Am Diet Assoc* 92(4):441, 1992.
72. McMurray MP et al: Family-oriented nutrition intervention for the lipid population, *J Am Diet Assoc* 91(1):57, 1991.
73. Shannon B et al: A dietary education program for hypercholesterolemic children and their parents, *J Am Diet Assoc* 91(2):208, 1991.
74. Boeckner LS et al: A risk-reduction nutrition course for adults, *J Am Diet Assoc* 90(2):260, 1990.

FURTHER READINGS

Fortmann SP et al: Effect of long-term community health education on blood pressure and hypertension control: The Stanford Five-City Project, *Am J Epidemiol* 132(4):629, 1990.

Hypertension Prevention Trial Research Group: The Hypertension Prevention Trial: three-year effects on dietary changes on blood pressure, *Arch Intern Med* 150:153, 1990.

Kaplan NM: New evidence on the role of sodium in hypertension: the Intersalt Study, *Am J Hypertens* 3:168, 1990 (brief 2-page commentary).

These three reports of studies covering many persons in the United States and other parts of the world provide ample evidence of the strong relation between hypertension and sodium, especially the monumental work of the Intersalt Study, which included centers in remote primitive areas of Brazil, Papua New Guinea, and Kenya and people from China, Russia, Iceland, Europe, and America. Principle investigators were Drs. Geoffrey Rose of England and Jeremiah Stamler of the United States.

Mata P et al: Effects of long-term monounsaturated- vs polyunsaturated-enriched diets in lipoproteins in healthy men and women, *Am J Clin Nutr* 55:846, 1992.
Trevisan M et al: Consumption of olive oil, butter, and vegetable oils and coronary heart disease risk factors, *JAMA* 263(5):688, 1990.

These two articles provide information to support more positive effects on CHD risk factors of diets using mono- and polyunsaturated fats than those using butter.

Owen AL: Dietary trends in fat and cholesterol consumption, *Top Clin Nutr* 5(3):48, 1990.

This review of changing consumer attitudes and practices in purchases and uses of food products with reduced amounts of fat, cholesterol, salt, sugar, and kcalories provides an excellent picture of how the American diet has changed substantially in the past few years.

CASE STUDY

The Patient with Myocardial Infarction

Edward Bennett is a 37-year-old sedentary executive seen for an annual physical examination 6 months ago. He had no complaints, other than feeling the "everyday pressures" of his job as a corporate attorney and head of the legal division. He admitted smoking two packs of cigarettes a day as a means of relieving stress.

Mr. Bennett is 175 cm (5 ft 10 in) tall and at the time of his examination weighed 83 kg (185 lb). His blood pressure was 148/90 and serum cholesterol 285 mg/dl. He was advised to quit smoking, exercise daily at a moderate pace, and lose 9 kg (20 lb).

He arrived in the hospital emergency room 3 months later complaining of severe chest pains and difficulty breathing. His wife reported that he had appeared pale that evening, had broken out into a cold sweat, and had vomited shortly after arriving home from work. Once regular breathing was restored by the emergency medical team and his pain subsided, a number of laboratory tests were ordered. These tests included serum glutamic-oxaloacetic transaminase (SGOT), lactate dehydrogenase (LDH), prothrombin time, lipid panel plus HDL-cholesterol, sedimentation rate, coagulation times, fasting blood sugar (FBS), blood urea nitrogen (BUN), and complete blood count (CBC). An electrocardiogram (ECG) was also ordered. The patient was then transferred to the coronary care unit for closer monitoring.

The tests results were elevated: SGOT, LDH, LDL and total cholesterol, triglycerides, glucose, prothrombin time, white blood cell count, and sedimentation rate. The HDL level was low. The ECG revealed an infarction of the posterior wall of the myocardium. The diagnosis was myocardial infarction, with underlying familial hypercholesterolemia.

In consultation with the clinical nutritionist the cardiologist ordered a liquid diet, increasing it to an 800-kcal soft diet with low saturated fats 2 days later. The nutritionist noted continued improvement in the patient's appetite accompanying recovery and recommended a full diet. A 1200 kcal low-saturated fat, low-cholesterol full diet was ordered by the end of the week. The nutritionist specified that the cholesterol be limited to 300 mg or less and that the total dietary fat content be limited to 25% of total kcalories with emphasis on use of unsaturated fats.

Two weeks later Mr. Bennett was discharged. During his convalescence the nutritionist and the nurse met with him and his wife several times to discuss his continuing care at home. At each follow-up clinical visit with the physician and with the nutritionist, Mr. Bennett showed good general recovery and enjoyment of his new modified fat and cholesterol food habits.

Questions for Analysis

1. What predisposing factors in Mr. Bennett's life-style place him in the high-risk category for coronary heart disease?
2. Why was moderate, consistent exercise originally recommended?
3. Explain the causes for Mr. Bennett's initial symptoms.
4. How does each laboratory test ordered in the emergency room relate to cell metabolism? Why were the results elevated?
5. What were the reasons for modifications in texture, fat, and total caloric levels in each diet prescribed for Mr. Bennett? Explain the association between the final diet order and his lipid disorder.
6. Outline a 1-day menu for Mr. Bennett that complies with the final hospital diet order.
7. What nondietary needs might Mr. Bennett have while convalescing at home? What community agencies might be of assistance?

Is Calcium a New Risk Factor in Hypertension Control?

If you had high blood pressure, what would you do—give up salt or drink more milk? This question may sound absurd to anyone familiar with traditional methods of hypertension control, which include a low-sodium diet. To them, giving up salt is the obvious reply. However, in the general public the question is being taken seriously, since a growing number of popular news articles state that persons with high blood pressure may need more calcium.

These reports are based on a number of studies showing that persons with hypertension drink less milk than those with normal blood pressures and also have lower serum calcium levels. These studies contradict the findings of earlier studies in which high serum calcium levels were observed in persons with high blood pressure. The latter results are to be expected because of calcium's known contractive effect on smooth muscle tissue such as blood vessels. Large amounts of calcium should cause blood vessels to contract, thus squeezing on the blood flow and bringing a buildup of pressure against arterial walls. The "new" research claims that persons with hypertension don't handle calcium normally. Some of these researchers believe that the sodium-calcium exchange system through which the calcium enters the cell when the sodium leaves it is defective. They tend to discredit the sodium theory because sodium reduction doesn't work for everyone with hypertension; even traditionalists realize that only about half of those with high blood pressure can control it through sodium reduction alone. Nonetheless there are problems with the calcium research:

- Most of the studies are based on a small number of subjects. For example, McCarron's study at the University of Oregon was based on only 23 subjects. Another study finding a different correlation of high blood pressure with high serum calcium was based on 9321 subjects.
- Although calcium researchers found low serum calcium levels in subjects with hypertension, total blood calcium levels did not vary with variable blood pressure readings in their study.
- In conditions characterized by high calcium levels, such as hyperparathyroidism, blood pressure levels are also high. As the condition improves and the serum calcium levels fall, blood pressure readings also fall.
- The calcium intake of subjects in the studies was based on oral 24-hour recall information on diet, which is not generally considered the most accurate method of determining nutrient intake.
- Assuming that the dietary information obtained is accurate, it indicated that subjects with hypertension may have consumed less milk but still obtained *adequate* amounts of calcium.

Another important point to remember is that most calcium-rich foods have higher than average sodium levels per serving. For example, 1 ½ oz of American cheese may provide 250 to 300 mg of calcium, but it also provides more than 400 mg of sodium.

Newer studies in many parts of the world, modern and primitive, have demonstrated a strong relationship between sodium and blood pressure. Unanswered questions remain about the effects of calcium, potassium, and many other factors on blood pressure. In any event the American Heart Association and other health organizations strongly advise the general public (1) to limit sodium intake and (2) to take in enough calcium to meet various needs for growth, bone and tooth maintenance, and muscle function.

REFERENCES

Kaplan NM: New evidence on the role of sodium in hypertension: the Intersalt Study, *Am J Hypertens* 3:168, 1990.

Law MR et al: By how much does dietary salt reduction lower blood pressure? *BMJ* 302:811, 1991.

McCarron DA, Morris CD: Blood pressure response to oral calcium in persons with mild to moderate hypertension, *Ann Intern Med* 103:825, 1985.

McCarron DA et al: Dietary calcium and blood pressure: modifying factors in specific populations, *Am J Clin Nutr* 54:215S, 1991.

McGregor GA: Sodium is more important than calcium in essential hypertension, *Hypertension* 7:628, 1985.

CHAPTER 9

Diabetes Mellitus

CHAPTER OUTLINE

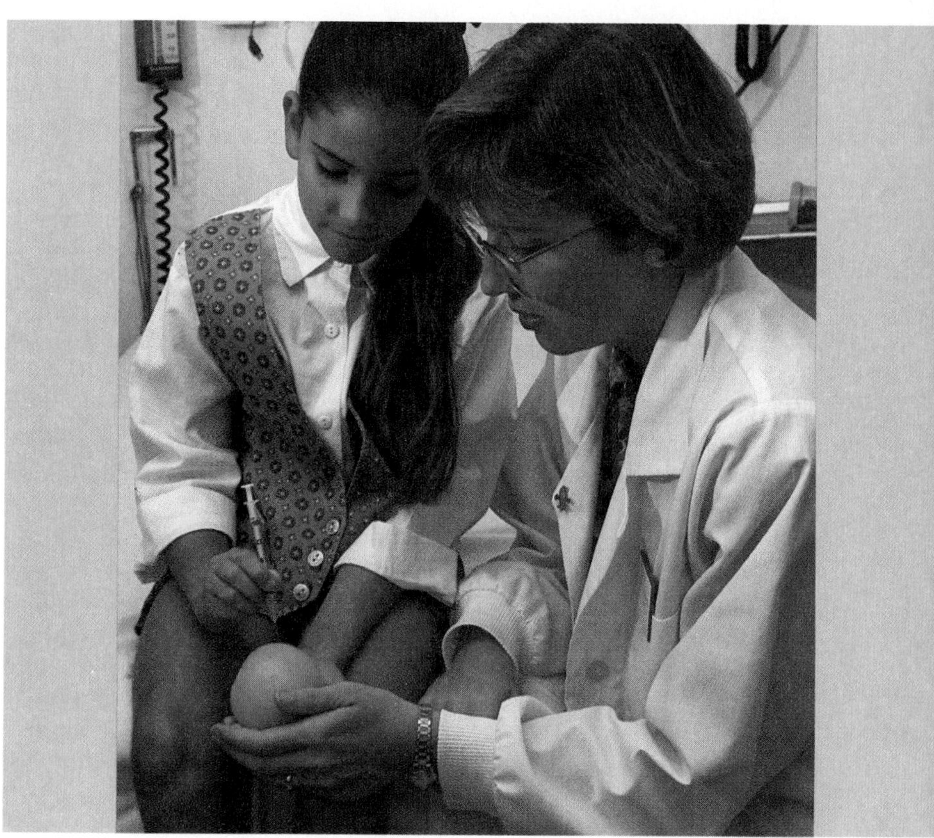

In our series of chapters on clinical nutrition, this chapter examines the problem of diabetes. We seek to understand its nature and how it can be managed to maintain good control and health and to avoid complications.

Nearly 11 million Americans have diabetes. One in 20 is afflicted with the disorder, but only about half are diagnosed. Of this total, 5% to 10% are insulin dependent and 80% to 95% are non-insulin dependent. In the North American population, diabetes complications have become the fifth-ranking cause of death from disease.

Until recently the traditional concept has been that the two major clinical forms of diabetes mellitus, insulin-dependent and non-insulin dependent, represent gradations of the same basic disease that result in metabolic abnormalities, only with quantitative differences in insulin insufficiency. Newer knowledge indicates that diabetes is a syndrome of many disorders characterized by hyperglycemia and in many persons by various complications.

Sound nutritional therapy remains the fundamental base of management for all persons with diabetes. Balancing tools for many are the newer insulins and self-monitoring of blood glucose levels.

Nature of Diabetes

History

The metabolic disease **diabetes mellitus** has both ancient roots and a rapidly expanding research base. Many current studies are helping to explain early observations of its nature and to develop better means of care. In the first century AD the Greek physician Aretaeus wrote of a malady in which the body "ate its own flesh" and gave off large quantities of urine. He gave it the name *diabetes,* from the Greek word meaning "siphon" or "to pass through." Much later, in the seventeenth century, the word *mellitus,* from the Latin word meaning "honey," was added because of the sweet nature of the urine. This addition distinguished it from **diabetes insipidus,** another disorder in which the passage of copious amounts of urine was observed.

Early Clinical Work: Diabetic "Dark Ages"

Diabetes mellitus has long been associated with weight and heredity. Early clinicians, Rollo in England and Boushardat in France, observed that diabetes improved in overweight patients who lost weight. Later the French clinician Lancereaux and his students described two kinds of diabetes: *diabete gras*—"fat diabetes"— and *diabete maigre*—"thin diabetes."[1] All these observations preceded any knowledge about insulin or a relationship between the pancreas and diabetes. Throughout these times, which have been aptly called the "diabetic dark ages," patients had short lives and were maintained on a variety of semistarvation regimens.[2]

Discovery of Insulin

In the following years, evidence began to grow pointing to the pancreas as a primary organ involved in the disease process. Paul Langerhans, a young German medical student, found special clusters, or islets, of cells scattered about the human pancreas that were different from the rest of the tissue. Although their function was still unknown, these islet cells were named for their young discoverer: the islets of Langerhans. Many researchers then focused their studies of diabetes on the pancreas. Finally in the period from 1921 to 1922 a University of Toronto team discovered and successfully used the pancreatic regulatory agent from the "island cells"—**insulin** (see *To Probe Further,* p. 180).[3]

Contributing Causes

Genetics: Insulin Activity

For some time insulin assay tests developed to measure the level of insulin activity in the blood have found insulin-like activity levels in early diabetes to be two or three times the normal insulin levels. Investigators postulated that the insulin was present but bound with a protein, making it unavailable. It is now evident that diabetes is a syndrome with multiple forms resulting from lack of insulin, as in insulin-dependent diabetes mellitus (IDDM), or from insulin resistance and subsequent pancreatic beta cell dysfunction, as in non-insulin-dependent diabetes mellitus (NIDDM).[4,5]

Diabetes has usually been defined in terms of heredity. However, increasing evidence indicates that *genetic* variation between those having IDDM and NIDDM is considerable. Studies of the underlying cause of IDDM have shown that an autoimmune attack of the body's insulin-producing cells is at fault, and scientists express growing confidence that within this decade continuing research will lead to safe preventive therapies.[6] Other current work has focused on ways of predicting the course of prediabetes by identifying disease-specific markers of islet cell antibodies or a predisease decreased growth velocity among unaffected high-risk children of persons with IDDM.

diabetes insipidus • A condition of the pituitary gland and insufficiency of one of its hormones, vasopressin or antidiuretic hormone, characterized by a copious output of a nonsweet urine, great thirst, and sometimes a large appetite. However, in diabetes insipidus these symptoms result from a specific injury to the pituitary gland, not a collection of metabolic disorders as in diabetes mellitus. The injured pituitary gland produces less vasopressin, a hormone that normally helps the kidneys resorb adequate water.

insulin • The hormone found in the islets of Langerhans B cells in the pancreas that is secreted when blood glucose and amino acids rise and assists their entry into cells. It also promotes glycogenesis and conversion of glucose into fat and inhibits lipolysis (fat breakdown). Commercial insulin is made from beef and pork pancreases or more recently from "artificial" human insulin products.

Insulin: Saga of a Success Story

TO PROBE FURTHER

On first glance, looking at numbers only, it appears that the development of insulin was a causal factor in changing the status of diabetes mellitus from a rare disease to one that affects over 10 million Americans. Closer inspection of the facts, however, reveals that the disease was thought to be rare only because its victims died young—fewer persons were around who had the disease. Today insulin enables over 2 million insulin-dependent individuals to live longer and enjoy productive lives.

The success story behind insulin lies not only in its ability to extend the life span of the person with diabetes but also in its own resilience. Insulin was discovered during the summer of 1921 at the University of Toronto by Frederick Banting, a surgeon who according to newspaper accounts of the day solved the mystery of insulin in his sleep, and Charles Best, a college graduate who was not yet enrolled in medical school. Their insulin was derived from the pancreas of dogs by tying off pancreatic ducts, waiting for the organ to "die," and then making an extract of the remaining tissue.

The extract worked fairly well in their tests with dogs. An extract that worked in humans was not developed for another 6 months, partly because their extract was originally given by mouth. Even when injected, their formula failed, which indicated that faulty purification methods may have been involved.

Finally in January of 1922 a successful extract was developed by a new member who joined the research team, J.B. Collip. Its effect on one patient's diabetic condition was not enough to counteract the effect of the treatment of the day—a diet that derived almost 71% of its kcalories from fat. The patient died at age 27 with atherosclerosis and coronary heart disease. However, the team was successful with their third patient. The young girl, who was first diagnosed as having diabetes when she was 11 years old, lived to be 73 years of age. After insulin therapy was initiated, she was taken off the popular "starvation" diet of the day, gained weight, and led a normal life.

Ironically, despite Collip's successful extraction procedure, his subsequent actions almost stopped their project. Jealousies developed, and with the permission of the head of the university's physiology department, Collip refused to share his purification methods with Banting. Then after his extraction product was a success, Collip conveniently "forgot" how to make it! As a result of this foolish battle, at least one patient died because the researchers ran out of the original extract.

Fortunately, Collip miraculously "remembered" how to make his extract the following May. Soon after, insulin was being mass-produced and made available to the growing number of persons who depended on it for their survival.

REFERENCES

Altman LK: The tumultuous discovery of insulin: finally, the hidden story is told, *New York Times*, pp. C-1 and C-6, 1982.

Bliss M: *The discovery of insulin*, Chicago, 1982, University of Chicago Press.

Nestle M et al: A case of diabetes mellitus, *N Engl J Med* 81:127, 1982.

With such screening tests, clinicians are studying possibilities of altering the course of prediabetes or preventing the onset of IDDM and its later devastating complications.[7,8] Meanwhile, because in the roughly 1 million people in the United States with IDDM pancreatic beta cells are destroying the body's own immune system, genetic engineers are making strides toward building a better beta cell through work with cloned laboratory cells. Their work has led to two promising future strategies for reducing the threat of complications: (1) transplanting human pancreatic tissue into persons with diabetes and (2) creating artificial beta cells.[9] In studies of insulin resistance in NIDDM, knowledge of underlying molecular defects has expanded with identification of three genes whose mutation and altered expression contribute to NIDDM.[10] These are (1) **islet amyloid polypeptide (IAPP),** the precursor of *islet amyloid*, the most common lesion seen in the pancreatic islets of diabetic subjects; and (2) **insulin receptor (IR)** and (3) **insulin-regulated glucose transporter (GLUT-4),** two genes that are expressed in insulin target tissues.

islet amyloid polypeptide (IAPP) • Precursor of islet *amyloid,* the most common pancreatic lesion of the islets of Langerhans in non-insulin-dependent diabetes mellitus (NIDDM). A mutant gene controlling synthesis of IAPP was recently discovered.

insulin receptor (IR) • Special body tissue cell receptor for insulin necessary for transporting insulin into target tissue cells for work of cell metabolism; if receptors are defective, insulin activity in cells is impaired. The gene controlling IR synthesis was recently discovered.

insulin-regulated glucose transporter (GLUT-4) • Insulin-controlled glucose transport system in body tissues necessary for normal insulin availability for cell metabolism; if the transport system is flawed, the glucose available for cell fuel is diminished. The gene controlling GLUT-4 synthesis was recently discovered.

TABLE 9–1

Comparison of IDDM and NIDDM

	IDDM	NIDDM
Other names	Type I Juvenile-onset Brittle diabetes Ketosis-prone	Type II Adult-onset Stable diabetes Ketosis-resistant Maturity-onset
Prevalence	5%-10%	80%-95%
Age of onset	Any age; usually less than 40 years	Any age; usually more than 40 years
Cause	Deficient or no insulin production, autoimmune disorder, viral infection	Insulin resistance, hyperinsulinemia, obesity
Symptoms at onset	Polydipsia, polyuria, polyphagia, weight loss	Often none; can have polydipsia, fatigue, blurred vision, symptoms of vascular or neural complications
Usual medical treatment:		
Medication	Insulin	Sulfonylureas (insulin required by some)
Diet	Required (timing and consistency critical)	Required (may be the only form of treatment for some)
Exercise	Recommended (to be integrated with other treatments)	Recommended (to be integrated with other treatments)

Environmental Role: "Thrifty" Gene

Environmental factors apparently play a role in unmasking an underlying diabetes genotype. A theory proposed earlier indicates that diabetes may be associated with genetic modifications for survival over time. The theory was based on the belief that in the past diabetes was a saving, or "thrifty," trait that provided better storage and metabolism of food during a time when our ancestors were living under more primitive and difficult survival conditions. Then as food supplies became plentiful, the negative aspects of the diabetic trait began to appear. Such is indeed the case, for example, with the experience of the Pima Indians of Arizona. Their ancient ancestors arrived on what is now the continent of North America in the Paleo-Indian migrations of the glacial period (about 23,000 to 12,000 BC), across the now submerged Bering land bridge that then connected Asia and North America. These hunter-gatherers pushed their way south through Canada about 12,000 years ago through a narrow ice-free tundra corridor that opened between the retreating glaciers and went south into Montana and the rest of North America. Archaeologic excavations in Arizona have revealed Paleo-Indian artifacts found with mammoth remains dated 1200 years ago, evidence that Indian ancestors were specialized hunter-gatherers who preyed on large game. As game disappeared this Indian group ate a limited diet mainly of carbohydrates rendered from primitive agriculture. Now, however, with the progress of civilization their modern-day descendents, the Pima Indians of Arizona, have become obese and *half* of the adults have NIDDM, the highest reported prevalence of this type in the world. This same pattern is seen among populations of urbanized Pacific Islanders as well as migrant Asian Indians. Thus the available evidence suggests that these groups have a genetic susceptibility to NIDDM (diabetic genotype) and that the disease is triggered by environmental factors. Subsequent study has reinforced the obesity-diabetes connection. Just as obesity may result from more than one genetic error, so too may diabetes.[11] As we commonly observe, diet may indeed interact with genetics to develop adult-onset diabetes.

Classification

Increasing evidence indicates differences between insulin-dependent and non-insulin-dependent diabetes, and epidemiologic studies have provided newer clinical and pathogenetic information. Based on this growing evidence an international work group sponsored by the National Institutes of Health proposed a classification for the diabetes syndrome based on whether insulin is needed for control. This basis is now used to designate the two main types—IDDM and NIDDM (Table 9-1).

Insulin-Dependent Diabetes Mellitus

In its insulin-dependent form, diabetes develops rapidly. It is more severe because of its lack of endogenous insulin to control blood glucose levels and the subsequent metabolic imbalances, and thus it is more unstable because of the difficulty in controlling blood glucose levels smoothly with exogenous insulin injections. As indicated, a variety of genetic, environmental, and immunologic influences selectively attack the insulin-producing beta cells of the islets of Langerhans, producing about 5% to 10% of all cases of diabetes in the United States. Peak ages of onset are between 6 and 11 years, affecting about 1 in every 600 school-aged children.[12,13] Rapid onset of excessive urination, thirst, and hunger accompanied by weight loss are standard clinical findings. Ketoacidosis, reflecting the metabolic imbalance, is fairly common.

Non-Insulin-Dependent Diabetes Mellitus

In its non-insulin-dependent form, diabetes shows a contrasting picture. It develops more slowly because some amount, although limited, of endogenous insulin is available, and thus the disease is usually milder and more stable. The obesity-diabetes genetic base plays a strong etiologic role, so that obesity and physical inactivity in adults are strong risk factors.[14-16] More recently it has been recognized that hypertension may also be associated with the development of insulin resistance and hyperinsulinemia in a number of population groups.[17-19] Because of the slow progression of NIDDM, the number of individuals with undiagnosed NIDDM is thought to be nearly the same as the number who have been diagnosed.[20] NIDDM occurs mainly in adults, and 80% to 90% of these individuals are obese. Because it is a milder metabolic form, ketoacidosis is infrequent. The majority of clients improve with weight loss and are maintained on nutritional therapy and exercise, which may sometimes be assisted by an oral hypoglycemic drug.

Symptoms

Initial observations at the onset of diabetes mellitus, or in its uncontrolled state, may include the following:

1. Polydipsia (increased thirst)
2. Polyuria (increased urination)
3. Polyphagia (increased hunger)
4. Weight loss (IDDM) or obesity (NIDDM)

Clinical laboratory test data reveal the following:

1. Glycosuria (sugar in the urine)
2. Hyperglycemia (elevated blood sugar)
3. Abnormal glucose tolerance tests

Other possible symptoms occur as the uncontrolled condition becomes more serious:

1. Blurred vision
2. Irritated or infected skin
3. Weakness, loss of strength

Continued metabolic consequences may occur as the uncontrolled condition becomes more serious:

1. Fluid and electrolyte imbalance
2. Acidosis (ketoacidosis)
3. Coma

Because the initial apparent symptoms of glycosuria and hyperglycemia are related to excess glucose, diabetes has been called a disease of carbohydrate metabolism. However, as more becomes known about the intimate interrelationships of carbohydrate metabolism with fat and protein metabolism, diabetes is increasingly viewed as a general metabolic disorder resulting from a lack of insulin (absolute, partial, or unavailable) affecting more or less each of the basic nutrients. It is especially related to the metabolism of the two fuels carbohydrates and fat in the body's energy system.

Metabolic Pattern of Diabetes

Normal Blood Sugar Controls

Control of the blood sugar within its normal range of 70 to 120 mg/dl (3.9 to 6.1 mmol/L) is vital to life. The cells may starve and die for want of enough of their major energy fuel. With too much, as in uncontrolled diabetes, the body's life-sustaining water, electrolyte, and acid-base balances no longer work.

A knowledge of the controls for maintaining a normal blood sugar level is essential to understand the impairment of these controls in diabetes. Review these normal controls as shown in Fig. 9-1. Entry of blood glucose from dietary carbohydrates, protein, and fat, as well as from liver glycogen through *glycogenolysis,* maintains a steady supply of blood glucose. To prevent a continued rise above 120 mg/dl (6.1 mmol/L), several routes of glucose use are active:

1. *Glycogenesis.* Conversion of glucose to glycogen for storage in the liver and muscle.
2. *Lipogenesis.* Conversion of glucose to fat and storage in adipose tissue.
3. *Glycolysis.* Cell oxidation of glucose for energy.

Regulatory Pancreatic Hormones

The nonrandom arrangement of the three types of glucoregulatory islet cells scattered in clusters throughout the pancreas indicates a closely interbalanced relationship. This arrangement of human islet cells is illustrated in Fig. 9-2. The largest portion of the islet cells is occupied by beta cells, or *B cells,* filling the central zone, or about 60% of the islet. The B cells synthesize *insulin.* Arranged around the outer rim of the islets are the alpha cells, or *A cells,* one to two cell layers thick, making up about 30% of the islet. The A cells synthesize **glucagon.** Interspersed between A

glucagon • A polypeptide hormone secreted by the A cells of the pancreatic islets of Langerhans in response to hypoglycemia. It has an opposite balancing effect to that of insulin, raising the blood sugar, and thus is used as a quick-acting antidote for the hypoglycemic reaction of insulin; stimulates glycogenolysis by activating the liver enzyme phosphorylase.

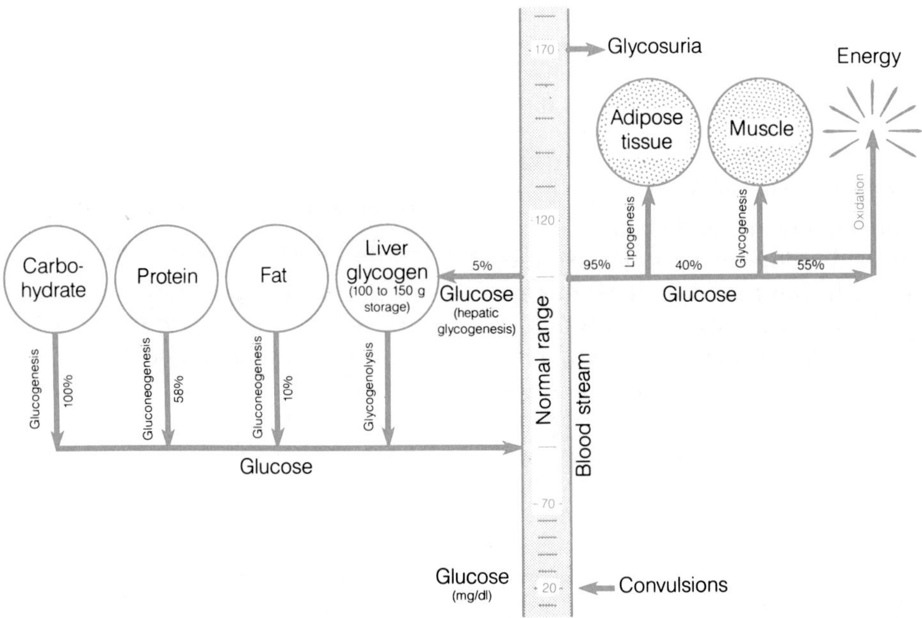

FIG. 9-1 Sources of blood glucose (food and stored glycogen) and normal routes of control.

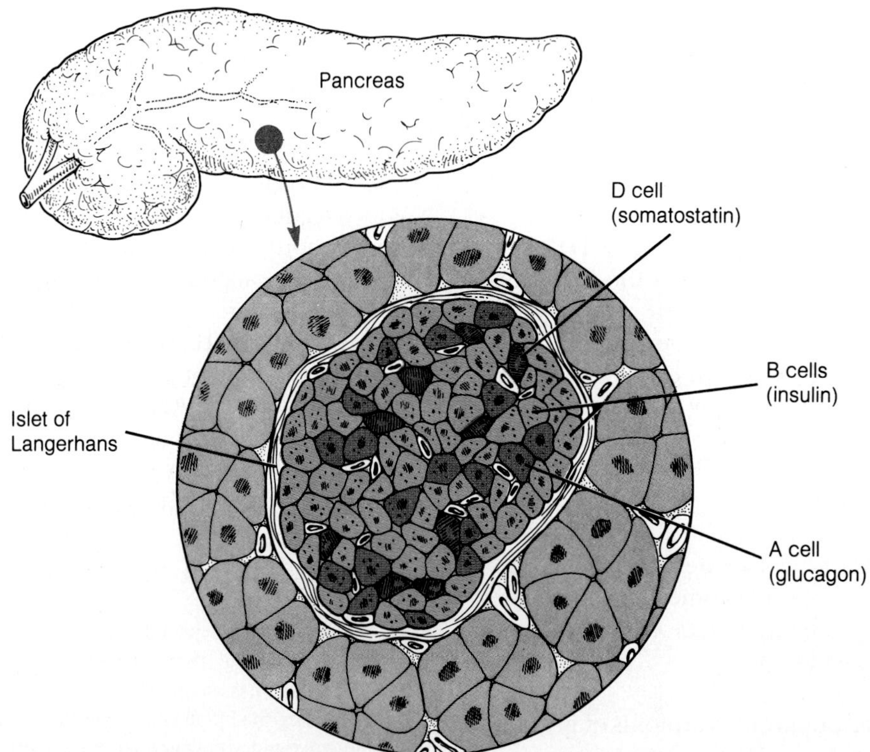

FIG. 9-2 Islets of Langerhans, located in the pancreas.

and B cells or occasionally between A cells are the delta cells, or *D cells*, the remaining 10% of the islet. The D cells synthesize **somatostatin.** Juncture points of the three types of cells act as sensors of the glucose blood concentration and its rate of change. They constantly adjust the rate of secretion of glucagon, insulin, and somatostatin to match whatever conditions prevail at any time.

Insulin

Although the precise mechanisms are not entirely clear in every case, insulin has a profound effect on glucose-control mechanisms. Insulin functions in several ways:

1. Insulin facilitates the transport of glucose through the cell's membrane by way of specialized insulin receptors. These receptors are located on the membrane of various insulin-sensitive cells, including those in adipose tissue, muscle tissue, and monocytes. A chemical linkage is formed between the insulin and another chemical compound on the target cell (the receptor site), causing an alteration of the cell membrane that allows the insulin coupled with the receptor to enter the cell. Researchers are reaching a better understanding of diabetes and how to treat the disease by studying insulin receptors.[10] These insulin receptors mediate all the metabolic effects of insulin. Research has shown that the cells of obese diabetics have fewer than the normal number of insulin receptors. These receptors increase as weight loss occurs and with physical exercise.
2. Insulin enhances the conversion of glucose or glycogen and its storage in the liver (glycogenesis).
3. It stimulates the conversion of glucose to fat (lipogenesis).
4. It inhibits fat breakdown (lipolysis) and the breakdown of protein.
5. It promotes the uptake of amino acids by skeletal muscles and increases protein synthesis.
6. It influences glucose oxidation through the main glycolytic pathway by aiding the necessary initial phosphorylation reaction catalyzed by the enzyme glucokinase.

Glucagon

The hormone glucagon, secreted by the A cells in the islets of Langerhans, functions as a coordinating antagonist to insulin. It rapidly mobilizes hepatic glycogen and to a lesser extent the fatty acids from adipose tissue. This action is designed to raise blood glucose levels to protect the brain and other tissues. Thus it helps maintain normal blood sugar levels during fasting and sleep hours. Its secretion is triggered by a lowering of blood glucose concentration, increased amino acid concentration, or sympathetic nervous system stimulation.

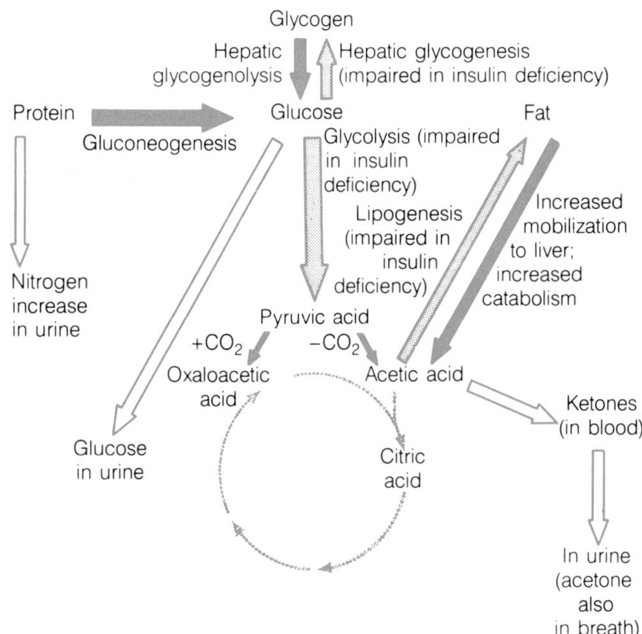

FIG. 9-3 Abnormal metabolism in uncontrolled diabetes. (*From Harper HA:* Review of physiological chemistry, *ed 10, Los Altos, Calif, 1963, Lange Medical Publications.)*

Somatostatin

The D cells are the major source of somatostatin, although this hormone is also synthesized and secreted in different regions of the body, including the hypothalamus. Somatostatin acts in concord with insulin and glucose to inhibit their reactions as needed to maintain normal blood glucose levels. It also accomplishes its glucoregulatory function by inhibiting the release of a number of other hormones as needed.

Metabolic Changes in Diabetes

In uncontrolled diabetes, insulin is lacking to facilitate the operation of normal controls of the blood sugar level (Fig. 9-3). As a result the glucose cannot be oxidized properly through the main glycolytic pathway in the cell to furnish energy; therefore it builds up in the blood (hyperglycemia). Fat formation (lipogenesis) is curtailed, and fat breakdown (lipolysis)

somatostatin • A hormone formed in the D cells of the pancreatic islets of Langerhans; a balancing factor in maintaining normal blood glucose levels by inhibiting the release of insulin and glucagon as needed.

increases, leading to excess ketone formation and accumulation (ketoacidosis). The appearance of the major ketone *acetone* in the urine indicates the development of ketoacidosis. Tissue protein is also broken down in an effort to secure energy, causing weight loss and nitrogen excretion in the urine.

General Management of Diabetes

Diagnosis

Glucose Tolerance

The guiding principles for treating diabetes are early detection and prevention of complications. Over a decade ago the National Diabetes Data Group of the National Institutes of Health and the Expert Committee on Diabetes of the World Health Organization proposed a change from the former 5-hour conventional oral glucose tolerance test, a change that subsequent studies have supported. Usually in the current procedure a 75-g dose of glucose is given and followed by two blood glucose tests: fasting and a 2-hour plasma glucose. A 2-hour plasma glucose value of 200 mg/dl (11.0 mmol/L) or above indicates diabetes, 140 mg/dl (7.8 mmol/L) being the upper limit of normal. Those values falling between 140 and 200 mg/dl (7.8 and 11.0 mmol/L) are labeled *impaired* glucose tolerance. Clinical experience indicates that persons in this latter group tend to progress toward diabetes at a rate about four times that of normal persons. Thus the initial study group recommended that both groups, those diagnosed as diabetic and those with impaired glucose tolerance, have follow-up nutritional therapy and monitoring for glucose management. These diagnostic and follow-up procedures are now usually followed in general clinical practice.

Glycosylated Hemoglobin A_{1c}

Another blood test used for diabetes screening and monitoring is that of glycosylated hemoglobin A_{1c} (Hb A_{1c}). Glycohemoglobins are relatively stable molecules within the red blood cell. During the 120-day life of the cell, glucose molecules attach themselves to the hemoglobin. This seemingly irreversible glycosylation of hemoglobin depends on the concentration of blood glucose. The higher the level of circulating glucose over the life of the red blood cells, the higher the concentration of glycohemoglobin. Thus the measurement of Hb A_{1c} relates to the level of blood glucose over a period of time. It provides an effective tool for evaluating long-term management and degree of control of the diabetic patient.

Treatment Objectives

The health team has three basic objectives in the care of the person with diabetes.

TABLE 9-2

The Facilitative Glucose Transporter Family

Glucose transporter	Tissue distribution
GLUT-1	All tissues, especially red blood cells, brain
GLUT-2	Pancreatic β-cells, liver, kidney, small intestine
GLUT-3	Brain, fat
GLUT-4	Muscle, fat
GLUT-5	Small intestine, kidney

Adapted from Unger RH: Diabetic hyperglycemia: link to impaired glucose transport in pancreatic β cells, *Science* 251:1200, 1991.
GLUT, Glucose transporter.

Maintain Optimal Nutrition

The first objective is a basic requirement for adequate growth and development and the maintenance of a desirable weight.

Avoid Hypoglycemia or Hyperglycemia

This objective is designed to keep the person relatively free of hypoglycemia or insulin reaction, which requires immediate countermeasures, or hyperglycemia, which if untreated contributes to more serious ketoacidosis or diabetic coma. Diabetic hyperglycemia is caused by impaired glucose uptake into pancreatic B cells by means of the glucose transporter *GLUT-2.*[10,21] The newly identified family of glucose transporters, including the insulin-regulated glucose transporter, GLUT-4, are numbered according to tissue distribution and are shown in Table 9-2.

Prevent Complications

The third objective recognizes the increased risk of developing complicating problems that reflect the tissue-damaging effect of chronic diabetes. These complications include the following:

1. *Retinopathy.* Early background lesions in capillaries of the eye usually result from (1) **microaneurysms,** minute sacs formed on the capillary membrane at points of membrane weakness caused by insufficient numbers of endothelial cells, and (2) hard exudates from capillary leakage. So-called cotton-wool spots, areas of tissue ischemia and infarction (tissue death from lack of oxygen caused by blood vessel blockage) of the neuroepithelial layer, occur later as the condition progresses. New, leaky replacement vessels form that tend to grow into the vitreous body of the eye, leading to possible vitreous hemorrhage and retinal detachment. The development of diabetic **retinopathy** is a complex process involving many factors, including insulin resis-

tance, cardiovascular disease, and hypertension. In addition, diabetes-related events such as hyperglycemia, hyperinsulinemia, altered hemodynamics, abnormal platelet aggregation, genetic factors, and growth factors set in motion the pathway that transforms normal vessels into abnormal ones.[22,23] Of these diabetic factors, *hyperglycemia* is the early gate-opening event and thus a major focus of diabetes management with tight control of blood glucose.[24] About 10% of persons with IDDM who develop these retinal malformations in the eye eventually become blind. Older persons with NIDDM may also develop blindness from macular edema, with surrounding microaneurysms and hard exudates, even in the absence of the proliferating retinal malformations. In the United States diabetes accounts for 20% of new cases of blindness for those between the ages of 45 and 74 years.

2. *Neuropathy.* Persons with diabetes are especially vulnerable to the development of nerve damage and diminished transmission of nerve impulses that affect muscle function and sensory perception in various parts of the body. Studies of this diabetes complication have focused mainly on neuronal metabolic abnormalities as a cause, especially in the metabolism of sorbitol and myoinositol, and the effect of tight glycemic control.[24,25] Schwann cells forming the myelin sheath around axons of peripheral neurons are rich in the enzymes aldose reductase and sorbitol dehydrogenase, which convert glucose to sorbitol and fructose. These two glucose products diffuse poorly across cell membranes and thus are osmotically active. Drug therapy with an aldose reductase inhibitor has been used in patients with chronic diabetes and painful **neuropathy** to improve the symptoms. The metabolic abnormalities can be prevented or reversed with aggressive insulin therapy and tight blood glucose control. Foot problems easily occur from decreased function of nerves and blood circulation to and from the feet. This makes daily foot care a necessity for a person with diabetes, following a daily routine of preventive inspection and behavior that protects feet from pressure or contact injuries.[25,26]
3. *Nephropathy.* As with those of other organ systems involved, functional changes in the kidney's nephrons usually begin early in the chronic course of diabetes, but their clinical effects occur over time. Diabetic **nephropathy** develops gradually through several stages related to clinical and tissue findings. The earliest clinical sign of *microalbuminuria,* so called because the small excretion is detected only by sensitive laboratory assays, develops over time into clinical dipstick-detectable *albuminuria.*[26,27] The basement membrane of the nephron's glomerulus thickens and diffuse tissue involvement—glomerulosclerosis—follows (see Chapter 10). The process of microscopic capillary lesions and hyalinization of afferent and efferent glomerular arterioles characteristic of Kimmelstiel-Wilson disease may be present. However, studies indicate that the course of the disease before end-stage renal failure develops may be prevented or halted by *early* aggressive insulin therapy through multiple daily injections or continuous subcutaneous insulin infusion (CSII) by an insulin pump, each monitored by self-administered blood glucose tests.[24,27] Initial drug therapy with *angiotensin converting enzyme (ACE) inhibitors* (captopril, enalapril) is recommended instead of diuretics and beta-blockers for the accompanying hypertension therapy, because of their specific ability to lower the intraglomerular capillary pressure without undesirable effects on glucose control and plasma lipid levels.[27]
4. *Vascular disease.* Atherosclerotic vascular disease is a major cause of illness and death among persons with diabetes. Coronary artery disease

microaneurysm • A small sac formed by the widening of the wall of small blood vessels. Diabetic aneurysms may form in the basement membrane of capillaries throughout vascular beds, as in the eye.

retinopathy • A noninflammatory disease of the retina, visual tissue of the eye, characterized by microaneurysms, intraretinal hemorrhages, waxy yellow exudates, "cotton wool" patches, and macular edema; a complication of diabetes that may lead to proliferation of fibrous tissue, retinal detachment, and blindness.

neuropathy • The general term for functional and pathologic changes in the peripheral nervous system. In diabetes, a chronic sensory condition affecting mainly the nerves of the legs, marked by numbness from sensory impairment, loss of tendon reflexes, severe pain, weakness, and wasting of muscles involved.

nephropathy • A disease of the kidneys; in diabetes, renal damage associated with functional and pathologic changes in the nephrons, which leads to glomerulosclerosis and chronic renal failure.

glomerulosclerosis • Intercapillary degeneration of the nephron glomerulus, a cluster of capillary loops cupped at the head of each nephron, resulting in the degeneration of the entire nephron; a diabetic complication with symptoms of albuminuria, nephrotic edema, hypertension, and renal insufficiency.

(CAD) occurs in diabetics about four times as often as in the general population, and with IDDM and NIDDM the risk of CAD increases with lengthening duration of the diabetes.[28,29] Peripheral vascular disease occurs about 40 times as often in diabetics as in others. The mechanism by which diabetes produces increased damage in the large arteries more so than its incidence in the general population is not clearly understood. It is certainly an additive factor. However, studies have indicated the potential impact of improved control of hyperglycemia with diet and insulin regulation on plasma lipids, lipoproteins, and apolipoproteins in persons with diabetes.[29-31] Current nutritional recommendations of the American Diabetes Association recognize the added risk of vascular disease for persons with diabetes in their revised lipid-lowering dietary guidelines. These recommendations are similar to the Step 1 Diet of the National Cholesterol Education Program of the National Institutes of Health.

Self-Care Role of the Person with Diabetes

To control diabetes effectively the person with diabetes must of necessity have a central position. Daily self-discipline and informed self-care supported by a skilled and sensitive health care team are required for sound diabetes management. Ultimately in the final analysis all persons with diabetes must treat themselves. This is especially true with the tighter normoglycemic control currently being used in self-monitored blood glucose control. Thus the need now for comprehensive diabetes education programs that encourage self-monitoring and self-care responsibility is even greater.

The basic current principles of nutritional therapy for IDDM and NIDDM in balance with insulin or other drug therapy are outlined in the next section. Following the outline of these guiding principles, we discuss approaches to applying them in practical dietary management, including use of the revised food exchange system.

Principles of Nutritional Therapy

Care of Persons with IDDM

The core problem in diabetes is energy balance or regulation of the body's primary fuel, glucose. Based on this concept of balance, three basic principles of nutritional therapy emerge: total energy balance, nutrient balance, and food distribution balance. The fundamental underlying principle may be stated simply: *The diet for any person with diabetes is always based on the normal nutritional needs of that individual.* The personal diet is expressed in terms of (1) total requirement of kcalories for energy; (2) a ratio of kcalories in grams of carbohydrates, protein, and fat; and (3) a general food distribution pattern for the day.

Total Energy Balance

Kcalories

The kcalorie specification of the diet prescription for IDDM is based on needs for normal growth and development, physical activity, and maintenance of a desirable lean weight.

Weight Management

Since IDDM usually begins during childhood (average age is 11), the weight-height measure for children is an index to adequate growth. In adult years the maintenance of a lean weight is a continuing objective of care.

Nutrient Balance

The ratio of carbohydrates, protein, and fat in the diet is based on current recommendations of the American Diabetes Association and the American Dietetic Association concerning ideal glucose regulation and lower fat intake to reduce risks of complications such as cardiovascular disease.[13,20]

Carbohydrates

A more liberal use of carbohydrates, mainly complex forms, is needed for smoother blood sugar control. About 50% to 60% of the total kcalories is assigned to carbohydrates. However, several characteristics of carbohydrate foods need to be examined:

1. *Complex carbohydrates.* The majority of the carbohydrate kcalories, about 45% to 50% of the diet's total kcalories, should be used as complex carbohydrates (starches). In most cases these carbohydrates break down more slowly and release their available glucose over time.
2. *Glycemic index.* Modification of carbohydrate food to take into account the glycemic index of single foods and food combinations, at least in light of our current knowledge, provides little clinical assistance in designing meals for diabetic patients. In comparison with the Diabetes Food Exchange Lists, it less accurately predicts postprandial responses to carbohydrate foods in mixed meals.[32,33] However, most persons with IDDM have developed their own "glycemic index" list based on their individual experience of blood glucose response to specific foods and make insulin adjustments accordingly.
3. *Fiber.* The degree to which fiber is present in complex carbohydrates such as grains, vegetables, and other starches influences the rate of absorption of

TABLE 9–3

A Summary of Dietary Sweeteners

Sweetener	Commercial use	Comparative sweetness*	Effectiveness in carbohydrate metabolism and diabetes control	Problems
Nutritive sweeteners (provide 4 kcal/g)				
Aspartame Combination of two amino acids: aspartic acid and a methyl ester of phenylalanine	Soft drinks Chewing gum Powdered beverages Whipped toppings Puddings Gelatin Tabletop sweetener	180-200	Does not contribute significant amount of kcalories or carbohydrates	Possibly tumorigenic† Possible source of excess phenylalanine for PKU children
Fructose Naturally occurring monosaccharide found in honey, fruits, high-fructose corn syrup	Baked products Frosting mixes Tabletop sweetener Home food preparation	1.4 Enhanced by Use in liquids Low temperature Acidity Dilution	Absorbed more slowly than sucrose Does not require insulin for entry into cells Achieves similar level of sweetness with smaller amounts Contributes moderate amounts of kcalories and carbohydrates to prevent hypoglycemia Should not be used by poorly controlled, obese diabetics	Caloric, carbohydrate values must be considered in calculating diets and recipes Intake of more than 75 g/day increases risk of hyperglycemia
Sorbitol Sugar alcohol naturally occurring in fruits and vegetables	Baked products Sugar-free gum	0.67	Not generally recommended for diabetes control because large amounts are needed to sweeten foods Lack of insulin results in increased conversion to glucose‡	Doses of more than 50-60 g/day result in diarrhea
Xylitol "Wood sugar" found in straw, fruits, corncobs	Banned for commercial use in the United States in 1982	1.22		Tumorigenic
L-Glucose, L-fructose: mirror images (isomers) of D-glucose and D-fructose	Currently under study for possible commercial use	Same as D-glucose (0.72) and D-fructose (1.4)	Contributes no kcalories or carbohydrates because isomeric configuration prevents absorption	
Nonnutritive sweeteners (noncaloric)				
Saccharin	Baked products Soft drinks Tabletop sweetener	300-600	Contributes no kcalories or carbohydrates to the diet	Bladder cancer in test animals§
Cyclamate	Banned for commercial use in the United States in 1970			Bladder cancer in test animals

*The sweetness of sucrose is assigned the value of 1.
†A breakdown product of aspartame, diketopiperazine, is considered tumorigenic by some researchers.
‡Sorbitol is metabolized to fructose, then glucose.
§FDA plan to ban saccharin in 1977 failed because of saccharin's popularity.

the food mix components and alters their effect on the blood sugar. An increased fiber content in the diabetic diet—especially of soluble dietary fiber forms such as those found in oats, barley, fruits, and legumes—appears to have beneficial effects in lowering postprandial plasma glucose and insulin as well as lipids.[34] A fiber intake of about 40 g/day or 25 g/1000 kcal of food intake is a reasonable goal.

4. *Simple carbohydrates.* The small remainder of the carbohydrate kcalories, 5% or less of the total dietary kcalories, may be used as simple carbohydrates. In general, simple carbohydrates—the single or double sugars found in fruits, milk, and sucrose-sweetened food items—should be controlled in the diabetic diet, placing greater emphasis on the complex forms. However, research on the glycemic index of various foods has indicated that a small amount of sucrose or fructose (see *Issues and Answers,* p. 203) is not necessarily detrimental, but it needs to be carefully controlled and used in mixed forms with other foods. Honey is a form of sugar (mainly fructose) and is not a sugar substitute, as some persons may believe.
5. *Sugar substitute sweeteners.* A variety of sugar substitutes are available. Noncaloric sweeteners such as saccharin and aspartame are acceptable. The recently marketed agent aspartame is made from two amino acids, phenylalanine and aspartic acid, and is metabolized as such.[35] Caloric sweeteners such as fructose and sorbitol must be accounted for in the meal. However, many persons with diabetes are intolerant of sorbitol and experience significant diarrhea from its use.[36] A summary of dietary sweeteners is given in Table 9-3.

Protein

Normal age requirements for protein govern the amount indicated for persons with diabetes. In general, protein intake among Americans is excessive and may accelerate the development of nephropathy in persons with diabetes.[37] Thus the intake recommended is restricted to the adult RDA 0.8 g/kg body weight, approximately 12% to 20% of the total kcalories, for all persons with diabetes other than children and pregnant or lactating women.

Fat

Fat should always be used in limited amounts with greater attention given to the control of saturated fats and cholesterol. Total fat intake is lowered to less than 30% of the day's total kcalories. With this reduction all fat components according to degree of saturation should be reduced proportionally. Of the total kcalories, the recommended proportion is less than 10% polyunsaturated, less than 10% saturated, and 10% to 15% monounsaturated fat. The daily intake of cholesterol should be limited to 300 mg or less.

In addition, it is recommended that sodium intake should not exceed 3000 mg/day. Alcohol should also be limited to occasional use or no use; limit to 1 or 2 alcohol equivalents 1 to 2 times per week if used.[38,39]

Food Distribution Balance

General Rule

In general, fairly even amounts of food should be spread throughout the day and adjusted to regular blood glucose self-monitoring. Increased meal frequency also has metabolic advantages for persons with NIDDM.[40] In either case this spread helps avoid excessive intakes at some points with longer fasting periods between meals, eliminating the "peaks and valleys" in food intake and consequent blood sugar swings. This means that a regular schedule of meals at fairly consistent times throughout the day with interval snacks as needed is a basic pattern on which to build.

Daily Schedule Demands

Food distribution must be planned ahead and adjusted according to each day's scheduled activities, with practical consideration given to work, social events, and stress periods.

Exercise

It is especially important that any exercise period or additional physical activity of any kind be accommodated in the food distribution plan (Table 9-4).

TABLE 9-4

Meal-Planning Guide for Active People with Type I Diabetes Mellitus

Exchange needs for	Sample menus
Moderate activity	
30 minutes	
1 bread *or*	1 bran muffin *or*
1 fruit	1 small orange
1 hour	
2 bread + 1 meat *or*	Tuna sandwich *or*
2 fruit + 1 milk	½ cup fruit salad + 1 cup milk
Strenuous activity	
30 minutes	
2 fruit *or*	1 small banana *or*
1 bread + 1 fat	½ bagel + 1 tsp cream cheese
1 hour	
2 bread + 1 meat +	Meat and cheese sandwich +
1 milk *or*	1 cup milk *or*
2 bread + 2 meat +	Hamburger +
2 fruit	1 cup orange juice

Summary: Diet Prescription

In general, the basic principle guiding daily energy needs is sufficient kcalories to meet growth and development needs, physical activities, and maintenance of lean body weight. The nutrient allocation of total kcalories recommended is as follows:

1. *Carbohydrates.* Carbohydrates should provide 50% to 60% of the total kcalories with the main portion as complex carbohydrates and 5% or less as sucrose. Choose food items to achieve a fiber intake of about 40 g with a major portion as soluble fiber.
2. *Protein.* Protein should provide 0.8 g/kg of body weight for nonpregnant, nonlactating adults. Follow the general RDA standard for pregnant and lactating women and for children according to age and sex.
3. *Fat.* Fat should provide 30% or less of the total kcalories with proportions as follows:
   - Polyunsaturated, less than 10%
   - Saturated, less than 10%
   - Monounsaturated, 10% to 15%

Insulin Therapy

The current management goal for persons with IDDM is to maintain a normal blood glucose level as closely as possible. Strong evidence is accumulating that maintaining such a "normoglycemic" state helps prevent the chronic complications of long-term uncontrolled hyperglycemia.[15] This goal requires, of course, a well-trained and highly motivated patient and family and a team of expert professionals to guide, teach, and support the necessary balances among insulin therapy, dietary management, and physical exercise. Three basic tools are needed to manage insulin therapy: (1) insulins that differ in time of action as well as source (2) delivery system options for administering the insulin, and (3) testing procedures to monitor resulting glucose control.

Types of insulin. A number of insulin preparations are available for therapeutic use. According to time of action, they are rapid, intermediate, and long acting, although individual responses are highly variable.

1. *Rapid-acting insulins* go by various names, depending on the manufacturer: for example, Humulin R, Regular, Semilente, and Velosulin R. A number of variables influence absorption rate, such as site of injection, physical activity, skin temperature, and any circulating antiinsulin antibodies. Effect on blood glucose can be detected in about an hour, peaks at 4 to 6 hours, and lasts about 12 to 16 hours.
2. *Intermediate-acting insulins* include Humulin L, Lente, NPH, Insulatard N, and Insulatard. Effect is detected in about 2 hours, peaks at about 11 hours, and lasts about 20 to 29 hours.
3. *Long-acting insulins* include Humulin U and Ultralente. Their duration is somewhat longer than the intermediate-acting insulins. They are seldom used except in special needs because their slow onset and extended action is more difficult to predict or control.

According to commercial source, insulins may be produced from beef and pork pancreases, (Table 9-5), which has been the main U.S. source until recently. But these animal-derived insulins are immunogenic to humans, beef more so than pork. In time they induce antiinsulin antibodies that delay and blunt the effect of the insulin injected. Now, however, hu-

TABLE 9–5

Types of Insulins

Insulin	Onset (hours)	Peak action (hours)	Peak duration (hours)	Species	Appearance
Rapid-acting					
Regular Semilente	½-1	2-4	5-7	Beef, pork, human	Clear
Intermediate-acting					
Lente NPH Mixtard Novolin	1½-4	4-12	18-24	Beef, pork, human	Cloudy
Long-acting					
Ultralente PZI	2-6	10-30	36+	Beef, pork	Cloudy

man insulin is available from two sources: (1) biosynthesis by recombinant DNA technology through rapidly reproducing bacteria that have been given the human gene and (2) chemical substitution of the terminal amino acid on the beta-chain of pork insulin. Because they carry the human insulin structure, these newer insulins are almost nonimmunogenic. A summary of insulin action is given in Table 9-5.

Insulin delivery systems. Intensive insulin therapy for more normal blood glucose control requires multiple injections of rapid-acting insulin, alone or in combination with intermediate-acting insulin. This is accomplished either by regular injection with disposable syringes or by CSII with an insulin pump. The pump is not for everyone, but for many it has made life easier with a steady control of blood glucose level. It is a small device, easily worn on the belt with a subcutaneous needle in the abdomen and buttons the wearer pushes to obtain a fixed programmed flow of insulin in balance with food intake. A new delivery system using a "capsule" implanted under the skin is now being tried in selected individuals.

Testing methods for monitoring results. Three methods are used to monitor an intensive program of insulin therapy. Two methods are regular tools; the third serves for occasional backup.

1. *Self-monitoring of blood glucose.* For insulin doses to be administered in sufficient time intervals and amounts to maintain normal blood glucose, close monitoring of immediate blood glucose levels is mandatory. With advancing technology for producing materials and equipment, two basic methods are available. The first is a visually interpreted strip that may be chosen when the diabetes is relatively stable and less precise information is sufficient or when intellectual skill, manual dexterity, or financial resources are limited. A drop of capillary blood from the finger is placed on the reagent pad on the end of the strip, and the reaction is matched to a color chart. The second method is a reflectance meter providing a digital reading from the reagent strip that may be chosen by persons who require more precise information, those who need meticulous control of unstable glycemia, and those who are color-blind. The frequency of monitoring varies according to need for control and goal of care. More frequent testing is indicated for unstable forms of diabetes, persons using insulin pumps, and those persons who prefer close control and freedom of movement. Usually two to eight or more before- and after-meal tests are performed daily.
2. *Glycosylated hemoglobin A_{1c}.* The Hb A_{1c} test is also used for monitoring an intensive insulin therapy program. The physician uses this test every few weeks or monthly to measure blood glucose response over time. Since glucose attaches to the hemoglobin over the life of the red blood cell, the test gives an accumulated history of glucose levels over a period of time, providing an effective management tool for evaluating progress and making decisions about treatment changes.

Insulin and Exercise Balance

A number of studies have indicated that exercise increases insulin efficiency in persons with diabetes by increasing the number of insulin receptors on muscle cells. Thus exercise has long been established as a useful adjuvant to diet and insulin therapy.[41] However, physical activity must be regular to be effective.

In counseling diabetic clients, one should avoid the simplistic advice to "exercise more often." Rather, a detailed history of personal activity and physical exercise habits should be discussed.[42] This information is then used as a basis for planning together a wise program of *regular* moderate exercise. Guidelines for extra food to cover periods of heavier exercise or athletic practice and competition are included (Table 9-4). Most participants in such an exercise program feel better physically and psychologically.[43] This improved sense of well-being should not be underestimated in persons facing a chronic disease. Self-monitoring is also a regular procedure now used by most persons with IDDM and is a helpful means of determining the balance needed at any point in time between exercise, insulin, and food.

Care of Patients with NIDDM

By far the greater number of persons with diabetes, approximately 85% of the total, have NIDDM. This usually milder form of diabetes differs from IDDM in that insulin is being produced by the B cells in the islets of Langerhans, but the body cells are resistant to its action. Genetic and acquired defects in the genes governing synthesis of IAPP (which causes islet **amyloid** lesions in B cells), the diabetes-associated insulin receptor in B cells, and GLUT-4 in target tissues produce molecular defects in these important secretory cells and transport vehicles (Table 9-1). Thus normal functions are hindered, creating insulin resistance.[10,21]

Contributing Factors

Numerous investigators have indicated a number of factors contributing to the development of NIDDM. Among these are age, obesity, little physical activity, diet, toxins, and stress. The disorder usually appears

TABLE 9-6

Dietary Strategies for the Two Main Types of Diabetes Mellitus

Dietary strategy	IDDM (nonobese)	NIDDM (usually obese)
Decrease energy intake (kcalories)	No	Yes
Increase frequency and number of feedings	Yes	Usually no
Have regular daily intake of kcalories, carbohydrates, protein, and fat	Very important	Not important if average caloric intake remains in low range
Plan consistent daily ratio of protein, carbohydrates, and fat for each feeding	Desirable	Not necessary
Use extra or planned ahead food to treat or prevent hypoglycemia	Very important	Not necessary
Plan regular times for meals/snacks	Very important	Not important
Use extra food for unusual exercise	Yes	Usually not necessary
During illness use small, frequent feedings of carbohydrates to prevent starvation ketosis	Important	Usually not necessary because of resistance to ketosis

in later adult years after the age of 40, and 60% to 90% of the individuals are obese and sedentary. A greater degree of obesity maintained over a longer period substantially increases the risk of diabetes development. Stress and energy regulation are also closely related to the autonomic nervous system response to stress and the central nervous system control of insulin secretion, and in turn to obesity and diabetes. This related background gives us a greater understanding of the interaction of stress, the nervous system, appetite control, and diabetes, as well as an ability to define persons at risk for developing NIDDM. As knowledge of environmental risk factors becomes more complete, hope is increasing that a large percentage of the cases of NIDDM can be prevented.

Nutritional Therapy

The basic therapy principles described for the treatment of IDDM carry over to the care of NIDDM. However, because the two conditions differ in nature, there are some differences in diet therapy.

Energy balance. Because the large majority of persons with NIDDM are obese, the major focus for determining kcalorie requirements is that of weight reduction. Specific caloric requirements to facilitate weight reduction are calculated for each person to account for individual differences. A diet of about 1200 kcal for women and 1500 kcal for men brings about successful weight reduction.

Nutrient balance. Therapy for both types of diabetes is the same. The current nutritional recommendations are based on principles of blood glucose and blood lipid controls.

Food distribution balance. Since NIDDM does not require insulin, the timing of meals or interval snacks is not so important that it needs to be balanced with insulin activity. A summary of the comparative dietary strategies for the two types of diabetes is provided in Table 9-6.

Oral Antidiabetic Drugs

Oral antidiabetic drugs are sometimes used to treat hyperglycemia in NIDDM because they lower the elevated blood glucose. They act by stimulating the pancreas to produce more endogenous insulin. These drugs belong to a group of compounds called sulfonylureas and include agents such as tolbutamide and the newer glipizide, a substituted phenylsulfonylurea, which effectively lowers blood glucose at considerably lower doses than most of the sulfonylurea compounds.

Diet Planning with Food Exchanges

The important first principle in working with persons who have diabetes is that you must start where they are. Any food planning process must focus first on the unique individual person rather than on the "case" or disease. Numerous planning approaches are used by skilled and sensitive clinical dietitians who tailor their actions to the person's learning needs and abilities, nutritional needs, personal needs, and life-style

amyloid • A complex abnormal starchlike formation; a glycoprotein more like its protein component and related to immunoglobulins but forming abnormal lesions in pancreatic islet cells.

TABLE 9-7

Food Exchange Groups

		Composition				
Food group	Unit of exchange	Carbohydrate (g)	Protein (g)	Fat (g)	Kcalories	Characteristic items
Milk	1 cup					
Skim		12	8	—	90	Skim or very low fat
Low fat		12	8	5	120	
Whole		12	8	8	150	
Vegetables	½ cup	5	2	—	25	Medium carbohydrate
Fruit	Varies	15	—	—	60	Portion size varies with carbohydrate value of item
Bread	Varies; 1 slice bread	15	3	—	80	Variety of starch items, breads, cereals, vegetables; portions equal in carbohydrate value to 1 slice bread
Meat	28 g (1 oz)	—				Protein foods; exchange units equal to protein value of 28 g lean meat
Lean		—	7	3	55	
Medium fat		—	7	5	75	
Higher fat		—	7	8	100	
Fat	1 tsp					Fat food items equal to 1 tsp margarine (oil, mayonnaise, olives, avocados)
Polyunsaturated		—	—	5	45	
Monounsaturated		—	—	5	45	
Saturated		—	—	5	45	

issues. Members of the Diabetes Care and Education Practice Group of the American Dietetic Association, for example, have published a helpful monograph in which they discuss no less than eleven meal planning approaches according to an individual's needs and requirements, such as degree of literacy, structure, complexity, and area of emphasis on weight loss and glucose control.[44] Nutritional management strategies for IDDM and NIDDM are also well reviewed in two articles published by the same group.[13,20] However, since the Food Exchange System is the most widely used method of meal planning, it is the approach we use.

The Food Exchange System for planning diabetic diets is based on the concept of food equivalents. It has been developed jointly by the American Diabetes Association and the American Dietetic Association. In most cases initial instruction is provided by a professional diet counselor—a registered dietitian with extensive clinical experience. The diabetic client finds it a helpful tool for planning meals and snacks. Since its introduction the Food Exchange System as outlined or in modified form has been widely used for nutritional care and teaching. In combination with professional counseling it is a sound means of dietary regulation that is flexible enough to meet a wide variety of living situations.

Six food groups are listed in the Food Exchange System: starch/bread, meat, vegetables, fruit, milk, and fats. The revised food lists incorporate guides for modifying fat and salt and increasing fiber, as well as additional lists for free foods, combination foods, and foods for occasional use—all in a well-written and colorfully illustrated booklet for the counselor and the client.[45] These complete food lists are given in Appendix S. A brief description of these six food groups according to their general composition and characteristics is given in Table 9-7. In using the food groups as a guide, food items within any one group may be freely exchanged, since all foods in that group in the portions indicated are of approximately the same food value. These six food groups form the basis for calculating dietary needs and helping clients learn to make a variety of wise food selections and substitutions.

Planning an Individual Meal Pattern

Discovering Individual Needs

First, the clinical dietitian learns as much as possible about each client's needs through a comprehensive history (see Chapter 1). A wide range of areas are included in the discussion, such as personal and family needs, psychosocial development, social activities, and work and school commitments; a typical day's routine; food habits defined and described; and a full medical history with particular reference to the diabetes, its course, and the client's personal experience with it. Pertinent medical and nutritional status data include laboratory tests and anthropometric measures of weight, height, and body composition.

TABLE 9-8

Guidelines for Estimating Approximate Daily Energy Need for Persons with Diabetes Mellitus According to Age, Sex, and General Physical Activity*

Persons with diabetes	Daily energy intake kcal/lb	kcal/kg
Children		
1 year	55	120
1-10 years (gradual decline with age)	45-36	100-80
Males		
11-15 years	20-36 (average, 30)	50-80 (average, 65)
16-20 years		
Very active	20-22	50
Average activity	18	30
Sedentary	15	30
Females		
11-15 years	17	35
15 years	15	30
Adults		
Men, active women	15 × DBW* (lb)	30
Sedentary men, most women, adults over age 55	13 × DBW (lb)	28
Sedentary women, obese persons, sedentary adults over age 55	10 × DBW (lb)	20
Pregnant women		
First trimester	13-15	28-32
Second and third trimesters; lactation	16-17	36-38

Modified from Franz MJ: Diabetes and nutrition: state of the science and the art, *Top Clin Nutr* 3(1):1, 1988.
* *DBW*, Desirable body weight (reasonable body weight).

Determining Diet Prescription

Second, based on information gathered through the comprehensive nutritional assessment, determine the appropriate diet prescription for the patient. Use the American Dietetic Association's nutritional recommendations and principles to calculate the individual's energy needs and nutrient ratios. Other reference tools include RDA standards (inside book covers) and growth charts for children (Appendix P).

Energy. Using guidelines such as those provided in Table 27-8, calculate the individual's general energy needs expressed in kcalories, taking into account any particular needs for growth and development, levels of physical activity, and maintenance of desirable body weight.

Nutrient ratios. Using the list of recommended nutrient ratios (see p. 160), calculate the kcalories provided by each nutrient from the individual's prescribed total kcalories calculated using Table 9-8. Then convert each energy nutrient's kcalorie allowance into grams: divide each kcalorie allowance by the respective fuel factor—carbohydrates, 4; fat, 9; and protein, 4.

Food distribution pattern. The clinical dietitian may want to indicate a general food distribution pattern, spreading the foods throughout the day according to the individual's accustomed habit, or insulin-food balance experience for clients who are not newly diagnosed, in a fairly even pattern. For example, dividing meals and snacks into fractions of tenths, a common day's pattern would be breakfast 1/10, morning snack 1/10, lunch 3/10, midafternoon snack 1/10, dinner 3/10, evening snack 1/10 (notation for charting 113131/10). However, in the current practice of intensive insulin therapy and frequent self-testing of blood, the client learns to make individual adjustments in the distribution of foods. In any event, the dietitian can work out an individual initial basic pattern for meals and snacks with the client, fairly evenly divided throughout the day, and adjust it as needed with follow-up monitoring.

Calculating Meal Pattern

Use the diet prescription formulated as described previously, along with the Food Exchange System values indicated in Table 9-7, to calculate the individual food plan. A short method of calculation is illustrated in Table 9-9 and described next.

Carbohydrate exchanges. Estimate general use of the following carbohydrate food items: milk, vegetable, and fruit. Remember that milk and fruit contribute simple sugars, and use them in moderate amounts. The majority of the carbohydrates are from starch/bread items—complex carbohydrates. First, estimate moderate allowances for milk, fruits, and vegetables on a general caloric level of the diet, nature of the food item, and its use by the patient as revealed in the initial nutritional history. Then calculate full nutrient values for the number of estimated exchanges used thus far. Calculate the nutrient allowances in the order indicated in Table 9-7. First total the carbohydrate column and subtract the total amount of carbohydrates used thus far from the total carbohydrates prescribed for the day. Then use the remaining carbohydrate allowance as starch/bread exchanges: divide by the carbohydrate value of one starch/bread exchange (15 g/exchange) to get the number of starch/bread exchanges. Now you should have filled in all the derived nutrient values for each of the first four carbohydrate exchange groups. Next, by proceeding in the same manner with the remaining two food ex-

TABLE 9–9

Calculation of Diabetic Diet: Short Method Using Exchange System (2200 kcal)

Food group	Total day's exchanges	Carbohydrates: 275 g (50% kcal)	Protein: 110 g (20% kcal)	Fat: 75 g (30% kcal)	Breakfast	Lunch	Dinner	Snacks PM	Snacks hs
Milk (skimmed)	2	24	10		1				1
Vegetable	4	20	8			2	2		
Fruit	3	45			1	1		1	
		89							
Bread	12.5	187	37		3	3	3	2	1.5
		276	55						
Meat	8		56	40	1	2	4		1
			111						
Fat	7			35	2	2	3		
				75					

change groups, calculate meat and fat exchanges to fulfill prescribed protein and fat allowances.

Meat exchanges. To calculate the number of meat exchanges, add the amounts of protein in items used thus far in the carbohydrate exchanges (milk, fruit, vegetables, and starch/bread). Subtract this amount from the day's total allowance of protein. Use the remaining protein allowance in meat exchanges: divide the remaining amounts of protein by the protein value of one exchange (7 g/exchange) to get the number of meat exchanges. Fill in derived values for protein and fat from the meat exchanges and total these amounts. Finally, the last nutrient column for fat can be completed.

Fat exchanges. To calculate the number of fat exchanges, add the amounts of fat in items used thus far (milk and meat) and subtract from the day's total fat allowance. Use the remaining fat allowance in fat exchanges (5 g/exchange). Now the nutritionist has the total number of exchanges for the day from each food exchange group ready to be distributed in an appropriate meal and snack pattern for the client according to individual needs.

Determining the Individual Meal Pattern

The total number of food exchanges calculated for each food group is now distributed as food units into the day's meal pattern to provide the overall food distribution balance according to the type of insulin therapy being used; basic food habits; home, school, and work situations; and any specific exercise periods. Calculation of nutrient distribution in grams is neither realistic nor necessary at this point, since food value

TABLE 9–10

Sample Menu Prescription:
2200 kcal:
275 g carbohydrates (50% kcal)
+
110 g protein (20% kcal)
+
75 g fat (30% kcal)

Meal	Food item
Breakfast	
1 medium, sliced fresh peach Shredded Wheat cereal 1 poached egg on whole grain toast 1 bran muffin 1 tsp margarine 1 cup low-fat milk Coffee or tea	
Lunch	**Afternoon snack**
Vegetable soup with wheat crackers Tuna sandwich on whole wheat bread Filling: Tuna (drained ½ cup) Mayonnaise (2 tsp) Chopped dill pickle Chopped celery Fresh pear	10 crackers with 2 tbsp peanut butter Orange
Dinner	**Evening snack**
Pan-broiled pork chop (trimmed well) 1 cup brown rice ½-1 cup green beans Tossed green salad Italian dressing (1-2 tbsp) ½ cup applesauce 1 bran muffin	3 cups popped, plain popcorn 1 oz cheese 1 cup low-fat milk

TABLE 9-11

How to Modify a Diabetic Meal Plan for Sick Days

Usual food intake	Exchange	Carbohydrates (g)
½ chicken breast, roasted	3 meat	0
1 tsp margarine	1 fat	0
½ cup rice	1 bread	15
Tossed green salad, lemon wedge	Free food	0
¾ cup strawberries	1 fruit	15
1 cup skim milk	1 milk	12
		TOTAL 42

Sick day intake*	Exchange	Carbohydrates (g)
2 cups broth	Free food	0
½ cup gelatin	1 fruit	15
1 cup ginger ale (regular)	2 fruit	30
2 cups herbal tea	Free food	0
		TOTAL 45

*The objective is to provide required amounts of carbohydrates for times when the person with diabetes just does not feel like eating much.

tables are simply not that precise, nor are they intended to be. A general individualized pattern fairly evenly spread throughout the day as indicated provides an initial guide with follow-up modification as experience suggests. The pattern resulting from the diet calculation in Table 9-8 follows this general distribution plan.

Planning a Day's Menu

Use the food exchange lists for meal planning according to the scheme the nutritionist has developed with the client. Guide the client and family in using these food lists for making a variety of appropriate food choices to fulfill the individual food pattern. A sample food plan is shown in Table 9-10.

Adjusting the Plan to the Individual

Get feedback from the client in follow-up sessions to identify any areas that require adjustment of the original plan. The plan should be tailored to fit practical individual needs, living situation, and general eating habits. Counseling continues to determine any further adjustments or changes that are needed.

Planning for Special Needs

Sick Days

When general illness occurs, the food and insulin must be adjusted accordingly. The texture of the food may be modified as needed to use easily digested and absorbed liquid foods while still maintaining as much as possible the glucose equivalents of the usual food plan (Table 9-11).

Physical Activity

For any unusual physical activity the IDDM client needs to make special plans ahead. This is particularly true of a young "brittle" diabetic engaging in athletic competition or practice.

Travel

When a trip is planned, confer with the client to guide food choices according to what will be available. Self-monitoring of blood glucose levels and insulin therapy equipment and making food plans are as important on vacation or a business trip as they are at home.[46] The traveler always needs to plan ahead with the health care team (see the *Clinical Application*, p. 198).

Eating Out

Provide similar guidelines and suggestions for various situations when the client eats meals away from home. As a general rule the plan must be made ahead of time so that accommodations for what is eaten at home before and after the meal eaten away from home reflects continuing balance needs for the day.

Stress

Any form of emotional stress is reflected in variations of diabetes control. These variations are caused by hormonal responses, which act as antagonists to insulin. Help the client learn and plan a variety of useful stress-reduction activities.

Diabetes Education Program

Goal: Person-Centered Self-Care

In past years the traditional medical model has guided diabetes education in its methods, language, and respective roles assumed. The professionals have viewed themselves as having major authoritative roles and assigned to the person with diabetes the more passive role of "patient." With notable exceptions in certain places, this model has been followed in most cases. However, with the increasing movement toward changing roles of practitioners and consumers in the health care system, persons with diabetes are assuming a more active voice in planning and conducting their own care. Several barriers in our traditional system stem from three sources: (1) our culture, (2) our health care delivery system, and (3) our professional training habits. Essentially, much of the core problem centers on *communication.* For example, a list of words we too commonly use that are objectionable to persons with diabetes, along with some suggestions of preferred language, include the following:

1. *"Diabetic" used as a noun.* The word *diabetic* is an adjective and should not be used alone as a noun. Use instead the phrase *person with diabetes.*

CLINICAL APPLICATION

Travel and Illness: "Real-life" Diabetic Situations

Routine meal-planning tips are all well and good. But what do you do when your client with diabetes wants to travel or catches cold? In both cases the client has too many distractions to concentrate fully on planning the most ideal menu. The fact remains, however, that diabetes management relies heavily on the food plan and, in the case of IDDM, on a flexible meal and snack pattern that can be adjusted to meet changing demands.

The following are a few helpful hints you may want to offer clients for those all too common situations.

Travel

Promote confidence about meal-planning skills. Review the number and type of exchanges allowed at each meal. Encourage the client to practice measuring portion sizes. Review tips on eating out.

Learn about the foods that will be available. For a cruise the client should get a copy of the menu in advance. For air travel, advise the client to order diabetic meals in advance. If foreign travel is involved, the client should ask the travel agent for information about foods commonly served to tourists.

Select appropriate snacks. Extra carbohydrates and caloric needs must be met during extra physical activities such as hiking, swimming, skiing, and mountain climbing.

Plan for time. Extended driving time should be avoided. The client should plan to include about 20 g of carbohydrates for every 2 hours of travel. For emergencies and unexpected delays, food for two meals and two snacks, including nonperishable items and liquids, should be on hand.

Plan for time zone changes. The schedule may need to be changed. If so, discuss any necessary meal schedule revisions to balance with insulin activity pattern.

Prepare companions. The client's companions must be able to recognize signs and symptoms of hypoglycemia and hyperglycemia and know their treatment. Remind the client to carry quick-acting carbohydrates at all times.

To support the medical regimen of insulin-dependent clients, remind them (1) to carry an identification bracelet, pendant, or card at all times; (2) to ask their physician for a letter explaining the need for syringes; (3) to carry adequate supplies and equipment for maintaining a schedule for self-testing blood; and (4) to take a prescription for insulin and secure brand names used for insulin in the country to which they are traveling.

Sick-day survival

Nausea and diarrhea. Fluid and electrolyte replacement is crucial with nausea and diarrhea. Advise the client to use salted crackers, broth, or soups as tolerated to replace sodium. The client should use a cola drink such as Coca Cola (small amounts of high-sugar foods may be tolerated as replacement for short periods of time such as during illness), tea, broth, or orange juice to replace potassium. The client should drink something at least every 2 to 3 hours to replace liquids.

Gastrointestinal disturbances. The insulin dosage may have to be decreased. A clear liquid diet including fruit juices, fruit ices, and soups for adequate amounts of carbohydrates is recommended. Protein supplementation through elemental nutrition may be necessary if symptoms last longer than 72 hours. As food tolerance improves, the client should progress to a soft diet that includes milk drinks, custards, and eggs.

Colds and fever. Colds and fever are often treated with aspirin, which tends to lower the sugar level. The client must not skip meals. If necessary, regular meals may be subdivided into small, frequent snacks. Insulin must not be omitted. If the client is completely unable to eat, the physician should be contacted for advice regarding insulin dosage.

In summary, in all cases the client must be advised (1) to maintain a steady intake of food every day, (2) to replace the carbohydrate value of solid foods with that of liquid or soft foods as needed, (3) to monitor blood and urine frequently for sugar and acetone levels, and (4) to contact the physician if the illness lasts more than a day or so. ◆

---

2. *Compliance.* The word *compliance* raises red flags in the minds of persons with diabetes. It is a purely medical term and connotes an authoritative physician position. Instead use the word *adherence,* which has been adopted recently by national committees and associations working in the field of diabetes. The word *adherence* indicates placement of more decision-making responsibility on the person with diabetes to determine courses of action in varying situations, which is, of course, the necessity.
3. *Patient.* Use instead the phrase *person with diabetes.* Persons with diabetes as is any other person, are patients *only* when they are in the hospital or seeing a physician for an illness.
4. *Cheating.* A particularly abusive word in the minds of many persons with diabetes, especially parents of children and young people with diabetes, is the word *cheating.* This flagrant language abuse suggests dishonesty or failure to live up to an external code. By and large, persons with diabetes do not "cheat." They may kid themselves or they may be inaccurate in their reporting, but they do not cheat. Use instead phrases such as *having difficulty* or *having a problem with.*

Content: Tools for Self-Care

A plan for diabetes education must recognize the need for building self-sufficiency and responsibility within persons with diabetes and their families. It should provide practical guidelines that build on the necessary skills a person with diabetes must have for the best possible control, as well as additional surrounding factors related to life situation and psychosocial needs. Content areas include needs in relation to the nature of diabetes, nutrition and basic meal planning, insulin (or oral medication) effects and how to regulate them, monitoring of blood glucose and urine sugar and acetone levels, hypoglycemia control, and how to deal with illness. These educational needs may be organized on three levels: (1) survival level, (2) home management level, and (3) life-style level. The Diabetes Care and Education dietetic practice group has provided two such management guidelines, one for children and adolescents and one for adults.[13,20]

Educational Materials: Person-Centered Standards

A broad, confusing array of diabetes education materials is available. Some are excellent, and some should be discarded. We are wisely reminded, especially by parents of some of our young adolescent clients, that whatever we use should measure up to several basic person-centered requirements. They should do the following:

1. Give the intended receiver credit for having some intelligence and wanting new information.
2. Inform persons fully and completely, giving both sides when experts disagree—as surely they do on occasion.
3. Appeal to various levels of audience, ranging from basic to sophisticated.
4. *Never* be patronizing, dehumanizing, or childish.

In the last analysis, whatever methods or materials we use, one central fact remains: the person who has diabetes is the *most* important and *fully equal* member of the diabetes care team. Interdisciplinary approaches and strategies that involve this recognition can be developed. However, for a number of health care management reasons, a current assessment of the nutritional care and education for patients with diabetes in a number of general primary care clinics indicates that many health care facilities do not yet provide these standards.[47]

To Sum Up

Diabetes mellitus is a syndrome composed of many metabolic disorders collectively characterized by hyperglycemia and other symptoms. Despite the number of possible causes, treatment still relies heavily on a basic type of therapy—a carefully planned diet.

Diabetes mellitus is classified in two main categories: insulin-dependent (IDDM) and non-insulin-dependent (NIDDM). Approximately 15% of all persons with diabetes have IDDM, which develops rapidly, occurs more often in children than adults, and is more severe and unstable. NIDDM occurs mostly in adults who are usually obese. Acidosis is rare. Therapy centers on weight loss. Oral hypoglycemic agents are used occasionally.

Blood sugar levels are controlled primarily by the pancreatic hormones *insulin,* which facilitates the passage of glucose through cell membranes via membrane receptors; *glucagon,* which ensures adequate levels of glucose to prevent hypoglycemia; and *somatostatin,* which controls the actions of insulin and glucagon to maintain normal blood glucose levels.

The diabetic state results from inadequate insulin secretion or insulin resistance because of *amyloid* islet lesions and molecular defects in insulin receptors and transporters. Symptoms range from polydipsia, polyuria, polyphagia, and signs of abnormal carbohydrate metabolism to fluid and electrolyte imbalances, acidosis, and coma in seriously uncontrolled conditions.

Treatment of IDDM involves blood glucose self-monitoring, insulin administration, and scheduled meals to balance insulin activity. Exercise is important, but it must be timed to prevent hypoglycemia resulting from insulin activity or lack of food. The major complications of retinopathy, nephropathy, or neuropathy may occur over time in uncontrolled chronic diabetes.

Treatment of NIDDM consists of weight management through kcalorie modification and exercise. The food plan should be rich in complex carbohydrates and fiber, low in simple sugars and fats (especially saturated fats), and moderate in protein. Moderate regular exercise increases the number of insulin receptor sites on cell membranes and aids in weight control.

QUESTIONS FOR REVIEW

1. Describe the major characteristics of the two types of diabetes mellitus. Explain how these characteristics influence differences in nutritional therapy. List and describe medications used to control these conditions.
2. Identify and explain symptoms of uncontrolled diabetes mellitus.
3. Describe the three major complications of uncontrolled chronic diabetes and the current program of intensive individual therapy designed to maintain normal blood glucose and help avoid these complications.
4. Mr. Jones just found out that he has diabetes mellitus. He is a sedentary, 45-year-old man who is 170 cm (5 ft 8 in) tall and weighs 94 kg (210 lb). No medications were prescribed for him. What is his desirable lean body

weight? If a 1500 kcal diet is prescribed, how many grams of carbohydrates, protein, and fat should be included? If he decides to drink, how many grams of alcohol are allowed each day? Convert this amount to ounces. Which food exchange should be reduced to allow for it? Should he purchase sugar substitutes or diabetic foods? Defend your answer. Mr. Jones wants his children to reduce their chances of developing diabetes. What advice would you offer?

REFERENCES

1. Whitehouse FW: Classification and pathogenesis of the diabetes syndrome: a historical perspective, *J Am Diet Assoc* 81(3):243, 1982.
2. Nestle M et al: A case of diabetes mellitus, *N Engl J Med* 81:127, 1982.
3. Bliss M: *The discovery of insulin,* Chicago, 1982, University of Chicago Press.
4. Saad MF et al: A two-step model for the development of non-insulin-dependent diabetes, *Am J Med* 90:229, 1991.
5. Moller DE, Flier JS: Insulin resistance—mechanisms, syndromes, and implications, *N Engl J Med* 325(13):938, 1991.
6. Atkinson MA, Maclaren NK: What causes diabetes? *Sci Am* 263(1):62, 1990.
7. Chase HP et al: Prediction of the course of pre-type I diabetes, *J Pediatr* 118(6):838, 1991.
8. David R et al: Decreased growth velocity before IDDM onset, *Diabetes* 40:211, 1991.
9. Stone R: Building a better beta cell, *Science* 255(5042):282, 1992.
10. Bell GI: Molecular defects in diabetes mellitus, *Diabetes* 40:413, 1991.
11. Wendorf M, Goldfine ID: Archaeology of NIDDM—excavation of the "thrifty" genotype, *Diabetes* 40:161, 1991.
12. Powers MA: *Handbook of diabetes nutritional management,* Rockville, Md, 1987, Aspen.
13. Connell JE, Thomas-Doberson D: Nutritional management of children with insulin-dependent diabetes mellitus: a review by the Diabetes Care and Education dietetic practice group, *J Am Diet Assoc* 9(12):1556, 1991.
14. Colditz GA et al: Weight as a risk factor in clinical diabetes in women, *Am J Epidemiol* 132(3):501, 1990.
15. McKeigue PM et al: Relation of central obesity and insulin resistance with high diabetes prevalence and cardiovascular risk in South Asians, *Lancet* 337:382, 1991.
16. Dowse GK et al: Abdominal obesity and physical inactivity as risk factors for NIDDM and impaired glucose tolerance in Indian, Creole, and Chinese Mauritians, *Diabetes Care* 14(4):271, 1991.
17. Horton ES: Exercise and decreased risk of NIDDM, *N Engl J Med* 325(3):196, 1991.
18. Donahue RP et al: Hyperinsulinemia and elevated blood pressure: cause, cofounder, or coincidence? *Am J Hygiene* 132(5):827, 1990.
19. Tjoa HI, Kaplan NM: Nonpharmacological treatment of hypertension in diabetes mellitus, *Diabetes Care* 14(6):449, 1991.
20. Beebe CA et al: Nutrition management for individuals with noninsulin-dependent diabetes mellitus in the 1990s: a review by the Diabetes Care and Education dietetic practice group, *J Am Diet Assoc* 91(2):1991.
21. Unger RH: Diabetes hyperglycemia: link to impaired glucose transport in pancreatic β-cells, *Science* 251:1200, 1991.
22. Rand LI: Diabetes retinopathy: can we modify its course? *Am J Med* 90(suppl 2A):665, 1991.
23. Lebovitz HE, Vinik AI: Retinopathy, nephropathy, neuropathy, and tight control, *Am J Med* 90(suppl 2A):805, 1991.
24. Benson JW: Disorders of carbohydrate metabolism: diabetes mellitus. In Metz R, Larson EB, eds: *Blue book of endocrinology,* Philadelphia, 1985, WB Saunders.
25. Levin ME: The diabetic foot: pathophysiology, evaluation, and treatment. In Levin ME, O'Neal LW, eds: *The diabetic foot,* ed 4, St Louis, 1988, Mosby.
26. Selby JV et al: The natural history and epidemiology of diabetes nephropathy: implications for prevention and control, *JAMA* 263(14):1954, 1990.
27. Reddi AS, Camerini-Davalos RA: Diabetic nephropathy: an update, *Arch Intern Med* 150:31, 1990.
28. Krolewski AS et al: Evolving natural history of coronary artery disease in diabetes mellitus, *Am J Med* 90(suppl 2A):56, 1991.
29. Harris MI: Hypercholesterolemia in diabetes and glucose intolerance in the US population, *Diabetes Care* 14(5):1991.
30. Simonson DC, Dzau VJ: Lipids, insulin, diabetes, *Am J Med* 90(suppl 2A):85, 1991.
31. Hollenbeck CB et al: Comparison of plasma glucose and insulin response to mixed meals of high-, intermediate-, and low-glycemic potention, *Diabetes Care* 11:323, 1988.
32. Laine DC et al: Comparison of predictive capabilities of diabetic exchange lists and glycemic index of foods, *Diabetes Care* 10:387, 1987.
33. Braaten JT et al: Oat gum lowers glucose and insulin after an oral glucose load, *Am J Clin Nutr* 53:1425, 1991.
34. Anderson JW et al: Metabolic effects of high-carbohydrate, high-fiber diets for insulin-dependent diabetic individuals, *Am J Clin Nutr* 54:936, 1991.
35. Butchko HH, Kotsonia FN: Acceptable daily intake vs actual intake: the aspartame example, *J Am Coll Nutr* 10(3):258, 1991.
36. Badiga MS et al: Diarrhea in diabetics: the role of sorbitol, *J Am Coll Nutr* 9(6):578, 1990.
37. Narins RG: Diabetic nephropathy: can the natural history be modified? *Am J Med* 90(suppl 2A):70, 1991.

38. Chitwood M, Welch CB: Alcohol, alcohol, everywhere—but not a drop to drink? *Diabetes Forecast* 46(11):38, 1992.
39. Jenkins DJA et al: Metabolic advantage of spreading the nutrient load: effects of increased meal frequency in non-insulin-dependent diabetes, *Am J Clin Nutr* 55:461, 1992.
40. Dahl-Jorgensen K et al: Effect of near normoglycemia for two years on progression of early diabetic retinopathy, nephropathy, and neuropathy: the Oslo study, *Diabetes Spectrum* 1(2):98, 1988.
41. Franz MJ: Exercise and the management of diabetes mellitus, *J Am Diet Assoc* 87(7):872, 1987.
42. Helz JW, Templeton B: Evidence of the role of psychosocial factors in diabetes mellitus: a review, *Am J Psychiatry* 147:1275, 1990.
43. Gill G: Psychological aspects of diabetes, *Br J Hosp Med* 46:301, 1991.
44. Green J, Holler H: *Meal planning approaches in the management of the person with diabetes,* Chicago, 1987, American Dietetic Association.
45. American Diabetes Association, American Dietetic Association: *Exchange lists for meal planning,* Chicago, 1986, The Associations.
46. Jornsay DL, Lorber DL: Diabetes and the traveler, *Clin Diabetes* 6(3):49, 1988.
47. Wylie-Rosett J et al: Assessment of nutrition care provided to patients with diabetes in primary-care clinics, *J Am Diet Assoc* 92(7):854, 1992.

FURTHER READING

Beebe CA et al: Nutrition management for individuals with noninsulin-dependent diabetes mellitus in the 1990s: a review by the Diabetes Care and Education dietetic practice group, *J Am Diet Assoc* 91(2):196, 1991.

Connell JE, Thomas-Dobersen D: Nutrition management of children and adolescents with insulin-dependent diabetes mellitus: a review by the Diabetes Care and Education dietetic practice group, *J Am Diet Assoc* 91(12):1556, 1991.

Gallagher AM, Crawley C, eds: Applying new technology in diabetes management to nutrition counseling: meters, insulin, and insulin delivery systems, *On the Cutting Edge* 13(4):1-33, 1992.

These important materials from the Diabetes Care and Education dietetic practice group of the American Dietetic Association are vital reference resources. The first two articles from the Journal review current guidelines for care and education of persons with diabetes. In the third reference the Diabetes Care and Education practice group devotes an entire issue of its bi-monthly newsletter, *On the Cutting Edge,* to new technologies used in the care of diabetes. Copies of this excellent resource are available from the DCE group (Joanne Gibbons, DCE Administrative Assistant, 9212 Delphi Road, S.W., Olympia, WA 98512; $5.00 plus $0.75 shipping/handling; make check payable to The American Dietetic Association/DCE).

Badiga MS et al: Diarrhea in diabetics: the role of sorbitol, *J Am Coll Nutr* 9(6):578, 1990.

Butchko HH, Kotsonis FN: Acceptable daily intake vs. actual intake: the aspartame example, *J Am Coll Nutr* 10(3):258, 1991.

These two articles provide needed background information about two sweeteners, the acceptable uses of aspartame, and the dangers of diarrhea from excessive sorbitol.

Helmrich SP et al: Physical activity and reduced occurrence of non-insulin-dependent diabetes mellitus, *N Engl J Med* 325(3):147, 1991.

Horton ES: Exercise and decreased risk of NIDDM, *N Engl J Med* 325(3):196, 1991.

This article and editorial from a valued reference journal provide current background information for the important role of exercise in managing NIDDM, which may also be applied to the balanced care of IDDM.

CASE STUDY

Patient with Insulin-Dependent Diabetes Mellitus

Angela Delano is a 45-year-old woman diagnosed 2 years ago with insulin-dependent diabetes mellitus (IDDM). She has three children whose birth weights were in the range of 4.5 to 5.0 kg (10 to 11 lb). The children, now teenagers, show no signs of diabetes, and their weights are reported to be within normal limits, despite their mother's fondness for cooking. Her husband, an underpaid construction worker, is slightly overweight.

Six months ago, Mrs. Delano was seen with a complaint of a series of infections during the past 2 months that lasted longer than usual. At that time she was measured as 165 cm (5 ft 5 in) and 93 kg (205 lb). Her glucose tolerance test was positive. She was seen for follow-up twice during the following month, each time showing hyperglycemia and glycosuria. At the second follow-up, an oral hypoglycemic agent was prescribed, and she was referred to the nutritionist for weight management counseling.

Mrs. Delano did not keep this appointment or her subsequent medical appointment. She was not seen again until a month ago, when she was admitted with ketoacidosis. She responded well to treatment and was placed on a 1200-kcal diet and a mixture of intermediate- and rapid-acting insulin given in two injections a day. On discharge, she was again referred to the nutritionist for individual counseling and diabetes education classes.

Questions for Analysis

1. What factors do you think contributed to the ketoacidosis? Why? What relation do these factors have to diabetes control?
2. What additional information about Mrs. Delano is necessary to understand her major nutritional problems? Why? How could this information be obtained?
3. Based on the information provided, what nutritional problems can be identified? What is the scientific basis for each problem?
4. Determine an appropriate diet prescription for Mrs. Delano and calculate her diet using the exchange system and short method. Using this diet calculation as a guide, outline a meal plan and a schedule of self-monitoring of blood glucose for Mrs. Delano. Assume that she administers the insulin before breakfast and before the evening meal.
5. Identify any personal factors that may affect Mrs. Delano's follow-through with her treatment plan. Do you anticipate any problems? If so, how would you attempt to help her solve them? Outline a diabetes education plan for Mrs. Delano.

Questions from Persons on Diabetic Diets

Persons with diabetes have many questions about their diets, especially when they are newly diagnosed and anxieties are high. They don't want just a "Yes" or "No" answer. For any item of concern, they want to know if it can be used at all and if use is limited, why and how much. Questions about alcohol and various sweeteners are common.

Alcohol and Diabetes: Do They Mix?

Two shots of whiskey on an empty stomach lowers blood sugar dramatically. For this reason, alcohol has been a taboo for years for persons with diabetes. It definitely has some negative effects because of the following:

- Alcohol interferes with the body's ability to regulate insulin-induced hypoglycemia (persons in poor control are most susceptible to this effect).
- It increases serum cholesterol levels, although this effect is transient.
- Alcohol consumption leads to hyperlipoproteinemia in susceptible persons, including persons with diabetes, when it is excessive.
- Alcohol consumption leads to hyperglycemia when it is excessive, although this is a transient effect usually lasting only a few hours.
- Alcohol induces a diabetic condition when used in excess by a prediabetic individual (in such persons, however, the blood sugar returns to normal following total abstinence without the patient's having to resort to using insulin or oral hypoglycemic agents).

But alcohol may not be quite as bad as most people think for the person with diabetes, because it does the following:

- Alcohol does not require insulin for its metabolism.
- It enhances the glucose-lowering effect of hypoglycemic agents, including insulin, when used in *moderate* amounts.
- It raises the HDL-C levels when used in *moderate* amounts, thus possibly providing some protection against cardiovascular disease.

In the light of this information, it appears that diabetes and alcohol can mix—*if* shaken gently. For your clients who choose to use alcohol, you want to discuss the following items with them:

1. Carry personal diabetes identification at all times in case of a hypoglycemic attack induced by alcohol.
2. Ask the physician if there are any contraindications to using alcohol such as hypertriglycerides, gastritis, pancreatitis, some types of cardiac and renal disease, and any drug interactions (such as that occurring with the use of barbiturates or tranquilizers).
3. Always sip alcoholic drinks slowly.
4. Never drink alcohol on an empty stomach.
5. Limit alcohol use to no more than one or two alcohol equivalents per day about 2 or 3 days a week. One equivalent is found in the following:
   - 1½ oz (a shot glass) of distilled alcoholic beverage (whiskey, Scotch, rye, vodka, brandy, cognac, or rum)
   - 4 oz of dry wine
   - 2 oz of dry sherry
   - 12 oz of beer (preferably "light" or reduced-kcalorie)
6. Avoid sweet drinks (for example, liqueurs; sweet wines; drinks mixed with tonic, soda, or fruit juice; and other liquids that have a high concentration of sugar).

In addition, warn any clients taking oral hypoglycemic agents about some of the problems that may occur when they drink alcohol (for example, nausea, deep flushing, tachycardia, and impaired speech). The effect is slightly delayed, beginning 3 to 10 minutes after taking a drink, and lasting up to an hour or longer.

Warn clients receiving insulin they should *not* reduce their food intake. Persons with NIDDM must consider the caloric value of the alcohol and omit 2 fat exchanges for each drink. In contrast, persons with IDDM should continue to eat their full diet as prescribed because of their susceptibility to hypoglycemia induced by alcohol.

Can I Use Fructose in My Diabetic Diet?

How would you answer this question from your diabetic client? Fructose has been touted as a sweetener for persons with diabetes because it is a naturally occurring sugar that is as much as one to one and one-half times as sweet as sucrose. But can the person with diabetes use it safely?

Although fructose as a sweetener is not for all persons with diabetes, generally you can reply, "Yes, but with qualifications."

Fructose must be calculated in the diabetic diet. Advertising claims promoting fructose are sometimes so misleading that many consumers mistakenly believe that it can be used as a "free" food. However, fructose has the same nutritive value as other sugars—4 kcal/g. Especially those persons with IDDM should be instructed to use fructose as carefully as they use any other food with a caloric and carbohydrate value.

The quantity must be limited. If fructose is used, the maximum amount is 75 g a day.

Fructose should be used under specific conditions. Its sweetness varies with temperature, acidity, and dilution. It has been used satisfactorily in some cooked desserts. However, with high temperatures, a rise in pH, and increased concentration of solution, its sweetness is re-

Continued.

duced. This leads to overconsumption, which affects blood sugar levels.

Refined fructose should be used. Natural sources of fructose such as honey also contain considerable amounts of glucose. Thus in comparison, if it is used at all, the person with diabetes is better off using a measured amount of refined fructose.

The American Diabetes Association emphasizes that until further studies show any clinical advantages for using fructose instead of sucrose, fructose should be used only in its pure form, in small amounts, and only by those persons with well-controlled diabetes who are not overweight.

REFERENCES

Chitwood M, Welch CB: Alcohol, alcohol, everywhere—but not a drop to drink? *Diabetes Forecast* 46(11):38, 1992.

Franz MJ: Diabetes mellitus: considerations in the development of guidelines for the occasional use of alcohol, *J Am Diet Assoc* 83(2):147, 1983.

Laine DC: Are sucrose and fructose compatible with a diabetic diet? *Top Clin Nutr* 3(1):46, 1988.

Powers MA, Laine DC: Sweeteners. In Powers MA, ed: *Handbook of diabetes nutritional management,* Rockville, Md, 1987, Aspen.

CHAPTER 10

Renal Disease

CHAPTER OUTLINE

Physiology of the Kidney
Glomerulonephritis
Nephrotic Syndrome
Acute Renal Failure
Chronic Renal Failure
Renal Calculuses
Urinary Tract Infection

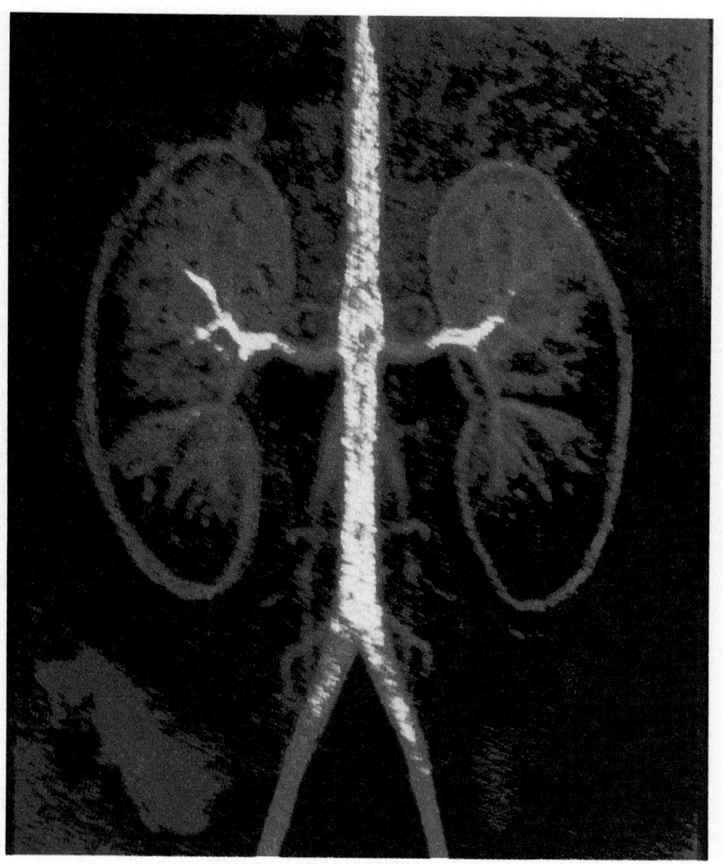

In this chapter we look at the vital structure and function of the kidney and its vast array of minute functional units, the nephrons. When disease attacks these tissues, serious functional problems develop.

Kidney diseases affect the lives of more than 8 million Americans and kill 60,000 a year. Another 3 million or more have related infections, many of which go undetected. In all, these kidney problems are a leading cause of lost work time and pay and are the fourth leading health problem in America today.

The recent advent of renal dialysis technology and kidney transplant techniques prolongs the lives of the 50,000 persons in the

United States who develop kidney failure each year. But this survival is not without great human and monetary cost. Although kidney disease may not be considered as much a killer as heart disease or cancer, it remains a serious national and personal health problem.

In this chapter we consider problems of infection, tissue breakdown, renal failure, and kidney stone formation. In each case we relate nutritional therapy to the nature of the illness and the renal functions impaired.

Physiology of the Kidney

Knowledge of the normal functions of the kidney forms an essential background for relating therapy in renal disorders to impaired functioning of the organ in disease. Major advances today in treating kidney disease are based on providing maximal support for these vital nephric functions (Fig. 10-1). We are endowed at birth with far more filtering-resorbing nephric units than we need, about 2 million of them, but we begin to lose them gradually after age 30.

To better understand the altered kidney functions in renal disease, an overview of kidney functions and structures is provided first.

Basic Renal Structures and Functions

The **nephron** is an exquisite example of a highly complex, minute tissue unit adapted in fine structural detail to its vital function of maintaining an internal fluid environment compatible with life. Important body fluids flow through the successive sections of some 1 million nephrons in each kidney. The nephrons *filter* most constituents from the entering blood, except red blood cells and protein; *resorb* needed substances as the filtrate continues along the winding tubules; *secrete* additional ions to maintain the acid-base balance; and finally *excrete* unneeded materials in a concentrated urine.

Several nephric structures perform unique homeostatic and metabolic tasks. These structures include the **glomerulus** and the tubules.

Glomerulus

At the head of each nephron, an entering or *afferent* arteriole breaks up into a group of collateral capillaries that rejoin to form the *efferent* or leaving arteriole. This tuft of looped collateral capillaries is held closely together in a cupped membrane, **Bowman's capsule.** This capsule is named for the young English physician, Sir William Bowman, who in 1843 first clearly established the basis of plasma filtration on this intimate relationship of blood-filled glomeruli and its enveloping membrane. The filtrate formed is cell-free and virtually protein-free. Otherwise, it carries the same constituents as it does when it enters the blood.

Tubules

Continuous with the base of Bowman's capsule, the nephron's tubule winds in a series of convolutions toward its terminal in the kidney pelvis. Specific resorption functions are performed by the various sections of the tubule.

Proximal tubule. Major nutrient resorption (that is, essentially 100% of the glucose and amino acids and 80% to 85% of the water, sodium, potassium, chloride, and most other substances) occurs in the proximal tubule. Only 15% to 30% of the filtrate remains.

Loop of Henle. This section of the tubule narrows at its midpoint, and its thin loop dips into the central renal **medulla.** Through a balanced system of water and sodium exchange in the limbs of the loop (the countercurrent system), important interstitial fluid densities are created in the medulla to concentrate the urine by osmotic pressure as it later passes through the collecting tubule.

Distal tubule. The latter portion of the tubule functions primarily in acid-base water balance with secretion of hydrogen ions. Sodium and water are conserved through the influence of the hormones aldosterone and vasopressin (also called antidiuretic hormone, or ADH).

Collecting tubule. In this final section of the nephron tubule, water is absorbed under the influence of vasopressin and the osmotic pressure of the surrounding interstitial fluid. The resulting volume of urine, now concentrated and excreted, is only 0.5% to 1.0% of the volume of the water and solutes originally filtered.

Renal Function in Disease

A number of disease conditions may interfere with the normal functioning of the nephrons.

Inflammatory and Degenerative Disease

Inflammation of the small blood vessels and membranes in the nephrons, the functional units of the kidneys, may be short-term, as in acute glomerulo-

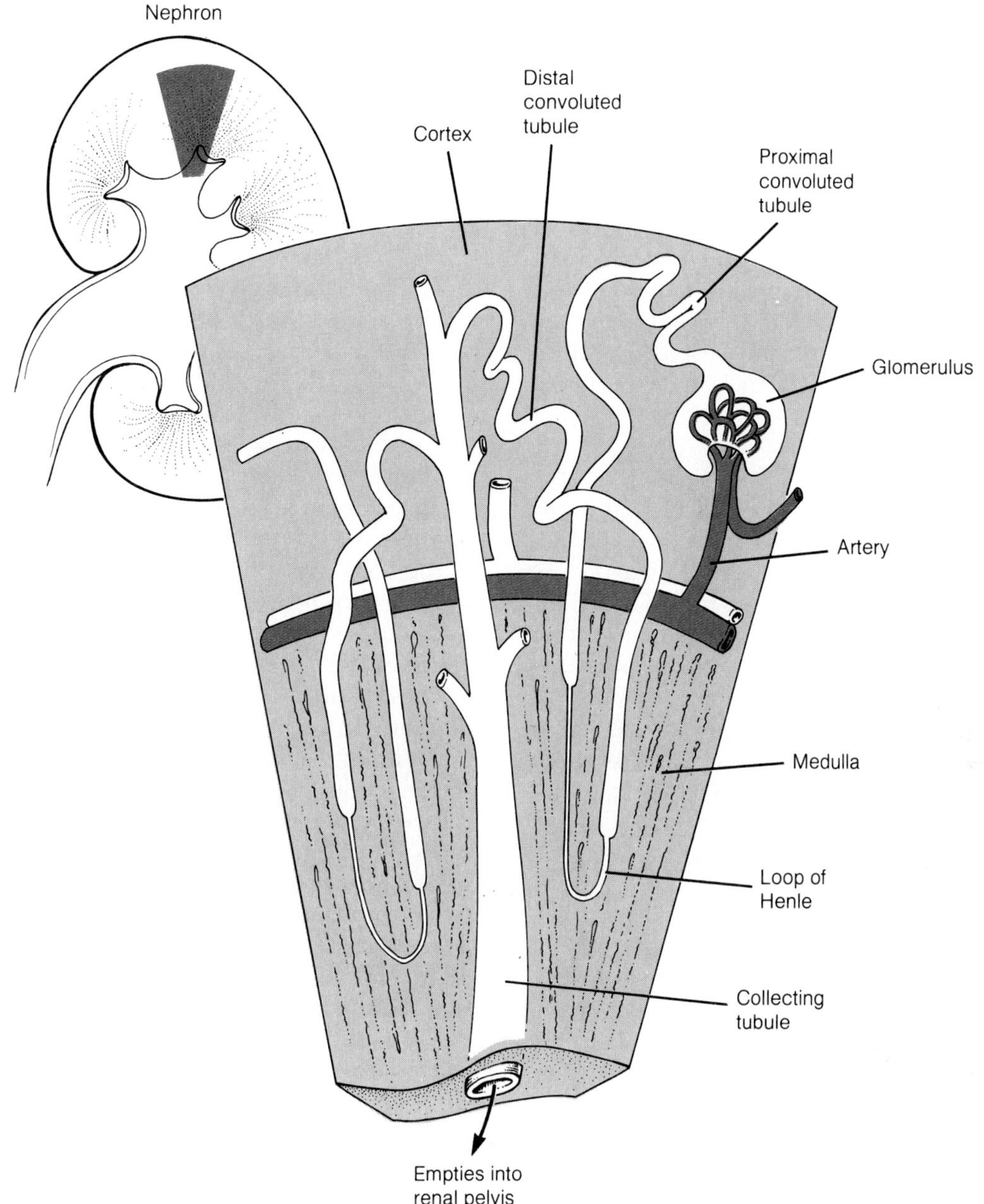

FIG. 10-1 The nephron—functional unit of the kidney.

nephritis. In other cases it may diffusely involve entire nephrons or nephron segments, disrupting normal function. Nephrotic lesions develop, leading to progressive chronic renal failure. Nutritional disturbances in the metabolism of protein, electrolytes, and water follow.

Infection and Obstruction

Bacterial infection of the urinary tract may range from occasional mild, uncomfortable bladder infections to more involved chronic, recurrent disease and obstruction from kidney stones. This obstruction in the uri-

nephron • A microscopic anatomic and functional unit of the kidney that selectively filters and resorbs essential blood factors, secretes hydrogen ions as needed for maintaining acid-base balance, then resorbs water to protect body fluids, and forms and excretes a concentrated urine for elimination of wastes.

medulla • The central portion of an organ. The renal medulla is the inner part of the kidney, holding the lower parts (loop of Henle and collecting tubule) of the nephron, which are organized grossly into pyramids with glomerular heads of the nephrons in the outer portion (cortex) of the kidney.

nary tract blocks drainage, causing further infection and tissue damage.

Damage from Other Diseases

Circulatory disorders such as prolonged hypertension, which are often associated with the renin-angiotensin-aldosterone mechanism, cause degeneration of the small renal arteries and curtail efficient function.[1,2] A vicious cycle ensues, since the demand on the kidneys in turn causes more hypertension and more damage. Other diseases, such as diabetes and gout, may also damage kidney function.[3,4] In addition, congenital abnormalities of the urinary tract may lead to poor function, infection, or obstruction.

Damage from Other Agents

Environmental agents such as insecticides, solvents, and similar materials are poisons that damage the kidneys.[5] Some drugs may also harm renal tissue.[6]

In the treatment of renal disease, nutritional therapy is based on impaired renal function and resulting clinical symptoms. In this chapter we focus primarily on the more serious degenerative processes of glomerulonephritis, nephrosis, and renal failure. Then we briefly review the more common conditions of obstructive kidney stones and urinary tract infection, or bacteriuria.

Glomerulonephritis

Etiology

Glomerulonephritis is an inflammatory process affecting the glomeruli, the small blood vessels in the head of the nephron. It is most common in its acute form in children 3 to 10 years of age, although 5% or more of the initial attacks occur in adults past age 50. The most common cause is a previous streptococcal infection. It has a more or less sudden onset, a brief course in its acute form, and is usually completely cleared in a year or two. In some cases it progresses to a chronic form, involving an increased amount of renal tissue and eventually requiring **dialysis** and other support treatments.

Immune Complex Disease

Immunologic techniques and electron microscopy have demonstrated the presence of a variety of antigens, antibodies, and complement fractions in this disease process. This knowledge has led the way to a new understanding of the origins and development of glomerular disease. *Antigen* is a term used for a "foreign invader" to the body that excites a response from the body's defense system to prevent its potentially harmful effects. An *antibody* is a substance produced by the body to ward off or neutralize the effect of the antigen. In glomerular disease the antigens are usually substances attacking the body from the outside: bacteria, viruses, and chemicals, including antibiotics and other drugs. Various factors determine the response to the invader. These include the origin, quantity, and route of entry of the antigen and the duration of its exposure to the body. The strength of the immune response to the antigen depends partly on the severity of the inflammation or the infection it excites and partly on the capacity of the body to respond through its *immunocompetency*. The excess of antigen and antibodies produced leads to the formation of *antigen-antibody complexes* in the circulation, which become trapped in the glomeruli as they are filtered through the nephron capillaries made permeable by the action of vasoactive amines. This antigen-antibody complex binds components of **complement,** a complex series of enzymatic proteins in the blood that serve as part of the body's immune system. The activated complement in turn provides active chemical factors that attract leukocytes, or white blood cells, whose lysosomal enzymes incite the resulting injury to the glomerulus.

These antigen-antibody complexes appear as lumpy deposits between the epithelial cells of the nephron capsule and the basement membrane of the glomeruli. As lesions develop, *fibrinogen* leaks into Bowman's capsule, with subsequent development of epithelial "crescents" in the space at the cupped interior of the capsule. These crescents then form scar tissue and obstruct the circulation through the glomerulus. Fatty degeneration and necrosis of the conjoined tubules follow, and ultimate destruction of the nephron results. The net result, if the disease becomes progressive, is a reduction in the number of functioning nephrons available in the kidneys.[7]

Clinical Symptoms

Classic symptoms of glomerulonephritis include gross **hematuria** and **proteinuria.** Varying degrees of edema may occur with shortness of breath as a result of sodium and water retention and circulatory congestion. Moderate **tachycardia** and mild or sharp elevation of blood pressure may occur. The patient generally is anorectic, which contributes to feeding problems. If the disease progresses to renal insufficiency, **oliguria** or **anuria** occurs, which signals development of acute renal failure.

Nutritional Therapy

In uncomplicated cases the general treatment is symptomatic and designed to provide optimal nutritional support. In short-term acute cases in children, pediatricians generally favor overall optimal nutrition with adequate protein, unless symptoms of oliguria or anuria develop. These complications usually last no more than 2 or 3 days and are managed by conservative treatment. Salt is usually not restricted unless complications of edema, hypertension, or oliguria become dangerous. Thus in most patients with acute uncomplicated glomerulonephritis, especially children with poststreptococcal glomerulonephritis, dietary modifications are not crucial. The main treatment centers on bed rest and antibiotic drug therapy. As a rule, the fluid intake is adjusted to output, including losses from vomiting or diarrhea.

If the disease process advances, however, more specific nutritional therapy measures are indicated. The nutrient factors most involved are protein, carbohydrates, sodium, potassium, and water.

Protein

If the **blood urea nitrogen (BUN)** is elevated and oliguria is present, dietary protein must be restricted. Usually the diet contains 0.5 g of protein/kg of ideal body weight. Some patients may use 1 g/kg as long as renal function is adequate to maintain a normal BUN level.

Carbohydrates

Carbohydrates should be given liberally to provide sufficient kcalories for energy needs. This also reduces the catabolism of protein and prevents starvation ketosis.

Sodium

The restriction of sodium varies with the degree of oliguria. If renal function is impaired, sodium is restricted to 500 to 1000 mg/day. As recovery occurs, sodium intake may be increased.

Potassium

With severe oliguria, renal clearance of potassium is impaired and potassium intoxication may occur, requiring dialysis. Thus potassium intake is monitored according to disease progression.

Water

Fluids are restricted in keeping with the ability of the kidney to excrete urine. If restriction is not indicated, fluids may be consumed as desired.

Nephrotic Syndrome

Etiology

Nephrotic syndrome, or **nephrosis,** is characterized by a group of symptoms resulting from kidney tissue damage and impaired nephric function. The most evident symptoms are massive *edema* and *proteinuria.* This condition may be caused by progressive glomerulonephritis. It may be associated with other diseases such as diabetes or with connective tissue disorders **(collagen disease).** It may result from drug reactions, from exposure to heavy metals, or even from a reaction to toxic venom following a bee sting.

The primary degenerative lesion is in the capillary basement membrane of the glomerulus, which permits the escape of large amounts of protein into the filtrate. The tubular changes that occur are secondary to the high protein concentration in the filtrate, with some protein uptake from the tubule lumen.

Clinical Symptoms

The cardinal symptom of massive edema is apparent. Ascites is common, and the abdomen becomes increasingly distended as fluid collects in the serous cavities. Often *striae* (stretch marks) appear on the stretched skin of the extremities.

dialysis • The process of separating crystalloids and colloids in solution by the difference in their rates of diffusion through a semipermeable membrane; crystalloids pass through readily and colloids pass through slowly or not at all.

complement • A complex series of enzymatic proteins occurring in normal serum that interact to combine with and augment (fill out, complete) the antigen-antibody complex of the body's immune system, producing lysis when the antigen is an intact cell; composed of 11 discrete proteins or functioning components activated by the immunoglobulin factors IgG and IgM (see Chapter 13).

hematuria • The abnormal presence of blood in the urine.

proteinuria • The presence of an excess of serum proteins such as albumin in the urine.

tachycardia • Excessively rapid action of the heart; usually applied to a heart rate above 100 beats per minute.

oliguria • The secretion of a small amount of urine in relation to fluid intake.

blood urea nitrogen (BUN) • The nitrogen component of urea in the blood; a measure of kidney function; elevated levels of BUN indicate a disorder of kidney function.

nephrosis • A nephrotic syndrome caused by degenerative epithelial lesions of the renal tubules of the nephrons, especially the *mesangium,* the thin basement membrane that helps support the capillary loops in a renal glomerulus; marked by edema, albuminuria, and decreased serum albumin.

collagen disease • A disease attacking collagen tissues, the protein substance of the white fibers (collagenous fibers) of skin, tendon, bone, cartilage, and other connective tissues; any of a group of diseases that are clinically distinct but have in common widespread pathologic changes in the connective tissue, such as rheumatoid arthritis, lupus erythematosus, scleroderma, and rheumatic fever.

The massive edema is largely caused by the gross loss of protein in the urine, some 4 to 10 g/24 hours or more. This means that the plasma protein is also greatly reduced. The albumin fraction, which is largely responsible for maintaining the capillary fluid shift mechanism and thus balance between tissue and circulating fluids, is decreased to less than 3 g/dl. The serum lipid levels are elevated, with cholesterol being over 300 mg/dl. Free fat, oval fat bodies, or fatty droplets are found in the urine. Protein losses are also indicated by the findings in the urine of globulins and specialized binding proteins for thyroid and iron, the loss of which sometimes produces signs of hypothyroidism and anemia. As the serum protein losses continue, tissue proteins are broken down and general malnutrition ensues. Fatty tissue changes in the liver and general sodium retention further contribute to the edema. The severe ascites and *pedal edema* mask the gross tissue wasting.

Nutritional Therapy

Nutritional therapy is directed toward the control of the major symptoms, edema and malnutrition.

Protein

In the past the standard recommendation for patients with nephrotic syndrome was a high-protein diet, sometimes as high as 3 to 4 g/kg body weight/day to restore the serum protein pool and prevent malnutrition. However, evidence has grown that high-protein diets may actually accelerate loss of renal function.[8-10] These studies indicate that patients on the standard high-protein diet had increased albumin excretion and lower serum albumin concentration than those on the lower-protein diet. However, although albumin synthesis was less on the lower-protein diet, it was offset by reduced protein losses in albuminuria and albumin catabolism, and no change occurred in the glomerular filtration rate.[11] Because of the increasing concern of investigators and clinicians that high-protein diets may accelerate progression of renal disease, patients with nephrotic syndrome are now being individually treated with a moderately restricted diet with protein intakes of 0.6 to 0.8 g/kg body weight/day (the adult RDA is 0.8 g/kg/day), plus 1.0 g/day of high biologic protein for each gram of urinary protein lost daily.[9,11]

Kcalories

Sufficient kcalories must always be provided to ensure protein use for tissue synthesis. High daily intakes of 35 to 60 kcal/kg of ideal body weight, depending on the patient's weight, are recommended. Since appetite is usually poor, much encouragement and support are needed. The food must be as appetizing as possible and in the form most easily tolerated.

Sodium

With diuretic drugs to help reduce the edema, moderate sodium restriction in the diet supports this tissue fluid management. Usually a 500- to 1000-mg sodium diet is sufficient to help initiate **diuresis.**

The dietary management is similar to that given for hepatitis, with the additional need for sodium restriction. Potassium restriction is not necessary. Iron and vitamin supplements may be helpful.

Acute Renal Failure

Acute renal failure signals sudden shutdown of renal function following metabolic insult or traumatic injury to normal kidneys. The situation is often life-threatening and is a medical emergency in which the clinical nutritionist and the nurse play important supportive roles.

Etiology

Severe Injury

Severe traumatic injury that causes widespread tissue destruction, such as extensive burns or crushing injuries, may lead to acute renal failure. In other instances the injury may result from traumatic shock, such as that following surgery on the abdominal aorta.

Infectious Diseases

In other cases the acute renal failure may be brought on by widespread infection such as peritonitis.

Toxic Agents

In some individuals, renal failure is caused by environmental agents such as carbon tetrachloride or poisonous mushrooms. In allergic or sensitive individuals, certain drugs such as penicillin may induce immunologic reactions that lead to renal failure.

Clinical Symptoms

The major clinical symptom of acute renal failure is *oliguria,* which is diminished urine output that may be precipitated by the underlying tissue problems that characterize acute renal failure. Usually tubular blockage is caused by cellular debris from tissue trauma or urinary failure with backup retention of filtrate materials. Vasomotor constriction of the afferent arterioles, as may occur in surgical shock, may result. Such a condition is called *vasomotor nephropathy* and is brought on by the reduced renal cortical blood flow. This lack of blood supply causes *ischemia* similar to that in a heart attack when the blood flow to the heart muscle is impeded.

Oliguria

Diminished urinary output is a cardinal symptom, often with proteinuria or hematuria accompanying the small output. Water balance becomes a crucial factor. The course of the disease is usually divided into an oliguric phase followed by a diuretic phase. The urinary output during the oliguric phase varies from as little as 20 to 200 ml/day.

Anorexia, Nausea, and Lethargy

During the initial phase of acute renal failure, the patient may be lethargic and anorectic and may suffer nausea and vomiting. Blood pressure elevation and signs of **uremia** may be present. Oral intake is usually difficult during this period.

Increasing Serum Urea Nitrogen and Creatinine Levels

During this initial catabolic period the serum urea nitrogen (SUN) level increases along with the creatinine level, which results from tissue breakdown of body muscle mass.[12] Blood potassium, phosphate, and sulfate levels also increase, and sodium, calcium, and bicarbonate levels decrease.

General Medical Management

Usually after initial conservative medical therapy, recovery occurs in a few days to 6 weeks. However, in more complicated cases in which the oliguria continues 4 to 5 days, more aggressive therapy, including **hemodialysis** and total parenteral nutrition (TPN), is used.

Nutritional Therapy

Oliguric Phase

The goals of initial nutritional therapy are to support overall medical management. These include reestablishing fluid and electrolyte balance, stopping the catabolic response, supporting tissue healing, and preventing infection. Thus in nutritional therapy the clinical nutritionist and the nurse pay close attention to fluid, electrolyte, and nutrient balances. The major challenge for nutritional therapy is the improvement of nutritional status, especially in patients who have significant catabolism.[12]

Fluids. Fluid intake is usually restricted to a basic allowance of 400 ml/day for the average adult. Any losses of fluids caused by vomiting, sweating, diarrhea, and other routes may be replaced with additional fluid. Allowance must also be made for the "water of combustion" resulting from the metabolism of fat, carbohydrates, and protein and from the catabolism of tissues that provide intracellular water. Children with acute renal failure especially require prompt, carefully monitored fluid resuscitation.[13]

Electrolytes. Electrolyte replacement is provided only for observed deficits. Special caution should be taken to avoid potassium administration, since serum potassium levels are usually elevated following massive tissue destruction.

Diet. Depending on the patient's condition, the nutrient intake may be oral or intravenous. In either case *no protein should be given* in this acute phase to limit nitrogen sources and potassium, phosphate, and sulfate levels. Carbohydrate intake should be increased to provide kcalories for energy demands of the illness and to prevent ketoacidosis and further protein catabolism. A daily intake of 100 to 200 g or more is indicated. Additional kcalories may be obtained from fat, either through oral feedings or lipid emulsions in intravenous feedings. Peripheral vein feeding of a 20% to 50% glucose solution may be administered continuously over 24 hours. B-complex vitamins and vitamin C should be provided to support the needed energy metabolism and tissue healing. If the patient is undergoing dialysis, TPN may be used as a feeding method (Chapter 4). In these cases a mixture of essential amino acids and nonessential amino acids, especially those that are partly synthesized in the kidney, supplemented by glucose and lipid emulsions is used to prevent excessive catabolism of tissue and to support healing and recovery of renal function.[12,14]

Monitoring. Daily records of fluid intake and output, as well as of weight, are essential to monitor fluid balance and tissue catabolism. Daily monitoring of serum electrolytes, particularly potassium, and creatinine is necessary.

Diuretic Phase

After successful initial therapy a diuretic phase follows. This represents the improved renal function and ability to excrete collections of the excess water and electrolytes that have gathered during the oliguric phase. At this time the fluid and dietary intake may be increased as the diuresis progresses until a normal intake is reached. However, protein should continue to be restricted until the BUN and serum creatinine levels decline toward normal. If the diuresis is accompanied by retention of sodium, dietary sodium must be restricted accordingly. Sufficient quantities of water and glucose also are needed to correct **hypernatremia.**

hemodialysis • The removal of certain elements from the blood according to their rates of diffusion through a semipermeable membrane, for example, by a hemodialysis machine.

hypernatremia • Excessive levels of sodium in the blood.

Aging Western Kidney

TO PROBE FURTHER

Renal disease typically follows a progressive downhill course. Why should this be? The work of Brenner's group at Harvard indicates that the stage may well have been set in our distant evolutionary past as an adaptation of the kidney to meet the nitrogenous excretion needs of our hunter-scavenger, meat-eating ancestors.

Because our ancestors were carnivores, their protein intake was transient and intermittent; they could only eat after a successful hunting expedition. Thus at these times of surfeit a large number of extra nephrons had to be available to meet their needs for the prompt excretion of waste products, largely urea, and the conservation of fluid and electrolytes until the next meal became available. They achieved this metabolic task mainly by *hyperfiltration* through increased use of their many extra superficial glomeruli, largely in the outer part (cortex) of the kidney, which normally maintains a resting state. It was only in the past 500 to 10,000 years, when population groups developed agriculture and herding, that a more continuous food intake pattern became possible. Now in many Western countries the adult diet averages approximately 3000 kcal and more than 100 g of protein, largely meat, *daily*.

Thus the answers to our initial questions—Why do we have far more nephrons than we seem to need? Why do we begin losing some of these nephrons through a "normal aging process" of glomerular sclerosis after age 30? Why is renal disease so inexorably progressive?—lie in a fundamental mismatch between the evolutionary design of our kidneys and the functional burden we place on them by our modern eating habits. Our sustained excessive protein levels in the blood, along with other solutes, impose demands for sustained increases in renal blood flow and glomerular filtration rates. This requires that our reserve glomeruli of the outer renal cortex be in more or less continuous use and predisposes even healthy persons to the observed progressive glomerular sclerosis over time, with deterioration of normal kidney function. In health this deterioration poses no problem because we have so many extra nephrons. But when renal disease occurs, the burden is compounded. The disease accelerates the deterioration process and makes coping impossible. The downhill course inevitably ensues. The aging and vulnerable kidney of people living in the Western countries thus seems to be related inevitably to our lifetime of large protein meals.

REFERENCES

Brenner BM et al: Dietary protein intake and the progressive nature of kidney disease, *N Engl J Med* 307(11):652, 1982.

Klahr S et al: The progression of renal disease, *N Engl J Med* 318(25):1657, 1988.

Mitch WE et al: *The progressive nature of renal disease,* New York, 1986, Churchill Livingstone.

With the skilled care of a trained team consisting of a physician, nutritionist, and nurse, the patient is supported until spontaneous healing occurs. After recovery, there is usually little residual impairment of renal function.

Chronic Renal Failure

Etiology

In the course of chronic renal failure the progressive degenerative changes in renal tissue bring increased depression of all renal functions.[7] Few functioning nephrons remain, and these gradually deteriorate (see *To Probe Further,* above). The symptom complex of advanced renal insufficiency is commonly though imprecisely called by its old term *uremia.*

Chronic renal insufficiency may result from a variety of diseases that involve the nephrons: (1) primary glomerular disease such as immune complex glomerulonephritis; (2) metabolic diseases with renal involvement such as diabetes mellitus, especially insulin-dependent diabetes mellitus; (3) exposure to toxic substances; (4) infections; (5) renal vascular disease; (6) renal tubular disease; (7) chronic pyelonephritis; and (8) congenital abnormalities of both kidneys. Depending on the nature of the predisposing renal disease, scarring of renal tissue is extensive and distorts the kidney structure and brings vascular changes from the prolonged hypertension involved.

Clinical Symptoms

Clinical symptoms result from the progressive loss of nephrons and the consequent decreased renal blood flow and glomerular filtration. As the nephrons are lost, the remaining nephrons have a decreasing ability to maintain body water balance, concentration of solutes in body fluids (osmolality), and electrolyte and acid-base balance. This continuing loss of nephrons brings many metabolic insults.

Water Balance

The increased load of solutes causes an osmotic diuresis. Increasingly the kidney cannot excrete a normal concentrated urine; dehydration follows and may become critical. On the other hand, water intoxication may occur if fluid intake is excessive.

Electrolyte Balance

A number of imbalances among the electrolytes result from the decreasing nephron function. The following are examples of the electrolytes affected:

1. *Sodium.* With the osmotic diuresis, sodium loss contributes to a decreasing extracellular fluid volume. As the plasma volume decreases, renal filtration declines further, worsening the renal failure. In this state the kidney cannot respond appropriately to maintain sodium balance. Any sudden increase in sodium intake cannot be excreted readily, causing increasing edema to follow.
2. *Potassium.* The balance of potassium usually is not impaired until the oliguria becomes severe or acidosis is increased. Hyperkalemia indicates severe advanced insufficiency.
3. *Phosphate, sulfate, and organic acids.* With reduced nephron function, reduced filtration and excretion of phosphate, sulfate, and organic acids caused by the metabolism of food occurs. Thus these anions become concentrated in body fluids, with subsequent displacement of bicarbonate ions. This imbalance contributes to the metabolic acidosis.
4. *Calcium and phosphate.* In health the normal levels of serum calcium and phosphorus are maintained in a direct relationship between the two elements. In chronic renal failure the metabolism of calcium and phosphorus is greatly disturbed as a consequence of renal tissue loss. Two metabolic functions of the kidney, the activation of vitamin D to its hormone form and the action of the parathyroid hormone to control serum calcium and phosphorus levels, cannot proceed at normal levels. The impaired vitamin D metabolism results in a bone disease called **osteodystrophy.** This disturbance brings bone pain, various bone deformities, an awkward gait, and impaired growth in children. Calcification of soft tissues may also result, further hindering renal function. These metabolic impairments interfere with normal controls of the serum calcium and serum phosphorus relationship, causing *hyperphosphatemia* and *hypocalcemia.*

Nitrogen Retention

The amounts of nitrogenous metabolites such as urea and creatinine are elevated with increasing loss of nephron function. The urea load results from dietary protein metabolism, and the creatinine load results from increasing catabolism of muscle mass.

Anemia

Another function of the normal kidney is participation in the production of red blood cells. The kidney mediates this production through release of an enzyme called *renal erythropoietic factor.* This enzyme acts on one of the plasma proteins, a globulin, to split away the glycoprotein molecule *erythropoietin.* Erythropoietin in turn circulates briefly for about 1 day in the blood and acts on the bone marrow to stimulate production of the red blood cells. The damaged kidney cannot accomplish this task, and depressed red blood cell production results. The red cells that are produced survive a shorter time but have a usual size and hemoglobin content.

Hypertension

As the blood flow to renal tissue is increasingly impaired, the resulting ischemia brings increasing hypertension through the close relationship of the nephrons to the renin-angiotensin mechanism. Hypertension in turn causes cardiovascular damage and further deterioration of the kidney.

Laboratory Findings

The major characteristic finding is **azotemia,** with elevated BUN, serum creatinine, and serum uric acid levels. Anemia and metabolic acidosis are evident.

Other Signs and Symptoms

The increasing loss of renal function brings progressive weakness, shortness of breath, general lethargy, and fatigue. Thirst, anorexia, weight loss, and general gastrointestinal irritability with diarrhea or vomiting result. The increasing capillary fragility causes skin, nose, oral, and gastrointestinal bleeding. The nervous system involvement results in muscular twitching, burning sensations in the extremities, or uremic convulsions. Cheyne-Stokes respiration (an irregular, cyclic type of breathing) signals acidosis. Ulceration of the mouth, persistent bad or metallic taste, and fetid breath are present. Malnutrition increases vulnerability to infection. Aching and pain in bones and joints continues as evidence of the osteodystrophy.

Nutritional Therapy

Treatment Goals

The variables of treatment center primarily on protein, sodium, potassium, phosphate, and water, with attention to adequate nonprotein kcalories. Levels of

osteodystrophy • A bone disease resulting from defective bone formation. The general term *dystrophy* applies to any disorder arising from faulty nutrition.

azotemia • An excess of urea or other nitrogenous substances in the blood.

each nutrient need to be individually adjusted according to the progression of illness, the type of treatment being used, and the patient's response to treatment. In general, however, basic therapy objectives are as follows:

1. Prevent protein catabolism and minimize uremic toxicity
2. Avoid dehydration or overhydration
3. Carefully correct acidosis
4. Correct electrolyte depletions and avoid excesses
5. Control fluid and electrolyte losses from vomiting and diarrhea
6. Maintain optimal nutritional status
7. Maintain appetite and stimulate morale and a sense of well-being
8. Control complications such as hypertension, bone pain, and central nervous system abnormalities
9. Retard progression of renal failure, thus postponing the ultimate necessity of dialysis

General Measures

Nutritional care plays a major role in many of these general therapy objectives, and the nutritionist becomes an indispensable member of the renal care team. Principles of therapeutic nutrition for chronic renal failure involve variable nutrient adjustments according to individual need.

Protein. The main problem is to provide sufficient protein to prevent tissue protein catabolism but to avoid an excess that elevates urea levels. In general, limitation of protein to 0.5 g/kg body weight/day helps reduce azotemia and hyperkalemia and control acidosis. Protein is usually adjusted according to creatinine clearance at rates below 40 ml/minute. Thereafter the dietary protein must be regulated according to declining renal function (Table 10-1).

TABLE 10–1

Protein and Nitrogen Needs in Chronic Renal Failure

Creatinine clearance (ml/min)	Nitrogen* (g/day)	Protein (g/day)
40 and above	Unrestricted	Unrestricted
10-40	9.6	60
5-20	6.4	40†
2-10	2.5-3.0 (+1.3-2.6)	20 (+ EAA/analogs)†
8 and below	Transplantation Dialysis	
5 and below	Dialysis	

Adapted from Bergstrom J: *Proceedings of the twelfth annual contractors conference,* Artificial kidney—chronic uremia program, National Institutes of Health, Bethesda, Md, NIH Pub No 81-1979, 1981.

*Total protein: 6.25.

†*EAA,* Essential amino acids; alpha-keto-acid and alpha-hydroxy-acid analogs of EAAs.

If the caloric requirements are liberally met, patients may be maintained in nitrogen equilibrium for prolonged periods on as little as 35 to 40 g of protein/day. When the blood urea level is high, however, the protein intake needs to be reduced to 20 g, with only essential amino acids supplied with milk and egg proteins. Thus the patient is not burdened with nonessential amino acids that make demands on the body for disposal of nitrogenous waste products and do little to counteract the tissue protein catabolism. In any event, protein must be closely controlled according to individual need, ranging in quantity from 20 to 70 g and having a high biologic value to supply essential amino acids.

Amino acid supplements. Promising approaches to protein replacement have been developed using mixtures of essential amino acids or of amino acid precursors such as alpha-keto-acid and alpha-hydroxy-acid analogs. Supplements have been developed containing nitrogen-free analogs of the branched-chain amino acids phenylalanine and methionine, which are known to be decarboxylated oxidatively in the liver, plus the remaining amino acids.

Kcalories. Adequate kcalories are mandatory. Carbohydrates and fat must supply sufficient nonprotein kcalories to spare protein for tissue protein synthesis and to supply energy. About 300 to 400 g of carbohydrates supply the average daily need. Sufficient fat, 75 to 90 g, is added to give the patient 2000 to 2500 kcal total daily. Patients are encouraged to consume all the carbohydrates and fats they can, since the end products of their metabolism, carbon dioxide and water, do not impose a burden on the progressive renal failure. If the kcalorie intake is inadequate, endogenous protein tissue catabolism to supply energy only further aggravates the existing renal failure.

Water. Total fluid intake must be guarded to avoid water intoxication from overloading or dehydration from too little water. The capacity of the damaged kidney to handle water is limited, and in many cases solids are excreted better with a controlled amount of water. In general with predialysis patients the fluid intake should be sufficient for urine volume. Sometimes the obligatory water loss may be high because of the large solute load in sodium and urea that must be excreted by an increasingly smaller number of nephrons.

Sodium. The need for sodium intake also varies. Severe restriction and excess are to be avoided. Since sodium is the chief determinant of extracellular fluid osmolarity, the dietary need is closely related to the patient's handling of water. In some cases sodium losses are sufficient to require a high salt intake of 4 to 5 g daily to achieve a balance. Weight loss and decreasing urine volume usually indicate a need for this additional sodium. If hypertension and edema are present, the sodium intake needs to be restricted. Usually, however, the sodium intake varies between 500 and 2000 mg.

Potassium. In renal failure the patient's potassium levels may be depressed or elevated. Guided by blood potassium determinations, the clinician adjusts the potassium intake to maintain normal levels. If significant losses of potassium occur with severe vomiting or diarrhea, *careful* supplementation with potassium may be needed. The damaged kidney generally cannot clear potassium adequately. Thus the daily dietary intake is kept at about 1500 mg.

Phosphate and calcium. As indicated, the patient with advanced renal disease exhibits hyperphosphatemia and hypocalcemia. These abnormal serum levels result from the secondary **hyperparathyroidism** in the damaged kidney function. Phosphate intake should therefore be restricted to slow down or prevent this developing imbalance, which leads to the complicating bone disease osteodystrophy. This restriction of phosphate should be started early, before symptoms of bone pain or deformity develop. Clinical studies of patients with early renal failure have indicated that a moderate dietary restriction of protein and phosphorus is an effective regimen for delaying progression of the functional renal deterioration.[14] To ensure control of phosphate levels, aluminum hydroxide gel may also be used to bind phosphate in the intestinal tract and thus prevent its absorption. A calcium supplement such as calcium lactate tablets relieves the hypocalcemia and its resultant tetany. In some cases calcium carbonate is used because it also buffers the accompanying metabolic acidosis.

Vitamins. In more restricted protein diets supplementary vitamins are usually advisable, since a diet supplying 40 g or less of protein does not contribute the full daily spectrum of all vitamins. A multivitamin tablet or capsule is usually added to the diet of renal patients on protein restriction. An activated form of vitamin D_3, 1-alpha-25-dihydroxycholecalciferol, may be used with caution to help correct the bone disease present.

hyperparathyroidism • Abnormally increased activity of the parathyroid gland resulting in excessive secretion of parathyroid hormone, which normally helps regulate serum calcium levels in balance with vitamin D hormone; excess secretion occurs when the serum calcium level falls below normal, as in chronic renal disease or in vitamin D deficiency.

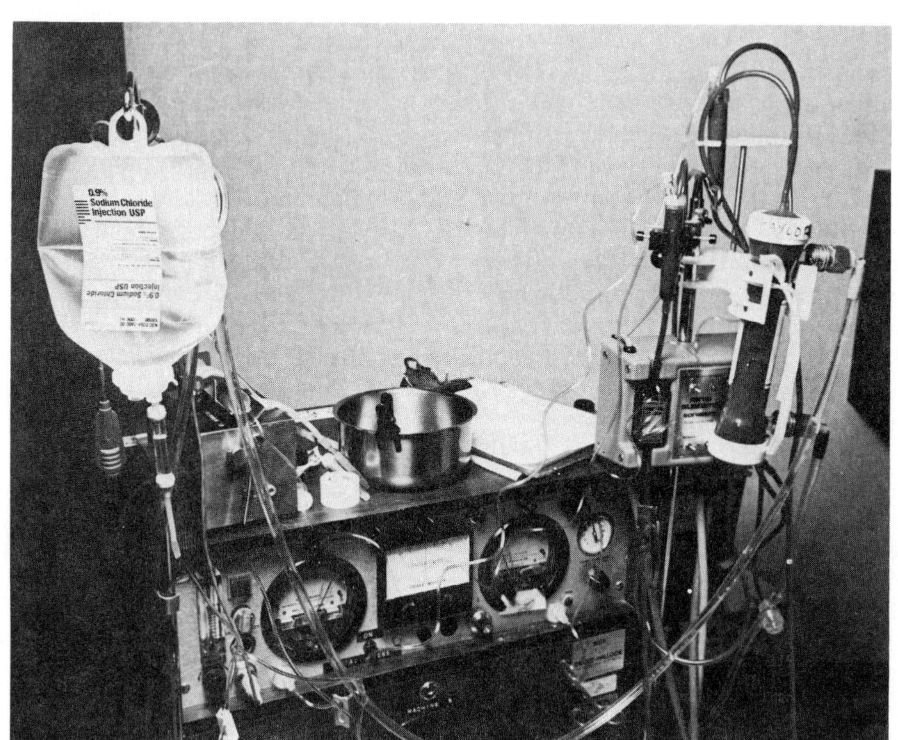

FIG. 10-2 Renal dialysis machine.

Maintenance Kidney Dialysis

With the advent of the artificial kidney machine a number of kidney dialysis centers have been established for the treatment of progressive chronic renal insufficiency (Fig. 10-2). Home units are also available, although considerable skill is required to operate them. These treatments, however, are expensive. The combined costs of the dialysis machine, replacement materials, various drugs, and trained personnel in dialysis centers is from $20,000 to $35,000 per year or more. The home treatment runs between $5,000 and $15,000 per year. Currently much of the cost is now paid under a provision of Medicare that covers chronic kidney disease. Some 18,000 to 20,000 patients receive this needed artificial kidney care.

To prepare the patient for *hemodialysis* therapy, a surgical fistula is made by joining an artery and a vein on the forearm just beneath the skin. After this attachment is healed, a needle is inserted through the healed tissue and connected by tubes to the dialysis machine. A patient with chronic renal failure usually requires two or three treatments per week, each treatment lasting 4 to 8 hours. During each treatment the patient's blood makes a number of round trips through the dialysate solution in the artificial kidney, "laundering" it to maintain normal blood levels of life-sustaining substances that the patient's own kidney can no longer accomplish. With this hemodialysis system, good patient survival rates over the years have been achieved. In selected cases, an alternate form of **peritoneal dialysis** is practical for long-term ambulatory therapy (see the *Clinical Application*, p. 217).

The process of *dialysis* operates on the principles of osmosis and diffusion. These processes occur when two solutions are separated by a porous membrane. The particles in solution and the water molecules pass through the pores in either direction until the two solutions reach equilibrium or equal strength. In the artificial kidney machine are two compartments: one contains blood from the patient carrying all the excess fluids and waste materials, and the other contains the *dialysate,* a solution that may be thought of as a "cleaning fluid." The two compartments are separated by cellophane, a porous material with thousands of holes per square inch. As in normal capillary function the blood cells are too large to pass through the pores in the cellophane. The remaining smaller molecules in the blood, however, pass through and are carried away by the dialysate. If a patient's blood is deficient in certain materials, these may be added to the dialysate. Today these artificial kidney machines maintain thousands of patients, enabling them to lead relatively full, productive lives for many years.

The diet of a patient on kidney dialysis is an important aspect of maintaining biochemical control. Several basic objectives of each individually tailored diet are (1) to maintain protein and kcalorie balance, (2) to prevent dehydration or fluid overload, (3) to maintain normal potassium and sodium blood levels, and (4) to maintain acceptable serum phosphorus and calcium levels. Control of infection is a basic goal. An underlying zinc deficiency, exhibited in impaired taste acuity, is often reported in chronic dialysis patients and improved with a supplement of 25 mg of zinc/day, thus enabling them to eat a better diet.[15]

Protein

For most adult dialysis patients a protein allowance of 1 g/kg lean body weight provides for nutritional needs, maintains positive nitrogen balance, does not produce excessive nitrogenous waste, and replaces the amino acids lost during each dialysis treatment. At least 75% of this daily protein allowance should consist of proteins of high biologic value, such as eggs, meat, fish, and poultry but little if any milk. Milk is restricted because it adds more fluid and has a high content of potassium, sodium, and phosphate.

Kcalories

Carbohydrates are supplied in generous amounts to provide the primary source of needed energy for daily activities and to prevent tissue protein breakdown. Fats are used for another source of energy in varying amounts, depending on blood lipid levels. Individuals on maintenance hemodialysis often have elevated triglyceride levels. The exact cause of these lipid changes is unknown, although a deficiency of *carnitine,* the amino acid that carries free long-chain fatty acids into cell mitochondria, is suspected. A carnitine deficiency may occur because of carnitine losses into the dialysate. Researchers have been able to reduce elevated blood triglyceride levels in hemodialysis patients by giving them carnitine.[16] The usual energy prescription during maintenance hemodialysis is 40 kcal/kg lean body weight. In selecting carbohydrate foods a majority of the kcalories should be supplied by simple carbohydrates, with control of complex carbohydrates. The complex carbohydrates contribute protein of lower biologic quality and should not take up a large amount of the protein allowance.

Water Balance

Fluid is usually limited to 400 or 500 ml, plus an amount equal to urinary output, if any. The total in-

peritoneal dialysis • Dialysis through the peritoneum into and out of the peritoneal cavity.

CLINICAL APPLICATION

Continuous Ambulatory Peritoneal Dialysis: Nutritional Needs of Clients on Portable Dialysis Machines

Persons with end-stage renal disease used to spend up to 18 hours a week on hemodialysis machines in a hospital or dialysis center. Now approximately 2800 Americans undergo dialysis 24 hours a day, 7 days a week, without spending 1 minute in a hospital room.

These individuals use continuous ambulatory peritoneal dialysis (CAPD), a home dialysis process that introduces dialysate directly into the peritoneal cavity, where it is exchanged for fluids that contain the metabolic waste products. This is done by attaching a disposable bag containing the dialysate to a catheter permanently inserted into the peritoneal cavity, waiting 20 to 30 minutes for the solution exchange, then lowering the bag to allow the force of gravity to cause the waste-containing fluid to drain into it. When the bag is empty, it can be folded around the waist or tucked into a pocket, allowing the user mobility.

The exchange takes place by osmosis and diffusion, the rate being determined by the amount of dextrose in the solution. The most common dialysates are 1.5%, 2.5%, or 4.25% dextrose in 1.5 to 2.0 L of solution. Most CAPD users require three to five exchanges each day. They are not only free to move, but with good self-care they are also free from some of the following extensive dietary restrictions placed on hemodialysis patients:

- *Protein and amino acid* losses are usually minimal and easily replaced by diet. High losses were more common in early CAPD systems because of peritonitis, a common problem associated with the need to replace bags frequently.
- *Potassium* requirements depend on the number of solution exchanges that take place each day. The fewer the number of exchanges, the greater the chance of developing high serum potassium levels. Also, patients who stop using CAPD must immediately reduce their potassium intake, since serum levels rise rapidly.
- *Phosphorus*-binding antacids are not needed as much because of improved control of phosphorus blood levels with CAPD use.
- *Sodium* restriction is not necessary. In patients susceptible to hypotension, high-sodium diets have even been recommended.
- *Fluid* restriction is unnecessary, since 2000 to 2200 ml of fluid may be removed with two 1.5% plus two 4.25% dextrose solutions used in one day. Some CAPD users even become dehydrated easily.

CAPD does pose a few nutrition-related problems, mainly because of the amount of dextrose in the dialysate. A study of patients given three 1.5% and two 4.25% dextrose solutions in one day revealed an intake of more than 800 kcal above the energy value of their regular diets. In addition to posing possible weight management problems, the extra dextrose may lead to elevated triglycerides and low density lipoprotein (LDL) levels and depressed levels of protective high density lipoproteins (HDL), thus increasing the risk of coronary heart disease in long-term users.

Nutritionists and nurses who counsel patients being transferred from hemodialysis to the CAPD regimen are faced with a special problem: patients are often reluctant to give up their special diets. To help the individual with end-stage renal disease make the transition to CAPD as trouble-free as possible, you may find it useful to explain clearly some of the possible effects of a restricted diet for persons on CAPD: (1) **hypotension** and dizziness from sodium depletion; (2) nausea, vomiting, muscle weakness, irregular heartbeat, or listlessness from **potassium depletion;** and (3) **dehydration** caused by rapid fluid removal.

You may find it helpful to use the following dietary regimen followed by nutritionists at a number of clinics as a guide for patient counseling:

- Increase protein intake to provide 1.2 to 1.5 g/kg body weight.
- Limit phosphorus intake to 1200 mg/day by restricting phosphorus-rich foods, such as nuts and legumes, to one serving a week; and dairy products and eggs to a half-cup portion or one egg or its equivalent each day.
- Increase potassium intake by eating a wide variety of fruits and vegetables each day.
- Encourage liberal fluid intake to prevent dehydration.
- Avoid sweets and fats to control triglyceride and HDL levels.
- Maintain lean body weight by incorporating the kcalories provided by the dialysate into the total meal plan.

Another important factor to keep in mind is that hemodialysis patients often lose their appetite. Thus the most basic aspect of your efforts to help CAPD clients adjust to this new system is to encourage them to eat. ◆

REFERENCES

Bannister DK et al: Nutritional effects of peritonitis in continuous ambulatory peritoneal dialysis (CAPD) patients, *J Am Diet Assoc* 87(1):53, 1987.

Blumenkrantz MJ et al: Metabolic balance studies and dietary protein requirements in patients undergoing continuous ambulatory peritoneal dialysis, *Kidney Int* 21(6):849, 1982.

Bodnar DM: Rationale for nutritional requirements for patients on continuous ambulatory peritoneal dialysis, *J Am Diet Assoc* 80(3):247, 1982.

take must account for additional fluids in the foods consumed and in water derived from the catabolism or oxidation of foods, as well as fecal fluid losses. Even with this restriction a mild fluid retention occurs between treatments, with a daily weight gain in that period of about 0.45 kg (1 lb).

Potassium

Potassium restriction is imperative to prevent hyperkalemia, which may become a problem. Potassium accumulation easily causes cardiac arrhythmias or cardiac arrest. Therefore a daily dietary restriction of 1500 to 2000 mg is usually followed.

Sodium

Sodium intake is limited to 1000 to 2000 mg daily to control body fluid retention and hypertension. This restriction helps prevent pulmonary edema or congestive heart failure from fluid overload.

Vitamins

During the dialysis treatments, water-soluble vitamins from the blood are lost in the dialysate. A daily supplementation of all the water-soluble vitamins is therefore usually given. However, the fat-soluble vitamins, especially vitamins A and D, may build up, and thus the multivitamin preparations used usually exclude these vitamins.

Peritoneal Dialysis

Indications for Use

An alternate form of dialysis, **peritoneal dialysis,** allows dialysate solutions to flow directly through a catheter port established through the abdominal wall into the abdominal cavity. The presence of this hyperosmolar solution causes waste materials to diffuse across the saclike **peritoneum** lining the abdominal cavity. Then this dialysate collection of waste materials flows back into the dialysate bag for disposal. The peritoneum serves as the filtering mechanism. This procedure is indicated for use in certain cases[17]:

- Short periods in acute renal failure
- In combination with conservative management of chronic renal disease for short periods during a brief infection
- Preoperative maintenance of a patient awaiting a kidney transplant
- Maintenance of a predialysis patient waiting to enter a chronic hemodialysis program
- Longer-term home care of chronic renal disease, especially for elderly persons and children and for persons with diabetes or systemic diseases

Types of Procedures and Dietary Management

Peritoneal dialysis may be given in any one of three procedures: (1) *intermittent peritoneal dialysis (IPD)* that is given usually at night, 10 hours each time, four times a week; (2) *continuous ambulatory peritoneal dialysis (CAPD)* in which a dialysate solution in a plastic pouch is infused and drained by gravity each day, five times at 4-hour intervals; and (3) *continuous cyclic peritoneal dialysis (CCPD)* in which three or four machine-delivered exchanges are given at night, about 3 hours each, leaving about 2 L of dialysate solution in the peritoneal cavity for 12 to 15 hours during the day.

Dietary management in each case is based on nutritional requirements and protein intake sufficient to cover any losses, with individual monitoring of need. As an example, details of the management of CAPD are given in the *Clinical Application,* p. 217. Special medical foods designed specifically to provide balanced enteral nutrition for renal disease patients, either orally or by tube-feeding, are available (Ross Laboratories): Suplena, a low-protein feeding for predialysis patients providing 30 g of protein/L; and Nepro, a moderate-protein feeding for dialysis patients providing 70 g of protein/L.

Clearly, all of the dietary factors play a role in the progression of renal disease. Although the relative importance of each factor varies depending on the underlying cause of the disease and the stage and mechanism of its progression, findings such as those reviewed by Ahmed do indicate that nutritional therapy helps decrease the rate of renal function deterioration in patients with chronic renal disease.[18] For many appropriate candidates, this delayed progression provides the needed time and nutritional status to prepare for the alternative decision of possible kidney transplant.

Kidney Transplant

Kidney transplantation has become a widely accepted treatment of chronic renal failure, with approximately 9000 kidney transplants being performed each year in the United States and about 14,000 persons awaiting transplants.[19] Previously the transplantation of kidneys from one person to another had been limited because of the rejection of the foreign organ by the recipient in many cases, except when the donor and the recipient were identical twins. Continued experience with various immunosuppressive drugs improved this situation. When the donor is a parent or an HLA *(human lymphocyte antigen complex)*-matched sibling, recipient survival with the first transplant still functional after 2 years has been 80% or greater.

Drug therapy is currently providing even more success with organ transplants. The drug *cyclosporine* helps suppress those cells in the recipient's immune system that attack the transplanted kidney, but it does not suppress those immune cells that a recipient needs to fight off infections. Thus cyclosporine not only supports the success of the transplant but also helps cut

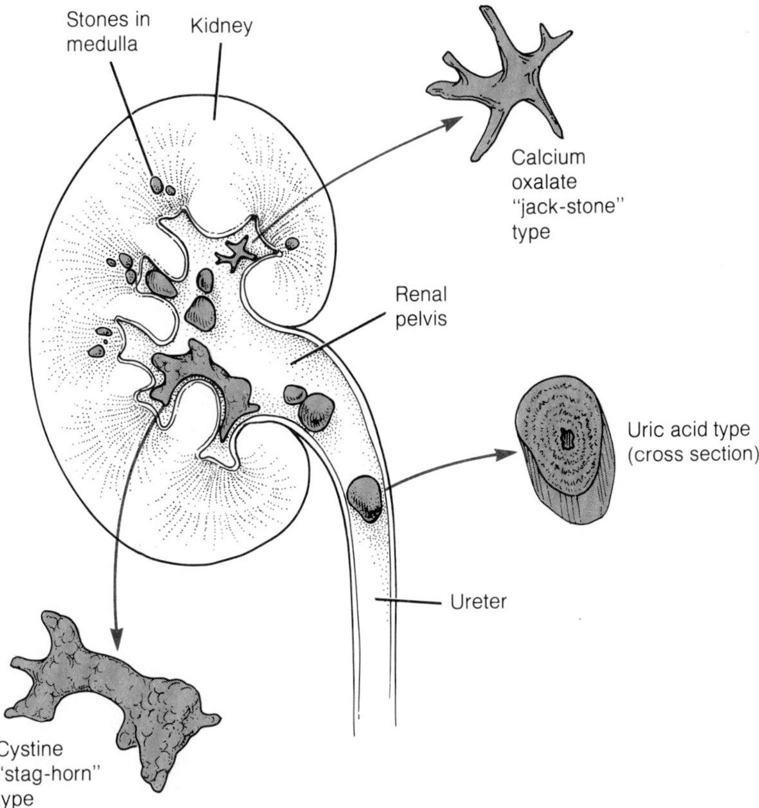

FIG. 10-3 Renal calculuses: stones in kidney, pelvis, and ureter.

down on infections. As a bonus, because of fewer rejections and infections, patients taking cyclosporine have had to pay less in extended hospital care costs. Nutritional support for the surgical procedures is an important adjunct to therapy. In general this care is complex and individual and best provided by a dietitian specialist in renal disease. Consideration is given to the optimal protein and energy intake, with relative restriction of simple sugars, total fat, cholesterol, and saturated fat.[20] Successful kidney transplantations have given new life to many patients with chronic renal failure. The quality of this extended life becomes a part of patient and family counseling (see *Issues and Answers*, p. 226).

Renal Calculuses

Etiology

Since the days of Hippocrates, kidney stone disease has appeared in medical documents. It continues to be a prevalent health problem. In North America, some 5% to 10% of the population suffers from kidney stones, 70% to 80% of which are composed of calcium oxalate with or without phosphate.[21] Kidney stone disease is chronic and recurrent.

Although the basic cause of renal calculuses is unknown, many factors contribute directly or indirectly to their formation. These factors relate to the nature of the urine itself or to the conditions of the urinary tract environment. The major stones formed, according to the particular concentration of urinary constituents, are calcium stones, struvite stones, uric acid stones, and cystine stones (Fig. 10-3).

Calcium Stones

Most renal stones are composed of calcium compounds, usually calcium oxalate or calcium oxalate mixed with calcium phosphate.[22] The normal daily excretion of calcium for persons on a moderate calcium diet of about 400 mg is 100 to 175 mg. With an average adult intake of 800 mg or more of calcium, homeostatic mechanisms regulate the amount of cal-

> **peritoneum** • A strong smooth surface; a serous membrane lining the abdominal and pelvic walls and undersurface of the diaphragm, forming a sac enclosing the body's vital visceral organs within the peritoneal cavity.

TABLE 10–2

Food Sources of Oxalates

Fruits	Vegetables	Nuts	Beverages	Other
Berries, all	Baked beans	Almonds	Chocolate	Grits
Currants	Beans, green and wax	Cashews	Cocoa	Tofu
Concord grapes	Beets	Peanuts	Draft beer	Soy products
Figs	Beet greens	Peanut butter	Tea	Wheat germ
Fruit cocktail	Celery			
Plums	Chard, Swiss			
Rhubarb	Chives			
Tangerines	Collards			
	Eggplant			
	Endive			
	Kale			
	Leeks			
	Mustard greens			
	Okra			
	Peppers, green			
	Rutabagas			
	Spinach			
	Squash, summer			
	Sweet potatoes			
	Tomatoes			
	Tomato soup			
	Vegetable soup			

cium excretion. In some persons, however, hyperexcretion of calcium occurs. This is called *idiopathic hypercalciuria* and accounts for 30% to 40% of the stone formers. In this condition the urine produced is supersaturated with crystalloid elements. Apparently in persons who form stones, which is a familial tendency, the normal urine substances that prevent agglomeration of these crystals are lacking. Excessive urinary calcium stones may result from the following:

1. *Excess calcium intake.* Prolonged use of large amounts of milk, alkali therapy for peptic ulcer, and use of a hard water supply contribute to excess calcium loads.
2. *Hypervitaminosis D.* Excess vitamin D may cause increased calcium absorption from the intestine as well as increased calcium withdrawal from bone.
3. *Prolonged immobilization.* Body casting or immobilization in illness or disability may lead to withdrawal of bone calcium and increased urine concentration.
4. *Hyperparathyroidism.* Primary hyperparathyroidism causes excess calcium excretion. About two thirds of the persons with this endocrine disorder have renal stones, but this disorder accounts for only about 5% of the total of persons with calcium stones.
5. *Renal tubular acidosis.* Excess excretion of calcium is caused by defective ammonia formation.
6. *Idiopathic calciuria.* Some persons, even those on a low-calcium diet, for unknown reasons may excrete as much as 500 mg of calcium daily.
7. *Oxalate.* Because of a metabolic error in handling oxalates, about half of the calcium stones are compounds with these materials. Oxalates occur naturally in only a few food sources (Table 10-2).
8. *Animal protein.* A diet high in animal protein, for example, the typical American diet, has been linked to increased excretions of calcium, oxalate, and urate.[23] A vegetarian-type diet has been recommended as a wise choice for stone-forming patients.
9. *Dietary fiber.* Added dietary fiber has been found to reduce risk factors for stone formation, especially calcium stones.[21]

Struvite Stones

Next to calcium stones in frequency are **struvite stones** composed of a simple compound, magnesium ammonium phosphate ($MgNH_4PO_4$). These are often called infection stones because they are associated with urinary tract infections. The offending organism in the infection is *Proteus mirabilis.* This is a urea-splitting bacterium that contains urease, an enzyme that hydrolyzes urea to ammonia. Thus the urinary pH becomes alkaline, and in the ammonia-rich environment struvite precipitates and forms large, staghorn calculuses. Surgical removal is usually indicated.

Uric Acid Stones

Excess uric acid excretion may be caused by a derangement in the intermediary metabolism of purines, as occurs in gout. It may also result from rapid tissue breakdown in the wasting diseases.

Cystine Stones

A hereditary metabolic defect in renal tubular resorption of the amino acid cystine causes this substance to accumulate in the urine, a condition called cystinuria. Since this disorder is of genetic origin, early onset age and a positive family history characterize patients with it. Formation of cystine stones is one of the most common metabolic disorders associated with renal stones before puberty.

Urinary Tract Infections

The physical changes in the urine and the organic stone matrix provide urinary tract conditions conducive to the formation of renal stones.

Physical Changes in the Urine

Physical changes in the urine that predispose susceptible persons to stone formation include the following:

1. *Urine concentration.* The concentration of urine may result from a lower water intake or from excess water loss, as in prolonged sweating, fever, vomiting, or diarrhea.
2. *Urinary pH.* Changes in urinary pH from its mean 5.85 to 6.0 may be influenced by diet or altered by the ingestion of acid or alkali medications.

Organic Stone Matrix

Formation of an organic stone matrix provides the core or nucleus (nidus), which acts as a seed crystal for precipitation. This organic matrix is a mucoprotein-carbohydrate complex in which galactose and hexosamine are the principal carbohydrates. Some possible sources of these organic materials include (1) bacterial masses from recurrent urinary infections; (2) renal epithelial tissue of the urinary tract that has sloughed off, possibly because of vitamin A deficiency; and (3) calcified plaques (Randall's plaques) formed beneath the renal epithelium in hypercalcinuria. Irritation and ulceration of overlying tissue cause the plaques to slough off into the collecting tubules.

Clinical Symptoms

Severe pain and numerous symptoms may result, with general weakness and sometimes fever. Laboratory examination of urine and chemical analysis of any stone that is passed help determine treatment.

Treatment

Fluid Intake

A large fluid intake produces a more dilute urine and is a hallmark of therapy. The dilute urine helps prevent concentration of stone constituents.

Urinary pH

An attempt to control the solubility factor is made by changing the urinary pH to an increased acidity or alkalinity, depending on the chemical composition of the stone formed. An exception is calcium oxalate stones, since the solubility of calcium oxalate in urine is not pH-dependent. Conversely, however, calcium phosphate is soluble in an acid urine.

Stone Composition

When possible, dietary constituents of the stone are controlled to reduce the amount of substance available for precipitation.

Binding Agents

Materials that bind the stone elements and prevent their absorption in the intestine cause fecal excretion. For example, sodium phytate is used to bind calcium, and aluminum gels are used to bind phosphate. Glycine and calcium have similar effects on oxalates.

Nutritional Therapy

Nutritional therapy is directly related to the stone chemistry.

Calcium Stones

For the patient with calcium stones a low-calcium diet of about 400 mg daily is usually given. This amount is half of an average adult intake of 800 mg. This lower level is achieved mainly by removing milk and dairy products. Other calcium food sources affected are leafy vegetables and whole grains. If the stone is calcium phosphate, phosphorous foods are also reduced. This is also accomplished mainly by removal of milk and dairy products. Sometimes a test diet of 200 mg of calcium may be used to rule out hyperparathyroidism as an etiologic factor.

Since calcium stones have an alkaline chemistry, an acid ash diet may also be used to create a urinary environment less conducive to precipitation of the basic stone elements. The classification of food groups is based on the pH of the metabolic ash produced (Table 10-3). An acid ash diet increases the amount of meat, grains, eggs, and cheese. It limits the amounts of vegetables, milk, and fruits. An alkaline ash diet outlines the opposite use of these foods.

The use of cranberry juice has been promoted to assist in the acidification of urine. Some past studies have reported finding significant decreases in mean urinary pH with the use of cranberry juice. However,

TABLE 10-3

Acid and Alkaline Ash Food Groups

Acid ash	Alkaline ash	Neutral
Meat	Milk	Beverages (coffee, tea)
Whole grains	Vegetables	
Eggs	Fruits (except cranberries, prunes, plums)	
Cheese		
Cranberries		
Prunes		
Plums		

TABLE 10-4

Summary of Dietary Principles in Renal Stone Disease

Stone chemistry	Nutrient modification	Dietary ash (urinary pH)
Calcium	Low calcium (400 mg)	Acid ash
Phosphate	Low phosphorus (1000-1200 mg)	
Oxalate	Low oxalate	
Struvite ($MgNH_4PO_4$)	Low phosphorus (1000-1200 mg) (associated with urinary infections)	Acid ash
Uric acid	Low purine	Alkaline ash
Cystine	Low methionine	Alkaline ash

the concentrations and volumes of juice used in such studies are not practical for clinical use. The commercially prepared cranberry juices on the consumer market are too dilute to be effective, since they contain only about 26% cranberry juice. Thus an inordinate volume is required to achieve any consistent effectiveness as a urinary acidifying agent. Instead most physicians rely on drugs to effect a sustained acidification of urinary pH.

Calcium oxalate stones, resulting from *hyperoxaluria,* are treated by avoiding foods high in oxalates (Table 10-2). Persons with calcium oxalate stones should avoid taking vitamin C supplements because about one half of ingested ascorbate is converted to oxalic acid. However, this is not always the case, and more studies of patients with renal calculuses are needed before precise conclusions can be reached.

Uric Acid Stones

Uric acid stones comprise about 4% of the total incidence of renal calculuses. Since uric acid is a metabolic product of purines, dietary control of this precursor is indicated. Purines are found in active tissue such as glandular meat, other lean meat, meat extractives, and in lesser amounts in plant sources such as whole grains and legumes. An effort to produce an alkaline ash to increase the urinary pH is indicated.

Cystine Stones

About 1% of the total stones produced are cystine, since their formation is a relatively rare genetic disease. Cystine is a nonessential amino acid produced from the essential amino acid methionine; therefore a diet low in methionine is initiated. This diet is used with high fluid intake and alkaline diet therapy.

The nutritional therapy principles in renal stone disease are outlined in Table 10-4. Dietary guides for each of these kidney stone conditions are provided in Appendix W.

Urinary Tract Infection

The term *urinary tract infection (UTI)* refers to a wide variety of clinical infections in which a significant number of microorganisms are present in any portion of the urinary tract.[24] A most common form is **cystitis,** an inflammation of the bladder prevalent in young women. At least 20% of women experience a UTI during their lifetime, the vast majority of which are cases of uncomplicated cystitis.[25] The condition is called recurrent UTI if three or more bouts are experienced in a year.

Etiology

The majority of cases of UTI are caused by aerobic members of the fecal flora, especially *Escherichia coli.* The presence of these organisms in the urine is termed *bacteriuria.* When urine is produced by the normal kidney, it is sterile and remains so as it travels to the bladder. In UTI, however, the normal urethra has microbial flora, so that any voided urine in normal persons contains many bacteria. Bacteriuria is said to be present when the quantity of organisms is more than 100,000 bacteria/ml of urine. The female anatomy is more conducive to entry of these bacteria into the urinary tract. Recurrent cystitis occurs mostly in young and otherwise healthy women who have infections that usually correspond with sexual activity and who are diaphragm users. In most cases simply having the diaphragm refitted to a smaller size or changing to another birth control method solves the problem.

Treatment

Antibiotic treatment in UTI has now been cut back a great deal. Clinical experience indicates that a single dose of antibiotic is just as effective as the usual 7- to 10-day course treatment in 90% of all women who have uncomplicated cystitis. General nutritional measures include acidifying the urine by taking vitamin C, since cranberry juice is not effective, and drinking plenty of fluids to produce a dilute urine. Control of UTI is an important measure, since it is a risk factor in stone formation.

To Sum Up

Through its unique functional units, the nephrons, the kidneys act as a filtration system, resorbing substances the body needs, secreting additional ions to maintain a proper pH balance in the blood, and excreting unnecessary materials in the urine.

Renal function may be impaired by a variety of conditions. These include inflammatory and degenerative disease; infection and obstruction; chronic diseases (hypertension, diabetes mellitus, and gout); environmental agents (insecticides, solvents, and toxic substances) and some medications; and trauma. Some clinical conditions affecting the structure and function of the kidney include glomerulonephritis, nephrotic syndrome, acute and chronic renal failure, renal calculuses, and urinary tract infections. In many cases except nephrotic syndrome, dietary protein may need to be reduced as part of the nutritional care plan. Water, electrolyte, and kcalorie intakes are also closely monitored to match individual needs.

Chronic kidney disease at its end stage, end-stage renal disease (ESRD), is treated by *dialysis, peritoneal dialysis,* or *kidney transplant.* Dialysis patients must be monitored closely for protein, water, and electrolyte balance. Nutritional support of transplant patients is needed primarily as support for the surgical procedure; a normal diet is often tolerated well after surgery and convalescence.

Most serious renal diseases have predisposing factors: *streptococcal* infection often precedes glomerulonephritis in children, *progressive glomerulonephritis* may lead to nephrotic syndrome, and untreated *urinary tract infections* may lead to renal calculuses. The Western diet is suspect as a predisposing factor in the development of *chronic renal failure.* Excess protein intake may overtax human nephrons, which were not originally designed to handle a steady diet of protein-rich foods.

QUESTIONS FOR REVIEW

1. For each of the following conditions, outline the nutritional components of therapy, explaining the impact of each on kidney function: glomerulonephritis, nephrotic syndrome, acute renal failure, and chronic renal failure.
2. Identify four clinical conditions that impair renal function. Give an example of each, describing its effect on various structures in the kidney.
3. List the nutritional factors that must be monitored in individuals undergoing hemodialysis.
4. Outline the medical and nutritional therapy used for patients with various types of renal calculuses, including a description of each type of stone and explaining the rationale for each aspect of therapy.
5. For what condition is a urinary tract infection a predisposing factor? What general nutritional principles are recommended in the treatment of such infections?

REFERENCES

1. Weir MR, Wolfsthal SD: Hypertension and the kidney, *Prim Care* 18(3):525, 1991.
2. Guyton AC: Blood pressure control—special role of the kidneys and body fluids, *Science* 252(5014):1813, 1991.
3. Brouhard BH, LaGrone L: Effect of dietary protein restriction on functional renal reserve in diabetic nephropathy, *Am J Med* 89:427, 1990.
4. Baldree LA, Stapleton FB: Uric acid metabolism in children, *Pediatr Clin North Am* 37(2):391, 1990.
5. Abuelo IG: Renal failure caused by chemicals, foods, plants, animal venom, and misuse of drugs: a review, *Arch Intern Med* 150:505, 1990.
6. McDonald BR et al: Acute renal failure associated with the use of intraperitoneal carboplatin: a report of two cases and review of the literature, *Am J Med* 90:386, 1991.
7. Klahr S et al: The progression of renal disease, *N Engl J Med* 318(25):1657, 1988.
8. Kaysen GA et al: Effects of dietary intake on albumin homeostasis in nephrotic patients, *Kidney Int* 29:572, 1986.
9. Coggins CH, Cornell BF: Nutritional management of nephrotic syndrome. In Mitch WE, Klahr S, eds: *Nutrition and the kidney,* Boston, 1988, Little, Brown.
10. Kopple JD: Nutrition, diet and the kidney. In Shils ME, Young VR, eds: *Modern nutrition in health and disease,* ed 7, Philadelphia, 1988, Lea & Febiger.
11. DiChiro J: Can nutritional therapy alter the course of renal disease? *Dietetic Currents* 18(2):1, 1991.
12. Feinstein EI: Total parenteral nutritional support of patients with acute renal failure, *Nutr Clin Prac* 3(1):9, 1988.
13. Feld LG et al: Fluid needs in acute renal failure, *Pediatr Clin North Am* 37(2):337, 1990.
14. Hak LJ, Raasch RH: Use of amino acids in patients with acute renal failure, *Nutr Clin Prac* 3(1):19, 1988.
15. Reid DJ et al: Effects of folate and zinc supplementation on patients undergoing chronic hemodialysis, *J Am Diet Assoc* 92(5):574, 1992.
16. Bartel LL et al: Effects of dialysis on serum carnitine, free fatty acids, and triglyceride levels in man and the rat, *Metabolism* 31(9):944, 1982.
17. Zeman FJ: *Clinical nutrition and dietetics,* ed 2, New York, 1991, Macmillan Publishing.

18. Ahmed FE: Effect of diet on progression of chronic renal disease, *J Am Diet Assoc* 91(10):1266, 1991.
19. Schanbacher B: An overview of development on the field of organ transplantation, *Kidney* 6:4, 1989.
20. Edwards MS, Doster S: Renal transplant diet recommendations: results of a survey of renal dietitians in the United States, *J Am Diet Assoc* 90(6):843, 1990.
21. Firth WA, Norman RW: The effects of modified diets on urinary risk factors for kidney stone disease, *J Can Diet Assoc* 51(3):404, 1990.
22. Metheny N: Renal stones and urinary pH, *Am J Nurs* 82:1372, 1982.
23. Menon M, Krishnan C: Evaluation and medical management of the patient with calcium stone disease, *Urol Clin North Am* 10(4):595, 1983.
24. Sobel JD: Bacterial etiologic agents in the pathogenesis of urinary tract infection, *Med Clin North Am* 75(2):253, 1991.
25. Ronald AR, Pattullo ALS: The natural history of urinary infection in adults, *Med Clin North Am* 75(2):299, 1991.

FURTHER READING

Abuelo IG: Renal failure caused by chemicals, foods, plants, animal venoms, and misuse of drugs, *Arch Intern Med* 150:505, 1990.

This experienced physician provides an excellent overview, complete with many tables of examples, of the many common substances around households and communities that are nephrotoxins and that cause severe kidney damage.

Ahmed FE: Effect of diet on progression of chronic renal disease, *J Am Diet Assoc* 91(10):1266, 1991.

Dr. Ahmed of the Food and Nutrition Board provides a helpful review of the literature concerning the impact of diet on the course of chronic renal disease and how nutritional management is used therapeutically to treat persons with renal insufficiency.

Bellisle F et al: Perceptions of and preferences for sweet taste in uremic children, *J Am Diet Assoc* 90(7):951, 1990.

Reid DJ et al: Effects of folate and zinc supplementation on patients undergoing chronic hemodialysis, *J Am Diet Assoc* 92(5):574, 1992.

These two articles relate problems of zinc metabolism associated with depressed taste acuity in children and adults with renal failure who are undergoing hemodialysis and the value of zinc supplementation to improve taste sensation and consequent food energy intake.

Curtis JA: *The renal patient's guide to good eating: a cookbook for patients by a patient,* Springfield, Ill, 1989, Charles C Thomas.

Gillit D et al: *A clinical guide to nutrition care in end-stage renal disease,* Chicago, 1987, American Dietetic Association.

These two guides by renal patients and renal dietitians who care for them provide a great amount of practical and professional guidance to help persons with chronic renal disease eat wisely but well.

CASE STUDY

Patient with Chronic Renal Failure

Aaron Steinberg is 36 years old, married, and works as a city planner for a large municipal government. He cited a recent history of nausea, anorexia, hematuria, and swollen ankles during an initial physical examination. His wife reported that he had been tiring more easily than usual during the past year. A history of previous illnesses proved negative, except for a severe case of influenza with sore throat 10 years before during an epidemic when he was stationed overseas with the Army. Tests were ordered, and the patient was advised to return in a week for review of the test results and sooner if his symptoms changed.

Mr. Steinberg did return, with additional symptoms of headaches and occasional blurred vision. At that time his blood pressure was 160/98, his temperature was 37.5° C (99.6° F), and he had lost 4 kg (8¾ lb). The laboratory tests showed albumin and red and white blood cells in the urine, with an elevated BUN; a test for phenolsulfonphthalein indicated a reduced filtration rate. The diagnosis was chronic renal failure.

The physician discussed the diagnosis and its serious prognosis with Mr. and Mrs. Steinberg, giving them the advantages and disadvantages of hemodialysis and kidney transplantation. Antihypertensive medication was prescribed along with other drugs to minimize discomfort.

During the following weeks Mr. Steinberg continued to lose weight, had increasing joint pain, and became anemic. He found it increasingly difficult to maintain his hectic schedule of frequent meetings, conferences, and public speeches because of gastrointestinal bleeding, increasing nausea, and occasional muscle spasms. Small mouth sores made eating difficult.

Finally the Steinbergs informed the physician of their decision to accept the kidney transplant as a means of controlling the disease process. They were referred to the clinical nutritionist for renal dietary counseling to control protein, sodium, potassium, phosphate, and fluids, as well as to ensure adequate kcalorie intake. After discussing these needs for nutritional maintenance before surgery, the nutritionist helped them develop a meal plan based on Mr. Steinberg's food preferences. Food selection and preparation were discussed in detail, with many ideas for building in as much variety and taste appeal as possible.

The Steinbergs' follow-up with the food plan was excellent. One month later the laboratory values were almost normal, blood pressures averaged 140/88, the headaches and blurred vision had virtually disappeared, and Mr. Steinberg had gained 3.2 kg (7 lb) of his lost weight. The nutrient supplements, including the amino acid analogs, were taken each day as instructed.

Fortunately a kidney donor was soon found, and with the aid of drug control of immune responses, the transplantation was apparently a success. Mr. Steinberg convalesced well at home, kept all follow-up visits with the health care team, and has continued to be asymptomatic 1 year following surgery.

Questions for Analysis

1. Identify a metabolic imbalance caused by renal failure that may account for each symptom presented by Mr. Steinberg.
2. What are the objectives in care of renal failure such as what Mr. Steinberg was experiencing?
3. What factors affect the amount of protein needed by persons with chronic renal failure? What amounts are usually used? Why? What are the amino acid analogs used with the low-protein diet and why are they used?
4. What factors affect the amount of sodium needed by persons with chronic renal failure? How much is usually recommended?
5. Why is it important to control potassium levels? How much is recommended? What clinical signs presented by Mr. Steinberg may indicate that he had not been getting enough potassium?
6. Why is control of phosphate important in the diet for chronic renal failure? What additional means may be used to control it?
7. What factors affect fluid balance in chronic renal failure? How much is usually allowed?
8. What is the basic principle of the low-protein dietary regimen? List and explain each factor in the diet and potential problems in its management.
9. Outline a general teaching plan you would use to instruct the Steinbergs about the preoperative and postoperative dietary needs.

Renal Disease: Technology versus the Quality of Life

Imagine spending up to 18 hours a week hooked up to a machine to which you literally owe your life. Imagine having a 40% chance of never being able to work outside the home again and leading a life of poverty and restricted mobility all because of that machine.

This is probably hard for most of us to conceive. Yet for approximately 55,000 Americans on maintenance dialysis, and the number of patients with end-stage renal disease requiring hemodialysis is increasing, this is the reality of their everyday lives. The medical-nutritional-nursing renal care team must also deal with this reality daily in working with these persons and their families. This sensitivity is especially needed in nutritional counseling and teaching. Food is tied up with so many personal values that when it must be drastically changed, or when choice is gone altogether, it's as if a part of the self has been diminished.

Researchers, physicians, and patients are becoming increasingly concerned with the *quality* of life rather than merely the *length* of life available to the person on dialysis. The only alternative currently available is kidney transplantation. On the surface this method is considered preferable to hemodialysis or even peritoneal dialysis because it frees the individual from any mechanical device. However, researchers are beginning to investigate the quality of life a transplant provides to determine whether either method is preferable to the other.

The first issue of greatest concern is the effect of the treatment on the person's life span. Mortality rates for individuals on dialysis (8% to 15%) are in the same range as for those receiving their first kidney transplant from a parent or sibling (10% to 15%). However, rates among young dialysis patients with no extrarenal disease drop as low as 2%, in contrast with rates that soar to 30% among individuals receiving kidneys from cadavers. Still, some persons believe that the benefits of increased mobility outweigh the drawbacks of a possible reduction in life span.

Life quality measures (sleep habits, food habits, energy level, sexual activity, changes in income and employment, satisfaction with marriage, and so on) in one study were examined among individuals undergoing dialysis or with successful and unsuccessful transplant operations. As expected, subjects who had successful operations reported a near-normal quality of life; they were less tired, were less inconvenienced by frequent medical treatments, and had better incomes or more full-time employment following renal failure than other renal patients.

Also as expected, individuals whose transplant operations were not successful indicated that the quality of their lives was the lowest of all subjects. For example, none of these subjects reported full-time employment since renal failure. They were mainly recipients of kidneys from cadavers; thus this process is assumed to be the least desired of all possible alternatives.

A surprising result of this study was that dialysis patients who never received a transplant thought that the quality of their lives was also near normal. Researchers admit that the reason for this probably includes denial or accommodation. However, they also acknowledge that human response to life experiences is an extremely complex issue, one that is difficult to assess with current "immature" research methods available for evaluating the quality of life in general.

The health care team members responsible for the patient with renal failure may have their own set of parameters for determining the quality of life each mode of treatment may provide. The results of this study suggest that the patient's own evaluation of life may involve factors much more complex than those to which the professional has been exposed. The study serves as a reminder that professionals must be open to the concerns and viewpoints of the individual faced with such major choices in treatment and must relate care planning in all areas to these personal concerns.

REFERENCES

Collins AJ et al: Changing risk factor demographics in end-stage renal disease patients entering hemodialysis and impact on long-term mortality, *Am J Kidney Dis* 15:422, 1990.

Husbye DG et al: Psychosocial, social, and somatic prognostic indicators in old patients undergoing long-term dialysis, *Arch Intern Med* 147:1921, 1987.

Johnson PJ et al: The quality of life of hemodialysis and transplant patients, *Kidney Int* 22(3):286, 1982.

CHAPTER 11

Nutrition and Surgery

CHAPTER OUTLINE

Nutritional Needs of General Surgery Patients
Special Nutritional Needs for Head and Neck Surgery Patients
Special Nutritional Needs for Gastrointestinal Surgery Patients
Special Nutritional Needs for Burn Patients

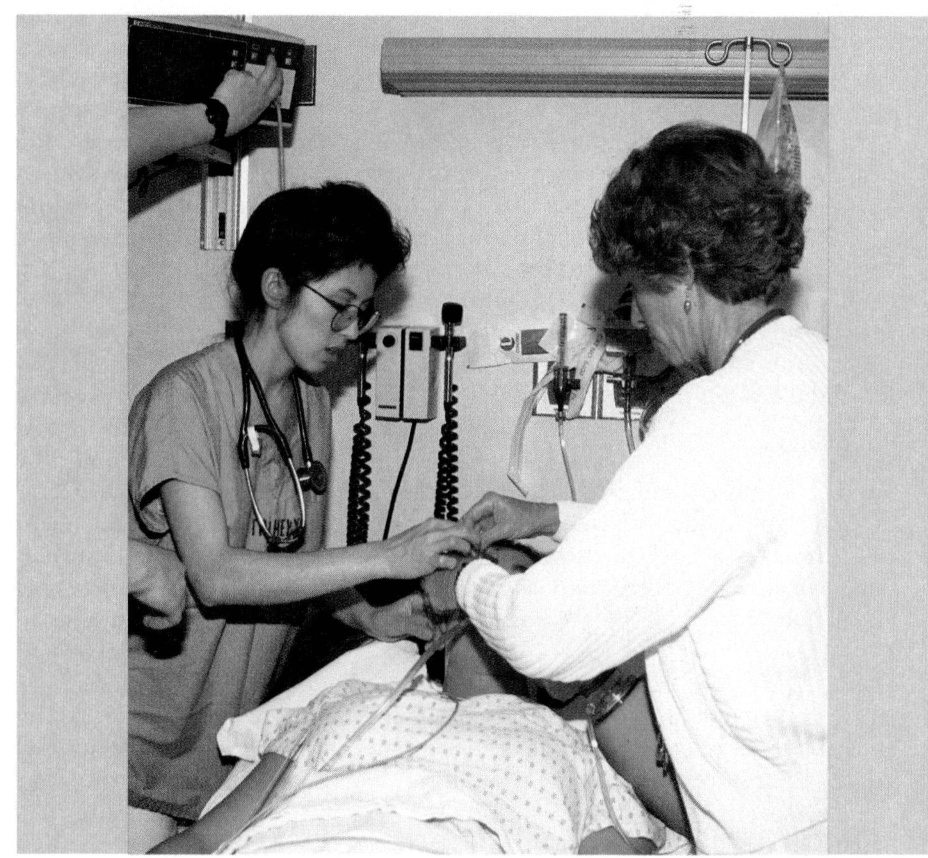

In this chapter we look at the needs of patients undergoing various surgical procedures for treatment of medical problems or injuries. A major focus is on gastrointestinal surgeries, which affect modes of feeding to meet nutritional requirements for healing and must accommodate resulting changes in the normal gastrointestinal tract.

A primary underlying need is the prevention of malnutrition. A large number of the malnourished patients observed in hospitals are surgical patients. Numerous American and European surveys of hos-

pitalized patients indicate that nearly 50% of surgical patients have clinical evidence of protein-energy malnutrition.

In this chapter we see how careful attention to preoperative nutritional preparation, together with vigorous postoperative nutritional support, reduces complications and provides resources for better healing and more rapid recovery.

Nutritional Needs of General Surgery Patients

Preoperative Nutrition

Preoperative malnutrition is often associated with poor postoperative outcome. Thus when surgery is planned, prompt attention to nutritional status is a primary task.[1] Nutritional resources fortify the patient for the demands of surgery. Preparation should correct any nutrient deficiencies and should also provide reserves for the surgery itself and for the immediate postoperative period until feedings are resumed (see the *Clinical Application,* p. 229).

Protein

The most common nutritional deficiency related to surgery is that of protein. Essential tissue and plasma reserves fortify the patient for blood losses during surgery and tissue catabolism in the postoperative period.

Energy

Sufficient kcalories should be provided to build up any weight deficit. Carbohydrates are needed for glycogen stores and to spare protein for tissue synthesis.

Vitamins and Minerals

Normal tissue stores of vitamins are needed for metabolism of carbohydrates and protein. Any deficiency state such as anemia needs to be corrected. Water and electrolyte balance should be maintained; any dehydration, acidosis, or alkalosis should be corrected.

Immediate Preoperative Period

Usually nothing is given by mouth for at least 8 hours before general surgery so that the stomach has no retained food at the time of the operation. In case of emergency surgery, if the patient has recently eaten a meal, gastric suction is used to remove it. Food in the stomach may be vomited and aspirated during surgery or during recovery from anesthesia. Any food present may also increase the possibility of postoperative gastric retention and gastric dilation. It may also interfere with the procedure itself, especially in abdominal surgery. Before abdominal or gastrointestinal surgery a low-residue or residue-free diet may be followed for several days to clear the operative site of any residue. Low-residue, chemically defined formulas, or **elemental formulas,** provide a complete diet in liquid form. Such formulas, if palatable enough, are taken orally in sufficient amounts to restore or maintain nutritional resources; otherwise, they may be fed by tube (see Chapter 3).

Postoperative Nutrition

Healthy body tissues undergo continuous turnover, with small physiologic losses being constantly replenished with nutrients eaten from food. In disease, however, especially surgical disease, losses are greatly increased. Replacement nutrients from food are diminished or even absent for a brief or extended period. Therapeutic nutritional support therefore becomes all the more significant as a means of aiding recovery.

Protein

In the postoperative recovery period, adequate protein intake is a primary therapeutic concern to replace losses and supply increased needs. A catabolic period with progressively increasing protein deficiency is common in surgical patients. Negative nitrogen balances of as much as 20 g/day may occur. This amount of nitrogen loss represents an actual loss of tissue protein of more than 1 lb/day. In addition, plasma protein is lost through hemorrhage, wound bleeding, and **exudates.** Increased metabolic losses result also from extensive tissue inflammation, from infection and trauma, or from immobilization and poor caloric intake. If any degree of prior malnutrition or chronic infection has existed, the patient's protein deficit may become even more severe and cause serious complications. A number of reasons exist for this increased protein demand.

Tissue synthesis in wound healing. Tissue proteins are synthesized only by amino acids brought to the tissue by circulating blood. These necessary amino acids must come from either ingested protein or intravenous feeding. Tissue protein deficiencies are best met by oral feedings whenever possible. When appetite is poor, palatable concentrated liquid drinks or commercial formulas may be useful (see Chapter 3). During early feeding periods or with the extremely malnourished patient, only small amounts of protein foods may be tolerated. However, increased intake is needed as early as possible to achieve the amount of protein required to restore lost protein tissues and to

CLINICAL APPLICATION

Energy and Protein Requirements in General Surgery Patients

General surgery patients have a variety of nutritional needs depending on individual nutritional status. The status dictates the therapy. The following are a few examples.

Adequately nourished preoperative patient. For the patient with energy and nitrogen balance, approximately 40 kcal/kg/day and 1.5 g of protein/kg/day should keep the prospective surgery patient in energy and nitrogen balance.

Adequately nourished postoperative patient. Energy requirements do not increase significantly after surgery (40 kcal/kg/day), but increased nitrogen losses from decreases in protein synthesis increase protein needs to 1.8 to 1.9 g protein/kg/day.

Nutritionally depleted, non-stressed patient. The patient requires repletion of body fat stores and lean body mass. Nutrient needs are similar to those of the adequately nourished postoperative patient, with 40 kcal/kg/day and 1.8 to 1.9 g of protein/kg/day producing moderate gains in fat and protein.

Nutritionally depleted, stressed patient. This patient has depleted energy and protein stores. These losses need to be matched *and* extra protein (2.0 to 2.2 g/kg/day) is necessary for repletion. Part of the kcalorie load (45 kcal/kg/day) should be given as fat. A 50:50 glucose-fat mix is recommended.

Adequately nourished, stressed patient. This patient has the highest requirements for energy (50 kcal/kg/day) and protein (2.5 g/kg/day), although the aim is to prevent loss, not to replenish. Glucose is not utilized sufficiently to provide adequate energy intake, so some of the energy needs to be provided as fat (50:50 glucose-fat mix). ◆

REFERENCES

Hill GL: The perioperative patient. In Kinney JM et al, eds: *Nutrition and metabolism in patient care,* Philadelphia, 1988, WB Saunders.

Hill GL, Church JM: Energy and protein requirements of general surgical patients requiring intravenous nutrition, *Br J Surg* 71:1, 1984.

synthesize new tissue at the wound site. Although tissue protein is broken down more rapidly during stress, it fortunately is also built up more rapidly, provided sufficient amino acids are present to supply the anabolic demand.

Avoidance of shock. Reduced blood volume—hypovolemia—from a loss of plasma proteins and a decrease in circulating red blood cell volume contributes to the potential danger of shock. Protein deficiencies enhance this danger.

Control of edema. When the serum protein level is low, edema develops. This condition is caused by loss of colloidal osmotic pressure to maintain the normal shift of fluid between capillaries and surrounding interstitial tissues. Even before clinical edema is evident, considerable excess fluid may collect in the interstitial spaces and affect heart and lung action. Local edema at the surgical site also delays closure of the wound and hinders the normal healing process.

Bone healing. In orthopedic surgery extensive bone healing is involved. Protein is essential for proper **callus** formation and calcification. A sound protein matrix must be present for the anchoring of mineral matter in bone tissue.

Resistance to infection. Amino acids are necessary constituents of the proteins involved in body defense mechanism: antibodies, special blood cells, hormones, and enzymes. Tissue integrity itself is the first line of defense against infections.

Lipid transport. Proteins are necessary for the transport of lipids in the body. They provide essential material to form lipoproteins, the transport form of fat in the body. Proteins thus protect the liver, a main site of fat metabolism, from damage caused by fatty infiltration.

Multiple clinical problems may easily develop following surgery when protein deficiencies exist. There may be poor wound healing, or **dehiscence;** delayed

elemental formula • A nutritional support formula composed of simple elemental nutrient components that require no further digestive breakdown and are thus readily absorbed.

exudate • Various materials such as cells, cellular debris, and fluids, usually resulting from inflammation, that have escaped from blood vessels and are deposited in or on surface tissues; protein content is high.

callus • Unorganized meshwork of newly grown, woven bone developed on a pattern of original fibrin clot (formed after fracture or surgery) and normally replaced in the healing process by hard adult bone.

dehiscence • A splitting open; the separation of the layers of a surgical wound, partial or superficial or complete, with total disruption requiring resuturing.

healing of fractures; anemia; failure of gastrointestinal stomas to function; depressed pulmonary and cardiac function; reduced resistance to infection; extensive weight loss; liver damage; and increased mortality risks.

Energy

A sufficient caloric intake is essential and often critical to the successful outcome of surgical procedures. Adequate amounts of carbohydrates ensure the use of protein for necessary tissue protein synthesis and supply the energy required for increased metabolic demands. As protein is increased, the total kcalories must be increased as well. About 2800 kcal/day must be provided before protein is used for tissue repair and not diverted to help provide energy. In acute stress, as in extensive surgery or burns, when protein needs may be as high as 200 g/day, 4000 to 6000 kcal may be required. In addition to the protein-sparing action, carbohydrates also help to avoid liver damage from depletion of glycogen reserves. Fat must be adequately but not excessively supplied to maintain body tissue fat reserves.

Fluid

During the postoperative period large fluid losses may occur from vomiting, hemorrhage, exudates, diuresis, fever, sweating, and increased metabolism. Where drainage is involved, still more fluid loss occurs. Table 11-1 indicates the general magnitude of water requirements for surgical patients. Intravenous therapy supplies initial needs, but oral intake should begin as soon as possible. Water intake must be maintained in sufficient quantity, according to individual need, to avoid extremes of dehydration or of water intoxification. Daily weight measurement of the patient provides a guideline for meeting fluid requirements.

TABLE 11–1

Daily Water Requirements of the Surgical Patient

Type of case and fluid needs	Average fluid required (ml)
Uncomplicated cases	
For vaporization	1000-1500
For urine	1000-1500
TOTAL	2000-3000
Complicated cases (sepsis, elevation of temperature, humid weather, renal damage)	
For vaporization	2000-2500
For urine	1000-1500
TOTAL	3000-4000
Seriously ill patients with drainage	
For vaporization	2000
For urine	1000
For replacement of body fluid losses	
Bile drainage	1000
Wangensteen drainage	3000
TOTAL	7000

Vitamins and Minerals

All of the vitamins play important roles in the healing process. Vitamin C especially is imperative for wound healing. It is necessary for the formation of cementing material in the ground substance of connective tissue, in capillary walls, and in the building up of new tissue. Extensive tissue regeneration as in burns or radical surgeries usually requires additional vitamin C supplementation. As kcalorie and protein intake is increased, the B vitamins must also be increased. They provide essential coenzyme factors for protein and energy metabolism. Vitamin K is essential to the blood-clotting mechanism.

Replacing mineral deficiencies and ensuring continued adequacy is essential. In tissue catabolism, potassium and phosphorus are lost. Electrolyte losses, especially sodium and chloride, accompany fluid losses. Iron deficiency anemia may develop from blood loss or from faulty iron absorption.

General Dietary Management

Oral Feeding

Because ordinary postoperative intravenous solutions cannot supply full nutrient needs or compete with oral feedings, the majority of general surgery patients can and should progress to oral feeding as soon as possible to provide adequate nutrition. Routine postoperative intravenous fluids are intended to supply hydration needs and electrolytes, not to sustain nutritional needs. Of a 5% dextrose solution, 1 L contains 50 g of sugar, with an energy value of only 200 kcal. Thus 3 L/day at best supplies only 600 kcal and no protein. The basal energy requirement alone is much more, without taking into consideration the increased metabolic stress demands of surgical illness.

Parenteral Feeding

In cases of major tissue trauma or damage or when a patient is unable to obtain sufficient nutrients orally, parenteral feeding may be needed (see Chapter 4). It provides nutritional support with solutions containing a higher percentage of glucose, as well as amino acids, electrolytes, minerals, and vitamins. Such solutions may be fed for brief periods by peripheral vein feeding or for longer periods or more severe nutritional needs by central vein feeding—total parenteral nutrition (TPN).

Particularly in cases of major surgery, aggressive nutritional support with enteral and parenteral means (see Chapters 3 and 4) is often a primary factor determining the outcome. The nutritional status of the patient is a critical focus in avoiding postoperative complications and improving morbidity and mortality rates. As many as 50% or more of the patients awaiting or recovering from surgery are malnourished.[2] Studies repeatedly show that malnourished patients have higher postoperative morbidity and mortality than well-nourished patients do and that comprehensive nutritional assessment and vigorous therapy support a positive outcome.[1-3] Strong nutritional support is essential for the skilled work of the surgeon to have its best outcome.

Routine Postoperative Diet

Generally as soon as intestinal peristalsis returns, water and clear liquids such as tea, coffee, broth, and juice may be given to help supply important fluids and some sodium and chloride. These initial liquids also help stimulate normal gastrointestinal function and early return to a full diet. Progression to full liquids should soon follow. Milk and milk products, including puddings, cream soups, high-protein beverages, and ice cream, begin to supply vital protein and carbohydrates. Each patient progresses to solid foods in soft to regular diets according to individual tolerances. Oral intake of solid foods should be encouraged and supported as soon as possible to hasten recovery.

Special Nutritional Needs for Head and Neck Surgery Patients

Surgery involving the mouth, throat, or neck requires modification of the manner of feeding, since the patient usually cannot chew or swallow in the normal way.

Oral Liquid Feedings

Concentrated feedings in liquid form need to be planned. These feedings may consist of special enteral formulas with protein hydrolysates or amino acids, with added carbohydrates, fat, vitamins, and minerals (see Chapter 3). Milk-based beverages, soups, fruit juices, or special supplemented formulas supply reinforced oral nourishment and may be given as tolerated.

Tube-Feeding

Patients who are comatose or severely debilitated or who have undergone radical neck or facial surgery may require tube-feeding. New developments in small-bore feeding tubes have made this method of feeding easier. In cases of long-term need, rapid development of sophisticated delivery systems and standardized formulas has made continued home enteral nutrition possible for many patients. These advances are discussed in detail in Chapter 3. Whatever the type of formula or mode of feeding, personal needs require constant sensitive support. Although long-term tube-feeding may well meet physiologic needs for the patient, it also contributes to psychologic stress, so personal support is an important part of patient care planning.

Special Nutritional Needs for Gastrointestinal Surgery Patients

Gastric Resection

Nutritional Problems

A number of nutritional problems may develop following gastric surgery, depending on the type of surgical procedure (Fig. 11-1) and the patient's response. A partial distal gastrectomy may create little postoperative difficulty, but a total gastrectomy, which involves excision of the stomach and joining of the remaining portion of the esophagus to the jejunum *(anastomosis),* involves more problems. This resectioning may produce serious nutritional deficits and thus require careful diet planning. When a vagotomy is also performed, increased gastric fullness and distention occur.[4] The stomach becomes atonic and empties poorly, so that food fermentation follows, producing flatus and diarrhea. After gastric surgery, especially with total gastrectomy, about 50% of the patients fail to regain weight to optimal levels. The nutritional care of patients who have had gastric surgery primarily falls into two periods: the immediate postoperative period and a later period involving "dumping syndrome."

Immediate Postoperative Period

In traditional practice following surgery, frequent, small oral feedings are gradually resumed according to the patient's tolerance. A typical pattern of simple dietary progression may cover about a 2-week period. The basic principles of such general dietary therapy for the postgastrectomy period are (1) size of meals (small and frequent) and (2) type of food (simple, easily digested, mild, and low in bulk). Increasingly, however, surgeons are using recently developed techniques and equipment such as a needle-catheter jejunostomy procedure at the time of the gastric resection to provide earlier nutritional support with an elemental formula.

Later Period: "Dumping Syndrome"

After patients have recovered from surgery and begin to eat food in greater volume and variety, they may experience increasing discomfort following meals. About 10 to 15 minutes after the meal, cramping and a full feeling occur. The pulse is rapid and is accompanied by weakness, cold sweating, and dizziness. Nausea and vomiting frequently follow. Such distressing reactions to food intake increase anxiety, so the person eats less. Weight loss and increasing malnu-

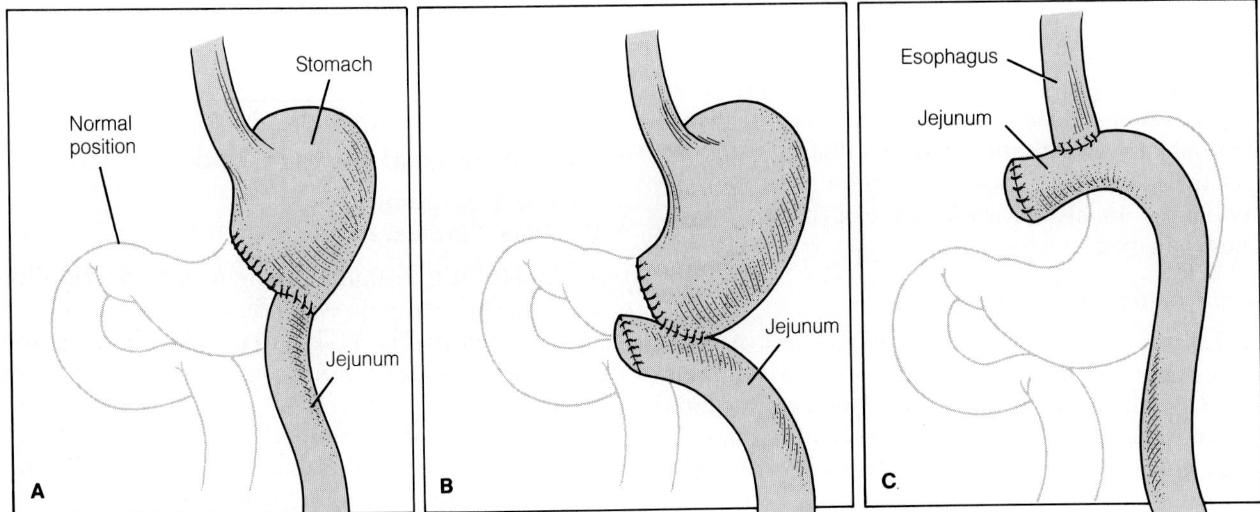

FIG. 11-1 Gastric surgery. **A,** Partial gastrectomy, Billroth 1. **B,** Partial gastrectomy, Billroth 11, **C,** Total gastrectomy.

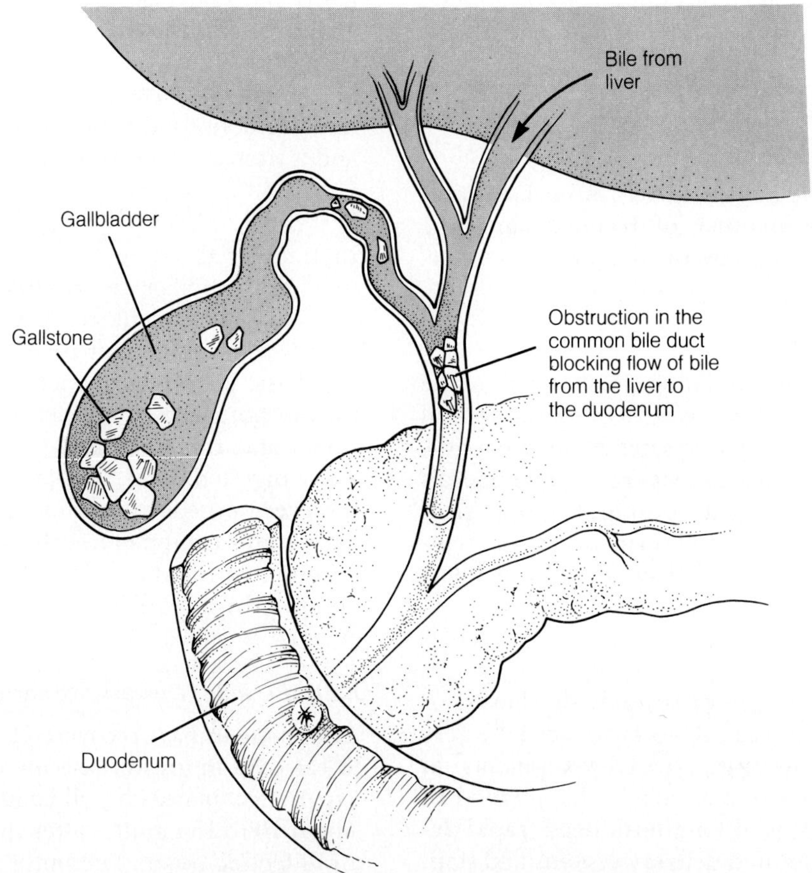

FIG. 11-2 Gallbladder with stones (cholelithiasis).

trition follow. This postgastrectomy complex of symptoms is commonly called the *dumping syndrome*. A more precise term used by some clinicians is *jejunal hyperosmolic syndrome*. This difficulty is more likely to occur in patients who have had a total gastrectomy. The symptoms of shock result when a meal containing a high proportion of readily hydrolyzed carbohydrates rapidly enters the jejunum. This entering food mass is a concentrated hyperosmolar solution in relation to the surrounding extracellular fluid. To achieve osmotic balance, water is drawn from the blood into the intestine, causing a rapid decrease in the vascular fluid compartment. As a result the blood pressure drops, and signs of cardiac insufficiency appear—rapid pulse, sweating, weakness, and tremors. A second sequence of events may follow about 2 hours later. The concentrated solution of simple carbohydrates is rapidly absorbed, causing a **postprandial** rise in the blood glucose. The glucose load then stimulates an overproduction of insulin in response, which in turn leads to an eventual drop in the blood sugar below normal fasting levels. Symptoms of mild hypoglycemia result.

Careful control of the diet often brings dramatic relief of these distressing symptoms and leads to a gradual regaining of lost weight. Carbohydrate intake, especially simple sugars, is kept to a minimum to prevent rapid passage of food and formation of a concentrated hyperosmolar solution. Protein and fat are increased to provide tissue-building material and retard emptying of the food mass into the large intestine. Meals are small, frequent, and dry, with fluid between them. There is less bulk to stimulate motility and less water for rapidly forming nutrient solutions. A summary of this dietary regimen is given in Table 11-2. Lost weight is usually recovered and nutritional deficiencies are corrected.

TABLE 11–2

Diet for Postoperative Gastric Dumping Syndrome

General description

- 5 or 6 small meals daily
- Relatively high fat content to retard passage of food and help maintain weight
- High protein content (meat, egg, cheese) to rebuild tissue and maintain weight
- Relatively low carbohydrate content to prevent rapid passage of quickly used foods
- No milk; no sugar, sweets, or desserts; no alcohol or sweet carbonated beverages
- Liquids between meals only; avoid fluids for at least 1 hour before and after meals
- Relatively low-roughage foods; raw foods as tolerated

Meal pattern

Breakfast
- 2 scrambled eggs with 1 to 2 tbsp butter or margarine
- ½ to 1 slice bread or small serving cereal with butter or margarine
- 2 crisp bacon strips
- 1 serving fruit*

Midmorning sandwich as follows:
- 1 slice bread
- Butter or margarine
- 56 g (2 oz) lean meat

Lunch
- 112 g (4 oz) lean meat with 1 or 2 tbsp butter or margarine
- Green or colored vegetable† with butter or margarine
- ½ to 1 slice bread with butter or margarine
- ½ banana or other solid fruit*

Midafternoon
- Same snack as midmorning

Dinner
- 112 g lean meat with 1 or 2 tbsp butter or margarine
- Green or colored vegetable† with butter or margarine
- ½ to 1 slice bread with butter or margarine (or small serving starchy vegetable substitute)
- 1 serving solid fruit*

Bedtime
- 56 g meat or 2 eggs or 56 g cheese or cottage cheese
- 1 slice bread or 5 crackers
- Butter or margarine

*Fruit choice: applesauce, baked apple, canned fruit (drained), banana, or orange or grapefruit sections

†Vegetable choice: asparagus, spinach, green beans, squash, beets, carrots, or green peas.

Cholecystectomy

For patients suffering from acute *cholecystitis* and *cholelithiasis* (Fig. 11-2), the treatment is usually **cholecystectomy,** surgical removal of the gallbladder.

Nutritional Problems

Following cholecystectomy, control of fat in the diet remains essential to wound healing and comfort. The presence of fat in the duodenum continues to stimulate the *cholecystokinin mechanism,* which causes contraction and pain in the surgical area. A period of adjustment to the more aqueous supply of liver bile for the preparation of fats for digestion also follows.

Dietary Management

Depending on individual tolerance and response, a relatively low-fat diet may need to be followed for a brief time, with moderate fat use thereafter.

Ileostomy and Colostomy

In cases of intestinal lesion or obstruction or when chronic inflammatory bowel disease (see Chapter 6) involves the entire colon, the treatment of choice is usually resection of the intestine to remove the dis-

postprandial • Occurring after a meal.

cholecystectomy • Surgical removal of the gallbladder.

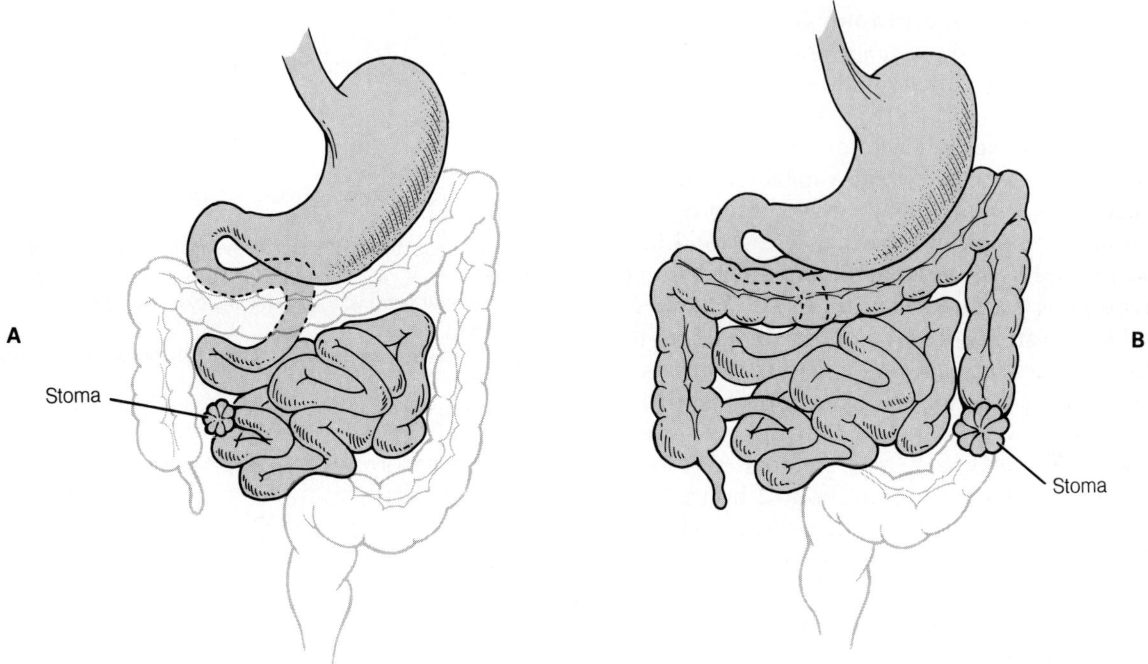

FIG. 11-3 **A,** Ileostomy. **B,** Colostomy.

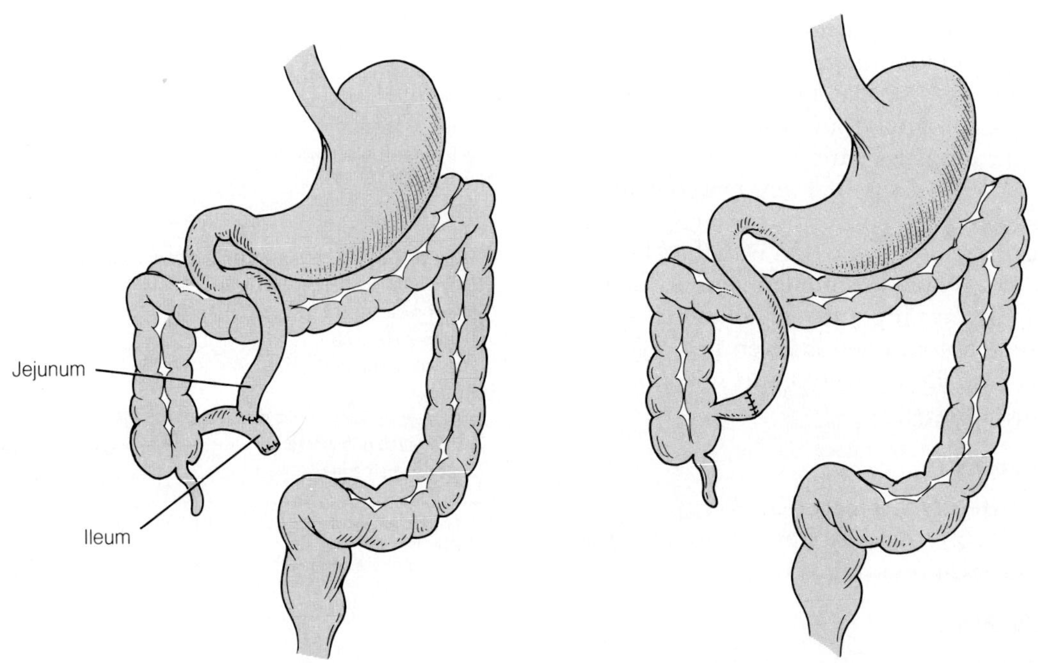

FIG. 11-4 Jejunoileostomy.

eased portion. A temporary or permanent *ileostomy* may also be established. In this procedure the end of the remaining small intestine, the ileum, is attached to an opening in the abdominal wall, and a **stoma** is formed to provide for discharge of the intestinal contents (Fig. 11-3, *A*). In a *colostomy* the left side of the colon is resected, and a stoma is made with the proximal sigmoid, or descending, colon (Fig. 11-3, *B*). In other cases a *jejunoileostomy* may be performed (Fig. 11-4).

Nutritional Problems

An ileostomy and a colostomy produce different problems for nutritional management. The intestinal contents at the point of the ileus are unformed, irritating, and even erosive to the skin. The standard Brooke ileostomy (Fig. 11-3, *A*), with outside pouch or appliance, drains freely and almost continuously.[5] Thus establishment of controlled functioning is difficult. Many patients, however, do develop a reasonable degree of regularity in regard to meals. The modified Koch pouch, an internal abdominal reservoir, has served as an alternative procedure. The surgeon forms a reservoir inside the abdominal cavity out of intestinal tissue and a one-way valve holds the collection until periodically the patient inserts a catheter to empty it.[5,6] This method was the first procedure that eliminated the need for the usual exterior plastic appliance. A recently developed attractive alternate procedure, the J-pouch–anal anastomosis, done in connection with a total colectomy provides an interior ileoanal reservoir and channel for elimination through the regular anal route.[5,7] Establishment of the ileoanal reservoir is done in two stages. First, a total **proctocolectomy** is done, usually indicated by progressive inflammatory bowel disease or colon cancer, and then the ileoanal reservoir is formed from loops of ileum placed in the rectal vault and a temporary loop ileostomy is created to allow healing of the new ileoanal reservoir.[5,7,8] Second, about 3 months later, the loop ileostomy is closed and the new ileoanal reservoir is used for bowel movements. Stool frequency, although greatly reduced to approximately eight bowel movements per day, remains a personal concern.

Dietary Management

The dietary therapy challenge centers on management of bowel output. In general, patients with ostomies should eat regular diets of foods that agree with them, sufficient in quantity and nutritive value to maintain proper weight and energy. Recent study of patients with ileoanal reservoirs has shown that individual control is best achieved by (1) consuming no more than three meals a day, (2) eating the last meal at least 2 hours before bedtime, and (3) evaluating individual bowel pattern to determine how long after a meal one can safely leave home. The basis of the diet is a well-balanced regular plan of only three meals, including a variety of foods and noting individual food tolerances. Despite its drawbacks, the ileoanal reservoir is an increasingly popular surgical alternative to stoma formation.[5] However, a colostomy is the more manageable of the ostomies. The normal contents of the intestine at this point in the colon are solid or semisolid, since more water and electrolytes have been absorbed by the proximal colon. The consistency of the discharge and its less irritating nature create fewer control problems. Often a sigmoid colostomy can be adequately controlled by simple dietary measures and periodic irrigation, so that in many cases no protective appliance is needed. Coping with any of these surgical procedures is difficult at best, however, and patients need much support and practical help and resources for learning about self-care.[5-7]

Rectal Surgery

Nutritional Problems

For a brief period following rectal surgery, *hemorrhoidectomy,* there is pain on elimination, and bowel movement is delayed until initial healing is begun.

Dietary Management

A clear fluid or nonresidue diet is indicated for initial use. The basic foods used are almost completely digested and absorbed in the small intestine, leaving minimal residue for elimination by the colon. An outline of foods used in such a diet is given in Table 11-3. In some cases a nonresidue commercial elemental formula that is completely absorbed may be used for the initial postoperative period.

Special Nutritional Needs for Burn Patients

Nutritional Support Base

A major concern of therapy for the patient with extensive burns is rigorous nutritional support. The clinical dietitian on the burn team is in a most strategic position to assess, plan, implement, and monitor the nutritional care for the burn patient.[9,10] Three important factors guide this important nutritional care: large catabolic losses, essential anabolic healing demands, and deep personal support needs.

Treatment and Prognosis

The plan of care and its outcome depend on several factors: (1) age—elderly persons and very young children are more vulnerable; (2) health condition—the presence of any preexisting condition, such as diabetes, cardiovascular or renal disease, or any other associated injuries complicates care; and (3) burn severity—the location and severity of the burn wounds and the time elapsed before treatment influence the outcome of care.

stoma • The opening established in the abdominal wall, connecting with the ileum or colon, for elimination of intestinal wastes after surgical removal of diseased portions of the intestinal tract.

proctocolectomy • Surgical removal of the rectum and colon.

TABLE 11-3

Nonresidue Diet and Postsurgical Nonresidue Diet

General description—nonresidue diet

- This diet includes only those foods free from fiber, seeds, and skins and with the minimal amount of residue.
- Fruits and vegetables are omitted, except for strained fruit juices.
- Milk is omitted.
- The diet is adequate in protein and kcalories, containing approximately 75 g protein, 110 g fat, 250 g carbohydrates, and 2260 kcal. It is likely to be inadequate in vitamin A, calcium, and riboflavin.
- If patients remain a long time on this diet, supplementary vitamins and minerals should be given.

	Allowed	Not allowed
Beverages	Carbonated beverages, coffee, tea	Milk and milk drinks
Bread	Crackers, melba, or rusks	Whole grain bread
Cereals	Refined, as Cream of Wheat, farina, fine cornmeal, Malt-o-Meal, pablum, rice, strained oatmeal, corn flakes, puffed rice, Rice Krispies	Whole grain and other cereals
Cheese		None allowed
Desserts	Plain cakes and cookies, gelatin desserts, water ices, angel food cake, arrowroot cookies, tapioca puddings made with fruit juice only	Pastries and all others
Eggs	As desired, preferably hard cooked	Fried eggs
Fats	Butter or substitute, small amount cream	None
Fruits	Strained fruit juices	All others
Meat, fish, poultry	Tender beef, chicken, fish, lamb, liver, veal, and crisp bacon	Fried or tough meat, pork
Potatoes or substitute	Only macaroni, noodles, spaghetti, refined rice	Potatoes, corn, hominy, unrefined rice
Soup	Bouillon and broth only	All others
Sweets	Hard candy, fondant, gumdrops, jelly, marshmallows, sugar, syrup, and honey	Other candy, jam, marmalade
Vegetables	Tomato juice	All others
Miscellaneous	Salt	Pepper

General description—postsurgical nonresidue diet

- This diet is slightly higher in residue but has greater variety, including potatoes, white bread products, processed cheese, sauces, desserts made with milk, and cream for coffee and cereal.
- The average daily menu contains 85 g protein and 2300 kcal and is slightly higher in vitamins and minerals.

Selection of foods

To the list add the following:
Cheese: processed cheese, mild cream cheeses
Potatoes: prepared any way, no skin
Bread: any kind without bran, white bread, rolls, pancakes, waffles
Fats: 2 oz of cream or half-and-half per meal, cream sauce, cream gravy
Desserts: all desserts, except those containing fruit and nuts
Condiments: as desired

Degree and Extent of Burns

The depth of the burn wound affects the healing process (Fig. 11-5). Burns are usually classified by degree: (1) first degree—**erythema** with cell necrosis above the basal layer of the epidermis; (2) second degree—erythema and blistering with necrosis within the dermis; and (3) third degree—loss of skin, including the fat layer. First-degree or partial-thickness burns regenerate new skin tissue from the epithelial cells lining the skin appendages, such as hair follicle, sweat glands, and **sebaceous** glands. Second- and third-degree, or full-thickness, burns do not leave sufficient skin for healing purposes; thus they heal only from the skin margins. Small area burns heal in this manner, but extensive full-thickness burns require skin grafting.

The body surface area injured by the burn is a basic factor in calculating nutritional support needs. Generally the burn team estimates body surface area involved by the so-called rule of nines or by a more accurate calculation using prepared charts. Second- and third-degree burns covering 15% to 20% or more of the total body surface, or even 10% in children and elderly persons, usually cause extensive fluid loss and

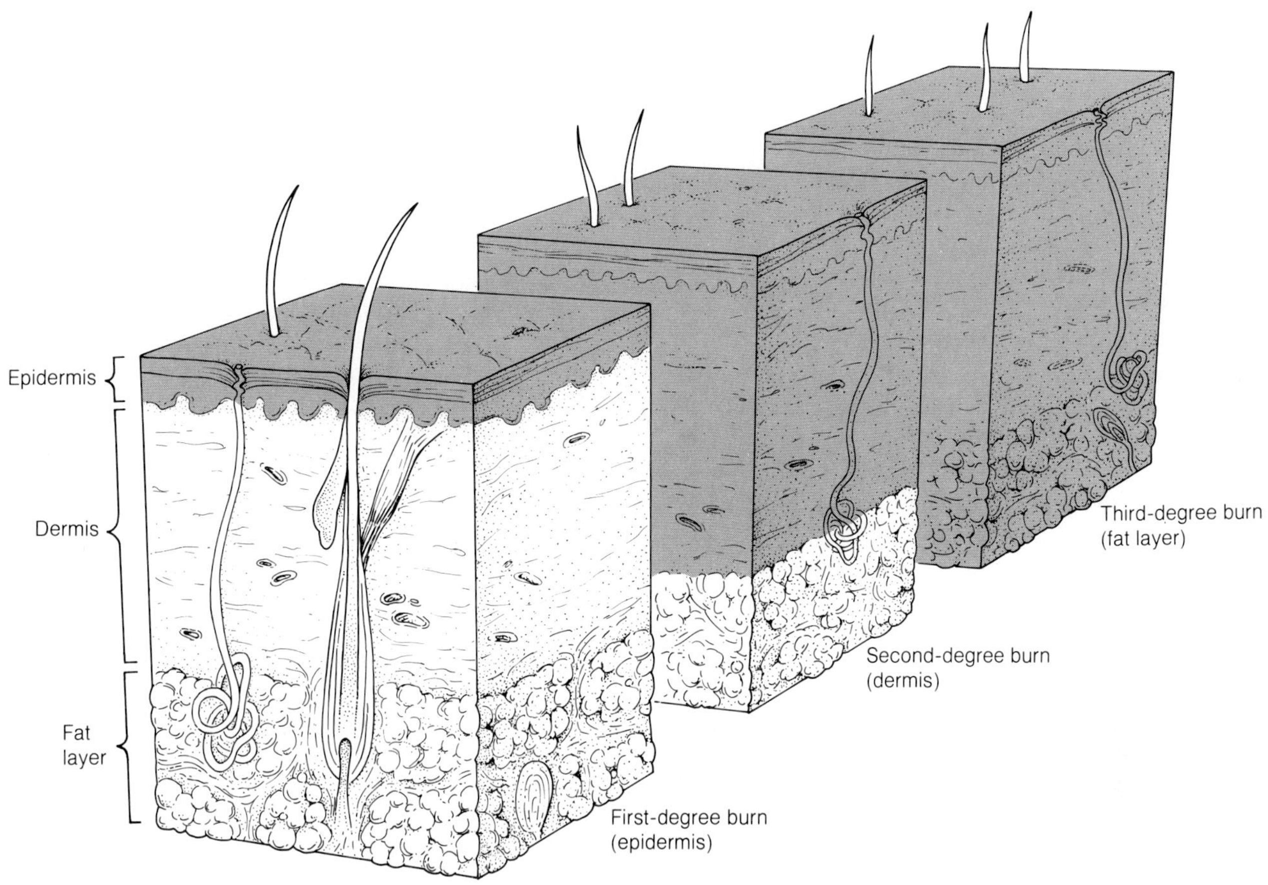

require intravenous fluid therapy. Burns of severe depth covering more than 50% of the body surface area are often fatal, especially in infants and older persons. Patients with major burn injuries are usually transferred immediately to a specialized burn care facility.

Stages of Nutritional Care

The nutritional care of the patient with massive burns is adjusted to individual needs and responses. At all times attention to amino acid needs is vital, in addition to critical fluid-electrolyte balance and energy (kcalorie) support. Generally three stages of care may be identified: the shock, recovery, and reconstruction periods.

"Ebb" or Shock Period

During the first 12 to 24 hours following injury, patients with major burns require rapid replacement of lost fluid and electrolytes. The inflammatory process associated with the injury increases the permeability of the vascular endothelium. Thus during this immediate time a **colloid** solution such as albumin or plasma is not effective, since most of it passes out into the extravascular fluids. Initially, therefore, a balanced salt solution such as **lactated Ringer's solution** is used to correct *hypovolemia* and prevent metabolic acidosis from inadequate tissue perfusion. Individual respon-

erythema • Redness of the skin produced by coagulation of the capillaries; results from a variety of causes; for example, radiant heat or burns.

sebaceous • Subcutaneous glands that secrete the fatty lubricating substance *sebum.*

colloid • Glutinous, gluelike; a dispersion of matter throughout a liquid.

lactated Ringer's solution • Sterile solution of calcium chloride, potassium chloride, sodium chloride, and sodium lactate in water given to replenish fluid and electrolytes; developed by English physiologist Sydney Ringer (1835-1910).

ses govern treatment. Usually vascular endothelial permeability returns to normal after the first day, and colloid solutions are then used to help restore plasma volume. During this initial period of resuscitation and hemodynamic stabilization, no attempt is made to meet nutritional requirements in protein and kcalories. Glucose-free, balanced electrolyte solutions are needed, because infusion of glucose at this time may result in hyperglycemia. Moreover, an adynamic ileus develops after the injury and precludes any use of the gastrointestinal tract (see *To Probe Further*, p. 239).

The full effort of the burn team during these initial hours following injury focuses on counteracting the stress-induced neurohormonal and physiologic responses that accelerate the body's metabolism. Rapid and effective fluid and electrolyte therapy is essential. A rapid series of events follows.

A massive flooding edema occurs at the burn site during the first hours to about the second day. Loss of enveloping skin surface and exposure of extracellular fluids lead to immediate loss of interstitial water and electrolytes, mainly sodium, and large protein depletion. In a homeostatic effort to balance the loss, body water shifts from extracellular spaces in other parts of the body, only to add to the continuous loss at the burn site. As a result of these initial shifts and losses, vascular fluid is decreased in volume and pressure. Hemoconcentration and diminished urine output follow. Then cellular (hypertonic) dehydration occurs as intracellular water is drawn out to balance extracellular fluid losses. Cell potassium is also withdrawn, and circulating serum potassium levels rise. Immediate intravenous fluid therapy replaces water and electrolytes by use of a saline solution such as lactated Ringer's solution. With such immediate care, shock can be prevented. Renal failure is a rare occurrence when resuscitation is started early.

"Flow" or Recovery Period

After about 48 to 72 hours, tissue fluids and electrolytes are gradually resorbed into the general circulation, and excess fluid is excreted. The patient returns to preinjury weight by about the end of the first week. Fluid balance is gradually reestablished, and the pattern of massive tissue loss is reversed. During this time there is a sudden diuresis. A careful check of fluid intake and output is essential, with constant checks for signs of dehydration or overhydration. Also toward the end of the first week, adequate bowel function returns and a vigorous feeding period must ensue. The vastly increased nutritional demands at this time provide the basis for a challenging and critical period of dietary management.

Nutritional demands. At this point, despite the patient's depression and anorexia, life may well depend on rigorous nutritional therapy. Several factors necessitate this increased intake:

1. Tissue destruction. The massive burn injury has brought large losses of protein and electrolytes that must be replaced.
2. Tissue catabolism. Tissue protein breakdown has followed the injury, with consequent loss of lean body mass and nitrogen.
3. Increased metabolism. Increased metabolic demands arise from additional needs. **Sepsis** or fever make extra kcalories necessary for energy needs. Extra carbohydrates and B vitamins are needed for energy as the body resources mobilize to meet increased basal metabolic requirements. Tissue regeneration requires extra protein and key vitamins such as ascorbic acid and minerals such as zinc.
4. Skin grafting. Optimal tissue health is necessary for subsequent skin grafting to be successful.

Principles of nutritional therapy. Successful nutritional therapy is based on vigorous energy and protein therapy as follows:

1. *High energy.* A 3000 to 5000 kcal amount with a high percentage of carbohydrates is necessary to spare protein essential for tissue regeneration and to supply the greatly increased metabolic demands for energy. The amount of kcalories required by an individual patient may be calculated from the following formulas[9,11]:

Adults: (25 kcal × preburn body weight [kg]) + (40 kcal × percent BSA burned)

Children: 30 to 100 kcal [RDA for age] × preburn body weight [kg]) + (40 kcal × percent BSA burned)

BSA is body surface area, and RDA is recommended dietary allowance.

Another method of determining energy need is (1) to calculate the basal energy expenditure (BEE) by the classic Harris-Benedict equations[12] (see Chapter 4) and (2) to multiply the BEE by the appropriate metabolic activity factor (MAF) according to the degree of metabolic stress involved (Table 11-4).[13] Adjustment of kcalories is necessary on an individual basis in relation to weight changes or complications such as infection, which change energy requirements.[14]

2. *High protein.* Depending on the extent of the burn injury, individual needs for protein vary from 150 g to as high as 400 g, depending on the extent of catabolic losses. Children require two to four times the normal RDAs of protein for age. Individual adult requirements may be calculated by the following formula:

Metabolic Response to Injury

TO PROBE FURTHER

Two distinct phases of injury response may be identified—the "ebb" and the "flow." The initial ebb phase occurs immediately after the injury and is associated with shock. It is characterized by the following specific metabolic events:

- Decreased oxygen consumption and cardiac output
- Decreased body temperature
- Increased blood glucose accompanied by normal glucose production
- Increased lactate and free fatty acid production
- Increased catecholamine, glucagon, and cortisol levels
- Decreased insulin production and insulin resistance

If the patient survives, the ebb phase evolves into the flow phase. This recovery period is characterized by the following:

- Increased oxygen consumption and cardiac output
- Increased body temperature
- Increased nitrogen excretion
- Mild elevation of blood glucose accompanied by increased glucose production
- Normal lactate level and mild increase of free fatty acid level
- Increased catecholamine, glucagon, and cortisol levels
- Increased insulin production and insulin resistance

Clinical efforts in the ebb phase are focused on maintaining cardiovascular performance and tissue perfusion. The flow phase is a period of hypermetabolism that demands appropriate nutritional support.

REFERENCE

Bessey PQ, Wilmore DW: The burned patient. In Kinney JM et al, eds: *Nutrition and metabolism in patient care,* Philadelphia, 1988, WB Saunders.

TABLE 11–4

Added Energy Cost of Metabolic Stress in Illness and Trauma, the Metabolic Activity Factor

MAF according to degree of stress	Examples of conditions
BEE × 1.25: minimal stress	Nutritionally sound, little stress
BEE × 1.30: moderate stress	Cancer, inflammatory bowel disease, skeletal trauma, minor surgery
BEE × 1.50: severe stress	Cancer chemotherapy or radiation, burns, major sepsis
BEE × 1.75-2: extreme stress	Acquired immunodeficiency syndrome (AIDS), major trauma or burns

Modified from Konishi CD: Metabolic support teams as nutrition educators: who supports whom? *Top Clin Nutr* 1(4):51, 1986.
MAF, Metabolic activity factor; *BEE,* basal energy expenditure.

1 g protein/kg preburn weight +
(3 g protein × percent BSA burned)

In general, most adults require an increased amount of protein, 2 to 3 g/kg of body weight, to achieve nitrogen balance.

3. *High vitamin.* From 1 to 2 g of vitamin C may be needed for tissue regeneration. Increased amounts of thiamin, riboflavin, and niacin are necessary to supply oxidative enzyme systems to metabolize extra carbohydrates and protein.

To provide the nutritional therapy necessary to satisfy the increased metabolic demands of the burn patient, enteral or parenteral therapy may be required.

Enteral Feeding. To achieve the necessary intake of nutrients during enteral feeding, an intake record must be carefully maintained. Because the nutritional needs are vital, this record of protein and kcalorie values in the amount of food consumed is a necessary tool for planning continuous care. Oral feedings are desirable if at all tolerated by the patient. Concentrated oral liquids must be given using protein hydrolysates or amino acids to ensure adequate intake. Commercial formulas are usually used to supply large amounts of nourishment. Gradual introduction of solid foods according to individual food preferences is done by about the second week. Initial tube-feeding may be required by some patients to ensure adequate intake. Low-bulk defined formula solutions may be given through small-bore feeding tubes (see Chapter 3). Continuous individual support and encourage-

sepsis • Presence of pathogenic microorganisms or their toxins in the blood or other tissues; conditions associated with such pathogens.

ment are necessary to help the patient eat the food required. The food should be made as attractive and appetizing as possible; items particularly liked should be encouraged and disliked foods should be avoided.

Parenteral Feeding. For some patients oral intake and tube-feedings may be inadequate to meet the accelerated demands or may be impossible because of associated injuries or complications. In these cases parenteral feeding is needed to provide essential nutritional support. Details of this often life-saving procedure are given in Chapter 4.

Reconstruction Period

In the reconstruction period, continued vigorous nutritional support is essential to maintain tissue integrity for successful skin grafting or plastic reconstructive surgery. In addition, the principles of rehabilitation care discussed in Chapter 13 apply in the case of burned patients. The patient needs not only physical rebuilding of body resources but also much emotional and social support to rebuild the human spirit and will, because there may be disfigurement and disability. The burn team members can do much to help instill the courage and confidence the patient must have to face the future again. Whatever the future demands, however, optimal physical stamina gained through persistent, supportive care—medical, nutritional, and nursing—helps the patient build the personal resources needed to cope.

To Sum Up

The nutritional demands of surgery begin before the patient reaches the operating table. Preoperatively the nutritionist and the nurse are concerned about correcting any existing deficiencies and building an optimal nutrient reserve to meet surgical demands. Postoperatively they are concerned with replacing losses and supporting recovery. The additional task of encouraging eating is often required during this period.

Specific preoperative nutritional requirements include protein, which is associated with tissue breakdown and infection when plasma levels are low; kcalories, which are required for energy reserves; and vitamins and minerals, which are necessary in adequate amounts to prevent deficiencies. During the postoperative stage, nutritional requirements frequently focus on (1) protein, again to account for losses; (2) kcalories, preferably as carbohydrates because of the protein-sparing effect and efficient use as an energy source; (3) fluids, to prevent dehydration and counteract losses caused by vomiting, hemorrhage, diuresis, or fever; (4) minerals, to replace sodium and chloride lost with fluids, as well as others required to combat tissue catabolism; and (5) vitamins such as vitamin C that are required for wound healing.

Preoperative and postoperative feedings are given in a variety of ways. Although the oral route is always preferred, damage to the intestinal tract or a poor appetite may require enteral or parenteral feedings. Foods are provided in a variety of consistencies, not only to match the feeding method but also the patient's desire or ability to handle foods mechanically. Patients progress as rapidly as possible from clear to full liquids and then from soft to regular foods as their recovery progresses.

Diets are modified according to the type of surgical procedure performed. They have to accommodate a reduction in length of the alimentary tract, thus diminished absorption capacity, as well as counterbalance catabolism and fluid loss. Gastrointestinal surgery and massive burn injuries require special nutritional care.

QUESTIONS FOR REVIEW

1. Describe the general impact of imbalances of the following nutritional factors during the preoperative, immediate postoperative, and postoperative periods: protein, kcalories, vitamins and minerals, and fluids.
2. Describe the major surgical effects for which nutritional therapy must be planned following these procedures: mouth, throat, or neck surgery; gastric resection; cholecystectomy; and rectal surgery.
3. Write a 1-day meal plan for a person experiencing the postgastrectomy dumping syndrome. What general dietary guidelines are used?
4. Describe the difference in care between an ileostomy and colostomy. What are the dietary implications of each?
5. Outline the nutritional care of a burn patient from the immediate shock treatment through recovery and tissue reconstruction.

REFERENCES

1. Campos ACL, Meguid MM: A critical appraisal of the usefulness of perioperative nutritional support, *Am J Clin Nutr* 55:117, 1992.
2. Mughal MM, Meguid MM: The effect of nutritional status on the morbidity after elective surgery for benign gastrointestinal disease, *J Parenter Enteral Nutr* 11(2):140, 1987.
3. Church JM, Hill GL: Assessing the efficacy of intravenous nutrition in general surgical patients: dynamic nutritional assessment with plasma proteins, *J Parenter Enteral Nutr* 11(2):135, 1987.
4. Sachdeva AK et al: Surgical treatment of peptic ulcer disease, *Med Clin North Am* 75(4):999, 1991.
5. Tyns FJ et al: Diet tolerance and stool frequency in patients with ileoanal reservoirs, *J Am Diet Assoc* 92(7):861, 1992.

6. Rathgeber MG: Nutrition and ostomies, ADA practice group, *Dietitians in Nutrition Support Newsletter* 8(6):5, 1987.
7. Lerch MM et al: Post operative adaptation of the small intestine after total colectomy and J-pouch-anal anastomosis, *Dis Colon Rectum* 32:600, 1989.
8. Miedema BW et al: Absorption and motility of the bypassed human ileum, *Dis Colon Rectum* 33:829, 1990.
9. Ireton-Jones CS, Baxter CR: Nutrition for adult burn patients: a review, *Nutr Clin Prac* 6(1):3, 1990.
10. Hustler DA: Nutrition monitoring of a pediatric burn patient, *Nutr Clin Prac* 6(1):11, 1991.
11. Luterman A, Adams M, Curreri W: Nutritional management of the burn patient, *Crit Care Q* 7:34, 1984.
12. Harris JA, Benedict FG: *Biometric study of basal metabolism in man,* Pub No 279, Washington, DC, 1919, Carnegie Institute of Washington.
13. Konishi CD: Metabolic support teams as nutrition support educators: who supports whom? *Top Clin Nutr* 1(4):51, 1986.
14. Goran MI et al: Estimating energy requirements in burned children: a new approach derived from measurements of resting energy expenditure, *Am J Clin Nutr* 54:35, 1991.

FURTHER READING

Cerra FB: How nutrition intervention changes what getting sick means, *J Parenter Enteral Nutr* 14 (suppl 5): 164, 1990.

This article provides a good review of three basic factors that influence what is observed in experimental or clinical investigations at the bedside when considering the effects of nutritional intervention: the disease process inherent in the metabolic response to injury, the presence of starvation, and the presence of nutritional intervention. The author explores each of these factors and how they interact when viewed from the aspect of the nutritional intervention with current and future therapies.

Hall JC: Use of internal validity in the construct of an index of undernutrition, *J Parenter Enteral Nutr* 14(6):582, 1990.

This article discusses the development of an index of protein-energy undernutrition from a cross-sectional study of 200 general surgical patients that is independent of the incidences of adverse clinical events.

Glatzer H: Burned: how I saved my house—and got 46 days in the hospital, This World, *San Francisco Chronicle,* March 15, 1992, Chronicle Publishing.

Hal Glatzer, San Francisco journalist, gives a moving first-person account of his journey through pain and recovery from first-, second-, and third-degree burns. He gives the reader unforgettable insight from the patient's point of view.

Hutsler DA: Nutritional monitoring of a pediatric burn patient, *Nutr Clin Prac* 6:11, 1991.

This experienced dietitian-specialist on a burn center team provides a case report of a young boy who sustained mostly full-thickness burns over 56% of his total body surface area. She describes in detail the challenge of initial evaluation and therapy, constant close monitoring, and appropriate responses to changing needs.

CASE STUDY

Patient with a Gastrectomy

Walter Reilly is a 42-year-old male admitted for a total gastrectomy 4 weeks ago. He had a history of repeated episodes of pain and bleeding, for which he had been hospitalized twice during the last 6 months.

Surgery proceeded smoothly, with an anastomosis established between the jejunum and esophagus. Mr. Reilly received nothing orally for 48 hours postoperatively but received TPN to provide nutritional support. He was then given ice chips and water, for which he gradually developed a tolerance.

Two days later Mr. Reilly was able to tolerate 30 to 60 ml (1 to 2 oz) of milk between sips of water. This amount increased, as did his appetite. He was graduated to servings of a single soft food (eggs, cereal, custards, or potato) offered once or twice a day. By the end of the second week he was tolerating a full soft diet on six small feedings daily. He was cautioned to use liquids in moderation during a discharge diet counseling session conducted 1 week later.

At a later follow-up visit with his physician, Mr. Reilly complained of general discomfort and cramping following meals. Other symptoms included tachycardia, dizziness, nausea and vomiting, and breaking into a cold sweat. He had also begun to lose weight, and appeared slightly emaciated. His physician referred him to the clinical nutritionist to explore any problem with eating habits. Mr. Reilly seemed to accept most of her recommendations. One week later he telephoned to explain that all symptoms had subsided and that he was tolerating the diet well.

Questions for Analysis

1. Do you think that the surgical procedure performed was warranted? Defend your response.
2. Explain the physiologic rationale for the refeeding program as planned.
3. What nutrient would you emphasize in this patient's diet? Why? What is its significance with surgery?
4. Why was some fluid limitation recommended?
5. Account for the symptoms that followed eating. What dietary recommendations would you make to control them?

New Methods for Assessing Nutritional Status?

Traditional methods used to assess nutritional status and needs rely heavily on the use of *objective* measures such as anthropometry, clinical criteria, laboratory tests, and in some instances indirect calorimetry. But how does *subjective* evaluation relate? What role does it play in getting the whole picture of the patient's situation and its effect on health and illness?

Canadian researchers seeking some answers to these questions have been studying the relationships between these two basic assessment approaches. Working with hospitalized surgery patients, they demonstrated a subjective clinical assessment of nutritional needs based on the history and physical examination, which they called a "subjective global assessment" (SGA). They have found that this subjective approach is highly correlated with assessments made using the usual objective measures. They also found that with SGA, postoperative infections could be predicted as well as or better than with objective measures.

In follow-up study the investigators applied SGA to 202 patients before gastrointestinal surgery and examined the effect of individual characteristics on the SGA ratings. This study confirmed the validity of SGA as a technique of nutritional assessment. SGA ratings are based on five features of the patient history:

- Weight changes (loss) in the past 6 months and changes in the past 2 weeks
- Changes in dietary intake
- Gastrointestinal symptoms (nausea, vomiting, diarrhea, and anorexia) that have persisted over 2 weeks
- Functional capacity (ambulatory or bedridden)
- Presence of disease and its relation to nutritional needs

Four features of the physical examination are rated as normal, mild, moderate, or severe for five parameters:

- Loss of subcutaneous fat (triceps and chest)
- Muscle wasting (quadriceps and deltoids)
- Ankle and sacral edema
- Ascites

On the basis of these features of the history and physical examination, health team members identify an SGA rank which indicates the patient's nutritional status: well nourished, moderate or suspected malnutrition, or severe malnutrition.

The researchers feel that a major advantage of SGA is its flexibility in capturing subtle patterns of change in clinical variables and relating them to the effects of disease or surgical stress.

REFERENCE

Detsky AS et al: What is subjective global assessment of nutritional status? *J Parenter Enteral Nutr* 11(1):8, 1987.

CHAPTER 12

Nutrition and AIDS

CHAPTER OUTLINE

Evolution of HIV and the AIDS Epidemic
Nature of the Disease Process
Medical Management
Nutritional Management

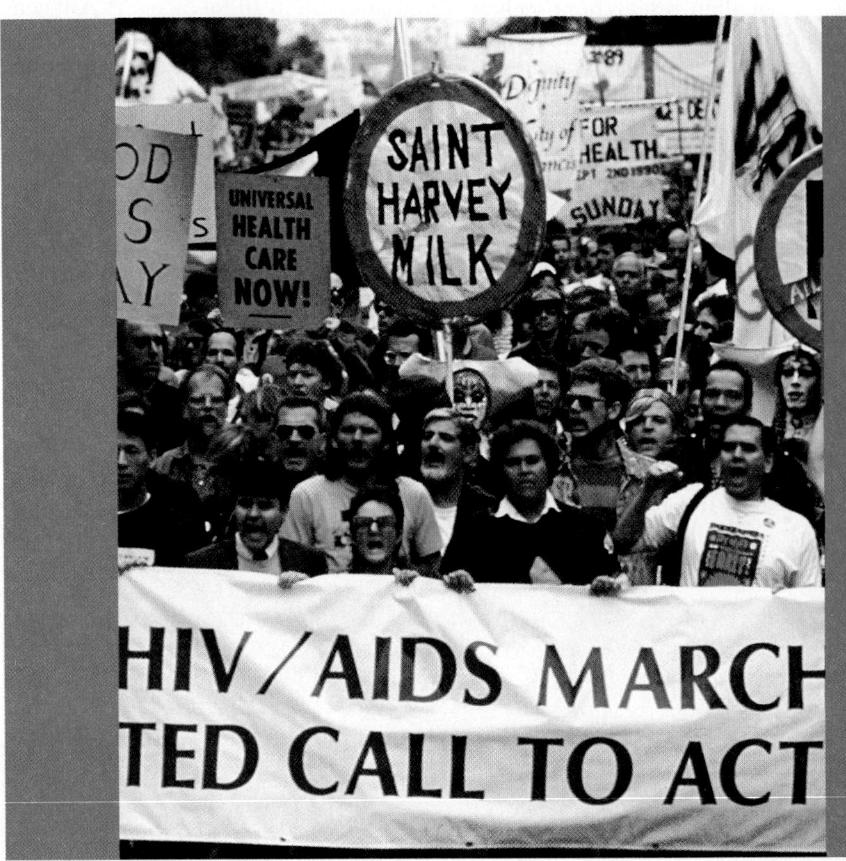

In this chapter of our clinical nutrition series we focus on AIDS, acquired immunodeficiency syndrome. This modern-day plague has thus far eluded modern medical science's search for a cure and left countless numbers of infected and dying young adults and children in its wake.

Worldwide, more than 12 million people are infected with human immunodeficiency virus-1 (HIV-1), the more virulent form. More than one million of these persons are North Americans. As knowledge of the disease process has grown over the past decade, it has become increasingly evident that nutritional support plays a vital role in the care of HIV-infected and AIDS patients.

Here we will examine the background of the AIDS epidemic, the nature of the human virus, and its effect on the body's immune system, leaving it vulnerable to various infections and cancers that lead to death. Then we will review the current state of medical management, especially the component of nutritional support and its relation to nutritional status and the course of the disease. Throughout we will see the important roles of both education and prevention in helping to stem the tide of this deadly disease.

Evolution of HIV and the AIDS Epidemic

In the late 1970s physicians on the East and West coasts of the United States, centered in New York City and San Francisco, became puzzled about an uncommon medical problem appearing among some of their patients.[1] These patients, in whom no known cause of immune suppression could be found, were nonetheless suffering and dying from complications of common infections, largely pneumonia, ordinarily handled easily by the human immune system and the usual antibiotics or other antibacterial drugs. To add to the puzzle, these and other patients seen from June 1981 to January 1983 with the similar immune-suppression condition of unknown cause were coming from quite diverse social and medical backgrounds—active homosexual men, intravenous drug users, recipients of transfused blood and blood products, including children with **hemophilia,** and also heterosexual men and women and their babies. What was this devastating disease? Its **virus** source and **pandemic** effects were soon to become alarmingly evident worldwide.

Early Viral History and Spread

Rapid Pandemic Spread

After the first U.S. cases were reported in 1981, an alarming decade of frustration and death followed.[2] Some highlights of that deadly decade include the following events:

- *June 1981.* Reports of an unexplained type of immune system failure among gay men start to surface in the United States; news of similar conditions among heterosexual men and women begins to increase from other parts of the world, especially central Africa.
- *July 1982.* The new disease is now found in hemophiliacs; named AIDS (acquired immunodeficiency syndrome) by American scientists.
- *January 1983.* Heterosexuals are also declared at risk after several women, whose sexual partners have AIDS, contract the disease.
- *May 1983.* A French scientist and leading pioneer of AIDS research, Luc Montagnier reports that he and his team at the Pasteur Institute in Paris have isolated the infectious agent now known as HIV (human immunodeficiency virus).
- *September 1984.* The first report of HIV infection is found in Thailand, which has subsequently developed one of the world's highest infection rates due in part to its open thriving sex industry.
- *March 1985.* The first test to detect HIV antibodies in the blood is approved in the United States.
- *March 1987.* The first drug, AZT (azidothymidine, now known as zidovudine), developed to fight the AIDS virus is approved for experimental use by the U.S. Food and Drug Administration (FDA).
- *April 1990.* The first U.S. Congressional action, named for Ryan White, a young hemophiliac who received HIV-infected blood transfusions as a child and died at age 18 of AIDS, provides funds to cities hardest hit by the disease.
- *October 1991.* The second anti-AIDS drug, dideoxyinosine (ddI), is approved by the U.S. FDA.
- *June 1992.* British scientists predict a 20% drop over the next decade in the population growth rate of the central African country of Uganda, where AIDS apparently first gained its hold and spread.
- *June 1992.* The third anti-AIDS drug, dideoxycytosine (ddC), is approved by the U.S. FDA.

Evolution of HIV

Social Change

Where did this new deadly virus come from and how did it gain such strength? From their studies thus far, scientists are beginning to find some answers. Apparently, as biologist Paul Ewald at Amherst College in Massachusetts argues in a forthcoming book, HIV

hemophilia • A hereditary hemorraghic disease due to deficiency of blood coagulation factor VIII; characterized by spontaneous or traumatic bleeding; transmitted as an X-linked (maternal) recessive trait to male children. This X-linked deficiency of factor VIII has played a major role in the history of royal families of Europe.

virus • A minute infectious agent, characterized by lack of independent metabolism and by the ability to reproduce with genetic continuity only within living host cells; ranges in size from about 200 nm (nanometers, also called millimicrons) to 15 nm—a linear measure equal to one-billionth of a meter. Each particle (virion) consists basically of nucleic acids (genetic material) and a protein shell which protects and contains the genetic material and any enzymes present.

pandemic • Widespread; distributed throughout a region, continent, or the world and affecting an exceptionally high proportion of the population as an epidemic.

represents not a new virus but an old one that has just recently grown deadly in humans as it gained strength during the social upheavals of the 1960s and 1970s.[3] The uprooting effect of this rapid social change and urbanization allowed the virus to spread rapidly through world populations and reproduce aggressively in its human host.

Parasite Nature of Virus

No virus can have a life of its own. All viruses by their structure and nature are the ultimate **parasites.** They are mere shreds of genetic material, a small packet of genetic information encased in a protein coat, containing a small chromosome of nucleic acids (RNA or DNA), usually with fewer than five genes (see Chapter 13). They can only live through a host, whom they invade and infect, hijacking the host's cell machinery to run off a multitude of copies of themselves, their purpose just to make as many self-copies as they can. The viruses of today are those that succeeded in that survival task over time and are, like all plants and animals, simply descendents of earlier forms. Most scientists agree that the human immunoviruses HIV-1 and HIV-2, which are genetically similar to viruses found in African primates (SIV, simian immunodeficiency virus), were probably transmitted to humans in an earlier age as ancient hunters cut themselves while butchering their kills for food. The rapidly increasing social-sexual changes and world travel of the past few decades have sped HIV-1 transmission and rapid multiplication. Its current deadly strength results from its aggressive growth within an increasing number of hosts.

Extent of Current Problem

Current Spread

Today, more than 12 million people throughout the world are infected with HIV. The great majority live in central Africa, south of the Sahara desert where the first cases appeared. Now, however, Southeast Asia with its increasing urbanization seems poised to become the plague's new epicenter. Currently infected populations are spread in nine main areas of the world[3,4]:

- Sub-Saharan Africa: 7.5+ million
- Southeast Asia: 1.5 million
- Latin America (Caribbean): 1.0 million
- North America: 1.0+ million
- North Africa, Middle East: 750,000
- Western Europe: 500,000
- Eastern Europe, Central Asia: 50,000
- East Asia, China, and Japan: 25,000
- Australasia: 25,000+

These official numbers are horrifying enough, but they tell only part of the story. Some developing world countries report only 5% to 10% of the actual number of cases.[4]

Projected Future Course

Epidemiologists and others studying the rapid spread of AIDS project gloomy numbers for the future course of the disease during the next decade, before the breakthroughs in curative drugs and population vaccines can eventually take effect. Reports at the Eighth International Conference on AIDS, meeting in Amsterdam, the Netherlands in July 1992, indicated two new areas of concern: (1) an increasing incidence of AIDS in heterosexual women with the accompanying risk of fetal transmission, and (2) the increasing spread of tuberculosis as an opportunistic pathogen in HIV-infected persons.[5] Over the next decade, Southeast Asia is expected to surpass central Africa in numbers of HIV-infected persons, especially among young women and their babies resulting from the open expanding sex industry of the region, especially in Thailand.[2] In the United States by the end of 1994, the Centers for Disease Control in Atlanta estimates that between 415,000 and 535,000 new cases of AIDS will have been diagnosed and well over a quarter of a million persons will be living with severe HIV disease at that time.[5] Although the future course of the worldwide HIV epidemic is difficult to predict, the sobering forecast of the World Health Organization (WHO) is that a minimum of 30 to 40 million people will be infected by the end of the decade.

Disease Progression

The individual clinical course of HIV infection varies substantially. However, three distinct stages mark the progression of the disease and are usually referred to as (1) primary HIV infection and extended asymptomatic incubation, (2) AIDS-related complex (ARC), and (3) terminal AIDS.

Primary HIV Infection

About 2 to 4 weeks after initial exposure and infection, a mild mononucleosis- or flu-like syndrome lasting about 1 week, may or may not occur. This brief response corresponds to the process of seroconversion during which initial antibodies to the viral infection are produced, and subsequent HIV testing will be positive. Signs of enlarged lymph nodes may occur, and an extended asymptomatic "well" period usually continues for the next 8 to 10 years. However, this relatively "well" period can be deceiving. New research indicates that it is actually a crucial stage in the underlying growth of the virus. Two independent study groups, one at National Institutes of Health (NIH), Laboratory of Immunoregulation, and the other at the University of Minnesota at Minneapolis, Department of Microbiology, report new findings that this extended period is a critical stage of viral incubation.[6,7] These researchers found that during this long time when the virus appears to be inactive, in reality it is hiding away in lymphoid tissues, such as lymph nodes, spleen, adenoid glands and tonsils, multiplying constantly in its parasite lifecycle within its host, taking over an increasing amount of white blood cells and gaining strength.[6-9]

In addition, new reports at a spring 1993 U.S. symposium of researchers further reinforced the findings of the virus in lymph tissue. Current research reported on the symposium topic "Frontiers in HIV Pathogenesis" added strength to the deception of the "inactive" period of HIV infection. They found even greater masses of infected cells in lymph tissues than were measured before with standard assays, leading them to issue buttons aptly summarizing the meeting's major theme with the blunt message: "It's the virus, stupid."[10] The researcher's newly developed amplified assay-testing process enabled them to routinely detect HIV in as many as 1 in 10 special T helper white blood cells (CD4+), a much greater viral load than had been thought, because the amplification limit in previous techniques could only find HIV in as few as 1 in 10,000 cells. Also, additional symposium reports of HIV in primate studies indicated that as CD4+ lymphocyte counts drop in the blood, they remain high in the lymph nodes, and the immune system only crashes when the CD4+ levels drop sharply in the lymph tissue.[10]

Some of the scientists have likened this apparently quiet period before the storm to the active life of a volcano, its inactive period a mountain of still beauty masking its actual interior cauldron developing strength for the inevitable blast. New research findings demonstrate the complexity and strength of this disease and the problems presented in finding a solution to stem the epidemic tide. These researchers and their colleagues underscore the crucial nature of this incubation period and the importance of earlier treatment intervention after HIV-seropositive detection, to slow this viral-strengthening hiatus while targeting drug development to combat its steady progression.

AIDS-Related Complex

After the extended asymptomatic HIV-positive stage, which may last as long as 10 years, a period of associated opportunistic infectious illnesses begins. This AIDS-related complex (ARC) of "opportunistic" illnesses is so-named because the HIV infection has now killed a sufficient number of the host protective white T cells (mainly T helper or CD4+ lymphocytes) to severely damage the person's immune system and lower the body's normal disease resistance. This gives even the most common of everyday infections an open opportunity to take root and grow. Common symptoms observed during this pre-AIDS period include persistent fatigue, thrush (oral *Candida albicans*), night sweats, diarrhea, fever over 100° F, unintentional weight loss of 5 kg (11 lbs) or more, remarkable headache, new skin rash, new or unusual cough, sore throat or mouth, unusual bruises or skin discoloration, and shortness of breath.[11]

Final Stage of AIDS

The terminal stage of HIV infection, commonly designated as AIDS, is marked by declining T helper lymphocyte counts from the normal healthy level of about 1000 such cells in every cubic millimeter of blood (1000/mm^3). HIV-infected persons usually experience a decline of these cells by an average of about 40 to 80/mm^3 every year.[12] Generally, when the falling T helper lymphocyte counts are roughly between 200 and 500/mm^3, diseases such as tuberculosis or Kaposi's sarcoma, the most common AIDS-associated malignancy, occur; at counts below 200/mm^3, *Pneumocystis carnii* pneumonia and *Toxoplasma gondii*, protozoan parasites able to infect a number of body organs, appear; and at counts under 50/mm^3, cytomegalovirus (CMV) or **lymphoma** can flourish.[1] When the virus finally kills enough white cells to overwhelm the weakened immune system resistance to the disease complications, death follows.

Public Health Service Responsibilities

In any major epidemic, the Public Health Service and its related agencies have the major task of monitoring and stopping the disease from spreading. Thus they carry responsibilities in two major areas: (1) surveillance, including testing and counseling; and (2) community education and prevention through interrupting its spread, vaccine research, and treatment.

Surveillance

Throughout the AIDS epidemic, as knowledge of this new disease and its nature has grown, the U.S. central control agency, Centers for Disease Control (CDC) in Atlanta, has worked in partnership with state and territorial health departments, and in constant worldwide knowledge exchange, to conduct accurate and comprehensive AIDS surveillance in the United States, including blinded (unlinked to individuals) research data gathered in large at-risk population surveys.[14] Since the middle 1980s such seroprevalence studies have provided a massive amount of information about HIV spread in various population groups, and helped CDC develop early classification guidelines for medical teams caring for HIV-infected pa-

parasite • An organism that lives on or in an organism of another species, know as the host, from whom all lifecycle nourishment is obtained.

lymphoma • A general term applied to any neoplastic disorder (cancer) of the lymphoid tissue.

tients (Table 12-1). The periodic CDC revisions of surveillance criteria reflect advances in the care and understanding of disease caused by HIV infection. For example, in accord with current knowledge and the evolution of the HIV epidemic among demographic groups, CDC has expanded the AIDS surveillance definition to include any HIV-seropositive person with a CD4+ (specific T lymphocyte subset analysis) cell count of less than 200 cells per microliter of blood.[14,15]

Because of the tremendous life-changing import of a positive HIV-1 test result to the patient and the patient's family and loved ones, public health testing programs have developed a coordinated pre- and post-test counseling component, especially in clinics serving high-risk areas.[16] First, a brief pretest interview assesses personal knowledge of HIV infection, provides risk-reduction education, and offers the HIV test. Then those who accept the HIV testing are given a two-week return appointment for a longer follow-up review of test results and counseling concerning health care and personal needs. Also, in addition to regular HIV-1 testing, sentinel testing for the initial African strain HIV-2 in clinics serving high-risk clients recently arrived from endemic HIV-2 areas has begun to detect the presence of this second form of the virus in the United States.[17]

Education and Prevention

The U.S. Department of Health and Human Services, through its Public Health Service and Food and Drug Administration divisions, has provided national health promotion and disease prevention objectives for the year 2000 that call for the expansion of HIV education and prevention efforts.[18] Wide community involvement in the community-based process of developing any health promotion/disease prevention program is essential for its successful outcome.[19] This need has been shown, for example, in the mobilizing of community leadership and resources to plan and implement interventions in other health problems such as heart disease and hazards such as smoking. The community support need is particularly true with HIV infection, which despite its burdening social stigma is now reaching into all communities in some form, cutting short the lives of children, adolescents, and young adults in ever increasing numbers. The Harvard Global AIDS Policy Coalition estimates that by the year 2000 between 38 million and 110 million adults and more than 10 million children will be infected worldwide.[20] Such a deadly pandemic epidemic warrants mobilizing and coordinating the most realistic and effective preventive strategies possible for all ethnic and socioeconomic community groups, to change sexual risk-taking behavior at all levels—local, national, and international.

Nature of the Disease Process

Action of HIV on the Immune System

HIV-1 and HIV-2 are members of a class of viruses called **retrovirus,** from their unique life cycle that involves a reverse transcription of RNA into DNA in

TABLE 12–1

Centers for Disease Control Classification System for HIV Infected Patients

Group	Classification and description
I	Acute HIV infection: Patients with transient signs and symptoms of HIV infection.
II	Asymptomatic HIV infection: Patients without previous signs or symptoms leading to classification in Group III or IV.
III	Persistent generalized lymphadenopathy (PGL): Patients with lymph nodes > 1 cm in diameter that persisted for > 3 months at two or more extrainguinal sites.
IV	Other HIV disease: *Subgroup A (constitutional disease):* patients with one or more of the following: fever > 1 month, involuntary weight loss > 10%, diarrhea > 1 month. *Subgroup B (neurological disease):* patients with dementia, myelopathy, or peripheral neuropathy. *Subgroup C (secondary infectious disease):* patients diagnosed with infectious disease from the following categories: *Category C-1:* 1 of 12 specified diseases listed in the CDC surveillance definition of AIDS—*Pneumocystis carinii* pneumonia, chronic cryptosporidosis, toxoplasmosis, extraintestinal strongyloidiasis, isosporiasis, candidiasis (esophageal, bronchial, or pulmonary), cryptococcosis, histoplasmosis, mycobacterial infection with *Mycobacterium avium* complex or *M. kansasii,* cytomegalovirus infection, chronic mucocutaneous or disseminated herpes simplex virus infection, and progressive multifocal leukoencephalopathy. *Category C-2:* symptomatic or invasive disease with oral, hairy leukoplakia, multidermatomal herpes zoster, recurrent salmonella bacteremia, nocardiosis, tuberculosis, or oral candidiasis. *Subgroup D (secondary cancers):* patients diagnosed with cancers known to be associated with HIV infection: Kaposi's sarcoma, non-Hodgkin's lymphoma (small, noncleaved lymphoma or immunoblastic sarcoma), or primary lymphoma of the brain. *Subgroup E (other conditions in HIV infection):* patients exhibiting clinical findings which may be due to HIV disease: chronic lymphoid interstitial pneumonitis, constitutional symptoms not meeting Subgroup IV-A, patients with infectious diseases not meeting Subgroup IV-C, and patients with neoplasms not meeting subgroup IV-D.

Adapted from Centers for Disease Control: Classification system for human T-lyphotropic virus type III/lymphadenopathy-associated virus infections. *MMWR* 35:334, 1986 and Raiten, DJ: Nutrition and HIV infection: a review and evaluation of the extant knowledge of the relationship between nutrition and HIV infection, *Nutr Clin Prac* 6(3):1S, 1991.

the cell nucleus, which is then integrated into the host cell DNA.[1] The virus consists of an outer envelope with attached surface proteins covering the outer protective shell and an inner shell that contains the small strands of ribonucleic acid (RNA) genetic material and enzymes, including the reverse transcriptase. Of the virus's nine genes, four apparently less essential ones are poorly understood. After entering the body, the virus attaches to host cells, mostly the actively replicating T helper (CD4+) white blood cells, major lymphocytes of the body's immune system. There it integrates itself into the host cell's DNA copying system, infecting and eventually killing the host cell. Rapidly increasing masses of virus particles erupt from the dying cells in small buds to immediately infect new cells.

Methods of Transmission and Groups at Risk

Throughout the world sexual behavior is central to the epidemic spread of HIV and AIDS. An estimated 71% of HIV infection worldwide is a result of heterosexual behavior and 15% to homosexual behavior, and only a relatively small proportion to intravenous drug use with contaminated needles.[20] In the United States as of 1992, reported AIDS cases by type of transmission were approximately 58% by homosexual behavior, 29% by intravenous drug use with shared blood-contaminated needles, 6% by heterosexual behavior, 3% by blood transfusions, and about 4% from other sources such as health care worker contact with blood of infected patients, a relatively rare event, and vertical transmission from infected mothers to their babies during pregnancy or at birth, which is a growing concern.[2,21,22]

Current worldwide studies of HIV-seropositive newborns indicate a maternal-fetal transmission rate of about 30%, with a low rate of 12.9% reported in the European Collaborative Study Group and a high rate of 45% in Nairobi, Kenya.[22] Infection is believed to occur predominately during the intrapartum period of labor and delivery, rather than earlier during pregnancy, and documented records show that such infected newborns require frequent hospitalizations during their first year of life.[22,23] The increase in pediatric cases of HIV infection brings more concern, and care of these children requires special considerations (see *Issues and Answers*, p. 261). Further, a study of young, sexually active women attending public family planning clinics in New York indicated that the greater disproportionate burden of HIV infection among these potential mothers was carried by non-Hispanic Blacks and Hispanics, whose HIV infection rate was about six times higher than the rate for non-Hispanic Whites.[24]

Overall, current U.S. reports are now in flux, with a rising proportion of cases coming from heterosexual contact. The fastest growing subgroup of new heterosexual cases is among women, with the proportion among younger women and adolescent girls alarmingly high.[20]

Groups at Risk

Persons at greatest risk of HIV infection, as previously indicated, are those who, if they are sexually active, are not consistently practicing responsible and safe sexual behavior, which consists of: (1) consistent and correct condom use for protection, the regular latex male sheath and the new female polyurethane condom, a cervical cap recently approved for use by the Food and Drug Administration[25-27]; and (2) avoidance of multiple sex partners and having sex with persons at risk for HIV. Others at risk are intravenous drug users who share contaminated needles. However, since the public donated blood supply for transfusions is now thoroughly cleared of HIV infection by a rigorous double-testing program, this route of infection risk by blood units for medical purposes has virtually been eliminated.[1]

Diagnosis of HIV Infection

Testing Procedures

Diagnosis of HIV infection is made by detection of the virus or serologic response to the virus. HIV infection can be identified by detection of specific antibodies as is also done in the routine screening of blood and blood products for transfusion and in most epidemiologic studies. The recommended procedure for virus detection is a two-step process.[1] The first step is enzyme-linked immunosorbent assay (ELISA) screening. In the second step, suspected positive samples from the ELISA screening are followed by *Western blot* testing for confirmation. Both of these tests are highly sensitive and specific, and both are used to confirm the results before informing the individual. Because a positive test is such a personal and life-changing event, most experienced physicians involved in the care of HIV infected patients repeat all positive tests again, even when they have been confirmed by Western blot, before informing the individual. Requirements for the testing procedure include pre- and post-test counseling to cover such issues as[1,28]:

- *Medical significance* of the test, whether positive or negative
- *Limitations* of the test

retrovirus • Any of a family of single-strand RNA viruses having an envelope and containing a reverse coding enzyme that allows for a reversal of genetic transcription from RNA to DNA rather than the usual DNA to RNA, the newly transcribed viral DNA then being incorporated into the host cell's DNA strand for the production of new RNA retroviruses.

- *Information* about HIV-1 and AIDS, how it is spread, and how to prevent its spread
- *Medical, nutritional, and psychosocial care* availability
- *Confidentiality* concept involved with documentation in the medical record; possible social and legal results of testing, personal needs, and support system

Clinical Symptoms and Illnesses

The early clinical symptoms that may follow initial exposure to the virus add further confirmation to the HIV-seropositive testing procedures. These initial symptoms, as well as possible associated illnesses and diseases that characterize the later ARC and AIDS stages, have been generally described above in discussing the basic disease progression. Some examples of these common infectious complications of AIDS and their clinical problems are listed in Table 12-2.

TABLE 12–2

Common Infectious Complications of AIDS

Microorganism	Clinical manifestation
Parasites	
Pneumocystis carinii	Pneumonia
Toxoplasma gondii	Focal encephalitis, pneumonia
Cryptosporidium	Malabsorption, diarrhea
Isospora belli	Diarrhea
Microspora	Malabsorption, diarrhea
Entamoeba histolyitica	Diarrhea
Giardia lamblia	Diarrhea
Acanthamoeba	Meningoencephalitis
Bacteria	
Campylobacter	Diarrhea, bacteremia
Legionella	Pneumonia
Listeria monocytogenes	Meningitis, bacteremia
Mycobacterium avium-intracellulare	Tuberculosis, diarrhea, other mycobacterium
Norcardia	Pneumonia, encephalitis
Pneumococcus	Pneumonia
Salmonella	Diarrhea, bacteremia
Shigella	Diarrhea, bacteremia
Haemophilus influenzae	Pneumonia
Streptococcus pneumoniae	Pneumonia
Staphylococcus aureus	Pneumonia
Fungi	
Aspergillus	Fungemia, pneumonia
Candida albicans	Thrush, stomatitis, esophagitis, pneumonia
Cryptococcus neoformans	Meningitis, pneumonitis
Histoplasma capsulatum	Pneumonitis, skin lesions
Coccidioides immitis	Pneumonitis
Viruses	
Cytomegalovirus	Esophagitis, pneumonitis, diarrhea
Herpes simplex virus	Ulcerative mucocutaneous lesions, stomatitis, esophagitis, pneumonia
Epstein-Barr	EBV-positive nonHodgkin's lymphomas, oral hairy leukoplakia
Hepatitis B	Nausea, vomiting, fever, antigenemia
Herpes zoster	Multiple dermatomal zoster
Papillomavirus	Oral hairy leukoplakia

Adapted from Gold, JWM: HIV-1 infection: diagnosis and management, *Med Clin North Am* 76(1):1, 1992; Bernard EM et al: Pneumocystosis, *Med Clin North Am* 76(1):107, 1992; and Ralten, DJ: Nutrition and HIV infection: a review and evaluation of the extant knowledge of the relationship between nutrition and HIV infection, *Nutr Clin Prac* 6(3):1S, 1991.

Basic Role of Nutrition in HIV Disease Process

Nutrition support plays a vital role throughout the HIV disease process in two basic areas. First, it is a vital component of care for the involuntary weight loss and body tissue wasting caused by the disease effects on metabolism, reflected in the severe state of protein-energy malnutrition. Then second, and fundamental in all conditions associated with the body's basic immune system (see extended discussion in Chapter 13), nutrition is an intimate and integral component of care through the specific roles of key nutrients in maintaining the body's immunocompetence. Further, for many of the associated diseases, individual nutritional status influences the impact of morbidity and mortality irrespective of the disease process.[29]

Medical Management

Basic Current Goals

The medical management of HIV-1 infection in all stages is constantly evolving as medical research seeks

TABLE 12–3

Initial Evaluation of Newly Diagnosed HIV-Infected Patients

Routine history and physical examination include:
- History of exposure to infectious complications of AIDS
- Assessment of baseline mental status

Baseline laboratory studies
- CBC, differential, platelets
- Biochemistry screening profile
- Urinalysis
- Chest x-ray
- Tuberculin test with anergy panel
- Serologic test for syphilis
- Toxoplasma serology
- T-lymphocyte subsets
- Hepatitis B serology (optional)

Nutritional assessment, counseling, support, and follow-up

Psychosocial and financial status assessment

Referral to and involvement in psychosocial support include:
- Social worker, nurse, psychologist or psychiatrist, patient support group, community support group, and agencies

Rehabilitation program for substance abusers

Planning for family members and children, including issues of testing and providing for their care

Adapted from Gold, JWM: HIV-1 infection: diagnosis and management, *Med Clin North Am* 76(1):1, 1992.

to eliminate, or at least suppress, the virus. Intensive current research is aimed at preventing the progressive immunodeficiency, stopping HIV-1 transmission to uninfected persons, and restoring depressed immune function to normal to prevent AIDS-associated complications. Thus present basic medical management objectives are threefold: (1) delay progression of the infection and improve the patient's immune system; (2) prevent opportunistic illnesses; and (3) recognize the infection early and provide rapid treatment for any complications of immune deficiency, including infections and cancers.

Initial Evaluation: AIDS Team

The initial medical evaluation of a newly diagnosed HIV-infected patient is critical in beginning and continuing the ongoing comprehensive care by the AIDS team of professional medical, nutritional, nursing, and psychosocial health care specialists. Table 12-3 outlines an initial evaluation guide for beginning the care of a person with newly identified HIV-1 infection. These guidelines emphasize the special coordinated care by all members of the AIDS team and the importance of personal nutritional and psychosocial support. A basic approach to ongoing medical management, in which all AIDS team members participate, is outlined in Table 12-4.

Antiretroviral Drug Therapy

Following the initial discovery and identification of HIV-1, research began in earnest to develop effective antiretroviral drugs to inhibit the replication of the virus. However, the problems involved are complex and the task has been frustrating. One of the earliest findings in this drug research effort was that certain members of a class of compounds called **dideoxynucleosides** effectively inhibited HIV-1 replication in the laboratory.[30] Subsequent clinical trials with HIV-infected patients have shown that in human cells, dideoxynucleosides are metabolized to a triphosphate group, which is believed to be the active agent against HIV. As triphosphates, dideoxynucleosides act as competitive inhibitors at the level of the virus's necessary enzyme for replicating itself, *HIV reverse transcriptase,* thus effectively preventing viral increase. The first drug in this class to be used in clinical trials, azidothymidine (AZT) or zidovudine, is currently the only antiretroviral drug thus far to be approved by the Food and Drug Administration. Several others, including dideoxyinosine (ddI), dideoxycytidine (ddC), d4T (dideoxythymidinene, didehydrothymidine), and azido-dideoxyuridine (AZdU), are in their preliminary stages of clinical trials.[30] However, toxic side effects of these drugs, as shown in Table 12-5, have created problems requiring additional attention. Some of these side effects, such as nausea, may be helped by diet modifications (see Chapter 13).

AZT's results in patient therapy have been found to diminish over time as the virus, confronted by the drug, readily mutates into slight variations out of the drug's range, making the virus slightly less efficient with each mutation. However, researchers on a Boston team at Massachusetts General Hospital are studying ways of using combinations of these drugs—in one experiment, AZT, ddI, and pyridinone—to achieve effective results over longer periods of time.[3] As more is constantly being learned about the biochemistry and molecular biology of HIV-1 and HIV-2, agents targeted at blocking specific steps in the replicating lifecycle of HIV, and at the same time are less suppressive of the bone marrow and create fewer side effects, are being developed.[30] For example, drugs now in clinical evaluation include agents that (1) block viral binding to the surface of susceptible cells (CD4 receptor and derivatives), (2) alter viral components and their assembly (glucosidase inhibitors), and (3) interfere with viral HIV release or budding (interferons).

Continuing Research and Future Developments

Continuing research for a long-awaited vaccine against HIV is nearing the stage of international trials. Although it has been a bumpy road with some rough spots still ahead, organizations of researchers and pol-

TABLE 12-4

Medical Treatment of HIV-Infected Patients

Evaluation for antiretroviral therapy and prophylaxis for *Pneumocystis carinii* pneumonia by monitoring T-helper lymphocyte count and clinical status.
- T cell count < 500 is an indication for zidovudine
- T cell count < 200 is an indication for PCP prophylaxis
- Hx of tuberculin reactivity, TB exposure, or chest x-ray compatible with old TB should lead to evaluation for prophylaxis

Education to improve general health knowledge and to avoid possible sources of infection.

Discussion of applicable research protocols.

Regular follow-ups to alert physician to earliest signs of AIDS-related complications.

Consideration of antiretroviral therapy failure in patient on prolonged treatment who develops new or recurrent symptoms and to rule out AIDS-related complications.

Adapted from Gold, JWM: HIV-1 infection: diagnosis and management, *Med Clin North Am* 76(1):1, 1992.

dideoxynucleosides • A class of drugs used to treat HIV-infected persons; a nucleoside is a combination of a sugar (a pentose) with a purine or pyrimidine (two types of compounds that provide the cross-linking "ladders" of the double strands of DNA) base.

TABLE 12–5

Toxicities of Dideoxynucleoside Drugs

AZT (azidothymidine, zidovudine, 3′-azido-2′, 3′-dideoxythymidline)

Bone marrow suppression. Anemia with increased mean corpuscular volume. Leukopenia and thrombocytopenia often dose-limiting
Nausea and vomiting
Headache
Malaise, fatigue, fever
Myalgias
Seizures (rare, but reported to be fatal)
Confusion, tremulousness
Wernicke's-like encephalopathy
Bluish pigmentation of finger and toenails
Hepatic transaminase elevation
Stevens-Johnson syndrome

ddI (dideoxyinosine, 2′,3′-dideoxyinosine)

Painful peripheral neuropathy
Sporadic pancreatitis (may be fatal)
Hyperamylasemia, hypertriglyceridemia
Headache
Insomnia, restlessness
Hepatic transaminase elevations (occasional hepatitis)
Hyperuricemia (with high doses)

ddC (dideoxycytidine, 2′,3′-dideoxycytidine)

Painful peripheral neuropathy
Aphthous stomatitis
Maculopapular rash (occasionally pseudovesicular)
Fevers
Arthralgias, edema
Thrombocytopenia

d4T (2′, 3′-dideoxythymidinene, 2′,3′-dideoxy-2′, 3′-didehydrothymidine)

Painful peripheral neuropathy
Anemia
Hepatic transaminase elevations

Adapted from Pluda, JM et al: Hematologic effects of AIDS therapies, *Hematology/Oncology Clin North Am* 5(2):229, 1991.

icy makers, as well as involved drug companies, indicate that sites are being selected in representative epidemic areas, such as central Africa, southeast Asia, Brazil, United States, and others, with clinical trials probably ready to start about 1995.[31-33] The central question seems no longer to be "Can we make a vaccine that works?", but rather "How do we speed it up?"[32]

There is no question that the epidemiology and treatment of HIV-1 infection will change rapidly over the next few years. Patients will live longer and with improved quality of life. Nonetheless, with longer life and treatment for known complications, it is likely that new complications will appear, such as uncommon infections, neurologic disease, or wasting syndromes.[1] The medical management of AIDS will continue to require involved health care professionals and patients.

Nutritional Management

Basic Approach: Individual Status and Needs

Although answers will soon come to many of our puzzling questions, as yet HIV infection is an elusive epidemic terminal disease and its treatment varies according to individual status and needs—medical, nutritional, and psychosocial. Research breakthroughs will help light our course, but in every case health care professionals and patients must remain highly involved, seeking the best possible individual care each step of the way.

There are many causes of malnutrition in HIV infection. Thus at any point, nutritional recommendations and support must be individual and integrated with other therapies. These nutritional care plans must provide a comprehensive view of the disease process through each of its stages, specific drug use, and the patient's wishes. All patients diagnosed as HIV infected should be considered to be at nutritional risk. Although the patient may be in an earlier asymptomatic period, the disease process, its complications, or treatments will begin to take their toll on the person's nutritional status. There are numerous ways in which the nutritional status of any HIV-infected person may be compromised. At all times, each patient must be viewed within the context of his or her own disease and individual lifestyle.

Wasting Effects of HIV Infection on Nutritional Status

Severe Malnutrition and Weight Loss

A fundamental effect of HIV infection is major weight loss, which eventually leads to extreme cachexia similar to that observed in cancer patients (see Chapter 13). Such serious weight loss was recognized in the Centers for Disease Control classification of body weight loss over 10% of usual weight, with more than 30 days of constitutional symptoms in an HIV-positive person, as a primary diagnosis of AIDS.[34] This serious characteristic body-wasting resulting from HIV infection then also becomes a cofactor in the development of the full disease syndrome in infected persons as the malnutrition itself suppresses cellular immune function. So striking is this chronic, relentless body wasting of AIDS that in Africa it has been given the name "slim disease."[35] Body wasting in AIDS is characterized by loss of body cell mass, primarily muscle protein; death occurs when body weight reaches ⅔ of normal weight and body cell mass reaches ½ of normal values.[36] This designation implies that death may be more often due to malnutrition, specifically negative nitrogen balance, than to the direct effects of infection or malignancy.[37] Also, the attendent diseases of the wasting process play a major role in the decreased quality of life, the debilitating weakness and fatigue, seen in AIDS patients.

TABLE 12–6

Outline of Nutritional Assessment in Persons with HIV Infection and AIDS

I. Estimated daily kcalorie and protein requirements for adults

A. Kcalories (total kcal)

Male/female: 35-40 kcal/kg

B. Protein (g)

Male/female: 2.0-2.5 g/kg

II. Calculated daily kcalorie and protein requirements for adults

A. Kcalories (total kcal) for weight maintenance

Male = (66.5 + (13.7 × wt [kg]) + (5 × ht [cm]) − (6.7 × age [yr])) × AF* × IF† + 500 kcal
Female = (665.1 + (9.6 × wt [kg]) + (1.8 × ht [cm]) − (4.7 × age [yr])) × AF* × IF† + 500 kcal

NOTE: Add 500 kcal to the equations above for weight gain.

B. Protein (g):

$$\text{Male/female} = \text{Total kcal} \times \frac{\text{g nitrogen}}{\text{150 kcal}} \times \frac{\text{6.25 g protein}}{\text{g nitrogen}}$$

III. Nutritional assessment parameters

	Extent of malnutrition		
	Mild	Moderate‡	Severe‡
Albumin (g/dL)	2.8-3.2	2.1-2.7	<2.1
Transferrin (mg/dL)	150-200	100-150	<100
Total lymphocyte count (cells/mm³)	1200-2000	800-1200	<800
Creatinine-height index (%) (actual/ideal × 100)	60-80	40-60	<40
Ideal body weight (%)	80-90	70-80	<70
Usual body weight (%)	85-95	75-85	<75
Weight loss/unit time	<5%/mo <7.5%/3 mo <10%/6 mo	<2%/wk >5%/mo >7.5%/3 mo >10%/6 mo	>2%/wk
Skin tests (no. reactive/no. placed)	4/4 (Normal)	1-2/4 (Weak)	0/4 (Anergic)
Anthropometry	Normal male	Normal female	
Triceps skinfold (mm)	12.5	16.5	
Mid-arm circumference (cm)	29.3	28.5	

Adapted from Hickey, MS: Nutritional support of patients with AIDS, *Surg Clin North Am* 71(3):645, 1991.
*Activity factors (AF): Confined to bed = 1.2, ambulatory = 1.3, fever factor = 1.13/°C>37
†Injury factor (IF): Surgery = 1.1-1.2, infection = 1.2-1.6, trauma = 1.1-1.8, sepsis = 1.4-1.8
‡Nutritional therapy indicated

Causes of Body Wasting

The characteristic body wasting of HIV infection may be due to any of the following processes, alone or in combination[37]:

- *Inadequate food intake.* Both clinicians and AIDS patients indicate, from their combined clinical observations and personal experience, that an important factor in the profound weight loss is severe anorexia, which is probably related to both the patient's personal life-changing situation and the body's physiologic changes from the disease. Recently encouraging results have come from the use of the drug *megesterol acetate* (Megase), a synthetic hormone similar to the natural hormone progesterone, which improves appetite and food intake, leading to weight gain.[38] Anorexia and its resulting decreased food intake, insufficient to meet body needs, clearly contributes to the body wasting.
- *Malabsorption of nutrients.* From early reports, as well as continuing clinical experience, diarrhea and malabsorption have been common in AIDS.[39,40] These malabsorptive symptoms have been related to both drug-diet interactions and progressive effects of HIV-infection. An "AIDS enteropathy" in the early stages of infection has been described, characterized by blunting of the intestinal villi, abnormal intestinal enzymes that cause clinical malabsorption, and HIV infection of infiltrating lymphocytes as well as enterocytes.[41-42] In later stages, the intestine is infected more frequently with opportunistic organisms

CLINICAL APPLICATION

The ABCDs of Nutrition Assessment in AIDS

The initial nutrition assessment visit with an HIV-infected patient is an important beginning point for the continuing nutritional care that is to follow. This encounter serves both informational and relational functions. It provides the necessary baseline information for planning practical individual nutrition support. But more importantly, it establishes the essential provider-patient relationship, the human context within which this continuing nutritional care and support will be provided as needed. The basic ABCDs of nutrition assessment will provide a practical guide (see Chapter 1), with special EFs added for HIV infection patients.

Anthropometry

- Age, sex, height
- Weight: current, usual, % usual, ideal, % ideal, weight loss over defined time period
- Mid–upper-arm measures: circumference, triceps skinfold thickness; calculated mid-arm muscle circumference

Biochemical indices

- Serum proteins: albumin, prealbumin, transferrin
- Liver function test (evaluate liver function)
- Blood urea nitrogen, serum electrolytes (evaluate renal function)
- Urinary urea nitrogen excretion over 24 hours (nitrogen balance)
- Creatinine height index
- Complete blood count (evaluate for anemia)
- Fasting glucose (evaluate for hyperglycemia or hypoglycemia)

Clinical observations

- General signs of nutritional status (see Table 1-2)
- Drug effects

Diet evaluation

- Usual intake, current intake, restrictions, modifications (use both 24-hour recall and food diaries)
- Nutrition supplements, vitamin-mineral supplements
- Food allergies, intolerances
- Activity level (general kcalories expended per day)
- Support system (care givers to help with nutrition care plan)

Environmental, behavioral, and psychologic assessment

- Living situation, personal support
- Food environment, types of meals, eating assistance needed

Financial assessment

- Medical insurance
- Income, financial support through care givers
- Current medical and other expenses
- Ability to afford food, enteral supplements, added vitamins-minerals ◆

REFERENCES

Ghiron L et al: Nutrition support of the HIV-positive, ARC, and AIDS patient, *Clin Nutr* 8(3):103, 1989.

Trujillo EB et al: Assessment of nutritional status, nutrient intake, and nutrition support in AIDS patients, *J Am Diet Assoc* 92(4):477, 1992.

such as *mycobacterium avium intracellulare (MAI), cryptosporidium parvum,* and the microsporidium *Enterocytozoon bieneusi.*[43] These and other such opportunistic infections result in more severe diarrhea and malabsorption.

- *Disordered metabolism.* In the final stage of weight loss in AIDS, changes in metabolism occur, including hypermetabolism and altered energy metabolism, usually associated with end-stage effects of the HIV infection as well as increased spread of opportunistic infections such as MAI or cytomegalovirus (CMV). There is progressive depletion of lean body mass as well as increased resting energy expenditure (REE).[44] Energy metabolism is altered as a futile cycling of fatty acids is associated with increased serum triglycerides, catabolism of skeletal muscle as an endogenous source of energy, and elevated levels of the cytokine alpha-interferon.[44,45] This metabolic picture is unlike simple starvation in which body fat is oxidized for energy.

Nutrition Assessment

The initial nutrition assessment must be comprehensive to provide the baseline information necessary for beginning and continuing nutritional care. Table 12-6 provides guidelines for calculating daily kcalories and protein needs, assessing weight changes, as well as evaluating biochemical data. The calculations and evaluations are especially required for those selected patients on special nutritional support therapies, enteral or parenteral.[46] Further person-centered nutritional care all HIV-infected patients require is evident in the ABCDs of nutrition assessment outlined in the *Clinical Application* above. This type of detailed initial nutrition interview includes investigation of the patient's medical history, physical and anthropometric data, biochemical indices, medications, living situation, dietary intake, general socioeconomic status, and assistance needs. All patients, at first contact with a health professional, should be referred for screening by the AIDS team clinical dietitian for nutrition problems, so that together with the patient, a continuing plan for ongoing nutritional care and support can be initiated.

Nutrition Intervention

Experienced clinical dietitians working with AIDS patients build nutrition care plans with each client or patient for appropriate nutrition intervention and

TABLE 12–7

Planning Nutrition Care for Patients with AIDS

Type of problem	Possible causes	Patient care plan considerations
Food intake		
	Anorexia	Patient, caregiver roles
	Drug, food interaction	Motivation, patient decision-making
	HIV, other infection	Education, counseling
	Taste alteration	Resource materials
	Food intolerances, allergies	Nutrition supplements
	Lack of access or ability to prepare food	Vitamin, mineral supplements
	Depression	Drug/food reactions
		Special enteral/parenteral nutrition support
		Monitoring, adjustments as needed
Nutrient absorption		
	HIV related infections or cancers	Treatment of underlying disease or disorder
	Diminished gastric HCl secretion	Pancreatic enzymes supplement
	Altered mucosal absorbing surface	Drug/nutrient reactions
	Organ Involvement: liver, pancreas, gallbladder, kidney	Special enteral/parenteral nutrition support, appropriate formula design
	Drug/nutrient interaction	Monitoring, adjustments as needed
Altered metabolism, excretion		
	HIV infection	Review of drug dosage, schedule
	Associated infections, diseases	Modification of diet, meal pattern
	Drug/nutrient interactions	Treatment of infection, symptoms
	Altered hormonal function	Review of diet nutrients, increase or decrease
	Organ dysfunction	Special enteral-parenteral nutrition support, appropriate formula design
		Monitoring, adjustments as needed

Adapted from Newman CF: *Practical guidelines for improving nutritional status in HIV-related disease,* University of California, Davis Medical School Fifth Annual Conference on Clinical Nutrition, Nutrition in the Treatment of Serious Medical Problems, Feb 28-29, 1992.

guidance.[47] This planning is continually adjusted as needed according to the disease progression and personal needs. It focuses on identifying food-nutrient problems, developing a plan of action for each problem, and outlining the form of nutrition support needed. Suggested guidelines for developing such patient-centered care plans are outlined in Table 12-7. For those persons receiving nutrition support in special enteral or parenteral forms, the dietitian will work with other members of the nutrition support team to develop an appropriate formula and feeding mode, using oral or tube-fed enteral means or intravenous feeding by peripheral or central veins (see Chapters 3 and 4). Hickey[46] has provided particular guidelines for nutritional support of patients with ARC or AIDS.

Nutrition Counseling, Education, and Supportive Strategies

Counseling Principles

An adolescent client once aptly defined a counselor as "someone to talk to while I make up my mind." Client-centered counselors in the care of persons with HIV infection must be just that. Professionals and patients must remain involved throughout the progressive course of the disease because the patient's wishes and needs are ultimately paramount in various treatments and decisions about care. The basic goal of nutrition counseling is to make the fewest possible changes in the person's lifestyle and food patterns necessary to promote optimal nutritional status while providing maximum comfort and quality of life.[47,48] In this person-centered care process, several counseling principles are particularly pertinent:

- *Motivation.* Changed behavior in any area requires motivation, the desire and the ability to achieve one's goals. Until the patient perceives food patterns and behaviors as appropriate goals, it is best to wait for a better time and begin with establishing a general supportive climate in which to continue working together. Any specific obstacle raised by the patient, such as time, physical limitations, money, or increased anxiety, can be met with related suggestions to think about. Priorities among needs should be recognized in the care plan and items introduced according to order of importance and immediacy of the patient's nutritional problems.
- *Rationale.* Any diet or food behavior change, with possible benefits and risks, must be clearly ex-

Are AIDS Patients Targets for Nutritional Hucksters?

TO PROBE FURTHER

When diseases such as acquired immunodeficiency syndrome (AIDS) lack curative therapy and have poor prognosis, many persons afflicted with such a disease are susceptible to claims of unproven, alternative therapies, that is, nutrition quackery. Some of the alternative therapies and approaches that are being touted as treatments for HIV infection include the following questionable practices.

Megadoses of nutrients

Large doses of vitamins A, C, E, B_{12}, selenium, and zinc have been recommended to restore cell-mediated immunity by increasing T cell number and activity. The value of such large doses has not been established by controlled clinical studies. In fact, the opposite is true; megadoses of these nutrients can be dangerous. Chronic intakes of vitamin A in excess of 50,000 IU/day can produce toxicity. Chronic intakes of excess zinc, as little as 25 mg/day, can cause gastrointestinal distress, nausea, and impaired immune function. Selenium is also toxic in high chronic doses, but the level at which this toxicity occurs is uncertain.

Dr. Berger's immune power diet

In his book, Berger (1985) states that poor health is caused by "immune hypersensitivity" to many foods such as milk, wheat, corn, yeast, soy, sugar, and eggs. He suggests a 21-day elimination diet for foods believed to cause allergies, followed by a reintroduction phase, then a maintenance diet to prevent food sensitivities and "revitalize" the immune system. The usefulness of this diet has not been tested or proven by scientific studies. The diet promoted in Berger's book (high in fruits and vegetables and low in fat and calcium) may produce undernutrition, and the suggestion that moldy food be consumed to test for allergy to molds may be dangerous to persons who are immunocompromised.

AL 721

AL 721, developed in Israel and approved by the FDA for clinical trials, is composed of "active lipids" (AL) mixed in a ratio of 70% neutral lipid, 20% lecithin, and 10% phosphatidylethanolamine—hence the 721 designation. It has been hypothesized that 721 can reduce or inhibit HIV infection. Clinical trials found little toxicity but no consistent trends in T cell quantitation or HIV cultures. Increases in body weight, serum total, and HDL and LDL cholesterol levels were noted. AL 721 can be made at home from soy or egg yolk lecithin or obtained already mixed, but is of unknown purity and can spoil easily if stored improperly.

Butylated Hydroxytoluene

Claims that Butylated Hydroxytoluene (BHT) kills HIV by attacking the "coating" on the virus are unfounded and unproven. The safety of its use is also questionable.

---

plained to the patient. The question "Why?" is always important to everybody.

- *Provider-patient agreement.* In the best interests of all concerned, the patient and health care provider must agree to the change. Any change should be structured around daily routines and include any care-givers as needed, and the counselor should provide any needed information and encouragement throughout the process.
- *Manageable steps.* All information given and actions agreed on should proceed in manageable steps, as small as need be, in order of complexity and difficulty. Information overload turns anyone off, but the particular stress load at any point here can be too intolerable for the patient to bear. At such points of stress, patients are also more vulnerable to the lure of unproven HIV therapies (see *To Probe Further* above).

Personal Food Management Skills

The patient's living situation and general practical skills in planning, purchasing, and preparing food must be considered. Information and guidance in developing skills in any aspect of procuring food, or in sources of needed help, should be provided.

Community Programs

Information may be needed about any available community food programs, such as Meals on Wheels for delivery of prepared meals at times the patient is too ill to get out for food. Also, information about food assistance programs, (Food Stamps or Food Commodities), for which the lower income person may qualify, may need to be provided.

Psychosocial Support

In the last analysis, every aspect of care provided should be given within a form and context that also provides genuine psychosocial support. All health care providers working with HIV-infected patients must be particularly sensitive to the special psychologic and social issues that confront persons with AIDS. Major stress areas may include issues relating to autonomy and dependency, a sense of uncertainty

"Maximum immunity diet"

Any value for megadoses of vitamin C to strengthen the immune system has not been established. Rebound scurvy has occurred upon cessation of the megadoses.

Laetrile

When used in combination with a strict vegan diet and vitamin supplements, laetrile is supposed to destroy a tumor enzyme (B-glucuronidase). In addition to being proven ineffective, this low-energy diet may supply inadequate amounts of calcium, iron, niacin, and vitamin B_{12}, and excessive amounts of thiamin, vitamins A and C, and zinc.

Gerson method

This program restricts all foods other than oatmeal and uncanned fresh fruits and vegetables, and advocates regular enemas, especially coffee enemas, to create an internal environment hostile to malignant cells. Efficacy has not been proven, not to mention the inadequacy of the diet.

Kelley regime

The Kelley regime excludes meat, milk in all forms except yogurt, and peanuts from the diet to overcome supposed pancreatic enzyme deficiency. Almonds are substituted for meat, and nutritional supplements including vitamins and minerals are recommended. Deficiencies of protein and calcium and fluid and electrolyte losses are possible in addition to possible vitamin A toxicity.

Yeast-free diet

The exclusion of high-carbohydrate and yeast-containing foods is supposed to prevent opportunistic yeast infections such as candidiasis. The underlying theory behind this has been characterized as speculative and there is a possibility that undernutrition may result.

Macrobiotic diet

A macrobiotic diet is based on oriental philosophy that it will restore balance and harmony between yin and yang forces and thereby improve health. However, it is very low in fat and high in fiber: 50% (by volume) whole grain cereals, 20%-30% vegetables, 10%-15% cooked beans or seaweed; and 5% miso (fermented soy paste) or tamari broth soup. This regimen can produce protein-kcalorie malnutrition, and provides inadequate intake of riboflavin, niacin, calcium in adults as well as pyridoxine and vitamins B_{12} and D in children (in addition to those nutrients mentioned for adults).

While it is conceivable that there are nutrients and other dietary substances than may improve some of the symptoms associated with HIV infection, it is still too early in our understanding of the disease process to make recommendations about supplementation. Alternative therapies require further study in controlled clinical trials.

REFERENCES

Dwyer JT et al: Unproven nutrition therapies for AIDS: what is the evidence? *Nutr Today* 23:25, 1988.

Raiten, DJ: Nutrition and HIV infection: a review and evaluation of the extant knowledge of the relationship between nutrition and HIV infection, *Nutr Clin Prac* 6(3):S1, 1991.

and fear of the unknown, grief, change and loss, fear of symptoms, fears of abandonment, and spiritual questions that arise when anyone is confronting a life-threatening illness.[48,49] Common emotions are hostility, denial, withdrawal, depression, anxiety, guilt, and confusion. All of these at one time or another may significantly influence treatment. Health care providers must always be aware and assess how the patient and caregivers are relating to the disease, using assistance of social workers, clinical psychologists, or psychiatrists as needed.[50,51] Stress reduction groups, including exercise training, are helpful, as they have proved to be in other life-threatening situations such as cancer and coronary heart disease.[52]

Most of all, however, health care workers must examine their own values and fears regarding sexual orientation, sexual behavior, intravenous drug use, and fears of AIDS transmission. Preconceived judgments are easily picked up by patients and threaten the provider-patient relationship. Before they can be effective with patients, all health care workers must first deal with their fears and prejudices and learn to let go such judgmental behavior.

To Sum Up

The viral evolution and current worldwide spread of human immunodeficiency virus (HIV) infection has reached epidemic proportions and is still growing. The disease progression follows three distinct stages of HIV infection, AIDS-related complex (ARC) with associated opportunistic illnesses, and full-blown acquired immunodeficiency syndrome (AIDS) with complicating diseases leading to death. This overall disease progression from initial infection to death lasts about 10 to 12 years. The Public Health Service and the Centers for Disease Control of the U.S. Department of Health and Human Services have responsibilities for monitoring the disease and providing leadership in research and treatment development in collaborative information exchange with scientists worldwide.

During the initial decade of the epidemic in the 1980s scientists learned the nature and lifecycle of the new mutation of HIV and its transmission modes and population groups at risk. Development of diagnostic testing procedures has enabled population surveillance and individual detection of disease and personal care to proceed. A fundamental role of nutrition support in this personal care of HIV-infected individuals has become evident.

Medical management of HIV infection, as yet without a vaccine or cure, involves supportive treatment of associated illnesses and complicating diseases. In the terminal HIV stage, as the virus eventually gains sufficient strength to destroy the host's immune system white cells, death follows. New drugs to slow the disease progression are developing.

Nutritional management centers on providing personal individual nutrition support to counteract the severe body wasting and malnutrition characteristic of the disease. The process of nutritional care involves comprehensive nutrition assessment and evaluation of personal needs, planning care with each patient and caregivers, and meeting practical food needs. Throughout the care process, nutrition counseling, education, and strategic services also help provide psychosocial support to each patient.

QUESTIONS FOR REVIEW

1. Describe the evolutionary history of the human immunodeficiency virus (HIV-1) and its current worldwide epidemic spread. How is it transmitted and why do you think it has spread so rapidly? Identify major population groups at risk.
2. Describe the nature of the AIDS virus and its action in the human body. What is a retrovirus?
3. Describe the progression of HIV infection in terms of its three basic stages of development from initial infection to death.
4. Identify some of the drugs currently used in medical management of HIV infection, and describe any associated actions, side effects, or toxicities that may relate to dietary management.
5. Outline basic parts of a comprehensive initial nutrition assessment of a patient with HIV infection and describe the reasons for each type of information and its evaluation.
6. Describe the general process of planning nutritional care on the basis of the patient assessment information and the main types of nutrition problems in HIV infection. Devise a related plan of action for each type of problem. Can you give an example of how you might follow-up to see what worked or did not work and make adjustments?

REFERENCES

1. Gold JWM: HIV-1 infection, *Med Clin North Am* 76(1):1, 1992.
2. Gorman C: Invincible AIDS, *Time* 140(5):30, 1992.
3. Cowley G: The future of AIDS, *Newsweek* CXXI(12):46, 1993.
4. Palca J: The sobering geography of AIDS, *Science* 252:372, 1991.
5. Castro KG et al: Perspectives on HIV/AIDS epidemiology and prevention from the Eighth International Conference on AIDS, *Am J Pub Health* 82(11):1465, 1992.
6. Pantaleo G et al: HIV infection is active and progressive in lymphoid tissue during the clinically latent stage of disease, *Nature* 362(6418):355, 1993.
7. Embretson J et al: Massive covert infection of helper T lymphocytes and macrophages by HIV during the incubation period of AIDS, *Nature* 362(6418):359, 1993.
8. Temin HM, Bolognesi DP: Where has HIV been hiding? *Nature* 362(6418):292, 1993.
9. Maddox J: Where the virus hides away, *Nature* 362(6418):287, 1993.
10. Cohen J: Keystone's blunt message: "It's the virus, stupid," *Science* 260(5106):292, 1993.
11. Hoover DR et al: The progression of untreated HIV-1 infection prior to AIDS, *Am J Pub Health* 82(11):1538, 1992.
12. Mills J, Masur H: AIDS-related infections, *Sci Am* 263(2):50, 1990.
13. Bayer R: The ethics of blinded HIV surveillance testing, *Am J Pub Health* 83(4):496, 1993.
14. Buehler JW: The surveillance definition for AIDS, *Am J Pub Health* 82(11):1462, 1992.
15. DesJarlais DC et al: Implications of the revised surveillance definition: AIDS among New York City drug users, *Am J Pub Health* 82(11):1531, 1992.
16. Otten MW et al: Changes in sexually transmitted disease rates after HIV testing and posttest counseling, Miami, 1988 to 1989, *Am J Pub Health* 83(4):529, 1993.
17. Onorato IM et al: Sentinel surveillance for HIV-2 infection in high-risk US populations, *Am J Pub Health* 83(4):515, 1993.
18. US Department of Health and Human Services, Public Health Services: *Healthy people 2000:* national health promotion and disease prevention objectives. DHHS Pub No 91-50212, Washington, DC, 1991, US Government Printing Office.
19. Wickizer TM et al: Activating communities for health promotion: a process evaluation method, *Am J Pub Health* 83(4):561, 1993.
20. Ehrhardt AA: Trends in sexual behavior and the HIV pandemic, *Am J Pub Health* 82(11):1459, 1992.
21. Weiss SH: HIV infection and the health care worker, *Med Clin North Am* 76(1):269, 1992.
22. Pizzo PA, Butler KM: In the vertical transmission of HIV, timing may be everything, *N Engl J Med* 325(9):652, 1991.
23. Glebatis DM et al: Hospitalization of HIV-seropositive newborns with AIDS-related disease within the first year of life, *Am J Pub Health* 81(suppl):46, 1991.
24. Stricof RL et al: HIV seroprevalence in clients of sentinel family planning clinics, *Am J Pub Health* 81(suppl):41, 1991.
25. Catania JA et al: Condom use in multi-ethnic neighborhoods of San Francisco: the population-based AMEN (AIDS in multi-ethnic neighborhoods) Study, *Am J Pub Health* 82:284, 1992.
26. Roper WL et al: Condoms and HIV/STD prevention: clarifying the message, *Am J Pub Health* 83(4):501, 1993.

27. Gollub EL, Stein ZA: The new female condom: item 1 on a woman's AIDS prevention agenda, *Am J Pub Health* 83(4):498, 1993.

28. New York Statewide Professional Standards Review Council: HIV testing policy. In Criteria manual for the treatment of AIDS, New York, 1990, *AIDS Intervention Management System.*

29. Raiten DJ: Nutrition and HIV infection: a review and evaluation of the extant knowledge of the relationship between nutrition and HIV infection, *Nutr Clin Prac* 6(suppl 3):13S, 1991.

30. Pluda JM et al: Hematologic effects of AIDS therapies, *Hematol Oncol Clin North Am* 5(2):229, 1991.

31. Cohen J: AIDS vaccine trials: bumpy road ahead, *Science* 251(4999):1312, 1991.

32. Cohen J: AIDS vaccine meeting: international trials soon, *Science* 254(5032):647, 1991.

33. Cohen J: AIDS vaccines: MicroGeneSys withdraws from trials, *Science* 259(5103):1821, 1993.

34. Centers for Disease Control: *Acquired immunodeficiency syndrome weekly surveillance report,* US AIDS Program, Centers for Disease Control, Center for Infectious Diseases, 1987.

35. Serwadda D et al: Slim disease: a new disease in Uganda and its association with HTLV-III infection, *The Lancet* 2:849, 1985.

36. Kotler DP et al: Magnitude of body-cell mass depletion and the timing of death from wasting in AIDS, *Am J Clin Nutr* 50:444, 1989.

37. Hellerstein MK et al: Current approach to the treatment of human immunodeficiency virus-associated weight loss: pathophysiologic considerations and emerging management strategies, *Semin Oncol* 17(6, suppl 9):17, 1990.

38. Tchekmedyian NS et al: Treatment of anorexia and weight loss with megesterol acetate in patients with cancer or acquired immunodeficiency syndrome, *Semin Oncol* 18(1, suppl 2):35, 1991.

39. Kotler DP et al: Enteropathy associated with the acquired immunodeficiency syndrome, *Ann Intern Med* 101:428, 1984.

40. Gillin JS et al: Malabsorption and mucosal abnormalities of the small intestine in the acquired immunodeficiency syndrome, *Ann Intern Med* 102:619, 1985.

41. Heise C et al: Human immunodeficiency virus infection of enterocytes and mononuclear cells in human jejunal mucosa, *Gastroenterology* 100:1522, 1991.

42. Ullrich R et al: Small intestinal structure and function in patients infected with human immunodeficiency virus (HIV): evidence for HIV induced enteropathy, *Ann Intern Med* 111:15, 1989.

43. Greenson JK et al: AIDS enteropathy: occult enteric infections and duodenal mucosal alterations in chronic diarrhea, *Ann Intern Med* 114:366, 1991.

44. Grunfeld C et al: Resting energy expenditures, caloric intake, and short-term weight change in human immunodeficiency virus infection and the acquired immunodeficiency syndrome, *Am J Clin Nutr* 55:455, 1992.

45. Grunfeld C et al: Circulating interferon-α levels and hypertriglyceridemia in the acquired immunodeficiency syndrome, *Am J Med* 90:154, 1991.

46. Hickey MS: Nutritional support of patients with AIDS, *Surg Clin North Am* 71(3):645, 1991.

47. Newman CF, Capazza CM: Home nutrition support in HIV disease, *J Home Health Care Prac* 3(2):25, 1991.

48. Ghiron L et al: Nutrition support of the HIV-positive, ARC, and AIDS patient, *Clin Nutr* 8(3):103, 1989.

49. Cleary PD et al: Depressive symptoms in blood donors notified of HIV infection, *Am J Pub Health* 83(4):534, 1993.

50. Antoni MH et al: Cognitive-behavioral stress management intervention buffers distress responses and immunologic changes following notification of HIV-1 seropositivity, *J Consult Clin Psychol* 59(6):906, 1991.

51. Jacobsberg LB, Perry S: Psychiatric disturbances, *Med Clin North Am* 76(1):99, 1992.

52. LaPerriere A et al: Aerobic exercise training in an AIDS risk group, *Int J Sports Med* 12(suppl 1):S53, 1991.

FURTHER READING

Hecker LM, Kotler DP: Malnutrition in patients with AIDS, *Nutr Rev* 48(11):393, 1990.

Tanowitz HB et al: Gastrointestinal manifestations, *Med Clin North Am* 76(1):45, 1992.

The two excellent review articles address two main areas of nutritional management, effects of HIV infection on (1) the gastrointestinal tract that hinder eating and absorption, and (2) the severe body wasting and malnutrition. The authors, experienced in clinical care and research concerning AIDS, provide background of these problems as a basis for providing relevant nutritional care.

Charny A, Ludman EK: Treating malnutrition in AIDS: comparison of dietitians' practices and nutrition care guidelines, *J Am Diet Assoc* 91(10):1273, 1991.

McCorkindale C et al: Nutritional status of HIV-infected patients during the early disease stages, *J Am Diet Assoc* 90(9):1236, 1990.

Trujillo EB et al: Assessment of nutritional status, nutrient intake, and nutrition support in AIDS patients, *J Am Diet Assoc* 92(4):477, 1992.

Ysseldyke LL: Nutritional complications and incidence of malnutrition among AIDS patients, *J Am Diet Assoc* 91(2):217, 1991.

These four articles from the Journal of the American Dietetic Association provide helpful information and nutritional care guidelines for developing nutritional care plans to meet the complicating factors of malnutrition and opportunistic diseases.

Weaver K: Reversible malnutrition in AIDS, *Am J Nurs* 91(9):25, 1991.

From her experiences as a nurse on the nutrition support team of a leading San Francisco Hospital providing care for many AIDS patients, this author gives practical and sensitive attention to quality-of-life problems inherent in progression of disease in the HIV-infected person.

CASE STUDY

HIV Infection in a Young Mother

Mrs. Theresa Stevens is a 25-year-old mother, admitted to the hospital with a history of weight loss, weakness, and watery diarrhea. She is married and has a 3-year-old son. Her husband is in a rehabilitation program for I.V. drug abuse. About one year ago she started to notice that she was becoming easily fatigued, but attributed it to taking care of a 2-year-old child. When her appetite began to wane and her weight dropped from 150 pounds to 90 pounds she went to her physician. In addition to the fatigue and weight loss, she reported fever and night sweats. Physical examination revealed swollen lymph glands, tongue lesions of herpes simplex, and perianal ulcers. Her physician admitted her to the hospital and further tests indicated depressed T cells and bronchial washings showed the presence of *Pneumocystis carinii* pneumonia. She was tested for HIV infection since *P. carinii* is uncommon in persons with healthy immune systems. Her blood test for HIV infection antibodies was positive.

While in the hospital, she developed symptoms of several infections: anorexia, fever, fatigue, nausea, vomiting, watery diarrhea, perianal ulcers, and rectal incontinence. Her temperature frequently registered 39.4° C (103° F) despite therapy with multiple antibiotics. The volume of diarrhea was measured to be 2500 ml/day and her vomiting necessitated intravenous hydration. She also began to receive treatment for *Pneumocystis carinii* pneumonia, esophageal candidiasis, oral and lingual herpes, and *Mycobacterium avium intracellulare* infection of the duodenum.

The patient did not tolerate a soft diet with nutritional supplements, continued to lose weight, and demonstrated severe anorexia, abdominal cramping, and bloating. Results of the nutritional assessment are as follows:

Height (cm)	100.1
Weight (kg)	40.9
Body weight (% ideal)	65
Body weight (% usual)	70
Triceps skinfold (% standard)	40
Mid-arm muscle circumference (% standard)	72
Serum albumin (g/dl)	2.2
Serum total protein (g/dl)	5.6
Serum total iron binding capacity (TIBC) (μg/dl)	192
Estimated resting energy expenditure (REE)	1750

Questions for Analysis

1. Name and describe several major clinical complications of the final stage of AIDS. How can these complicating diseases profoundly compromise a patient's nutritional status?
2. On the basis of the nutritional assessment, what is this patient's nutritional diagnosis?
3. What should be the goal of nutritional therapy based on the baseline nutritional assessment data and the patient's history?
4. By what route of feeding should nutritional support be administered?

REFERENCE

Rago RR, Feurer ID: Acquired immunodeficiency syndrome (AIDS). In Blackburn GL et al (eds): *Nutritional medicine: a case management approach,* Philadelphia, 1989, WB Saunders.

Special Consideration for Pediatric Patients with AIDS

Although limited, the available information on pediatric AIDS indicates that malnutrition, particularly undernutrition of kcalories, is a recurring problem. With adults, the disease alone impacts nutrition status, but in children, growth and development add to the impact of disease process.

Nutritional assessments should be performed routinely in pediatric patients with AIDS so any problems can be identified and treated as they occur and nutritional deficits can be minimized. Assessments should include anthropometry, plasma protein evaluation, complete blood counts, and evaluation of appetite and intake. Eating ability should be determined and the social situation evaluated.

Providing enough kcalories to maintain linear growth and weight gain is sometimes difficult. Increasing protein intake 50% to 100% over the RDA has been recommended. However, needs are individual and should be monitored. Suggestions to provide supplemental kcaloric and nutrient intake are listed below:

- Use a kcalorie-dense formula (24 to 27 kcal/oz) for infants. Add glucose polymers or medium-chain triglycerides to formulas or reduce the amount of water added to powdered formulas to boost kcalories.
- Try food supplements that are high in kcalories and protein.
- Add fats such as butter, margarine, or mayonnaise to foods to boost kcalories.
- Encourage nutrient-dense snacks such as raisins and peanuts or peanut butter.
- For the older, lactose-tolerant child, add skim milk powder to whole milk to boost kcalories and proteins.
- Make adjustments in diet consistency and temperatures to overcome eating difficulties associated with disease complications and any other eating problems.
- For lactose-intolerance, which occurs frequently in children with AIDS, use lactose-free, soy-based infant formulas instead of milk.
- Add Lactaid, a commercial preparation of lactose, to milk products to permit improved digestion.
- Use low-lactose dairy foods such as yogurt and mild cheddar cheese, if tolerated.

Vitamin and mineral supplements in amounts one or two times the RDA may offset possible deficits and contribute to meeting increased requirements during hypermetabolic states. Attention should also be given to drug-nutrient interactions and other effects of drugs on nutritional status.

Proper procedures and sanitary formula preparation must be followed for infants being bottle fed. Infants should not be put to bed with a bottle of milk or juice as they are easily contaminated. Unpasteurized milk and milk products should also be avoided as they may be a source of Salmonella and other microorganisms that can cause intestinal infections.

Children should never be fed any food directly from a jar to avoid possible bacterial contamination of the remaining food from the child's mouth. Fruits and vegetables should be peeled or cooked, and meats should be well cooked. All utensils and dishes should be washed in a dishwasher or in hot sudsy water and air dried.

REFERENCES

Bentler M, Stanish M: Nutrition support of the pediatric patient with AIDS, *J Am Diet Assoc* 87:488, 1987.

Berry RK: Home care of the child with AIDS, *Pediatr Nurs* 14:341, 1988.

Carrott Top Nutrition Resources: *Nutrition handbook for AIDS*, Aurora, Colo, 1988, Carrot Top Nutrition Resources.

Grossman M: Special problems in the child with AIDS. In Sande MA, Volberding PA (eds): *The medical management of AIDS*, ed 2, Philadelphia, 1990, WB Saunders.

Maring Klug R: AIDS beyond the hospital. II. Children with AIDS, *Am J Nurs* 86:1126, 1986.

Raiten DJ: Nutrition and HIV infection: a review and evaluation of the extant knowledge of the relationship between nutrition and HIV infection, *Nutr Clin Prac* 6(3):S1, 1991.

CHAPTER 13

Nutrition and Cancer

CHAPTER OUTLINE

Cancer Pathogenesis and Nutrition
Cancer Therapy and Nutrition
Nutritional Therapy and Cancer
Eating Problems in Cancer Patients

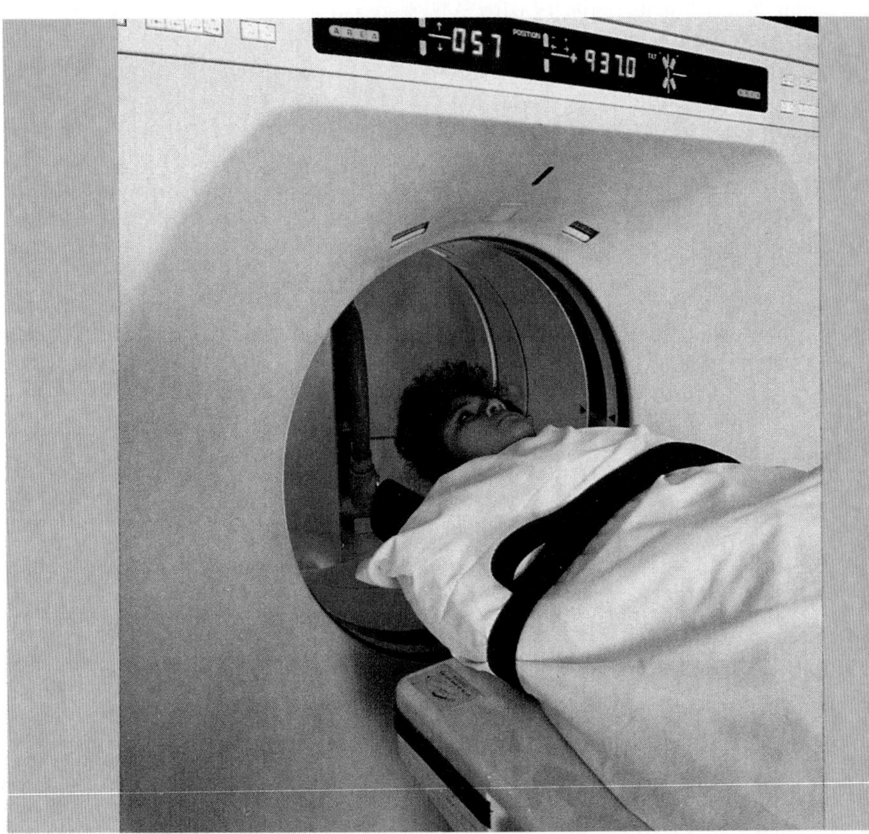

In this chapter we focus on cancer, one of the major diseases in the Western world. We examine the nature of the cancer process and its treatments and seek to relate these processes to the nutritional factors involved.

The U.S. Department of Health and Human Services estimates that about 510,000 Americans die of cancer each year, with 30% dying of lung cancer. In its multiple forms cancer has become one of our major public health problems, second only to heart disease, and accounts for about 20% of the total deaths in the United States each year.

In attempting to understand the nature of cancer and its relationship to nutrition, we immediately confront related problems of defi-

nition and study. The types of cancer are many and vary worldwide, and their definition changes with population migrations, multiple etiologies, and conflicting research results. We find that we are not dealing with a single entity, but rather with a wide range of malignant tumors collectively known as cancer. It is thus more correct to use the plural term cancers.

In this chapter we relate nutrition and cancer in two basic areas: (1) prevention, *through the environment and the body's defense system; and (2)* therapy, *through nutritional support for medical treatment and rehabilitation. To understand these nutritional relationships we must understand the nature of cancer as a growth process, the physiologic basis of cancer in the structure and function of cells, and the body's defense systems in immunity and in the healing process.*

Cancer Pathogenesis and Nutrition

The term **cancer** refers to the process of inappropriate malignant **neoplasms** (new growths), or tumors, forming in various body tissue sites. Since nutrition is fundamental to all tissue growth, we need to look briefly at the cancer cell to understand the relationship of nutritional factors to cancer. This "misguided cell" and its tumor tissue represent normal cell growth that has gone wild.

Cancer Cell

In adult humans some 3 to 4 million cells complete the normal life-sustaining process of cell division every second, largely without mistake, and guided by the genetic code. The central question in cell biology has been this: How are the process and rate of cell reproduction maintained so precisely in normal cells? The question in cancer research, based on the increased knowledge of normal cell physiology, follows: How and why is this normal, precise regulation of cell reproduction and function lost in cancer cells, and why do cancer cells then remain mutant and malformed, functionally immature, imperfect, and incapable of normal cell life?

Principles of Cancer Pathogenesis

Cells arise only from preexisting cells by division and carry the genetic pattern of the preexisting cell. As this knowledge is applied to disease and to problems in cancer pathogenesis, several key principles emerge.

Gene Control

Normally the various cell structures and functions operate in an orderly manner under the control of genes, which direct the specific processes of protein synthesis in the cell. Gene action may be switched on and off, depending on the position of a cell in the body, the stage of body development, and the external environment. Specific regulator genes control function by producing a repressor substance as needed to regulate operator genes and structural genes. This orderly regulation of induction and repression of cell activity may be lost with mutation of the regulatory genes. Control is also lost when a specific gene for some reason moves from its position to another location on the chromosome. A cell may become malignant when one of these potentially cancer-causing genes is then translocated and reinserted into a highly active part of the deoxyribonucleic acid (DNA) (Fig. 13-1). This has been shown to occur, for example, in patients with Burkitt's lymphoma and the blood cancer acute nonlymphocytic leukemia. Now apparently these root causes of damaged DNA and the impaired ability of the cell to repair it are joined by the recently discovered cellular genes called *proto-oncogenes,* which in their developed form of **oncogenes** cause neoplastic growth. The proliferation of normal cells is regulated by a counterbalance between growth-promoting proto-oncogenes and growth-restraining tumor suppressor genes.[1] This search for genetic damage and the explanation of how that damage affects biochemical function in the cell are key lines of current research holding much promise for further unfolding the mysteries of cancer.

Normal Cell Derivation

The cancer cell is derived from a normal cell that has lost control over cell reproduction and is thereby transformed from a normal cell to a cancer cell.

Cancer Tumor Types

Based on cell nature and differentiation, it is possible to classify cancer tumor types according to (1) originating tissue, with those arising from connective tissue

cancer • A malignant cellular tumor with properties of tissue invasion and spreading to other parts of the body.

neoplasm • Any new or abnormal cellular growth, specifically one that is uncontrolled and progressive.

oncogene • Any of various genes that, when activated as by radiation or by a virus, may cause a normal cell to become cancerous; viral genetic material carrying the potential of cancer and passed from parent to offspring.

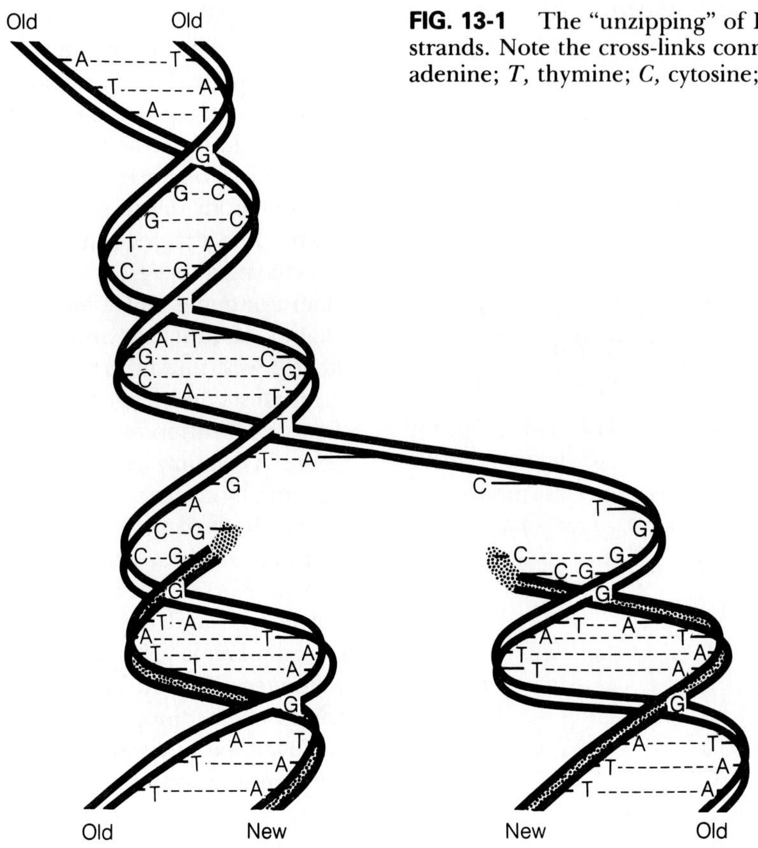

FIG. 13-1 The "unzipping" of DNA to form new RNA strands. Note the cross-links connecting the strands: *A*, adenine; *T*, thymine; *C*, cytosine; *G*, guanine.

called **sarcomas** and those from epithelial tissue called **carcinomas,** and (2) extent or degree of cell tissue change and differentiation, with stages defined according to rate of growth, degree of autonomy, and invasiveness.

Relation to the Aging Process

Since the incidence of cancer increases with age, a relationship exists between cancer genesis and the aging process in cells, tissues, and organ systems.

Causes of Cancer Cell Development

It is thus evident that the basic cause of cancers is a fundamental loss of control over normal cell reproduction. Researchers have discovered several interrelated causes contributing to this loss of cell control.

Mutations

Mutations result from loss of one or more regulatory genes in the cell nucleus. Such mutant genes may be inherited or released by exposure to some environmental agent.

Chemical Carcinogens

Chemical carcinogens interfere with the structure or function of regulatory genes. The greatest exposure to such agents that comes by individual choice is in cigarette smoking. Other exposure comes by general environmental substances such as natural and synthetic pesticide residues, water and air pollution, food additives and contaminants, and occupational hazards. However, many of our natural environmental agents carry more hazard, depending on the dose.[2] For example, a weak carcinogen such as saccharine may be a potential hazard if persons consume relatively large amounts of it; whereas a potent workplace carcinogen may pose little hazard to a worker who is protected and receives little exposure.[3] The principle that "the dose makes the poison" applies to all substances, including carcinogens, natural or synthetic. Possible cancer-causing actions of such substances may be mutation, effect on regulation of gene function, or activation of a dormant virus.

Radiation

Radiation that is sufficient to damage DNA causes breakage and incorrect rejoining of chromosomes. Radiation may be ionizing, such as from x-rays, radioactive materials, or atomic exhausts and wastes, or it may be nonionizing, such as from sunlight. Our current pursuit of the bronzed-god look has taken a large toll; sun-related skin cancer is rapidly on the rise in the United States and Europe, afflicting younger and younger persons. The common form on the head and neck is usually basal cell carcinoma and is easily cured by surgical removal. However, a far more lethal form, **malignant melanoma,** occurs in the skin cells that produce the pigment *melanin* and accounts for about 2% of all cancers. In the United States the incidence varies with latitude, from 22,500 cases/year in northern states to 65,000 cases in southern states. The rising incidence is probably due to increased recreational exposure to sunlight. The mortality rate is about 45%.

Oncogenic Viruses

Oncogenic, or tumor-inducing, viruses that interfere with the function of regulatory genes have been identified. Oncogenes involved are the focus of much current research related to cell growth factors and possible new therapies for blocking tumor cell growth.[1,4,5] Although oncogenes were first found in viruses, their evolutionary history indicates that they are also present and functioning in normal vertebrate cells. What leads to cancerous growth is their abnormal expression. A virus, which is little more than a packet of genetic information encased in a protein coat, contains a small chromosome of DNA or ribonucleic acid (RNA) with a relatively small number of genes, usually fewer than five and never more than several hundred. In contrast, cells of complex organisms have tens of thousands of genes. Generally when viruses produce disease, they act as parasites, taking over the cell machinery to replicate themselves. Continuing study indicates that viruses must be thought of as the second most important risk factor for cancer development, exceeded only by tobacco use.[6]

Epidemiologic Factors

Answers to the enigma of cancer have also been sought in epidemiologic studies of distribution and occurrence in relation to factors such as race, diet, region, gender, age, heredity, and occupation but with variable and conflicting results. It is becoming increasingly clear, for example, that racial differences in cancer incidence between blacks and whites in the U. S. are great, with more cancer among blacks than whites, and have nothing to do with race but have much to do with poverty, which has implications for nutritional status, health care, education, and resources.[7,8] The world incidence of cancer varies greatly from country to country, and that of specific cancer types varies from sixfold to 300-fold. Although our cancer incidence rates have not changed much over the past few decades, cancer is *endemic* in our population; the U.S. incidence rates are appreciably greater than those in many other countries.

Intriguing epidemiologic data have come from the changes in cancer observed in migratory populations. For example, in Japan, colon and breast cancer are low, and stomach cancers are high; the reverse is true in the United States. However, within two or three generations Japanese immigrants to the United States show a shift of cancer incidence from that of Japan to that of the United States as their native dietary habits slowly change to match those of American life. Although it has been difficult to pinpoint specific dietary factors in cancer etiology, worldwide epidemiologic studies show significant correlation of mortality from breast cancer with the consumption of dietary fats in countries around the world.

Epidemiologic evidence from case-control studies provides a basis for a primary prevention approach for reducing cancer risks.[9,10]

Stress Factors

The idea that emotions may play a part in malignancy is not new. The second century Greek physician, Galen, wrote of such relationships, as have many different kinds of "healers" since that time. Although these relationships are difficult to measure, that does not mean they do not exist. Even with great technologic and scientific advances in Western societies, medicine holds fast to the scientific method and its basic tenet that a thing must be measurable under controlled conditions to be said to exist. Nonetheless, observations made of relationships between cancer and less measurable stress factors are increasing. Clinicians and researchers have reported that psychic trauma, especially the loss of a central relationship, does seem to carry with it a strong cancer correlation. The answer to such a possible relationship to cancer may lie in two physiologic areas: (1) damage to the thymus gland and the immune system, and (2) hormonal effects mediated through the hypothalamus, pituitary gland, and adrenal cortex (see Chapter 2). This "cascade of physiologic events" may provide the neurologic currency that converts anxiety to malignancy. Such a stressful state may also make a person more vulnerable to other factors present, influencing the integrity of the immune system, food behaviors, and nutritional status.

sarcoma • A tumor, usually malignant, arising from connective tissue.

carcinoma • A malignant new growth made up of epithelial cells, infiltrating the surrounding tissue, and spreading to other parts of the body.

malignant melanoma • A tumor tending to become progressively worse; composed of melanin, the dark pigment of the skin and other body tissues; usually arising from the skin; and aggravated by excessive sun exposure.

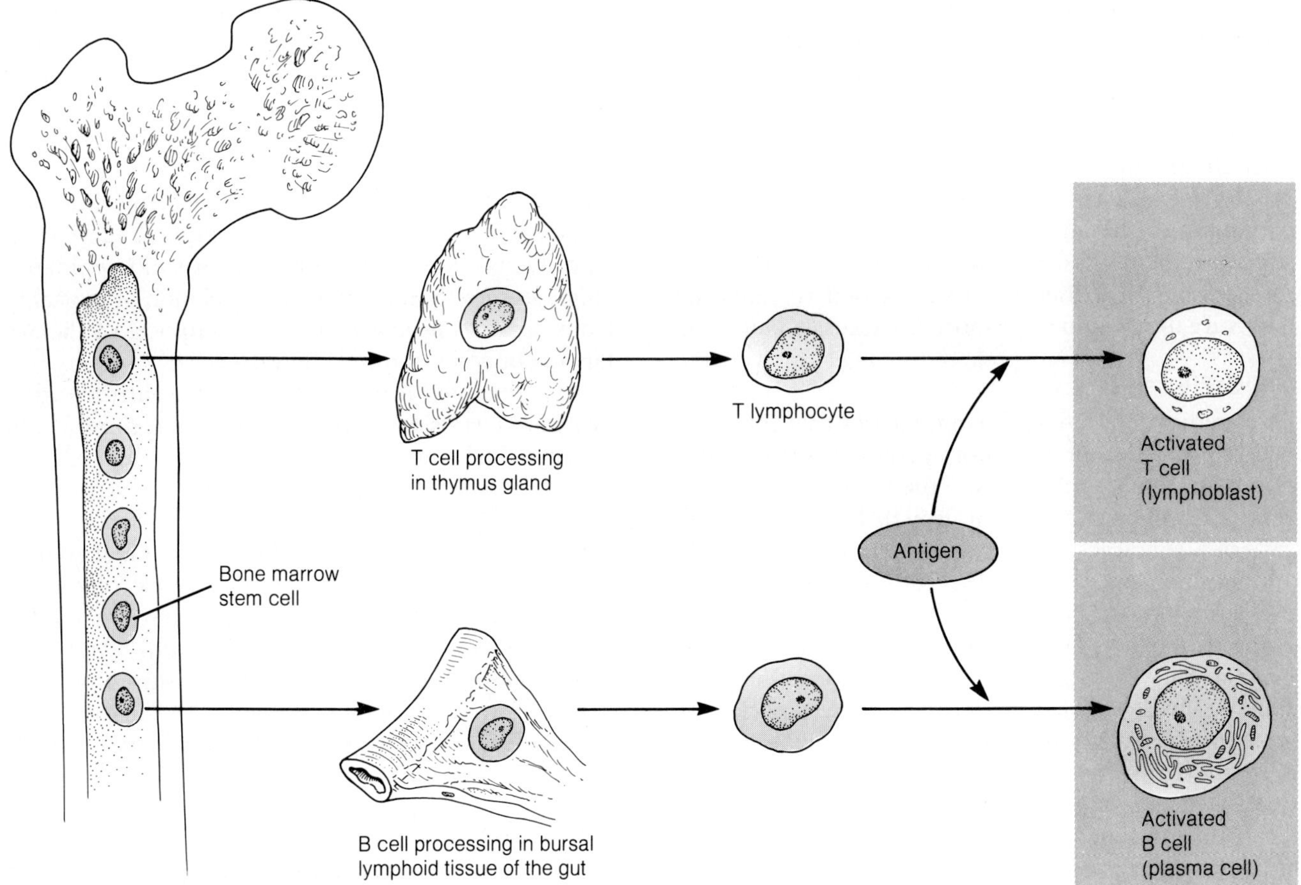

FIG. 13-2 Development of the T and B cells, lymphocyte components of the body's immune system.

Body's Defense System

We maintain a remarkably efficient and profoundly complex defense system. This normal immune response protects us not only against organisms such as bacteria and viruses that invade from outside the body but also against "alien" malignant cells from tumors that develop within the body, spreading invading cells into other body tissues and forming secondary tumors, or **metastases,** that become life-threatening.[11]

Components of the Immune System

The immune system consists of primary surveillance mechanisms to detect and destroy malignant cells arising daily in the body. Two major populations of lymphoid cells are involved, which in turn mediate specific **cellular immunity** and **humoral immunity** as well as supportive backup biologic systems. These two populations of lymphoid cells, or *lymphocytes,* a type of white blood cell, develop early in life from a common stem cell in the fetal liver and bone marrow (Fig. 13-2). They then differentiate and populate the peripheral lymphoid organs during the latter stages of gestation. They are called *T cells,* traced from thymus-derived cells, and *B cells,* traced from bursa-derived cells. Both T and B lymphocytes are derived from precursor cells in the bone marrow.

T Cells. After precursor cells migrate to the thymus, the T cell population is differentiated in this small gland, which lies posterior to the sternum and anterior to the great vessels partly covering the trachea. The thymus is a small organ, weighing about 14 g (½ oz) at birth, reaching its largest size of 37 g (1⅓ oz) at puberty, and shrinking in older age to a weight of 7 g (¼ oz). The T cells represent the majority of the circulating pool of lymphocytes in blood and lymph and in certain areas of the lymph nodes and spleen. These cells recognize invading antigens by means of specific specialized receptors on their surfaces. When T cells contact an *antigen*—a foreign intruder, a "non-self," or alien substance such as abnormal cancer cells—they proliferate and initiate specific cellular immune responses: (1) they activate the *phagocytes,* special cells of the reticuloendothelial system that have intracellular killing and degrading mechanisms for destroying invaders; and (2) they initiate the inflammatory response through chemical mediators released by the antigen-stimulated T cells. Scientists have now discovered that some T lymphocytes do even more, not only proliferating in response to an antigen but also attacking it. These special T cells are called "helper cell independent cytotoxic T lymphocytes," abbreviated *HIT cells.*

B Cells. The B cell population matures first in the bone marrow and then, following migration, in the solid peripheral lymphoid tissues of the body, lymph nodes, spleen, and gut. These cells are responsible for synthesis and secretion of specialized proteins known as *antibodies.* When the B cells contact an antigen, they proliferate, differentiate, and initiate specific humoral immune responses: (1) they start production of specific antibodies or *immunoglobulins* of the five major molecular classes (IgG, IgA, IgM, IgD, IgE) in the blood, and (2) they produce a specific form of immunoglobulin A (IgA) in secretions of the bowel and upper respiratory mucosa. A subsequent combination of antigen and antibody activates the complement system, which attracts phagocytes and initiates inflammation.

Integrity of the body's immune system components requires nutritional support. Members of severely malnourished populations show changes in the structure and function of the immune system with atrophy of the liver, bowel wall, bone marrow, spleen, and lymphoid tissue.[12,13] Thus the role of nutrition in maintaining normal immunity and in combating sustained attacks in malignancy is evident.

Nutritional Immunology

Integrity of body tissue and its capacity to maintain the healing process may be considered an added component of the body's overall defense system. Tissue protein synthesis requires optimal nutritional intake to support (1) the function and structure of the cell and all its parts, including DNA, RNA, amino acids, and proteins; and (2) the integrity of the immune system components.[12] Wise and early use of vigorous nutritional support for cancer patients has been shown to provide recovery of normal nutritional status, including immunocompetence, thereby improving their response to therapy and improving their prognoses. States of malnutrition, especially alcohol-induced, create a high risk of nutritional immunosuppression.[14]

Cancer Therapy and Nutrition

Current cancer therapy takes three major forms: *surgery, radiotherapy,* and *chemotherapy.* Nutritional support for any form of cancer therapy enhances its potential success.

Surgery

Early diagnosis of operable tumors has led to successful surgical treatment of a large number of cancer patients. As with any surgery and especially with hypermetabolic and frequently malnourished cancer patients, optimal nutritional status preoperatively and maximal nutritional support postoperatively are fundamental to the healing process. Nutrition contributes (1) support of the general healing process and overall body metabolism, and (2) specifically to the modification of nutrient factors, texture, or feeding mode according to the surgical site and organ function involved. Prevention of problems through early detection and surgical treatment has significantly increased cancer cure rates. Surgical treatment may also be used with other forms of therapy for removal of a single metastasis or for prevention and alleviation of symptoms.

Radiotherapy

Following the discovery of **radiation** in the nineteenth century, scientists soon found that it damages body tissue. Continued study of its use and control revealed that normal tissue could largely withstand an amount of radiation that would damage or destroy cancer tissue. The subsequent role of radiation in cancer treatment has developed around controlled use with two types of tumors: (1) those responsive to radiation therapy, or radiotherapy, within a dose level tolerable to health of normal tissue, and (2) those that may be targeted without damage to overlying vital organ tissue.

metastasis • The spread or transfer of disease from one organ or part to another not directly connected to the primary site.

cellular immunity • Specific acquired immunity in which the role of the T lymphocytes predominate.

humoral immunity • Specific acquired immunity in which the role of antibodies produced by the B lymphocytes and plasma cells predominate.

radiation • A form of cancer therapy using electromagnetic rays having both wave and particle functions; radio waves may span the entire spectrum from low-frequency through white light to high-frequency gamma rays.

Forms of Radiotherapy

Radiation used in cancer therapy is produced from three main sources:

1. *X-rays.* The oldest form of cancer treatment is with x-rays. These are electromagnetic waves similar to heat and light rays. Their penetration varies with the speed at which the electrons strike the target.
2. *Radioactive isotopes.* A number of elements occur in nature as radioactive materials, such as radium and uranium, and others are made radioactive by bombardment with high velocity atomic particles. These have been used for radiation therapy. Radioactive isotopes of these materials produce gamma rays as the unstable elements are broken down. One of the most common radioisotopes in present use is cobalt 60.
3. *Atomic particles.* Other atomic particles such as neutrons, protons, and electrons are accelerated to high velocities by accelerators and are being used to treat some cancers resistant to conventional types of radiation. These more recent developments of physics have enabled physicians to treat a larger number of cancer patients more effectively.

Effects of Radiotherapy in Cancer Management

Radiotherapy may be used alone or in conjunction with other therapies for curative and **palliative care** for some 50% of all cancer patients at some time during the course of their disease. Radiation effects influence nutritional status and therapy a great deal, depending on site and intensity of treatment.

Head and neck. Radiation to the head, neck, or esophagus affects the oral mucosa and the salivary secretions. It also influences taste sensations and sensitivity to food temperature and texture.

Abdomen. Radiation to the abdomen may produce denuded bowel mucosa, loss of villi and absorbing surface area, vascular changes from intimal thickening, thrombosis, ulcer formation, or inflammation. Obstruction, fistula formation, or strictures may further contribute to general malabsorption, compounded by curtailment of food intake resulting from anorexia and nausea.

Chemotherapy

Although chemotherapy has been recognized as a valid cancer therapy over the past few decades, the most effective agents currently in use have largely been developed only within the past few years.

Principles of Chemotherapeutic Action

Intensive research in the past few years has resulted in the development of a large number of effective *antineoplastic drugs.* Their therapeutic use is based on two general principles of rate and mode of action:

1. *Rate.* The so-called cell or log (logarithm) kill hypothesis of the action of chemotherapeutic agents on tumors indicates that a single dose may only be as much as 99.9% effective in killing the tumor cells. Thus if as large a tumor as is compatible with life—consisting of about 1 trillion cancer cells and weighing about 1 kg (2.2 lb)—may be treated with a drug tolerable at a toxicity level that is 99.9% effective, the tumor is reduced to a size of 1 billion cells, a 1-cm tumor. Successive doses causing this rate of "fractional killing" reduce the tumor to less than 100,000 cells and bring it within the capability of the body's own immune system to take over and make the final kill and cure. The smaller the tumor, either by early detection or by initial treatment by surgery or radiation, the greater the possible effectiveness of the chemotherapeutic agents. Also, two other principles of dosage rate for greater effectiveness are (1) aggressive use of maximal tolerable doses in repeated series and (2) use of several drugs together for a *synergistic* effect.
2. *Mode.* The relationship of the cell growth and reproduction cycle to mode of action of the various chemotherapeutic agents accounts for their combined effectiveness in controlling tumor growth and for their side effects. Nucleic acids provide the material essential for life of the cell: DNA produces RNA, which in turn guides amino acids into specific protein synthesis. Through the exquisitely interbalanced and regulated stages of the cell growth and the reproduction cycle of cell division, these materials carry out their orderly processes. The chemotherapeutic agents arrest the tumors by disrupting these cell processes, that is, some agents interfere with the production of the necessary nitrogenous bases of nucleic acids for normal DNA synthesis, whereas others disrupt the normal DNA structure and RNA replication. Still others prevent normal mitosis (or cell division), cause hormonal imbalances, or make specific amino acids necessary for protein synthesis unavailable. These modes of action help provide a basis for grouping agents into classes, as indicated in a following section. Those cells that reproduce most rapidly, such as cancer cells, are most responsive to these agents.

Toxic Effects of Chemotherapy

Chemotherapeutic agents have the same effects on rapidly reproducing normal cells as they do on rapidly reproducing cancer cells. Interference with normal function is most apparent in the normal cells of the bone marrow, the gastrointestinal tract, and the hair follicles, accounting for a number of the toxic side effects and problems in nutritional management:

1. *Bone marrow effects,* including interference with production of red cells (anemia), white cells (infections), and platelets (bleeding).

2. *Gastrointestinal effects,* including nausea and vomiting, **stomatitis,** anorexia, ulcers, and diarrhea.

3. *Hair follicle effects,* including alopecia (baldness) and general hair loss.

Classes of Chemotherapeutic Agents

According to their chemical nature or mode of action, the most commonly used cancer chemotherapeutic agents may be divided into the following six main classes:

1. *Alkaloids* (plant-derived agents) interfere with mitosis by disorganizing the chromosome spindles. Examples are the *Vinca* alkaloids vincristine and vinblastine derived from the periwinkle plant *(Vinca rosea).*

2. *Alkylating agents* interfere with cell division by binding to DNA, RNA, and certain cell enzymes, preventing their normal actions in control of cell reproduction. Examples are cisplatin and cyclophosphamide.

3. *Antibiotics* interfere with DNA structure or function, disrupting cell organization and actions. Examples are doxorubicin (Adriamycin), bleomycin, and mithramycin.

4. *Antimetabolites* interfere with DNA synthesis by blocking reactions that provide necessary precursors. Examples are methotrexate (limits the availability of folic acid), mercaptopurine, and 5-fluorouracil.

5. *Enzymes* interfere with reactions that make necessary amino acids available for protein synthesis. An example is L-asparaginase.

6. *Hormones* interfere with cell metabolism by altering the hormonal balance of the body with probable effects on the cell membrane. Examples are prednisone, estrogens, androgens, and progestins.

Modes of Chemotherapeutic Use

The cancer chemotherapeutic agents may be used in two ways:

1. *Combined therapy.* Combinations of drugs are used in a coordinated and sequential manner, allowing time between series for normal tissue recovery. An example is the so-called MOPP therapy, a combination of mechlorethamine (mustard), Oncovin (vincristine), procarbazine, and prednisone that is used for treatment of Hodgkin's disease.

2. *Adjuvant therapy.* Chemotherapy may be used in conjunction with other treatments such as surgery or radiotherapy to increase the cure rate.

Nutritional Therapy and Cancer

Numerous problems present needs for nutritional therapy and the care of patients with cancer. In general, nutritional therapy deals with two types of problems: (1) those related to the disease process itself and (2) those related to medical treatment of the disease process. Thus the basic objectives of nutritional therapy in cancer are (1) to meet the increased metabolic demands of the disease and prevent catabolism as much as possible and (2) to alleviate symptoms resulting from the disease and its treatment through adaptations of food and the feeding process.

Problems Related to the Disease Process

Problems forming the basic challenge to nutritional therapy are caused by general systemic effects of the neoplastic disease process and by specific responses related to the type of cancer.

General Systemic Reactions to Neoplastic Disease

Nutritional therapy in cancer is not so much concerned with specific nutrient-related etiologies and subsequent manipulations of these factors as it is with the overall systemic reactions of the body to the neoplastic disease process. Neoplastic disease is commonly associated with three basic systemic effects: *anorexia, hypermetabolic state,* and *negative nitrogen balance,* which are often accompanied by increasing weight loss. These effects may vary widely with individual patients according to type and stage of the disease from mild, scarcely discernible responses to the extreme forms of debilitating **cachexia** seen in advanced disease, and estimated to cause more than 50% of cancer deaths.[15,16] This extreme weight loss and weakness are caused by abnormalities in glucose and protein metabolism in which cancer patients cannot produce glucose efficiently from carbohydrates and instead "feed" off their own tissue protein and convert it to glucose.[15,17] The "new-old" drug hydrazine sulfate seems to correct this metabolic error, allowing patients to conserve more energy.[18]

Anorexia is frequently accompanied by depression or discomfort from normal eating. This contributes further to a limited nutrient intake at the time the disease process causes an increased metabolic rate and nutrient demand. Often this imbalance of decreased intake and increased demand creates a negative nitrogen balance, an indication of body tissue wasting. Sometimes a true tissue loss of protein is masked by outward nitrogen equilibrium as the growing tumor retains nitrogen at the expense of the host, further compounding the problem.

palliative care • Care affording relief but not cure; useful for comfort when cure is still unknown or obscured.

stomatitis • Inflammation of the oral mucosa, especially the buccal tissue lining the inside of the cheeks but also of the tongue, palate, floor of the mouth, and gums.

Specific Responses Related to Type of Cancer

In addition to the primary nutritional deficiencies induced by the disease, interrelated functional and metabolic problems that arise from specific types of cancer affect the body and further contribute to nutritional depletion. These secondary difficulties in ingestion and use of nutrients relate to specific tumors that cause obstructions or lesions in the gastrointestinal tract or adjacent tissue. Thus these conditions curtail intake of adequate nutrients.

Malabsorption. If the malignancy involves the pancreas, pancreatic duct, or common bile duct, normal secretory function of digestive enzymes and related materials such as bile salts is subsequently limited. Biliary obstruction also produces a deficiency of prothrombin, leading to blood-clotting problems and a deficiency of bile flow. This in turn interferes with normal digestion and absorption of fats and fat-soluble vitamins. A resulting vitamin D deficiency, for example, leads to further decreased calcium absorption and metabolism with subsequent osteomalacia. Protein and electrolyte absorption, as well as that of other nutrients, may also be diminished by solid tumor infiltration of the small intestine or by spread to lymph nodes.

Bypass problems. Abdominal tumors may also cause either gastrocolic or jejunocolic fistulas, which result in a bypass of the small intestine and contribute to subsequent malabsorption. Diarrhea, *steatorrhea,* and protein loss follow. Extensive protein may also be lost in exudates associated with various gastrointestinal enteropathies.

Fluid-electrolyte imbalances. Gastrointestinal lesions leading to general malabsorption also contribute to fluid and electrolyte losses. Ensuing vomiting and diarrhea not only bring loss of water but also cause loss of water-soluble vitamins. Tumors of the liver or metastasis involving heart muscle may bring liver or cardiac failure and consequent ascites and cardiac edema. Any urinary tract obstruction or renal involvement brings additional water imbalance. Any general obstruction of venous circulation or of the lymphatic drainage brings further edema. **Villous adenoma** and **adenocarcinoma** of the colon contribute to severe electrolyte imbalance.

Hormonal imbalances. Medullary carcinoma of the thyroid gland, with associated excess secretion of calcitonin and increased urinary sodium and phosphorus levels, contributes to *hyponatremia.* Intestinal malignancy and hyperadrenocorticalism contribute to *hypokalemia.* Osseous cancer and breast cancer with bone metastases contribute to *hypercalcemia.*

Anemia. The underlying problem of anemia may be compounded by a number of factors, including anorexia, with curtailment and malabsorption of dietary nutrients necessary for hemoglobin synthesis—iron, protein, folic acid, vitamin B_{12}, and vitamin C. Additional contributory factors may be increased hemolysis, bleeding of ulcerated lesions, or the presence of gastrointestinal fistulas.

Problems Related to Cancer Treatment

Medical treatments for cancer entail physiologic stress. These results include toxic tissue effects, often with damage to cell DNA structure, and changes in normal body function. Thus the benefit achieved is not without attendant problems. Nutritional support seeks to alleviate these problems.

Problems Related to Surgery

Beyond the regular nutritional needs surrounding any surgical procedure and its healing process, gastrointestinal surgery poses special problems for normal ingestion, digestion, and absorption of food nutrients. Head and neck surgery, or resections in the oropharyngeal area, are sometimes necessitated by cancer. Food intake is greatly affected in such cases, and a creative variety of food forms and semiliquid textures and modes of feeding must be devised. Often the mechanical problems of food ingestion make long-term tube-feeding necessary (see Chapter 3).

Gastrectomy may cause postgastrectomy "dumping syndrome" and necessitate frequent, small, low-carbohydrate feedings (see Chapter 11). **Vagotomy** contributes to gastric stasis. Various intestinal resections or tumor excisions may cause steatorrhea because of bacterial overgrowth in the afferent intestinal loop—blind loop syndrome, general malabsorption, fistulas, or **stenosis.** Pancreatectomy contributes to loss of digestive enzymes, induced insulin-dependent diabetes mellitus, and general weight loss.

Problems Related to Radiotherapy

Radiation to the oropharyngeal area often produces a loss of taste sensation with increasing anorexia and nausea and decreased appetite.[19] Other means of tempting appetite through food appearance, aroma,

villous adenoma • Epithelial tumor of the glandular structure forming a soft, large protrusion on the mucosa of the large intestine.

adenocarcinoma • Tumor arising from glandular tissue or in which tumor cells form glandular structures; usually classified according to a type of glandular cell arrangement.

TABLE 13–1

Medications Used to Control Nausea and Vomiting in Patients Receiving Chemotherapy

Antiemetic drug/ action	Cancer chemotherapeutic drug counteracted	Dosage used	Side effects	Comments
Phenothiazines Action: blocks CTZ* stimulation by dopamine Examples Compazine (prochlorperazine) Torecan (thiethylperazine) Phenergan (promethazine)	Moderate emetic-potential drugs	5-10 mg, orally or parenterally before chemotherapy; every 4-6 hr after for 24-48 hr	Sedation Orthostatic hypertension	Less effective when given on an "as needed" basis
Droperidol (Inapsine) Action: sedative and antiemetic	Cisplatin	0.5 mg intravenously 1 hr before chemotherapy; every 4 hr after chemotherapy	Somnolence	Some patients given up to 1.5 mg intravenously developed a tolerance for the drug
Corticosteroids	Cyclophosphamide			
Dexamethasone (Hexadrol, Decadron)	Doxorubicin	10 mg intramuscularly before chemotherapy	Perianal stinging if given too rapidly	Moderate to high relief in 70% of the patients
Methylprednisolone (Solu-Medrol)	Nitrogen mustard Mitomycin Methyl-CCNU†	250 mg intravenously every 6 hr for 4 doses beginning 2 hr after therapy	Swelling Facial rash Weakness, lethargy	Effects of methylprednisolone considered disappointing
Tetrahydrocannabinol (THC, marijuana)	Variety of agents studied Methotrexate 5-FU‡ Methyl-CCNU Cyclophosphamide Doxorubicin Nitrosoureas Mechlorethamine Cisplatin	10 mg/min^2	Somnolence Visual hallucinations	Patients (usually older) not used to THC refused to continue it because of CNS§ effects Response associated with extent of THC-induced "high" Most effective with fluorouracil, cyclophosphamide, methotrexate, doxorubicin "High" blocked by giving a phenothiazine
Metoclopramide (Reglan)	Cisplatin	Single 20-mg dose, given orally halfway through a 6-hr infusion of cisplatin (100 mg/min^2); higher doses might be possible intravenously (1-3 mg/kg/dose)	Sedation	Works well for patients who do not respond to other antiemetic drugs

Data modified from studies reported by Huber SL, Ballentine R: *Nutr Support Serv* 2(10):30, 1982.

* *CTZ,* Chemoreceptor zone (vomiting center in the brain).

† *Methyl-CCNU,*methyl-1-(2-chloroethyl)-3-cyclohexyl-1-nitrosourea.

‡ *5-FU,* 5-fluorouracil.

§ *CNS,* central nervous system.

and texture must be developed. Radiation to the abdomen may cause intestinal damage with tissue edema and congestion, decreased peristalsis, or **endarteritis** in small blood vessels. The intestinal wall may develop fibrosis, stenosis, necrosis, or ulceration. If these conditions continue, they may lead to hemorrhage, obstruction, fistulas, diarrhea, or malabsorption—all contributing to nutritional problems. The liver is somewhat more resistant to damage from radiation in adults, but children are more vulnerable.

Problems Related to Chemotherapy

The major nutritional problems during chemotherapy relate to (1) the gastrointestinal symptoms caused by the effect of the toxic drugs on the rapidly developing mucosal cells, (2) the anemia associated with effects on the bone marrow, and (3) the general systemic toxicity effect on appetite. The stomatitis, nausea, diarrhea, and malabsorption contribute to many food intolerances, although these responses are not true in all cases. Frequently before the chemotherapy is started for each series or course of treatment, an antiemetic drug such as prochlorperazine (Compazine) is used (Table 13-1). Such drugs act on the vomiting center in the brain to prevent the nausea response. Prolonged vomiting seriously affects fluid and electrolyte balance, especially in elderly persons, and needs to be controlled. Large scale controlled drug trials have reported successful antiemetic use of megestrol acetate (Megace) with breast cancer patients in whom the drug was tolerated well and who had increased appetites and food intakes accompanied by weight gains in true body mass rather than in fluid retention.[20] Megestrol, a synthetic female sex hormone similar to the natural hormone progesterone, was first noted to produce sharp increases in appetite and weight gain when used to treat advanced breast cancer and control metastasis.[21]

Special nutritional management has also been used during chemotherapy to improve food intake and reduce nausea and vomiting. In a pilot study with patients receiving a periodic treatment series of the drug cisplatin (Platinol), in comparison to the control group on full regular diets, the study group received a special diet of three planned meals a day of plain colorless, odorless foods, including items such as cottage cheese, applesauce, vanilla ice cream, and other predetermined foods.[22] The special diet was based on observations that chronic long-term cisplatin treatment cycles created conditioned, or learned, food aversions to odors and colors of foods and progressive malnutrition. Patients in the study group experienced far fewer episodes of nausea and vomiting, and greater food intake during the entire study period. The potential for developing conditioned food aversions while on long-term chemotherapy is diminished by use of food having little or no odor or color, because the drug-related *dysgeusia* and *dysosmia* are correlated with visual and olfactory stimulation factors.[22,23]

Certain chemotherapeutic drugs also have special effects. For example, monoamine oxidase inhibitors (MAOI) such as tranylcypromine sulfate (Parnate) and phenelzine sulfate (Nardil) may be used for pretreatment relief of mental or emotional depression or for palliative therapy. These antidepressant drugs cause well-known pressor effects when used with tyramine-rich foods (Table 13-2). Thus these foods should be avoided when using such drugs.

Principles of Nutritional Therapy for Cancer

Two important principles of nutritional therapy, which are vital in any sound nutritional practice but especially essential in the care of patients with cancer, provide the basis for planning nutritional care of each patient: (1) personal nutritional assessment and (2) vigorous nutritional therapy to maintain good nutritional status and thus support medical treatment.

Nutritional Assessment

The primary goal in nutritional care for cancer patients is to maintain a high level of body nutrition and prevent states of malnutrition. Since replenishing a malnourished patient is more difficult, initial assessment is imperative to determine individual status with vigorous follow-up care to maintain good nutrition. Therefore initial assessment for baseline data and regular monitoring thereafter are necessary. A detailed personal history is essential to determine individual needs, desires, and tolerances. To be valid the interview should be conducted as a conversation, using verbal and nonverbal probes and pauses rather than a cross fire of separate questions and answers.[24] (Review all of these procedures in Chapter 1.)

Nutritional Therapy and Plan of Care

Based on careful individual nutritional assessment, a plan for optimal nutrient therapy may be developed with each patient according to identified needs. Since *early,* vigorous attention to maintaining an optimal state of nutrition has proved to be essential to rates of success of medical treatment, primary care by the clinical nutritionist and the nurse on a regular basis is a necessary part of the oncology team practice. Working closely with the oncology nurse and physician, the clinical nutritionist assesses personal needs, determines nutritional requirements, plans and manages nutritional care, monitors progress and responses to therapy, and makes adjustments in care according to status and tolerances.

TABLE 13–2

Tyramine-Restricted Diet

General directions

- Designed for patients on monoamine oxidase inhibitors, drugs that have been reported to cause hypertensive crises when used with tyramine-rich foods. These include foods in which aging, protein breakdown, and putrefaction are used to increase flavor. Studies indicate that as little as 5 to 6 mg of tyramine may produce a response, and 25 mg is a dangerous dose.
- Food sources of other pressor amines such as histamine, dihydroxyphenylalanine, and hydroxytyramine are also avoided.
- Avoid all foods listed. Limited amounts of foods with a lower amount of tyramine, such as yeast bread, may be included in a specific diet.
- Avoid over-the-counter drugs such as decongestants, cold remedies, and antihistamines.

Foods to avoid		Additional foods to avoid
(Representative tyramine values in μg/g or ml)		Other aged cheeses
		Blue
		Boursault
Cheeses		Brick
New York State cheddar	1416	Cheddars (other)
Gruyère	516	Gouda
Stilton	466	Mozzarella
Emmentaler	225	Parmesan
Brie	180	Provolone
Camembert	86	Romano
Processed American	50	Roquefort
		Yeast and products made with yeast
Wines		Homemade bread
Chianti	25.4	Yeast extracts such as soup cubes, canned meats, and marmite
Sherry	3.6	
Riesling	0.6	Italian broad beans with pod (fava beans)
Sauternes	0.4	Meat
		Aged game
Beer, ale—varies with brand		Liver
Highest	4.4	Canned meats with yeast extracts
Average	2.3	Fish (salted dried)
Least	1.8	Herring, cod, capelin
		Pickled herring
		Other
		Chocolate
		Cream, especially sour
		Salad dressings
		Soy sauce
		Vanilla
		Yogurt

Nutritional Needs

Each of the nutrient factors related to tissue protein synthesis and energy metabolism requires careful attention. The increased needs for energy, protein, vitamins and minerals, and fluid are based on demands made by the disease and its treatment. Individual needs vary, but general guidelines are the same.

Energy

The total energy value of the diet must be increased to prevent excessive weight loss and to meet increased metabolic demands. Caloric density sufficient to counter catabolic or hypermetabolic states and to support necessary anabolism is necessary. Of this total dietary kcalorie value, carbohydrates must be sufficient to spare protein for vital tissue synthesis. For an adult patient with good nutritional status, about 2000 kcal provides for maintenance needs. A more malnourished patient may require 3000 to 4000 kcal, depending on the degree of malnutrition and body trauma. Carbohydrates should supply the majority of the energy intake, with fat restricted to 30% or less of the total kcalories. Numerous studies have related dietary fat to cancer risk, especially breast and colon cancer, and to cancer metastasis and effectiveness of cancer therapy.[25-27] The practical feasibility of dietary intervention programs to reduce fat intake has been demonstrated by recent studies of the National Cancer

Institute, a large multicentered pilot study, and the Women's Health Trial.[28,29] In these studies women with breast cancer and women at high risk for breast cancer were able to reduce their dietary fat from a baseline of approximately 40% of total kcalories from fat to 22% while increasing their intakes of all the vitamins and minerals. These results indicate that a nutritionally sound low-fat diet can be successfully implemented in highly motivated, free-living groups of individuals.

Protein

Additional protein is required to provide essential amino acids and nitrogen necessary for tissue regeneration, healing, and rehabilitation. A protein/kcalorie ratio sufficient to allow efficient use of protein and to prevent body protein wasting is important. An adult patient with good nutritional status needs about 80 to 100 g of protein to meet maintenance needs and to ensure anabolism. A malnourished patient needs more to replenish tissues and to ensure positive nitrogen balance.

Vitamins and Minerals

The need for key vitamins and minerals controlling efficient protein and amino acid metabolism and energy metabolism is basic. For example, the B-complex vitamins in general serve as necessary coenzyme agents in energy and protein metabolism. Vitamins A and C are important tissue-structuring materials. Vitamin A also has a significant role in protective immunity and cell differentiation; vitamin C has significant antioxidant, enzymatic, and immune biologic functions related to cancer.[30,31] Increased dietary consumption of vegetables and fruits is a primary means of obtaining these vitamins.[32] Recent studies of nutritional molecular carcinogenesis suggest also that the expression of certain oncogenes may be reduced by vitamins A, E, and D.[33] Vitamin D hormone ensures proper calcium and phosphorus metabolism in bone and in blood serum. Vitamin E protects the integrity of cell wall materials and hence tissue integrity. Many minerals function in structural or enzymatic roles in vital metabolic and tissue-building processes. Thus an optimal intake of vitamins and minerals, at least at recommended dietary allowance levels and augmented with supplements according to individual patient nutritional status, is indicated.

Fluid

Fluids are increased to counteract losses from gastrointestinal problems and any additional loss caused by infections and fever. Sufficient fluid intake is also necessary to help the kidneys rid the body of the breakdown products from destroyed cancer cells and from the drugs themselves. Increased fluid also helps protect the urinary tract from irritation and inflammation. For example, the use of some chemotherapeutic agents, such as cyclophosphamide (Cytoxan), requires 2 to 3 L of fluids daily to prevent hemorrhagic cystitis.

Eating Problems in Cancer Patients

The classic dictum of nutritional management given in Chapter 3 in the discussion of enteral nutrition support is also fundamental for patients with cancer: *"If the gut works, use it."* Oral and enteral feeding modes pose fewer problems, especially with cancer, than do alternate means. Faced with the need for increased nutrition in cancer therapy and attendant problems in food tolerances or ingestion, the nutritionist and the physician have a wide spectrum of feeding methods and materials available. From these they may select the most appropriate nutritional therapy for each patient, always basing clinical judgments on individual needs and circumstances. This spectrum of feeding modalities includes an oral diet amplified with nutrient supplements for increased protein, kcalories, vitamins, and minerals; enteral tube-feeding with several routes of entry; and parenteral nutrition through central and peripheral veins. Details of these modes of nutritional support are provided in Chapters 3 and 4.

If at all possible, normal ingestion of food with nutrient supplements as needed is most desirable. The diet must focus on protein and energy intake with optimal total nutrition. Based on individual nutritional assessment, including a personal interview, a personal food plan is developed with the patient incorporating desired food forms, tolerances, and family food patterns (see the *Clinical Application,* p. 275). Often the diet of the hospitalized patient is supplemented with familiar foods from home as the clinical nutritionist plans with the family. Food tolerances vary according to the current treatment and nature of the diseases. A number of adjustments in food texture, temperature, amount, timing, taste, appearance, and form are made to help alleviate symptoms stemming from common problems in successive parts of the gastrointestinal tract.

Difficulties in eating may be caused by loss of appetite, problems in the mouth, or swallowing problems.

Loss of Appetite

Anorexia is a major problem and curtails food intake when it is needed most. It is a general systemic effect of the cancer disease process itself. This loss of appetite is often further induced by the cancer treatment and may be progressively enhanced by anxiety, depression, and stress of the illness. Such a vicious cycle, if not countered by much effort, leads to more

CLINICAL APPLICATION

Promoting Oral Intake in Cancer Patients

Encouraging and maintaining adequate oral intake for cancer patients is one of the most difficult aspects of cancer treatment. It is time consuming and often frustrating, but may be one of the most rewarding experiences in patient care. By identifying feeding problems, initiating appropriate interventions, and providing individual education, adequate oral nutrition is promoted. The dietitian is the key figure for coordinating the nutritional program, but its success requires the full support and cooperation of the entire health care team, especially the nurse.

The patient interview is one of the most important parts of the nutritional assessment. Information that helps identify adequacy of current nutritional intake and potential nutritional problems is obtained during the interview. The following list of questions may assist in gathering accurate information about the patient's ability to obtain oral nutrition:

- How would you describe your appetite?
- Has it changed recently?
- Are you eating differently than you have most of your life?
- Do you usually eat three meals each day? Has this changed recently?
- Are you nauseated or experiencing vomiting? Is this food-related or medication-related? How long have you been experiencing this? How often do you vomit or feel nauseated?
- Do you have a bowel movement every day? Has this changed?
- Do you have diarrhea? If so, do you think this may be food-related?
- Do food smells or cooking odors bother you?
- Do you have difficulty chewing?
- Do your dentures (if any) fit? Do you wear them?
- Do you have difficulty swallowing?
- Is your mouth dry? Does your saliva seem to be different? Is it thicker or decreased in amounts?
- Do you find it easier to drink liquids than to eat solid foods?
- What were you able to eat yesterday? (Obtain a brief 24-hour dietary recall.)
- Are you unable to eat certain foods right now?
- Do some foods taste different to you? Can you give an example?
- Have you ever taken any high-kcalorie, high-protein supplements? When? What kind? How often? Were you able to tolerate them?
- Do you take a multivitamin supplement?
- Do you have any food allergies or intolerances? Are these new, or have you always experienced these intolerances?
- Do you prepare your own meals? If so, do you ever feel too tired to prepare something to eat?

The success of the interview depends on the dietitian's professional competence, interviewing skills, and bedside manner. If the dietitian establishes a feeling of comfort and trust with the patient, the opportunity to accomplish successful dietary interventions is great. ◆

REFERENCE

Nahikian-Nelms ML: Encouraging oral intake. In Bloch AS, ed: *Nutrition management of the cancer patient,* Rockville, Md, 1990, Aspen.

malnutrition and the well-recognized starvation "cancer cachexia." A program of eating *not dependent on the appetite for stimulus* must be planned with the patient and family. It is helpful sometimes to develop protein and caloric goals, discussing the role of nutrients and key foods in combating the disease and providing support for therapy. With such support the patient and family are better able to build a positive mental attitude toward the diet as an integral part of the treatment and a means of accepting responsibility for this aspect of therapy as much as possible. Often this positive attitude of the vital role patients play in their own treatment is a means of gaining some sense of control of their own lives, a sense frequently lost in the bewildering world of cancer and its therapy.

Many of the food suggestions given in this chapter for a variety of specific symptoms help improve appetite. The overall goal is to provide food with as much nutrient density as possible so that "every bite counts." Texture is varied as tolerated, with appeal to sensory perceptions of color, aroma, and taste to enhance the desire to eat. Often a series of small meals using a wide variety of food items is tolerated better than regular larger meals. If appetite is better in the morning, a good breakfast should be emphasized. Getting some exercise before meals and maintaining surroundings that reduce stress may also help in the eating process.

Mouth Problems

Various problems contributing to eating difficulties may stem from sore mouth, stomatitis, or taste changes. A sore mouth often results from chemotherapy or radiotherapy to the head and neck area. It is increased from any state of malnutrition or from infections such as **candidiasis** (thrush), with numer-

candidiasis • Infection with the fungus of the genus *Candida,* generally caused by *C. albicans,* so-named for the whitish appearance of its small lesions; usually a superficial infection in moist areas of the skin or inner mucous membranes.

ous ulcerations of the oral and throat mucosa. Frequent small meals and snacks soft in texture, bland in nature, and cool to cold in temperature are often tolerated better. Medications such as topical anesthetic liquids (lidocaine) used as sprays, mouth gels, or washes help relieve pain so that the patient may eat. Other simple water solutions with baking soda or salt help control irritation. Chemotherapy or radiotherapy to the head and neck may also cause alterations in the tongue's taste buds, causing taste distortion ("taste blindness") and inability to distinguish the basic tastes of salt, sweet, sour, or bitter with consequent food aversions. Since the aversion is often toward basic protein foods, a high-protein liquid supplement may be needed. Preparation of foods appealing in aroma and appearance and in small amounts should be continued. Since zinc deficiency is also related to diminished taste, sometimes a zinc supplement may be indicated.

Dental problems may also contribute to mouth difficulties. If brushing the teeth is painful, teeth may be cleaned with cotton swabs dipped in a 3% hydrogen peroxide solution diluted with warm water. Glycerin flavored with a few drops of lemon juice may be helpful as a mouth freshener, and sponge-tipped sticks impregnated with dentifrice are available. Attention to any dental work needed and moderation of concentrated sweets helps prevent dental problems.

Salivary secretions are also affected by cancer therapy, so foods with a high liquid content should be used. Solid foods may be swallowed more easily with the use of sauces, gravies, broths, yogurt, or salad dressings. A food processor or blender renders foods to semisolid or liquid forms and makes them easier to swallow. If the swallowing problem is especially severe because of tumor growth or therapy, guides for a special swallowing training program including progressive food textures, exercises, and positions may be followed.

Upper Gastrointestinal Problems

Eating difficulties in the upper gastrointestinal tract include nausea and vomiting, general indigestion, bloating, and specific surgery responses such as the postgastrectomy dumping syndrome (see Chapter 11). Nausea is often enhanced by foods that are hot, sweet, fatty, or spicy, so these things should be avoided according to individual tolerance. Frequent small feedings of cold foods, soft to liquid in texture, may be more appealing, and may be eaten slowly with rest in between. Eating dry foods such as crackers and dry toast on arising in the morning may be helpful. The physician may prescribe an antinausea drug such as prochlorperazine (Compazine) or megestrol acetate (Megase) to help with food tolerance.

Lower Gastrointestinal Problems

Food problems in the lower gastrointestinal tract include general diarrhea, constipation, flatulence, and specific lactose intolerance or surgery responses such as with intestinal resections and various ostomies. Helpful guidance for patients with colostomies, ileostomies, and ileoanal reservoirs is necessary (see Chapter 11). Lactose intolerance resulting from deficiency of the enzyme lactase calls for the avoidance of milk and milk products according to tolerance. The effect of chemotherapy or radiation treatment on the mucosal cells secreting lactase also contributes to this condition. In such cases a nutrient supplement formula with a soy protein base, which also has demonstrated anticarcinogenic activity, may be used.[34] To control diarrhea a diet of liquid or low-residue food with low-residue nutrient supplements is useful. As the condition improves, foods with more bulk may be added gradually in small, frequent meals. Constipation is helped by high-fiber foods, increased fluids, and naturally laxative foods such as prunes or juice.

Nutrient Supplements

A number of commercial nutrient supplement products are available. Their nutrient ratios should be studied carefully to make wise selections among them according to specific need. They are available in a variety of forms and flavors and may be used in different ways to enhance nutrient density, such as snacks between meals of regular food to add extra protein and kcalories or as additions to foods prepared. Some of the available formulas are elemental diets nutritionally complete for use when only low-residue liquids are used. A comparative review of these products provides the basis for developing a formulary in the hospital setting for a limited number of such products (see Chapter 3). A food processor may be used at home to produce creative solid and liquid food combinations from regular foods for interval liquid supplementation.

Involving cancer patients in their personal nutritional care plan is necessary for its success (see the *Clinical Application,* p. 275). They need to feel some sense of personal control. They participate in the choice of supplements and determine which products they prefer. By starting the patient with small quantities, the patient and the nutrition team then set goals for the quantities that need to be ingested. Individual patients may need to schedule their supplements as medications, which commits the entire health care team to the nutritional care plan. This team involvement helps the patient to understand the importance of adequate nutrition.[35]

Feeding in Terminal Illness

Although many advances have been made in the detection and treatment of cancer, mortality rates for some cancers have not declined and in some cancers have actually increased. For example, according to the National Cancer Institute, two decades ago 26.9

When Does Feeding Become an Ethical Issue?

TO PROBE FURTHER

Plato believed that the moral person and the physician both should abide by the Hippocratic principle of medicine, "Above all, do no harm." In recent times others have returned to Plato's use of this medical model of ethics.

Current writers assert that an ethic of care rests on the "premise of nonviolence—that no one should be hurt." The uniqueness of this outlook is that it insists that women have made a valuable contribution to ethical theory by stressing values associated with caring. These implications are profound, especially for professions comprised largely of women such as dietetics and nursing.

Technology such as enteral and parenteral nutrition may sometimes support a caring intent and compassionate spirit, while at other times such modern technology becomes a value in and of itself with its own standard of efficiency. Enteral and parenteral feeding techniques may be used to maintain indefinitely patients who are unable to take food orally.

Concerned ethical thinkers use the following moral principles for decisions in regard to life-sustaining treatment that encompasses enteral or parenteral nutrition: benefit to patient; respect for patient autonomy or self-determination; maintenance of moral integrity of health professionals; and justice in distributing scarce medical resources among eligible patients. They offer helpful views to guide clinicians in coming to a reasoned and defensible resolution of moral conflict.

- *Alternatives to artificial nutrition.* All options of nutritional support should be explored, not simply considering "Give food or fluids" versus "Do not give food or fluids." Dietitians are particularly useful in identifying alternative feeding strategies. The full range of therapeutic options should be carefully explored instead of assuming that the question is "Let the patient die" versus "Keep the patient alive."
- *Patient prognosis for recovery of functions.* A widely held ethically defensible view is that aggressive means of life prolongation becomes less morally desirable in proportion to the inability of the patient to regain what he or she considers to be useful function. The persistent vegetative state and permanent loss of consciousness are examples of extreme cases in which recovery of function is not possible. That accurately determining the prognosis for recovery is essential may be considered an understatement.
- *Total management plans and goals of therapy.* The patient's prognosis and nature of the illness might determine whether the goal of medical care is to attempt cure, to manage a chronic illness that cannot be cured so as to maintain maximal patient function, or to allow a terminally ill patient to die with maximal comfort and symptom control. Nutritional treatment may make excellent sense within one plan of care, but no sense at all in another.
- *Wishes of the patient or patient surrogate.* Legally and ethically acceptable is that in almost all cases the voluntary choice of an informed patient should be overriding. When the patient cannot choose, a surrogate or other substitute decision maker who is familiar with the patient's values and wishes may be consulted.
- *Ability of the patient to choose.* It is important to assess the patient's ability to make the particular medical care choice that is relevant to the matter at hand. In some circumstances, expert psychiatric or psychologic evaluation is needed to determine this.
- *Benefits and burdens of artificial treatment.* The medical team often tends to overestimate the benefits and underestimate the burdens of the treatments they use routinely. When the means of administering nutrition become invasive and painful, then the burdens may become substantial. Restraining the patient or repeated blood draws to monitor the effects of total parenteral nutrition may be deemed burdens unacceptable to the patient. Patients may feel that being kept alive by artificial means is an indignity itself and that life is no longer useful or meaningful to them. Spiritual and emotional burdens should be assessed equally with physical burdens in making accurate assessments of the moral obligations to patients.

Modern medical technology has produced circumstances that caregivers and patients alike have never faced before. Decisions regarding nutrition and hydration in terminally ill patients are becoming more frequent. Ethical and moral questions do not always have black or white solutions; they are often gray. The ethics task for dietitians may be to achieve balance between what works and who cares.

REFERENCES

Brody H, Noel MB: Dietitians' role in decisions to withhold nutrition and hydration, *J Am Diet Assoc* 91(5):580, 1991.

Dalton S: What are the sources and standards of ethical judgment in dietetics? *J Am Diet Assoc* 91(5):545, 1991.

Gilligan C: *In a different voice: psychological theory and women's development,* Cambridge, Mass, 1990, Harvard University Press.

The American Dietetic Association: Issues in feeding the terminally ill adult, *J Am Diet Assoc* 87:78, 1987.

women out of every 100,000 died of breast cancer; the rate by the end of the 1980s had grown to 27.5 per 100,000, and the trend seems to be heading upward.[36] Cancer is now the leading cause of death for women in the United States and if trends continue will be the leading overall cause of death in the United States by the year 2000.[9]

We feel these results in our work with cancer patients. We see the progressive weight loss and malnutrition that occurs, caused by the tumor and its metastasis, that leads to profound nutritional depletion and is a major cause of morbidity and mortality.[37] For some patients a time comes when the spread of the disease overcomes the body's resources to combat it. When the patient is no longer able to eat, enteral tube-feeding or parenteral feeding may be used. Ultimately, however, ethical questions about continued feeding efforts are faced in many such cases (see *To Probe Further,* p. 277). Answers lie with the patient, as long as possible, and with the family, but sensitive and supportive counseling is needed from the cancer team members, especially the clinical dietitian responsible for the nutritional support and the nurse responsible for administering the continued feeding and for personal care. These skilled professionals, along with the physician, the patient, and the family face these decisions together.[38]

To Sum Up

Cancer is a term applied to abnormal, malignant growth in various body tissue sites. The cancerous cell is derived from a normal cell but loses its control over reproduction. It is classified by its point of origin as a sarcoma (arising from connective tissue) or carcinoma (arising from epithelial tissue) and by stages according to the degree of cell tissue change, rate of growth, autonomy, and invasiveness.

Cancer cell development occurs via mutation, carcinogens, radiation, and oncogenic viruses. It is also apparently influenced by many epidemiologic factors such as diet, alcohol consumption, smoking, and physical and psychologic stress factors. Cell development is mediated by the body's immune system, primarily its T cells—a type of white cell found in blood, lymph, and certain parts of the lymph nodes and spleen—and B cells, which manufacture and secrete antibodies.

Cancer therapy consists primarily of surgery, radiotherapy, and chemotherapy. Supportive nutritional therapy for the cancer patient is highly individualized and depends on the response of each body system to the disease and to the treatment itself. It is based on a thorough nutritional assessment of energy, protein, electrolyte, and fluid needs and may be provided by a number of routes (oral, enteral, or parenteral). The oral route is preferred, if at all possible. In some cases nutrient and kcalorie supplements are required. These requirements must be designed for the specific physical and psychologic needs of the individual patient.

QUESTIONS FOR REVIEW

1. What is cancer? Identify and describe several major contributions to cancer cell formation.
2. How does your body attempt to defend itself against cancer? What nutritional factors may diminish this ability?
3. List and describe the rationale and mode of action of the types of therapies used to treat cancer.
4. Differentiate those factors challenging cancer recovery that are associated with the disease process versus the type of therapy used.
5. Outline a general procedure for the nutritional management of a cancer patient.

REFERENCES

1. Weinberg RA: Tumor suppressor genes, *Science* 254(5035):1138, 1991.
2. Ames BN et al: Ranking possible carcinogenic hazards, *Science* 236:271, 1987.
3. Report: Of interest to you: comparing possible hazards from natural and man-made substances, *J Am Diet Assoc* 92(5):597, 1992.
4. Aaronson SA: Growth factors and cancer, *Science* 254(5035):1146, 1991.
5. Marx J: Oncogenes evoke new cancer therapies, *Science* 249(4975):1376, 1990.
6. Hausen H: Viruses in human cancer, *Science* 254(5035):1167, 1991.
7. Gibbons A: Does war on cancer equal war on poverty? *Science* 253(5017):260, 1991.
8. Coates RJ et al: Race, nutritional status, and survival from breast cancer, *J Natl Cancer Inst* 82(21):1684, 1990.
9. Henderson BE et al: Toward the primary prevention of cancer, *Science* 254(5035):1131, 1991.
10. Wynder EL: Primary prevention of cancer: planning and policy considerations, *J Natl Cancer Inst* 83(7):475, 1991.
11. Liotta LA: Cancer invasion and metastasis, *Sci Am* 266(2):54, 1992.
12. Beisel WR: History of nutritional immunology: introduction and overview, *J Nutr* 122:591, 1992.
13. Chandra RK: Protein-energy malnutrition and immunological responses, *J Nutr* 122:597, 1992.
14. Watzl B, Watson RR: Role of alcohol abuse in nutrition immunosuppression, *J Nutr* 122:733, 1992.
15. Tayek JA, Chlebowski RT: Metabolic response to chemotherapy in colon cancer patients, *J Parenter Enteral Nutr* 16 (suppl 6):65, 1992.
16. Shaw JHF et al: Leucine kinetics in patients with benign disease, non-weight-losing cancer and cancer cachexia: studies at the whole-body and tissue level and the response to nutritional support, *Surgery* 109:37, 1991.

17. Tayck JA: A review of cancer cachexia and abnormal glucose metabolism in humans with cancer, *J Am Coll Nutr* 11:445, 1992.
18. Seligmann J, Witherspoon D: A new, old cancer drug, *Newsweek*, p 95, June 6, 1983.
19. Hearne BE et al: Enteral nutrition support in head and neck cancer: tube vs oral feeding during radiation therapy, *J Am Diet Assoc* 85:669, 1985.
20. Tchekmedyian NS et al: Nutrition in advanced cancer: anorexia as an outcome variable and target of therapy, *J Parenter Enteral Nutr* 16(suppl 6):88, 1992.
21. Tchekmedyian NS et al: High-dose megestrol acetate: a possible treatment for cachexia, *JAMA* 257:1195, 1987.
22. Menashian L et al: Improved food intake and reduced nausea and vomiting in patients given a restricted diet while receiving cisplatin chemotherapy, *J Am Diet Assoc* 92(1):58, 1992.
23. Darbinian J, Coulston A: Impact of chemotherapy on the nutritional status of the cancer patient. In Bloch A, ed: *Nutrition management of the cancer patient,* Rockville, Md, 1990, Aspen.
24. Jain M: Diet history: questionnaire and interview techniques used in some retrospective studies of cancer, *J Am Diet Assoc* 89(11):1647, 1989.
25. Djuric Z et al: Effects of a low-fat diet on levels of oxidative damage to DNA in human peripheral nucleated blood cells, *J Natl Cancer Inst* 83(11):766, 1991.
26. Erickson KL, Hubbard NE: Dietary fat and tumor metastasis, *Nutr Rev* 48(1):6, 1990.
27. Burns CP, Spector AA: Effects of lipids on cancer therapy, *Nutr Rev* 48(6):233, 1990.
28. Buzzard IM et al: Diet intervention methods to reduce fat intake: nutrient and food group composition of self-selected low-fat diets, *J Am Diet Assoc* 90(1):42, 1990.
29. Gorbach SL et al: Changes in food patterns during a low-fat dietary intervention in women, *J Am Diet Assoc* 90(6):802, 1990.
30. Ross C: Vitamin A and protective immunity, *Nutr Today* 27(4):18, 1992.
31. Henson DE et al: Ascorbic acid: biologic functions and relation to cancer, *J Natl Cancer Inst* 83(8):547, 1991.
32. Negri E et al: Vegetable and fruit consumption and cancer risk, *Int J Cancer* 48:350, 1991.
33. Prasad KN, Edwards-Prasad J: Expressions of some molecular cancer risk factors and their modification by vitamins, *J Am Coll Nutr* 9(1):28, 1990.
34. Messina M, Messina V: Increasing use of soyfoods and their potential role in cancer prevention, *J Am Diet Assoc* 91(7):836, 1991.
35. Nahikian-Nelms ML: Encouraging oral intake. In Bloch AS, ed: *Nutrition management of the cancer patient,* Rockville, Md, 1990, Aspen.
36. Marshall E: Breast cancer: statement in the war on cancer, *Science* 254(5039):1719, 1991.
37. Daly JM et al: Nutritional support in the cancer patients, *J Parenter Enteral Nutr* 14(suppl 5):244S, 1990.
38. Brody H, Noel MB: Dietitians' role in decisions to withhold nutrition and hydration, *J Am Diet Assoc* 91(5):580, 1991.

FURTHER READING

Ames BN et al: Ranking possible carcinogenic hazards, *Science* 236:271, 1987.

Dr. Ames provides results from his Berkeley laboratory studies on a wide variety of environmental carcinogens, explains why animal cancer tests cannot be used to predict absolute human risks, and supplies a large table ranking hazards.

Brody H, Noel MB: Dietitians' role in decisions to withhold nutrition and hydration, *J Am Diet Assoc* 91(5):580, 1991.
Dalton S: What are the sources and standards of ethical judgment in dietetics? *J Am Diet Assoc* 91(5):545, 1991.
Edelstein S, Anderson S: Bioethics and dietetics: education and attitudes, *J Am Diet Assoc* 91(5):546, 1991.
Wall MG et al: Feeding the terminally ill: dietitians attitudes and beliefs, *J Am Diet Assoc* 91(5):549, 1991.

These four articles in a single issue of the *Journal of the American Dietetic Association* provide guidance for facing difficult decisions involved in nutritional care of the terminally ill cancer patient.

Burkitt D: An approach to the reduction of the most common Western cancers: the failure of therapy to reduce disease, *Arch Surg* 126:345, 1991.

In his thought-provoking article Dr. Burkitt discusses cancer and environment, dietary changes, and the future of cancer research. He makes a strong case for primary prevention, indicating that there is no evidence that the incidence of any disease was ever reduced by treatment alone.

Bloch AS, ed: *Nutrition management of the cancer patient,* Rockville, Md, 1990, Aspen.

This helpful reference by an experienced oncology dietitian and her contributors provides a comprehensive background for a better understanding of the complexities of caring for cancer patients.

CASE STUDY

Patient with Cancer

Catherine Schofield is a 35-year-old mother of three young children. She was admitted to Green Hills Hospital 3 weeks ago with multiple enterocutaneous fistulas. She weighed 52 kg (116 lb) on admission and is 165 cm (5 ft 6 in) tall. Mrs. Schofield had undergone a hysterectomy 4 months before admission, following a recurrence of cervical cancer. During the chemotherapy that followed for 7 months, she had regular bouts with nausea and anorexia. Surgery was performed again. Her fistulas continued to drain for 2 weeks postoperatively, during which time she tolerated clear liquids only. An intravenous drip of 10% glucose and 0.45 normal saline was ordered to supplement fluids and kcalories. This week she developed peritonitis and has had a fever of 39° C (102° F) for the past 24 hours. Her weight has dropped to 41 kg (90 lb); drainage from the fistulas has become odorous. The patient was placed in isolation today and was advised by her physician that he intended to start her on total parenteral nutrition (TPN) and take some more tests to determine her progress.

Questions for Analysis

1. What types of nutritional assessment procedures would be used by the TPN team for planning Mrs. Schofield's nutritional therapy? Explain the purpose of each.
2. Calculate Mrs. Schofield's energy and protein needs, and account for increased needs.
3. Why did Mrs. Schofield develop nausea and anorexia during chemotherapy? What are the implications of this for recovery? Outline a plan for evaluating and controlling nausea and vomiting in patients undergoing chemotherapy.
4. What personal concerns would you expect Mrs. Schofield to have? What resources would you use to help her obtain the personal and physical support she probably needs?

Toward the Prevention of Cancer

Studies of geographic, socioeconomic, chronologic, and immigration patterns of cancer distribution indicate that the vast majority of cases of cancer are due primarily to environmental factors. The logical conclusion is that reduction of these causative factors may reduce or eliminate most forms of cancer.

The American Cancer Society suggests that two thirds of all cases of cancer in the United States are caused by only two factors: inhaled smoke and ingested food.

Tobacco, alone or in combination with alcohol, remains the most important cause of cancer, accounting for about one of every three cancer cases in the United States. Cigarettes are the most important cause of tobacco-related cancer, but other forms of tobacco (chewing tobacco and snuff) are also established carcinogens. The cancer risk of ex-smokers remains elevated compared to lifetime nonsmokers. However, quitting smoking, even late in life after heavy long-term abuse, greatly reduces cancer risk when compared with the risk had smoking been continued. Despite the rhetoric of tobacco companies, even regular smokers of low-tar cigarettes still have a much higher cancer risk than nonsmokers.

Alcohol, in addition to its synergistic effects with tobacco, increases risk of cancers of the oral cavity, pharynx, liver, and esophagus. Alcohol use has also been consistently linked to colorectal cancer and female breast cancer. Liquor, wine, and beer seem to be equal in effect on cancer risk.

Major incriminating dietary factors that appear now to be carcinogenic are the food changes that contrast current Western diets with those of our paleolithic hunter-gatherer ancestors. We have reduced the amount of energy we obtain from starchy foods by one half to two thirds. We have more than doubled the proportion of energy we derive from fat and changed from mostly unsaturated fats to saturated fats. We have increased our salt intake fivefold. And sugar now accounts for one fifth of our total energy intake. The diet of our ancestors was energy dilute, whereas our modern diet is energy dense.

Many studies link what we eat and don't eat to the development of cancer. Direct relationships between preserved or salty foods and nasopharynx and stomach cancer have been consistently observed in case-control and correlational studies. Generous use of fresh fruits and vegetables has consistently been found to decrease the risk of stomach cancer. Epidemiologic studies suggest a relation between high–animal fat, low-fiber intakes and colorectal cancer. The basis for this relationship lies in the decreased transit time through the colon associated with high-fiber diets, and the increased water content in the intestinal lumen that dilutes other nutrients such as animal fat.

Considerable, though not yet conclusive, evidence exists that ascorbic acid has a protective effect against cancer of the esophagus, larynx, and oral cavity. Nutrients such as vitamin A, beta-carotene, vitamin E, and ascorbic acid are thought to lower cancer risk in patients with elevated risk for cancers of the lung, esophagus, colon, and skin. Clinical and laboratory studies support findings that adequate intakes of vitamin D and calcium are associated with reduced incidence of colorectal cancer. These studies did not necessarily utilize supplemental amounts of these nutrients in addition to the RDAs but were based more on low levels of intake of these nutrients which would parallel the low levels of fresh fruit and vegetable intakes that are prevalent in our society.

The majority of the causes of cancer—such as tobacco, alcohol, animal fat, obesity, and ultraviolet light—are associated with life-style,—that is, personal choices and not environmental causes. This fact reinforces the basic truth that the best cure is prevention. Life-style changes are prevention.

REFERENCES

Burkitt D: An approach to the reduction of the most common Western cancers, *Arch Surg* 126:345, 1991.

Garland CF et al: Can colon cancer incidence and death rates be reduced with calcium and vitamin D? *Am J Clin Nutr* 54:193, 1991.

Greenwald P, Sondik EJ: Cancer control objectives, *J Natl Cancer Inst* 2:3, 1986.

Henderson BE et al: Toward the primary prevention of cancer, *Science* 254:1131, 1991.

Prasad KN, Edwards-Prasad J: Expressions of some molecular cancer risk factors and their modification by vitamins, *J Am Coll Nutr* 9(1):28, 1990.

Wynder EL: Primary prevention of cancer: planning and policy considerations, *J Natl Cancer Inst* 83(7):475, 1991.

CHAPTER 14

Nutritional Support in Disabling Disease and Rehabilitation

CHAPTER OUTLINE

Nutritional Support and Rehabilitative Care
Principles of Supportive Nutritional Care
Musculoskeletal Disease
Neuromuscular Disease
Progressive Neurologic Disorders

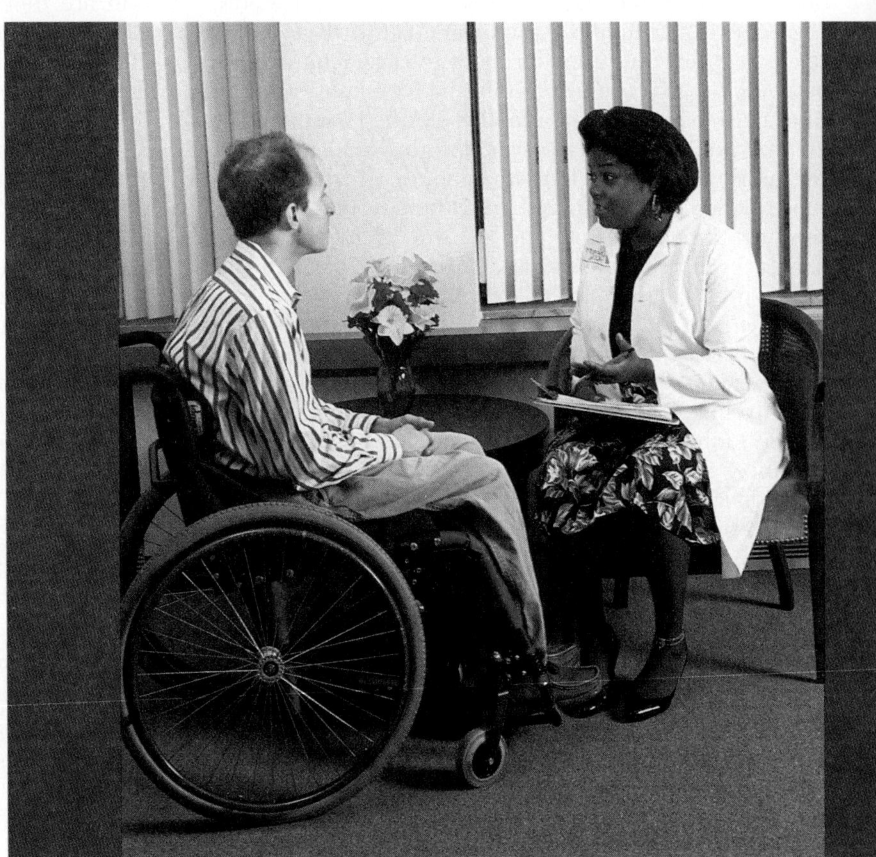

This chapter completes our clinical nutrition series. In addition to the primary care clinical problems we have reviewed in the preceding chapters, we conclude with a focus on long-term disabling disease requiring rehabilitative care.

Persons who have sustained severe injury or illness often require extended specialized care. These long-term needs result from the stress of disabling illness or injury, which carries added physical, mental, and social burdens. Such situations often involve profound trauma and devastating effects that call for tremendous coping resources from the patient and family.

In this final chapter we examine the supportive role of nutrition in the rehabilitative process following musculoskeletal disease such as arthritis; neuromuscular disease such as brain or spinal cord injury, stroke, or developmental disabilities; and progressive neurologic disorders, such as slowly developing Parkinson's disease or the catastrophic dementia of Alzheimer's disease. In each case we see that personalized nutritional care plays a vital role in the healing and restoring process. These traumatic situations demand special knowledge and skills and much personal strength.

Nutritional Support and Rehabilitative Care

Goals of Supportive Care

Positive goals guide care for those with disabling disease or injury. Successful support is rooted in a positive philosophy based on the optimal potential of each person affected. This approach requires a specialized team working together with the patient and family to meet individual needs. It is built on clearly defined *preventive* and *restorative* personal care objectives. To the greatest degree possible within each situation, two goals are fundamental in planning care: (1) to prevent further **disability** and (2) to restore potential function. Health workers and clients alike have developed many techniques of care to meet these two goals. Both of these key principles apply to nutritional care. Together with other specialized therapists on the rehabilitation team, the registered dietitian functions as the nutrition specialist and carries numerous nutritional care responsibilities[1]:

- *Nutritional assessment*—initial comprehensive evaluation and continuing reassessment at appropriate intervals
- *Nutritional therapy*—to meet fundamental nutrient and energy needs, as well as any special individual requirements
- *Eating or feeding assessment*—needs for self-help eating devices or food marketing and preparation
- *Assessment of dysphagia*—textural or other food or feeding modification needs
- *Coordination of community services*—referrals and communications to meet individual needs, home health care, rehabilitation, public health, vocational agencies, financial assistance, or other services
- *Nutritional education and counseling*—with the individual client, the family, and other caregivers

Team Approach Method

Through the health care system and its various resources and levels of care, how are these goals to be met? In some devastating cases obstacles may seem almost insurmountable. And in others, when an underlying disease may as yet lack a cure, the prognosis is poor. Nonetheless, these support goals remain valid, and everyone involved persists toward them. Often the patient's initial reaction is one of defeat and resignation or withdrawal. Certainly the patient and family cannot accomplish the necessary care alone. Such a complex and complicated process requires a strong *team approach*. A number of sensitive and skilled specialists lend their particular training, insights, and resources to identify specific personal needs and work with the patient and family to help develop some solutions. Rehabilitation team specialists include the physician (physiatrist), clinical nutritionist, nurse, occupational therapist, physical therapist, recreational therapist, psychologist, and social worker.

At all times, however, these health care specialists remember that the most important member of the team is the client. Goal setting is always personal and done *with*, not for, the client and family. These three partners—the professional specialists, the client, and the family—together form a greater health care team. It is always a shared, supportive undertaking, whatever the individual limitations or outcome (see *To Probe Further*, p. 284).

Socioeconomic and Psychologic Factors

Social Attitudes

The general attitudes of society toward disabled persons vary between extremes of overprotection and avoidance. These social attitudes result mainly from negative conditioning over years and are not easily changed. Some people are repelled by deformities or severe illness, perhaps because they sense their own vulnerability and mortality; others completely ignore them. Neither extreme approach is helpful. Overprotection robs persons of their sense of self and smothers the *will* to fight against surrounding odds and develop self-acceptance. But disabled persons do have varying special needs, and social avoidance of these needs creates additional problems in everyday living—doorways not made for wheelchairs, unmanageable stairs and street curbs, lack of access to public transportation, and many more daily barriers.

disability • Mental or physical impairment that prevents an individual from performing one or more gainful activities; not synonymous with **handicap**, which implies serious disadvantage.

Invisible Disability

TO PROBE FURTHER

Persons with obvious disabling conditions receive cues from others that help them adapt to their disabilities. Anyone with a disability undergoes some revision of self-concept, a disruption in familiar role patterns, and a period of adjustment to the limitations. This adjustment often involves stages of the classic mode of the "sick role": (1) exemption from normal responsibility, (2) wanting to get well, and (3) cooperation with health professionals.

However, the person with an invisible disability such as kidney failure, some types of cancer, cardiovascular disease, or diabetes is often denied these supportive cues and feedback in the difficult task of adjustment and is often denied obtaining employment. These conditions are not apparent or easily observed by casual acquaintances. Often this reinforces the use of denial of the actual limitations and more damage through poor self-care. The person is better able to avoid the sick role and ignore the condition's limitations. Yet these persons need rehabilitative support and training as much as those with more obvious disabilities.

These psychologic aspects of invisible disability carry implications for all members of the health care team. Because the loss is not tangible, the patient or client often lacks the support for living a normal life in the home or workplace, especially support for the initial grieving and adjustment needed for living with a chronic condition, which hinders adjustment. Health professionals must be aware of the psychodynamics of the adaptive process, must anticipate needs, must offer guidance, and must assist the client in mourning outwardly. Then the healing process may begin.

REFERENCES

Cross EW: Implementing the Americans with Disabilities Act, *J Am Diet Assoc* 93(3):273, 1993.

Falvo DR, Allen H, Maki DR: Psychosocial aspects of invisible disability, *Rehabil Lit* 43:2, 1982.

Economic Problems

Care of persons with disabling injury or severe illness is a long and costly process. A major area of exploration for the health care team is one of financial resources and assistance needed. Continuing long-term economic problems may also revolve around employment capabilities, earning capacities, or the means for providing care.

Living Situation

Disabled persons face many practical problems of everyday living. Whether a person needs long-term hospital care or maintains independent living, perhaps with an attendant, depends on a number of physical and situational factors. If, with help, the person can maintain a home, the necessary special equipment for maximal self-care and added care by the attendant must be provided (see *Issues and Answers,* p. 304).

Psychologic Barriers

Positive resolution of many practical and emotional problems requires tremendous psychologic adjustment. Each person struggles with self-image and physical body trauma, often withdrawing in defeat and exhaustion. Personality changes occur during rehabilitative processes that test inner strength and physical stamina. Depending on the nature of personal coping resources and defenses, the person may or may not be able to function. Much of the health team's keen insight and concern are directed toward supporting each person's efforts to meet individual needs. That many disabled persons do reach self-care goals in some measure is evident in the remarkable achievements some of them do attain despite, or perhaps because of, their difficulties.

Special Needs of Older Disabled Persons

America is aging. Population projections indicate that by the year 2000, 13% of the population will be over 65; by 2030, 22%. Over the next decade the most rapid population increase will be among those over 85 years of age.[2] And with older age comes an increased number of disabled elderly persons. The U.S. Rehabilitation Services Administration, using a baseline of 1 disabled American in 10, estimates that the odds of being disabled increase to 1 in 3 after age 65. Increased services, including rehabilitative services, are needed. But rehabilitative needs of older persons differ, of course, from those of younger persons. Three life-changing events of aging determine these needs: retirement, chronic illnesses, and general physical decline.

Vocational Rehabilitation

Without adequate planning ahead, many older persons experience stressful disorientation with retirement from a lifetime occupation of active involvement in a familiar working environment. Supportive activities focus on vocational planning and effective use of leisure time. At this point, many persons have not been accustomed to viewing leisure activities in a positive manner and need help in making this adjustment. In addition, vocational programs following retirement help persons find gainful employment or ways of contributing their wisdom and skills to others now working in their field. Such activity, in turn, enhances the health and social assets of the older person.

Residual Disabilities from Chronic Illnesses

In the age period of 60 to 75 (the young-old), rehabilitation must focus on problems remaining from heart disease, hypertension, cerebrovascular accident (CVA, stroke), or cancer. Chronic illnesses may be related to damaging health behaviors such as alcoholism, smoking, excessive eating of foods high in fat and salt, and a sedentary life. Survival after a heart attack or stroke may leave an older person with chronic disabilities. Early efforts at rehabilitation may be effective in preventing disability, avoiding complications, and restoring reasonable function.

Physical Decline in Aging

In persons between 75 and 85 years of age and older (the old-old), disability increases sharply. Much of this increase comes from falls and resulting fractures, chronic brain failure, disorders in locomotion, impaired senses of perception, and increased problems with drug reactions and interactions. Older persons may have multiple pathologic conditions and may take a number of different drugs or receive a variety of medical treatments. In this age group minor disabilities often result in major handicaps. Mental and physical dependency may require supportive care in the home or long-term care facility. Common health problems in the young-old and the old-old groups—including arthritis, depression, deficiencies because of poor dentition and fad diets, infections, skin and foot disorders, sensory deprivation, and cardiorespiratory and cardiovascular insufficiency—involve nutritional care as well.

In general, however, disease and disability do not affect only the young-old and old-old, nor are all of these age groups disabled. Many of the disabled are young persons, and many older adults continue to be fit and healthy. But the increasing age of the general population inevitably brings with it an increasing number of older adults with chronic diseases and various disabilities of aging. Even minor disabilities may cause major **handicaps** in everyday living, and minor injuries may bring major debilitating results. In any case the two goals of rehabilitative care continue to be prevention of further disability and the restoration of the maximal function available.

Principles of Supportive Nutritional Care

Prevention of Malnutrition

Kilocalories

The rehabilitative process of physical therapy involves hard work. The patient tires easily, and the energy intake must be sufficient to meet the energy output demands. Although excess kcalories must be avoided to prevent obesity, sufficient energy for tissue metabolism is essential.

Protein

General protein needs are based on maintaining strength of tissue structure and function. Tissue and organ integrity provides bulwark against catabolism, infections, negative nitrogen balance, and **decubitus ulcers.**[3] Dietary protein in optimal quantity and quality ensures the necessary supply of all the essential amino acids required for tissue synthesis. In addition to these general needs, severe trauma such as that involved in spinal cord injury brings special needs to meet the catabolic response (p. 290).

Carbohydrates

General energy needs are met by optimal dietary carbohydrates as the major fuel source. Severe trauma also requires maximal levels of carbohydrates, especially in the early stages following injury. More breakdown of tissue protein and fat occurs to provide needed energy, thus effectively adding to the negative nitrogen balance. Carbohydrate foods sufficient to provide the needed energy are therefore important.

Fat

At any point in rehabilitative care the diet must supply linoleic acid, the essential fatty acid, and a moderate amount of fat for the body's general metabolic activities and tissue integrity. The general dietary recommendation that fat supply about 30% of the total kcalories is sufficient. Some fat for food palatability also aids appetite, which tends to be poor in the course of long-confining illness.

Vitamins and Minerals

Optimal intake of vitamins and minerals for metabolic activity and nutritional maintenance is needed. The normal recommended dietary allowance (RDA) standards for age and sex are adequate in most cases, unless a deficiency state such as anemia indicates a need for supplementation. In some rehabilitation centers, however, multivitamin preparations are given routinely as insurance against deficiencies.

handicap • Mental or physical defect that may or may not be congenital that prevents the individual from participating in normal life activities; implies disadvantage.

decubitus ulcer • Pressure sores in long-term bed-bound or immobile patients at points of bony protuberances, where prolonged pressure of body weight in one position cuts off adequate blood circulation to that area, causing tissue death and ulceration.

Restoration of Eating Ability

Normal Development of the Eating Process

In the normal growth and development of a child the feeding and eating process develops through an overlapping and interdependent series of physical and physiologic stages. The usual activities of eating—swallowing, chewing, and hand and utensil use—gradually develop with motor ability, along with much practice and patience. With an understanding of these normal patterns, the disabled person works with the professional team of occupational and physical therapists, nutritionists, and nurses to find adaptive procedures to restore a basic eating ability. For each client, four aspects of the eating process require special individual attention: (1) the nature and degree of motor control, (2) eating position, (3) use of adapted utensils, and (4) supportive individual needs. For example, blind persons need a description of the food served, its placement on the plate named generally in a clockwise direction to help in remembering it, and a follow-up training course in preparing food with a number of assistive tools and techniques.

Nutritional Base

The personal food plan should fulfill basic nutritional needs. In addition, awareness of sensory stimuli such as variety in food texture, color, and flavor may enhance appetite and motivate learning of new adapted modes of eating. Providing "comfort foods" or familiar ethnic and well-liked foods also encourages the sometimes difficult process of relearning how to eat.

Independence in Daily Living

With each disabled person the goal is to achieve as much independence in daily living as possible. Maximum use is made of individual neuromotor resources and emotional reserves. These personal resources are aided by self-feeding devices as needed. A large number of these devices are available, many created by the inventive mind of a concerned occupational therapist.[4] For example, the catalog of Fred Sammons, Inc., currently containing over 1000 items, is well known to many dietitians and nurses and is in classrooms and on bookshelves across the country. It provides many ideas for developing and using tools for self-feeding and food preparation according to individual capacity and need. The Consulting Dietitians Practice Group of the American Dietetic Association, with Sammons' collaboration, has prepared a comprehensive training program for health care professionals, including a slide or tape presentation, a professional guide manual, and a feeding evaluation kit.

A number of representative disabling conditions illustrate various areas of need for supportive nutritional care. Next we briefly review examples of such conditions in three types of problems: (1) musculoskeletal disease, (2) neuromuscular disease, and (3) progressive neurologic disorders.

Musculoskeletal Disease

Rheumatoid Arthritis

Clinical Characteristics

Rheumatoid arthritis is a chronic, systemic inflammatory disease usually occurring in the young adult years. It is a severe type of *autoimmune* disorder in which the body's immune system acts against its own tissues, mainly the joints of the hands, arms, and feet, causing them to become extremely painful, stiff, and deformed. Although the precise triggering antigen is still unknown, a number of possible primary causes (a virus or several viruses) that stimulate the immune response in the immunogenetically susceptible host are under study.[5] The major clinical manifestations of rheumatoid arthritis in the joints involve tissue changes in the **synosheaths.** The disease primarily affects the small joints of the upper extremities, with rapidly progressing joint deformity and destruction. This disability dramatically affects activities of daily living, especially the fundamental necessity of obtaining and eating food. The hands and wrists are involved, including destruction of wrist ligaments and tendons, weakened finger and hand grip strength, and limited finger movement (Fig. 14-1), all of which limit ability to self-feed, shop for food, and prepare food.[6] Elbow and shoulder involvement also hinders bringing food to the mouth, and further tissue damage of the *temporomandibular joint (TMJ)* limits normal opening and closing of the mouth and alters chewing ability. Other nonjoint problems such as anemia of chronic disease, decreased salivary secretions, dysphagia, and bone disease further complicate nutritional problems leading to overall malnutrition.[6-8]

Medical Management

Medical treatment may involve a number of drugs for the control of the inflammatory process. These drugs include salicylates, nonsteroidal antiinflammatory agents, antimalarial agents, gold salts, D-penicillamine, steroids, and immunosuppressive agents.[5] Weekly low-dose therapy with the anticancer drug methotrexate, which acts as an antimetabolite to folic acid in DNA synthesis, is sometimes used but frequently causes the complicating viral condition **herpes zoster.**[9] Aspirin, as well as other nonsteroidal antiinflammatory drugs (NSAIDs), is still a mainstay of medical therapy, with use of enteric-coated preparations to avoid gastric irritation (see Chapter 6). When irreversible destruction of cartilage occurs in advanced stages of the disease, reconstructive joint surgery along with physical therapy and occupational therapy gives the best results.[5]

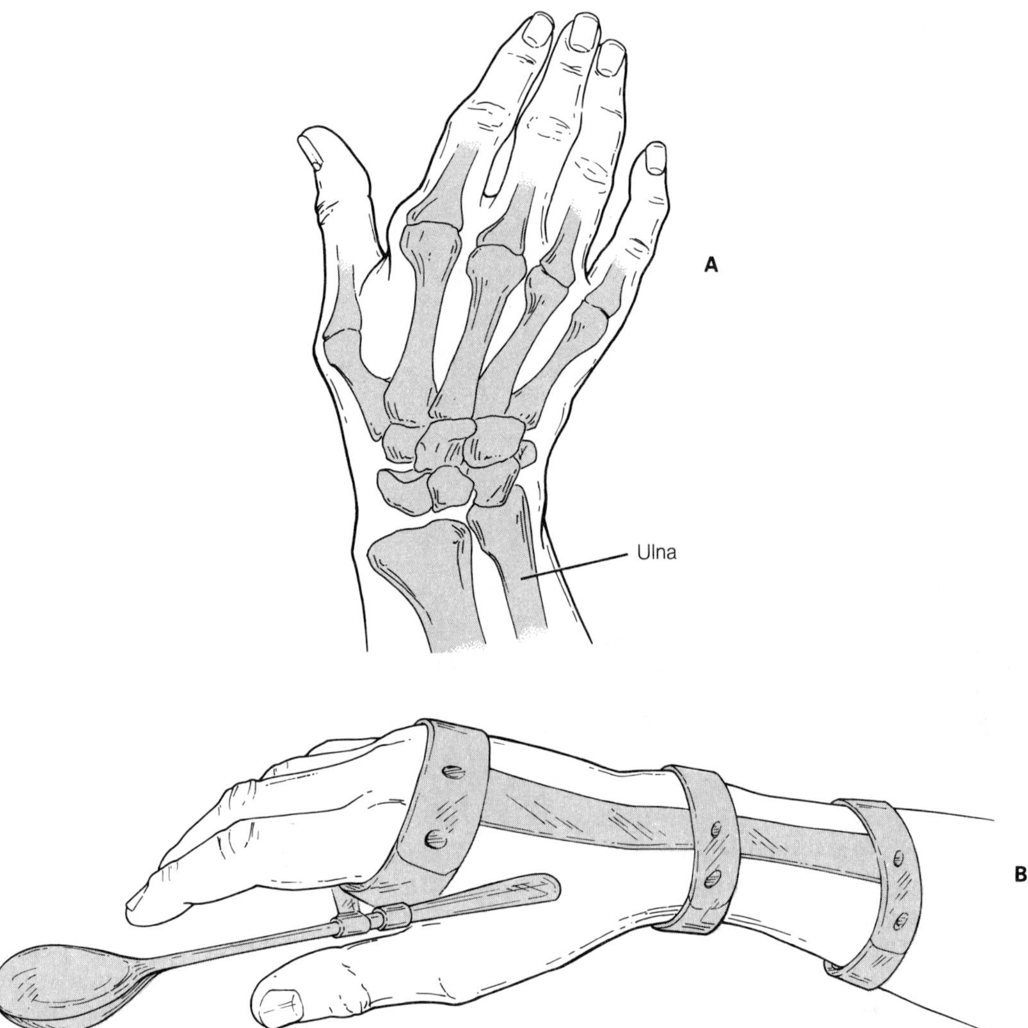

FIG. 14-1 **A,** Arthritic hand showing ulnar drift. **B,** Self-help device for stirring food during preparation and for eating assistance.

Nutritional Management

In all settings, approaches to planning appropriate nutritional support must begin with early assessment of individual patient status and needs, especially to detect any degree of malnutrition.[7,8] An initial history must thus assess potential drug-nutrient-food interactions (see Chapter 2) and their nutritional effects, as well as any of the numerous unproven regimens for arthritis that the patient may be using.[7]

In addition, attention may be given to dietary modifications under study that have shown promise in controlled trials. In separate studies, Endres et al[10] and Kremer et al[11] have provided evidence that dietary supplementation with the omega-3 fatty acids eicosapentaenoic acid (EPA) and docosahexaenoic acid (DHA) suppresses synthesis of *interleukin-1* and *tumor*

synosheath • Protective pliable connective tissue surrounding the bony-collagen mesh and fluid that come together in the synovial area between major bone heads in joints; it allows normal padded and lubricated joint movement and motion.

herpes zoster • An acute self-limiting viral inflammatory disease of posterior nerve roots causing skin eruptions in a lateral pattern across the back of the torso served by these nerves and accompanied by neuralgic pain; caused by the virus of chicken pox and commonly called *shingles.*

cytokines • Substances produced in tissues that cause inflammatory changes in tissue cells; for example, tumor necrosis factor and interleukin-1.

CLINICAL APPLICATION — Tilt and Swallow

The swallowing reflex is frequently diminished or absent in disabled persons. The reflex may be enhanced, however, by the use of an ice collar or by brushing the neck with a small brush, such as a paint brush, just before eating. The liquid or semisolid food should be placed behind the front teeth, and the patient should slowly tilt the head back and swallow. This routine may be learned as the helper uses the repeated statement, "Tilt and swallow. . . tilt and swallow. . . . " ◆

REFERENCE

Price ME, Dilorio C: Swallowing: a practice guide, *Am J Nurs* 90(7):42, 1990.

necrosis factor, two **cytokines** with potent inflammatory activities. Extensive studies warranted by this evidence of clinical improvement are continuing.[11,12] Other clinical studies have included investigation of food-induced allergic arthritis involving sensitivity to items such as milk, shrimp, and nitrates that occurs in about 5% of rheumatic disease patients.[13]

Special functional assessment of eating ability is also needed, including any swallowing problems involved in the lack of salivary secretions and dysphagia (see the *Clinical Application,* above).[14] Standard nutritional status assessment is essential (see Chapter 1). On the basis of these data, nutritional needs can be determined.

Energy. Energy needs may be estimated using the Harris-Benedict equations for basal energy expenditure (BEE), with the added multiple for metabolic activity factors (MAFs)—about 1.15 to 1.35 during active disease—for stress such as disease activity, sepsis, fever, skeletal injury, or surgery (see Chapter 11). If the client is receiving physical therapy, an additional physical activity factor of about 1.2 is used.[6,8] Increase kcalories as needed to achieve desirable weight gain. Follow-up monitoring indicates any needed adjustments in energy estimates.

Protein. Protein needs vary with visceral protein status, surgical therapy, proteinuria, and nitrogen balance. A well-nourished patient needs about 0.5 to 1.0 g of protein/kg/day during quiet disease periods. An increase to 1.5 to 2.0 g/kg/day, or a nonprotein kcalorie to nitrogen ratio of 150:1 (see Chapter 11), is needed during active inflammatory disease periods.

Vitamins and minerals. Standard recommendations for vitamins and minerals are used with only specific supplementation as needed, such as supplying calcium and vitamin D for bone disease.

Special enteral and parenteral feeding. Tube-feeding may be used either to supplement oral intake or to supply total nutritional support (see Chapter 3). Parenteral nutrition support is seldom used, except for preoperative and postoperative needs or when bowel rest is indicated.

The course of rheumatoid arthritis is unpredictable. Although the disease is usually progressive and some degree of permanent deformity may result, many patients after years of disease are capable of self-care with rehabilitation training and are fully employable. Continuing optimal nutritional support is important maintenance therapy.

Juvenile Rheumatoid Arthritis

A juvenile form of rheumatoid arthritis, sometimes called Still's disease, occurs in children under the age of 4. Usually it follows a less complicated course and clears up in adolescence. However, growth abnormalities are common and sometimes leave permanent deformities. Inflammatory effects cause anorexia that leads to adipose and muscle tissue breakdown.[15] Protein-energy malnutrition has been demonstrated in about 35% of patients with juvenile rheumatoid arthritis; 71.1% were reported to have a high "likelihood-of-malnutrition" score based on anthropometry, biochemical tests, and food diary results.[16] Continuing nutritional assessment and counseling for the child and family are essential to support growth needs.

Osteoarthritis

This type of arthritis is a different form of joint disease known as *degenerative arthritis* because inflammation is usually minimal. Osteoarthritis affects approximately 44% of persons over age 40 in the United States. It evolves in middle age, becomes chronic, and may be progressive in its course, mainly affecting hand and knee joints. Joint pain limits mobility and use of the hands. Although severe disability is not common, osteoarthritis may become a chronic disabling disease in the elderly.[17] As with rheumatoid arthritis, no cure is known for the disease process, which ultimately destroys cartilage between rubbing heads of bones in involved joints. However, damaged joints can be replaced. **Arthroplasty,** surgical replacement of a joint by metal or plastic components, has been available for hip replacements since the 1960s, and the technique is now being applied to other joints. Engineers and orthopedic surgeons are still refining replacements for the knee and shoulder, joints that are more complex than the hip.

In general medical management, appropriate pain-control medication including aspirin and NSAIDs such as ibuprofen (Advil, Motrin) or sulindac (Clinoril) helps relieve symptoms. Nutritional management seeks to ensure a well-balanced diet and to control excessive body weight and the painful pressure on weight-bearing joints. Dietary studies of ambulatory elderly persons with osteoarthritis have shown (1) deficiencies in food sources (dairy and grain groups) of calcium, vitamin D, thiamin, iron, and riboflavin; (2) an obesity rate of about 80% with an average weight gain since age 20 of approximately 60 lb; and (3) use of vitamin-mineral supplements by about 40% of the subjects.[17] Some subjects indicated that they took these supplements to deal with the arthritis, a practice without support of existing research but often suggested by lay publications.[18] Depending on degree of hand joint involvement, self-feeding devices may assist the activity of eating.

Osteoporosis

Osteoporosis, the metabolic bone disorder, is the most common skeletal disorder in the United States, affecting about 24 million individuals. Approximately one third of the postmenopausal women of the United States have osteoporosis and suffer from some 1.3 million associated fractures each year. Over age 70, osteoporosis affects men and women after a slow, steady rate of bone loss and increasing fracture potential develop over many decades. When the porous bone mass finally falls below a fracture threshold, fractures may occur spontaneously or with minimal trauma. These osteoporotic fractures in the elderly are a major cause of disabling illness and death. Bones of the vertebrae and the hip are most vulnerable, but hip fractures are more serious. The annual cost of treating patients with osteoporosis ranges from $7 to $12 billion.[19]

Medical treatment of menopausal osteoporosis in women is most effectively managed with estrogen replacement therapy. The slow, steadily developing form of osteoporosis in men and women responds more readily to nutritional therapy with a sound diet including a calcium intake of 1200 to 1500 mg/day, increased physical activity, and weight control. Newer medical treatments under investigation include the cyclic use of bisphosphonate (etidronate), a structural analog of the naturally occurring pyrophosphate, a component of the hydroxyapatite crystals forming bone.[19,20] The 2-week cycle with bisphosphonates depresses the osteoclast activity of resorbing bone. It is followed in turn by a 13-week cycle of a daily supplement of 500 mg of calcium and 10 μg of cholecalciferol (400 IU of vitamin D) to ensure that optimal mineralization occurs during osteoblast activity. The best approach, of course, is *prevention*—ensuring that the adolescent and young adult have sufficient dietary calcium for building bone mass, which reaches its peak by age 30, enhanced by physical activity. Then a continuing sound diet and physical activity help to sustain this normal bone mass.

Neuromuscular Disease

Growing Problem of Neurologic Injuries

In the United States traumatic injury is the leading cause of death in the first four decades of life and the third leading cause of death for all ages.[21,22] U.S. statistics indicate that in the year 1989 alone, 150,000 persons were killed outright by trauma from automobile and industrial accidents, gunshot wounds and homicides, and sports injuries.[21,23] Increasingly the strain on urban medical care centers comes into focus as special investigative reports in our local city newspapers remind us in bold front page Sunday headlines,"Trauma Care Crisis."[24] Further realization of the problem of traumatic injury comes from the fact that more Americans die from highway trauma each year than have died of AIDS (acquired immunodeficiency syndrome) since that disease was first identified in 1981, and in both conditions the majority of the victims are young males between 16 and 30 years of age.[21,25]

With current advancements in emergency medicine the number of persons surviving traumatic brain and spinal cord injury has increased dramatically. In the following discussion we review nutritional care of the injured patient in the acute care setting and follow-up nutritional management in rehabilitation.

Traumatic Brain Injury

After-Injury Metabolic Alterations

The brain is the control center of body functions and activities. Thus brain injury brings an immediate cascade of systemic metabolic responses that affect the

arthroplasty • Surgical procedure for replacing degenerated joints such as the hip with mechanical joints of metal or special plastic; formation of movable joint replacement developed by a team of biomedical engineers and orthopedists.

entire body as it mobilizes resources to protect itself. The systemic inflammatory response is activated and a sustained state of *hypermetabolism* develops. Ultimately, if the process continues unchecked, a sequence of organ failure follows. These hypermetabolic alterations include increased cardiac output and reduced vascular resistance, increased oxygen use, hyperglycemia, increased glucose use, and lipolysis. Any complication prolongs the hypermetabolic phase, and the increasing protein *catabolism* causes depletion of lean body mass.[26,27] Increased energy expenditure and urinary nitrogen excretion mark this increased metabolic demand in response to trauma.

Initial Nutritional Management

The immediate goals of the trauma team are control of the injury, maintenance of oxygen transport, and metabolic support.[26] Nutritional support as soon as possible is vital to meet the hypermetabolic drain on the body tissue resources for increased energy and protein demands.[27,28] Energy needs may be estimated by the traditional Harris-Benedict formula, multiplied by an MAF of 1.75 to 2.0 for the extreme stress of major trauma (see Chapter 11). However, since regular monitoring of energy needs is essential, often more than once a day, most trauma centers now use indirect calorimetry at the bedside with a mobile calorimeter unit such as the Beckman Metabolic Measurement Cart (Beckman Instruments, Anaheim, Calif.). Indirect calorimetry calculates energy production by measuring oxygen consumption and carbon dioxide production to provide a respiratory quotient.

Early nutritional support may be delivered by either the enteral or parenteral route (see Chapters 3 and 4). Successful use of enteral feedings as early as 2 to 3 days after injury has been reported, with a full caloric intake of 3020 kcal/24 hr achieved by day 7 (Vital HN by Ross: 10% fat, 16% hydrolyzed protein, 74% carbohydrates, continuous infusion) using a percutaneous endoscopic gastrojejunostomy through the abdominal wall with external Y-connector tubing at the gastric port for suctioning to prevent reflux and a jejunal J-tube placement and port for feeding.[29] Parenteral nutrition is an alternate option because it may be started within the first 24 hours after injury and may be immediately adjusted to the nutritional requirements of each patient according to daily metabolic profile and urinary nitrogen analysis.[30] Some trauma centers prefer a combination of early total parenteral nutrition (TPN) through a central vein catheter (see Chapter 4) within 24 hours, starting enteral nutrition as soon as it is tolerated, and gradually tapering the TPN and discontinuing it when the enteral feeding is considered adequate.[26]

Rehabilitative Nutrition

Nutritional rehabilitation of the person with traumatic brain injury presents a complex of individual problems that require skilled and sensitive nutritional management. To develop individual nutritional care plans the rehabilitation dietitian works closely with other team members, especially the nurse, occupational therapist, speech pathologist, cognitive rehabilitation therapist, and physical therapist to assess the degree of *dysphagia,* difficulty with chewing and swallowing, and level of language deficits and communication, as well as the ability to perform basic daily living skills including food preparation and eating. Yankelson[31] has provided helpful insights for assessing needs in a variety of injury effects, establishing short- and long-range goals and developing strategies to reach these goals, along with many practical suggestions for adapting food forms and textures to meet eating problems such as dysphagia.

Spinal Cord Injury

After-Injury Management

Each year catastrophic spinal cord injury in the United States affects some 10,000 trauma survivors between the ages of 16 and 30.[25,32] Over 200,000 quadriplegic and paraplegic patients now require lifetime care at an estimated patient cost of approximately $600,000, and because of advanced medical care, the number of survivors is increasing each year.[33,34] Most of these spinal cord injuries are from automobile accidents (48%); other factors include falls (21%), sports injuries (14%), and physical assaults (15%).[25,33] Injury and loss of neurologic function in the upper cervical area of the spinal cord results in *quadriplegia,* paralysis from the neck down. Injuries and loss of neurologic function in the lower thoracic, lumbar, and sacral areas of the spine result in *paraplegia,* paralysis of the lower portion of the body. This spinal cord damage disrupts nerve transmission of impulses from the brain to peripheral nerves and muscles so that muscle function below the level of injury is lost. Immobilization brings complicating illnesses. Metabolic changes include negative nitrogen balance, low serum albumin, increasing loss of calcium, bone and skin collagen loss, and weight loss. Protein-energy malnutrition is common. As many as half of the hospitalized patients and two thirds of the patients admitted to a rehabilitation unit have clinical signs of malnutrition.

Nutritional Management

Enteral feeding tubes placed beyond the pylorus usually make it possible to start nutritional support within 3 to 5 days. The patients are usually well-nourished at the time of the sudden injury. Thus the goal of starting the feeding process as early as possible is to counteract the initial acute phase of spinal shock and to prevent the onset of a malnutrition decline and secondary illnesses. Metabolic rates vary widely, as do energy needs, but they tend to be lower than those of other trauma patients because of the decreased metabolic activity of denervated muscle.[33] The higher the injury to the spinal column, the greater the denervated muscle mass and the lower the measure of energy expenditure. Because the spinal cord injury patient is susceptible to the ill effects of overfeeding, frequent measure of metabolic rate is an important nutritional assessment tool for determining kcalorie needs. If metabolic measures are not available, daily guidelines derived from studies may be used: 23 kcal/kg body weight for quadriplegics and 28 kcal/kg body weight for paraplegics.[35,33]

Rehabilitative Nutrition

When the acute phase passes and the patient is stabilized, usually within 2 to 3 months after injury, the extended rehabilitative training phase begins. This complex process of many parts is designed to restore the client to the best functional capacity possible to promote independent living.[36] It aims at the prevention and treatment of complications associated with spinal cord injury and uses combined therapies from the team of rehabilitation specialists: physiatrist, registered dietitian, registered nurse, physical therapist, occupational therapist, speech therapist, psychologist, social worker, and vocational counselor. Nutritional management involves individual assessment and care of (1) basic energy-nutrient needs and feeding capacities and (2) complications associated with the spinal cord injury.

Basic Nutritional Needs

Energy needs are based on sufficient kcalories to maintain an ideal body weight somewhat below that for a comparative person given in standard weight-height tables for healthy populations (see inside back book cover). For example, general weight goals for paraplegics have been recommended at 10 to 15 lb below standard body weight and for quadriplegics at 15 to 20 lb below standard weight.[36,37] Excess weight gain is common in spinal cord injury clients because of the decreased metabolic rate that persists from the preceding acute after-injury phase and the continued relative immobilization.[33] Reported weight gains by paraplegic and quadriplegic rehabilitation clients on uncontrolled diets have been 2.82 lb (1.28 kg) and 4.05 lb (1.84 kg) weekly, respectively.[35] Obesity contributes to medical problems and adds physical problems to the frequent turning in bed necessary to prevent bed sores and the transfers between bed to wheelchair. Adequate protein intake is essential for maintaining muscle mass and tissue integrity to prevent negative nitrogen balance, ulcer formation, or infection. Palatable high-protein supplements between meals may be needed to maintain an adequate intake. The client may be at risk for vitamin or mineral deficiencies if appetite and food intake are poor because of depression or fatigue. A standard multiple vitamin-mineral preparation is frequently recommended.

Associated Complications

Several nutrition-related complications in rehabilitation for spinal cord injury patients require special attention.

Pressure sores. Decubitus ulcers are caused by immobilization, loss of pressure sensation around bony prominences, decreased blood circulation, and skin breakdown. They are easily infected and difficult to heal. They occur in 60% of quadriplegic patients and 52% of paraplegics. Nutritional factors involved include anemia, which reduces oxygen supply to tissues, excessive weight loss, which reduces padding of bony prominences, and low levels of plasma proteins such as albumin, which lead to edema and loss of skin elasticity. The protein deficiency requires an increased protein intake. More severe ulcers require more intense nutritional intervention, with protein needs of 1.5 to 2.0 g/kg body weight. Other nutrients important to the healing process include supplements of vitamin C and zinc.

Hypercalciuria. Immobility leads to an imbalance in calcium metabolism with a loss of bone calcium and its increased excretion in the urine. In the long term this loss of bone calcium leads to osteoporosis, which has been found to be present and progressive in 88% of the patients with spinal cord injury, affecting the denervated musculoskeletal tissue below the level of injury.[33] A balance of calcium–vitamin D therapy and a prudent control of excessive protein intake that causes increased calcium withdrawal are indicated. Bone fractures result in about 7% of these patients.

Renal calculuses. The hypercalciuria also contributes to formation of renal calculuses. The neurogenic effects following spinal cord injury cause loss of normal bladder control, resulting in problems of urinary reflux, retention, incontinence, infection, and stone formation.[36] Regular catheterization is necessary to prevent accumulation of bacteria and solutes such as calcium and other particles that easily form stones. A high fluid intake of 2 to 3 L/day must be a part of the overall nutritional care plan to dilute the urine and reduce the solute concentration.

Neurogenic bowel. Gastrointestinal complications from loss of normal neuromuscular controls include decreased peristalsis and loss of bowel control. A regularly scheduled program for emptying the bowel is necessary. About 12 hours before the scheduled time, 4 oz (120 ml) of prune juice with a little lemon juice is taken. Then 20 to 30 minutes before the scheduled evacuation time, one or two glycerin suppositories are placed well above the anal sphincter, at least 2½ in (6.5 cm) into the rectum, against the rectal mucosa. The patient is then placed on the toilet or bedside commode and provided with adequate support. This daily schedule and recording of results continues with no interruption by enemas. The paraplegic patient is taught manual evacuation as part of the continuing care program at home. A vital part of this program is a high-fiber diet to provide added bulk and ample fluid intake to prevent impaction.

Depression. During the initial days of shock and survival after the injury, the full impact of the disability is not realized. When transfer to the rehabilitation unit occurs and the full extent of the disability is realized, a period of depression is a normal part of the personal grieving and healing process. Its severity and duration depend in large measure on the patient's personal strengths and resources, but it also requires the sensitive yet realistic support of family and the rehabilitation team for the serious and demanding work of rehabilitation to be successful. The nutritionist must help ensure that adequate energy, protein, and fluid intake is maintained with appetizing foods, especially when the patient's spirits are low. Even subtle improvements in muscle mass and function from nutritional care are a source of strength to mind and body.

Cerebrovascular Accident (Stroke)

Brain injury caused by a stroke also causes varying degrees of nerve damage and body paralysis (see Chapter 8). Cerebrovascular disease from underlying atherosclerosis ranks third as a cause of death and second as a cause of disability in the United States.[38] In recent years the incidence of strokes has declined, largely because of the improvement in control of hypertension and increased public education concerning hypertension. Nutritional management is detailed in Chapter 8. Rehabilitation care follows the same general goals and methods discussed in this chapter (see the *Case Study,* p. 303).

Developmental Disabilities

During the developmental period of childhood, neuromuscular conditions such as cerebral palsy, epilepsy, spina bifida, and Down syndrome cause eating problems that contribute to poor growth and delayed development.

Cerebral Palsy

Cerebral palsy is a general term for nonprogressive disorders of muscle control of movements and posture and has a multitude of etiologies. It results from brain damage that occurs largely before or at birth, probably ultimately caused by *hypoxia,* or poor oxygen supply to the brain.[39] Most affected children fall into one of two groups: (1) *spastic*—muscles of one or more limbs permanently contracted, making normal movements difficult if at all possible, and (2) *athetoid*—involuntary writhing movements. Mental retardation (an IQ below 70) occurs in about 75% of persons with cerebral palsy, mostly in the spastic group. Exceptions, however, occurring mostly among athetoid persons, are important, and some of these persons are highly intelligent. Some features of the condition during childhood change as the child grows older, often for the better with patience and skillful treatment.

Early nutritional management focuses mainly on feeding problems. When the infant or young child cannot obtain sufficient nourishment because of oral motor dysfunction or when satisfactory oral feeding is interrupted for a prolonged period because of illness or surgery, enteral nutrition support by nasoenteric or gastrostomy tube-feeding (see Chapter 3) may be necessary.[39] In such cases, transition to oral feeding is usually difficult. In any case, oral feeding poses numerous functional and behavioral problems. Recent studies of children with cerebral palsy ages 1 to 16 have revealed feeding problems in at least 50% of the children, resulting in poor energy and nutrient intakes and growth retardation.[40,41] Feeding problems of oral motor dysfunction (for example, difficulties in sucking, swallowing, or chewing), gross motor and self-feeding impairment, lack of appetite, food aversions, and alternate feeding practices of prolonged assisted feeding and use of pureed foods significantly reduce energy and nutrient intake.[41] Early and ongoing nutritional assessment, intervention, and counseling are essential components of rehabilitation team care. In cases where accurate height measures to assess growth are difficult because of joint contractures, spasticity, or inability to stand, reasonably accurate stature may be calculated from knee height measures (see Chapter 1) using the standard equations given in Table 14-1.[42,43] Studies of anthropometric and dietary data from adults with cerebral palsy indicate that the growth retardation seen in children persists with age and many still have feeding problems, but exercise helps promote better nutrition.[44] Among the adults studied, those who participated in regular exercise programs had more adequate diets and lower body

TABLE 14–1

Equations for Estimating Stature from Knee Height

Age/sex group	Equation
White males	
6-18 years	stature = (knee height × 2.22) + 40.54
19-59 years	stature = (knee height × 1.88) + 71.85
White females	
6-18 years	stature = (knee height × 2.15) + 43.21
19-59 years	stature = (knee height × 1.86) − (age × 0.05) ± 70.25

Adapted from Estimating stature from knee height. In *Directions for the Ross Knee Height Caliper*, Columbus, Ohio, 1990, Ross Laboratories.
Equations are based on normal, healthy individuals. Stature and knee height are measured in centimeters.

fat percentages than those who did not exercise regularly.

Epilepsy

Epilepsy, literally "seizures," is a neuromuscular disorder in which abnormal electric activity in the brain causes recurring transient seizures. Normally the brain regulates all human activities, thoughts, perceptions, and emotions through the regular orderly electric excitation of its nerve cells. But in an epileptic state during a seizure, an unregulated chaotic electric discharge occurs. Seizures often appear spontaneously, or in some cases they may be set off by some stimulus such as a flashing light. This brain dysfunction may develop for no obvious reason or there may be an inherited predisposition. In other cases, it may result from a wide variety of disease or injury, such as birth trauma, a metabolic imbalance in the body, head injury, brain infection (meningitis or encephalitis), stroke, brain tumor, drug intoxication, or alcohol or drug withdrawal states. Epilepsy occurs in about 1 person in 200; the number of epileptics in the United States is about 1 million. Usually the disorder starts in childhood or adolescence. About a third of these persons outgrow the condition and do not need medication. Another third find their seizures controlled well by drug treatment and require less medication over time. The remaining third find that their condition remains the same or becomes more resistant to drug therapy. Anticonvulsant drugs are the first line of treatment for epilepsy and in most cases do lessen seizure frequency.

Nutritional management of epilepsy functions in several areas of care. First, it helps to ensure an appropriate diet for normal growth during childhood and adolescence and for health maintenance in adulthood. Second, it seeks to ameliorate side effects of the anticonvulsant drugs used. Some of the most commonly used ones and their relation to food and nutrients are shown in Table 14-2. Third, if a *ketogenic* diet is used, the clinical nutritionist is responsible for its calculations and the education of the staff, patient, and family in its use. This special high-fat diet was developed to control epilepsy before current anticonvulsant drugs became widely available in the 1940s and has only had sporadic use since that time. However, as is sometimes the case with maintenance drugs used for long periods, some persons and types of the disease do not respond as well as others to the continued drug use. Intractable myoclonic epilepsy resists drug therapy, and persons with this form of epilepsy have responded well to the use of the traditional ketogenic diet control.[45] The diet, with minimal medication as needed to avoid drug side effects, is used for about 3 years and includes a terminal weaning period, after which additional medication is usually not required. In earlier use, the ketogenic diet has been most successful for young children 2 to 5 years old but has helped persons in a wide age range from 7 months to 38 years. Recently the effectiveness of ketogenic diets in treating epilepsy among children has been reconfirmed.[45,46] Absolute adherence is necessary for successful control, so the home environment must be supportive. Details of its strict calculations and food groups to achieve the necessary 4:1 or 3:1 ratio by weight of fat to carbohydrates plus protein may be found in a number of medical center diet manuals.[47]

Spina Bifida

Spina bifida is a congenital defect in the formation of the spine. It develops during early embryonic life when the neural tube, which forms the spinal cord, does not close completely, leaving part of one or more vertebrae of the spinal cord exposed at birth.[48] The vertebral canal usually closes within four weeks of conception. Thus this congenital defect often can be diagnosed early in the pregnancy by *ultrasound scanning* or by high levels of **alpha-fetoprotein** in the amnionic

spina bifida • Congenital defect in the fetal closing of the neural tube to form a portion of the lower spine, leaving the spine unclosed and the spinal cord open in various degrees of exposure and damage.

alpha-fetoprotein • A fetal antigen in amnionic fluid that provides an early pregnancy test for fetal malformations such as neural tube defect.

TABLE 14–2

Anticonvulsant Drugs Used to Control Basic Types of Epilepsy and Their Nutrition-Related Side Effects

Most commonly used drug	Drug trade name	Nutrition-related side effects
Grand mal (tonic/clonic) seizures		
Phenytoin (adults)	Dilantin	Nausea, vomiting, and constipation; reduced taste sensation; vitamins D and K catabolism; reduced serum calcium, B_6, B_{12}, folate, and serum magnesium levels; overgrowth of gums
Phenobarbitol	Luminal	Increased appetite or anorexia, nausea, vomiting, vitamins D and K catabolism, reduced bone density
Primidone	Mysoline	Gastrointestinal upset, weight loss
Carbamazepine	Tegretol	Nausea, vomiting, diarrhea, abdominal pain, xerostomia (dry mouth), glossitis (sore tongue), stomatitis (sore mouth), increased blood urea nitrogen
Petit mal (absence) seizures		
Ethosuximide	Zarontin	Gastrointestinal upset, nausea, vomiting, anorexia, weight loss
Valproic acid	Depakane, Depakote	Nausea, vomiting, indigestion, diarrhea, abdominal pain, constipation, anorexia and weight loss, or increased appetite and weight gain
Clonazepam	Klonopin	Hyperactivity, short attention span, impulsive behavior, weight gain
Partial seizures		
Phenytoin (adults)	Dilantin	Nausea, vomiting, and constipation; reduced taste sensation; vitamins D and K catabolism; reduced serum calcium, B_6, B_{12}, folate, and serum magnesium levels; overgrowth of gums
Phenobarbitol	Luminal	Increased appetite or anorexia, nausea, vomiting, vitamins D and K catabolism, reduced bone density
Carbamazepine	Tegretol	Nausea, vomiting, diarrhea, abdominal pain, xerostomia (dry mouth), glossitis (sore tongue), stomatitis (sore mouth), increased blood urea nitrogen

fluid or maternal blood, so that appropriate genetic counseling may be provided for the parents. The defect may occur anywhere along the spine but is more common in the lower back. The neurologic damage that occurs depends on the severity and level of the lesion on the spine.[49] The incidence is about one case per 1000 babies born but increases with either very young or old maternal age. A mother who has had one affected child is 10 times more likely than the average woman to have another affected child.

The three main forms of spina bifida are the following:

- *Spina bifida occulta.* This is the least serious and most common form. The name indicates an unseen cleft in the spine. It often goes unnoticed in otherwise healthy children save for a small dimple over the area of the underlying abnormality, but occasionally accompanying problems occur in the lower spinal cord such as leg weakness and urinary incontinence.
- *Myelomeningocele.* Also known as myelocele, this is the most severe form, and the child is usually severely disabled. The spinal cord (myelo) and its enveloping membranes (meninges) protrude from the spine in a sac (cele).[48] Sometimes the baby is born with just a raw swelling over the spine consisting of a malformed spinal cord that is not contained in a membranous sac. In either case, the legs are partially or completely paralyzed and sensation is lost in all areas below the level of the lesion. Paralysis of the bladder leads to urinary incontinence or retention, repeated urinary tract infections, and eventually kidney damage, so preventive use of an indwelling catheter is necessary. Paralysis of the anal area causes chronic constipation. *Hydrocephalus,* excess cerebrospinal fluid within the skull, is common and may result in brain damage.
- *Meningocele.* This form is less severe because the nerve tissue of the spinal cord is usually intact. Outer skin covers the bulging sac and therefore no functional problems usually occur. Ideally, necessary surgical repairs are performed in the first few days of life.

Nutritional management of children with spina bifida focuses on growth pattern and individual degree of problems with growth retardation and short stature, low muscle mass and weakness, deformities or paralysis of lower extremities, and reduced ability to control the bladder and bowels. Normal growth charts have been revised for use with nutritional assessment of these children.[48] Nutritional care plans give attention to the main problems of short stature and poor growth, increased weight, and constipation. Obesity is a particular problem because of several factors: (1) low basal metabolic rate related to lowered amount of lean body mass, (2) little physical activity related to the disabling condition and dependency on a wheelchair; and (3) use of food and overfeeding by parents or other caregivers to reward or show love or to counteract what is seen as frailty or weakness from the disability.[48,49] All of these factors become part of ongoing nutritional counseling.

Down's Syndrome

A chromosomal abnormality accounts for the mental retardation and characteristic appearance of children with Down's syndrome, a condition first described in the previous century by the British physician John L.H. Down (1828-1896). Its cause remained a mystery until 1959, when modern researchers discovered that persons with Down's syndrome had one too many chromosomes in each of their cells—47 instead of the normal 46. Because the extra chromosome is usually number 21, they gave it the alternate name of *trisomy 21*. The two parent chromosomes numbered 21 fail to go into separate daughter cells during the first stage of sperm or egg cell formation, and some eggs or sperm are thus formed with an extra number 21 chromosome. If one of these takes part in fertilization, the resulting baby has the extra chromosome and Down's syndrome. This event is more likely if the mother is over 35, indicating that defective egg formation, rather than sperm formation, is usually the cause. Down's syndrome occurs in about 1 in 650 babies born. The rate rises steeply with increased maternal age to about 1 in 40 among mothers over 40. The degree of mental retardation varies with an intelligence quotient anywhere from 30 to 80, but all children with Down's syndrome are capable of limited learning, and some can learn to read. These children are usually affectionate, cheerful, and friendly, and they get along well with family and friends. They thrive to their full potential in a loving family.

Nutritional needs center on delayed feeding skills; inappropriate, excessive, or inadequate intakes of food energy and nutrients; and poor eating habits. Studies indicate frequent obesity, possibly because of excessive fat, low physical activity, or both.[50] Diets need to be individualized because these children tend to gain excess weight if they are given the intakes recommended for most children, and plans need to be made for increasing physical activity.

Progressive Neurologic Disorders

Progressive neurologic disorders, especially through the middle and older years of adulthood, have disabling effects on the personal lives of many individuals. Examples are given in this section to illustrate some of these effects and the approaches to providing nutritional support.

Parkinson's Disease

Parkinson's disease is a long-known neurologic disease first described by the English physician James Parkinson (1755-1824) nearly two centuries ago, but its underlying origin remains unknown. Modern researchers speculate that the triggering cause may be related to some environmental factor such as a toxin.[51] Genetic factors are not the cause, but in some families, persons may be genetically predisposed to the disease. It is a common disorder reported in every race and region of the world, usually with onset of motor symptoms after age 40 and rising in incidence with advancing age. In the United States about 1 person in 200, mostly elderly, is affected by the disease, with some 50,000 new cases a year. Men are more likely to be affected than women.

The disorder affects the *basal ganglia,* a cluster of nerve cells at the central base of the brain. Signals from the brain's motor cortex pass via the brainstem *reticular formation* and the spinal cord to the muscles, which contract. Other signals pass through the basal ganglia, which provide a *damping effect* to help smooth and control the signal flow to the reticular formation and spinal cord, thus preventing uncoordinated muscle contraction responses. This damping effect is produced by the balancing action of two neurotransmitters: (1) *dopamine,* which is made in the basal ganglia and is necessary for the damping effect, stimulates the signal flow, and (2) *acetylcholine,* a widespread neurotransmitter in the body, inhibits it. In Parkinson's disease, degeneration of key parts of the basal ganglia causes a lack of dopamine within this part of the brain, thus preventing the basal ganglia from modifying nerve pathways that control muscle function.[52] The muscles become overly tense, causing joint rigidity and a general body stiffness, a fine constant tremor even at rest, and slow movements.

Medical Management

Although there is no cure for Parkinson's disease, drug management helps minimize symptoms for many patients. A dramatic change in treatment came in the 1960s with the advent of the drug levodopa, which the body transforms into the needed dopamine.[53] Levodopa is the most effective drug for symptomatic treatment of Parkinson's disease when it is given with a dopa decarboxylase inhibitor such as carbidopa. However, its beneficial effect wears off, so other drugs such as bromocriptine and amantadine are used, with levodopa successfully being reintroduced later. Dopamine itself cannot be used since it does not cross the blood-brain barrier as does levodopa.[52] New methods of drug delivery to achieve a slow, steady release and means of slowing down the progression of Parkinson's disease are the major goals of present research.[54] Current surgical research is investigating transplants of dopamine-secreting adrenal medulla tissue and the grafting of fetal brain dopamine neurons.[54,55]

Nutritional Management

Nutritional care centers on nutrition-related drug effects, eating problems, and malnutrition. Common side effects of levodopa include severe nausea that affects food intake. Excessive intake of vitamin B_6 should be avoided because it interacts with levodopa and reduces the drug's beneficial effect. Hand tremors make obtaining and preparing food, as well as carrying food from the bowl or plate to the mouth difficult. Thus, for example, soups should be avoided and more textured foods should be used that may be cut into pieces or formed into cohesive bites with the aid of the knife and pierced securely with the fork in the European fashion of eating. As the disease progresses, problems with chewing, swallowing, or aspiration of small food items such as peas or nuts, as well as discomfort from constipation, flatulence, or delayed gastric emptying may occur. Small frequent meals of increased carbohydrates and decreased fat, chewing thoroughly and eating slowly with special utensils as needed, and appropriate energy intake to maintain optimal weight and adequate fiber and fluid to prevent constipation are helpful.

Recent study indicates that a special diet of daytime protein restriction to about 10 g, with protein foods such as meat and dairy products to provide the remainder of the day's total RDA (0.8 g/kg/day) being reserved for use in the evening meal and later snack, has provided a helpful adjunct therapy for patients experiencing unpredictable motor-response fluctuations from levodopa.[56] These beneficial effects of steady symptom control appear to result from a decrease during the day in the plasma concentration of dietary protein-derived large neutral amino acids that compete with levodopa for transport into the brain.

Huntington's Chorea

First described by American physician George Huntington (1850-1916), Huntington's chorea is an uncommon genetic disease in which degeneration of the basal ganglia of the brain results in **chorea**—rapid, jerky, involuntary movements—and *dementia*—progressive mental impairment. Currently, after a decade-long search, a large group of scientists from six institutions have finally discovered the defective gene that causes the disease, opening the way to future therapies and possibly to an eventual cure.[57] Symptoms do not usually appear until about age 35 to 50; cases of symptomatic effects beginning in childhood are rare. This genetic disease is inherited in an autosomal dominant pattern with each child having a 50% chance of the condition developing. To illustrate the strength of this transmission pattern, the highest concentration of patients with Huntington's chorea in one family in the world has been found and its gene linkage studied in depth by Wexler et al[58] in the little village of San Luis on the shores of Lake Maracaibo high in the Andes mountains of Venezuela. For a recent nutritional evaluation, 75 affected persons in four generations of this family were studied, while 40 unaffected family members with no choreic descendants served as controls.[59] In the United States the disease develops in about 5 persons per 100,000. Generally the symptoms do not appear until middle adulthood, so affected persons may have children before knowing that they have the disease.

Medical Management

As a result of recent advances in genetics, a test is now available for young adults whose parents have Huntington's chorea to learn with 95% accuracy whether they carry the gene and thus have the disorder. This test then helps them decide whether to have children themselves. There is no known cure, so medical management helps to lessen the characteristic chorea that affects the face, arms, and trunk with random grimaces, twitches, and general clumsiness. The drug chlorpromazine (Thorazine), the most widely used antipsychotic drug for its tranquilizing effect (it suppresses brain centers that control abnormal emotions and behaviors), has been found useful. The mental impairment of Huntington's chorea is evident in personality and behavioral changes, difficulty making decisions, apathy, irritability, and memory loss.

Nutritional Management

The excessive muscular activity requires adequate energy and nutrient intake to prevent malnutrition and excess weight loss. As the disease progresses, patients may become cachectic and even with an adequate food intake show a progressively catabolic state. A recent study identified 55% of the patients in advanced stages of the disease who were malnourished despite receiving the same food intake as control subjects.[59] Nutritional counseling involves help in planning high energy–nutrient diets to combat malnutrition and assistance with dysphagia or feeding problems and the drug side effect of constipation.

Guillain-Barré Syndrome

This acute postinfectious polyneuritis was first described by two twentieth-century French neurologists, Georges Guillain (1876-1961) and Jean Alexander Barré (1880-1965). It is a rare form of damage to the peripheral nerves in which the **myelin sheaths** covering nerve axons and sometimes the axons themselves deteriorate, causing loss of nerve conduction and partial or complete paralysis.[60] Nerve inflammation occurs particularly where nerve roots leave the spine, impairing movement and sensation. Muscular weakness in the legs, often accompanied by numbness and tingling, progresses upward to trunk and arms and face and head. A low-grade fever persists, and there may be urinary tract infection, respiratory failure requiring a ventilator, and personality changes. This acute syndrome is an autoimmune reaction often following a viral infection and sometimes an immunization. In 1976 a U.S. epidemic occurred following a mass vaccination against swine flu. In general the U.S. incidence is about 15 cases per million persons per year.

Medical Management

Hospitalization for close monitoring of an acute condition is essential, especially if breathing difficulty occurs. In severe cases, *plasmapheresis*—in which blood plasma is withdrawn from the patient, treated to remove antibodies, and replaced—may be done. An early short course of intravenous steroid therapy with methylprednisolone has proved to be generally ineffective in recent trials but did reduce symptom disability time.[61] Most people recover completely without specific treatment other than general supportive care, but some are left with permanent weakness in affected areas.

Nutritional Management

During early acute phases, enteral or parenteral nutrition support may be necessary with attention to increased energy and protein needs in the formula solutions (see Chapters 3 and 4). Also, if respiratory distress occurs requiring ventilator assistance, increased use of fat for needed energy fuel rather than increased carbohydrates, such as is needed for patients with chronic obstructive pulmonary disease, is indicated (see Chapter 8). Food consistency and texture may need to be adjusted in early oral feedings to accommodate any chewing and swallowing problems from weak facial and throat muscles. Continuing attention to energy and nutrient needs during convalescence is required to restore lost body weight and muscle mass.

Amyotrophic Lateral Sclerosis

Amyotrophic lateral sclerosis (ALS), also known as Lou Gehrig disease for the famous U.S. baseball player who was struck down by ALS at the height of his successful major league career, is the most common of the motor neuron diseases.[62] In rare neuronal disorders such as ALS, nerves that control muscular activity degenerate within the brain and spinal cord. About 10% of ALS cases are genetic in origin; the remaining 90% are apparently sporadic.

Medical Management

Although current medical treatment of ALS is limited, a recent study by a large team of scientists from the United States, Canada, Belgium, and Australia working on the hereditary form of ALS among dozens of families reports the discovery of the gene causing a hereditary form of the disease.[63,64] The researchers identified the gene on the long arm of chromosome 21 and found that it controls the synthesis of an enzyme called *copper/zinc-binding superoxide dismutase,* which helps cells get rid of highly toxic and destructive superoxide free radicals that are produced by a variety of oxidative cell reactions.[64,65] If the enzyme were abnormal because of the defective ALS gene, free cell radicals might well build up, causing the death of the motor neurons affected in ALS. As it is now, the relentless nerve degeneration of ALS progresses to involve the muscles of respiration and swallowing, usually killing its victims in about 3 years.[64] This giant step of identifying the responsible defective gene will lead to more knowledge of how the progressive destructive course of ALS may be slowed, controlled, or prevented.

Nutritional Management

Nutritional care planning and counseling focuses on increased energy intake and adjusted nutrient needs as the disease progresses.[66] Weakness of hands and arms and problems with chewing, swallowing, delayed or absent response of the gag reflex, and risk of aspiration require that eating assistance be given and that food textures be modified. Frequent small meals

chorea • A wide variety of ceaseless involuntary movements that are rapid, complex, and jerky yet appear to be well-coordinated; characteristic movements of Huntington's disease.

myelin sheath • Covering of myelin, a lipid-protein substance with a high fat proportion to protein, surrounding nerve axons that serves as an electric insulator and speeds the conduction of nerve impulses, interrupted at intervals along the length of the axon by gaps known as Ranvier's nodes.

amyotrophic lateral sclerosis (ALS) • A progressive neuromuscular disease characterized by the degeneration of the neurons of the spinal cord and motor cells of the brainstem causing a deficit of upper and lower motor neurons; death usually occurs in 2 to 3 years.

may be better tolerated. In advanced stages, enteral and parenteral nutrition support supply needed energy and nutrients in a variety of individualized formulas (see Chapters 3 and 4).

Multiple Sclerosis

Multiple sclerosis (MS) is a progressive disease of the central nervous system in which scattered patches of insulating myelin, the fatty covering of nerve fibers in the brain and spinal cord that protects the neurons and facilitates the passage of neuromuscular impulses, are destroyed. In these denuded patches, the myelin is replaced by nonfunctional plaques of scar tissue so that the nerve fiber no longer conducts electric impulses normally. The severity of the condition varies greatly among the persons affected. The precise cause of MS is unknown, but it is an autoimmune disease in which the body's defense system begins to treat the myelin tissue in the central nervous system as a foreign substance and gradually destroys it with subsequent scarring. Ongoing studies are investigating triggering events for this mutiny in the immune system involving T cells and the protein antigens produced and the possibilities of using these autoimmune components as treatment strategies in a manner similar to that of vaccines.[67,68] An as yet unknown genetic factor is probably involved since relatives of affected persons are eight times more likely than others to develop the disease. Environment seems to play a role; MS is five times more common in temperate zones such as the United States and Europe than in the tropics, perhaps being induced by a virus picked up in a person's first 15 years of life in these temperate climates.[69] Approximately two thirds of the persons affected experience the beginning symptoms between ages 20 and 40; more women than men are affected at a 2:1 ratio; and MS is most commonly found in white populations. In the relatively high-risk temperate areas the incidence of MS is about 1 in every 1000 people. Depending on how extensive the tissue involvement and which parts of the brain and spinal cord are affected, the effects of MS vary widely from mild periodic feelings of tingling, numbness, constriction, or stiffness in any part of the body to more severe disabling disease. The role of dietary factors remains uncertain, but considerable investigation has implicated a high-fat diet as an agent.[69]

Medical Management

Physicians have lacked specific means of treatment while the search for a cure goes on. Corticosteroid drugs have been used to alleviate symptoms of an acute attack. Currently, however, a more specifically effective drug is being made available. An advisory panel of the U.S. Food and Drug Administration has approved use of the new drug *beta-interferon (Betaseron),* and it will probably be on the market by 1994. It is the first drug shown in testing to be effective in reducing the number and severity of symptomatic episodes of MS, although hundreds of drugs have been tried over the past decades. Betaseron is a genetically engineered drug containing beta-interferon, a type of protein that helps regulate the immune system. Adjunct physical therapy helps maintain muscle strength and the ability to remain mobile and independent.

Nutritional Management

General nutritional care responds to basic nutrition needs for adequate energy and nutrient intake to maintain or restore optimal nutritional status and assist with symptomatic gastrointestinal problems with eating and elimination, as occur with other neuromuscular diseases. If steroid therapy is used, dietary sodium is reduced. Low-fat foods are wise in any case in possible relation to disease control[69] and for healthy weight management. Nasoenteric or gastrostomy tube-feeding may be needed in advanced disease to provide enteral nutrition support.

Myasthenia Gravis

The neuromuscular disease **myasthenia gravis** occurs in about 1 of every 20,000 persons, causing the affected person to become paralyzed because of the inability of the neuromuscular junctions to transmit nerve fiber signals to the muscles.[52] It is an autoimmune disorder in which for unknown reasons the body's immune system attacks and gradually destroys the receptors in muscles that are responsible for picking up nerve impulses. As a result the affected muscles respond only weakly or not at all to nerve impulses. Only about 2 to 5 new cases of this rare disease per 100,000 persons are diagnosed annually. Myasthenia gravis affects more women than men in a ratio of 3:2, and although it may occur at any age, it usually occurs between ages 20 and 30 in women and 50 and 70 in men. Facial muscles are usually involved first, causing drooped eyelids, double vision, and sometimes a lack of facial animation with an absent stare appearance. Weak muscles of the face, throat, larynx, and neck cause difficulties in speaking and eating. As muscles in the arms and legs become involved, problems with other daily living activities such as food procurement and preparation, dressing, combing the hair, and climbing up stairs also develop. In severe cases, the respiratory muscles in the chest weaken and cause breathing difficulty.

Medical Management

Treatment may involve a thymectomy, removal of the thymus gland, a small gland in the upper chest thought to be partly responsible for the abnormal antibody activity, especially if a small tumor is found in it. Temporary relief may be obtained by regular plasmapheresis to exchange the patient's antibody-containing blood for antibody-free blood. These antibodies produced by the disease attack the receptors on the muscle cells that bind the acetylcholine neurotransmitter necessary for muscle contraction, thus effectively reducing stimulation of muscle cells and weakening muscle action. Drugs used to treat MS, such as neostigmine (Prostigmin) or pyridostigmine (Mestinon, Regonol), increase the amount of neurotransmitter at the nerve ending by blocking the action of the enzyme *acetylcholinesterase,* which normally breaks it down.[53] Usually this enzyme splits the transmitter acetylcholine into an acetate ion and choline, and choline is actively resorbed into the neural terminal to be reused in forming new acetylcholine. The blocking action of these drugs increases levels of the acetylcholine transmitter by allowing more of it to accumulate in the synaptic cleft between nerve and muscle fiber endings, thus permitting the remaining receptors to function more efficiently.

Nutritional Management

Nutritional care has three main goals: (1) to maintain optimal energy-nutrient intake for muscle strength and good nutritional status, (2) to meet any eating problems caused by the disorder by adjusting meal patterns to a major meal at breakfast when the patient is more rested and frequent small meals through the day and by modifying food texture and supplying supplemental enteral feedings as needed, and (3) to help counteract the drug side effects of nausea and vomiting. The drugs described should be taken with liquid or food to lessen stomach irritation.

Alzheimer's Disease

Alzheimer's disease was named for the German neurologist Alois Alzheimer[70] (1864-1915), who in 1907 first described the characteristic neurofibrillary tangles found in the postmortem brain of a 51-year-old demented woman. The disease is a form of progressive dementia in which nerve cells degenerate in the brain and the brain substance shrinks. The hallmark of the disease is the development of abnormal intracellular filaments in tangles of neurofibrils and extracellular deposits of **amyloid**-forming protein in senile plaques (amyloid plaques) and cerebral blood vessels, as first reported by Alzheimer.[71,72] The density of these plaques has become the basis for the postmortem diagnosis of Alzheimer's disease; there is no absolute diagnostic test for the disease during life. Alzheimer's disease accounts for 60% to 80% of dementia cases over the age of 65, and afflicts 5% to 11% of the population over the age of 65 and about half of the population over the age of 85.[71,73] In addition to its human cost to patient and family, it levies a tremendous social and financial burden. Currently more than 4 million Americans have been diagnosed, many of whom require institutional care at a cost that exceeds $50 billion a year and is expected to increase to $80 billion in the next few years.[71,72] With the rapidly increasing elderly population of persons over 85, the health care problem of Alzheimer's disease is assuming enormous proportions. Research into causes and treatment have greatly expanded in recent years, but the cause remains unknown and there is still no means of stopping the progressive years of mental and personal decline until death. This declining progression of Alzheimer's disease has been divided into three broad stages: (1) Stage I, the early period of increasing forgetfulness and anxious depression; (2) Stage II, a middle period of severe memory loss for recent events, disorientation, and personality changes; and (3) Stage III, the final period of severe confusion, psychosis, memory loss, personal neglect, being bedridden, feeding problems, full-time nursing care, and finally death from an infection such as pneumonia.[74]

Medical Management

No treatment exists for Alzheimer's disease itself, except for suitable day-to-day nursing and social care for the patient and the family. Keeping the patient well nourished, occupied, and exercised helps to lessen anxiety and personal distress, especially in the earlier stages when the person is sufficiently aware of his or her condition. Some use of tranquilizing medication often helps improve difficult behavior and enables the patient to sleep. Research into drug therapy continues. Family counseling and respite care are essential.

Nutritional Management

Nutritional care in each stage of Alzheimer's disease becomes increasingly difficult and challenging. Adequate nutrition throughout the course of the disease

myasthenia gravis • A progressive neuromuscular disease caused by faulty nerve conduction from the presence of antibodies to acetylcholine receptors at the neuromuscular junction.

amyloid • A glycoprotein substance, having a relation to starchlike structure but more a protein compound; an abnormal complex material forming characteristic brain deposits of fibrillary tangles always found in postmortem examinations of patients with Alzheimer's disease, the only means of definitive diagnosis. It is found in various body tissues that, when advanced, forms lesions that destroy functional cells and injure the organ.

TABLE 14-3

Progression of Alzheimer's Disease

Stage	General symptoms	Nutrition-related effects
Stage I (early)	Loss of memory Decrease in social and vocational skills Careless work, housekeeping, finances Easily lost Personality changes Recognition of faces Well-oriented to time	Difficulty in shopping, cooking Forgetting to eat Changes in taste and smell Unusual food choices Degeneration of appetite regulation
Stage II (middle)	Inability to recall names Disorientation to time Delusions Depression Agitation Language problems	Increased energy requirement from agitation Holding food in mouth Forgetting to swallow Losing ability to use utensils Using spoon only Eating with hands
Stage III (final)	Complete disorientation Forgetting own name Not recognizing family Loss of verbal skills Loss of basic self-care skills Urinary and fecal incontinence Bedridden	No recognition of food Refusal to eat or open mouth for feeding Need for nasogastric feeding

Adapted from Gray GE: Nutrition and dementia, *J Am Diet Assoc* 89(12):1795, 1989.

is essential to improve physical well-being, to help maximize the patient's functioning, and to improve the quality of life. Nutrition-related changes occur at each progressive stage of the illness, as shown in Table 14-3, and illustrate the major goals of maintaining adequate nutrition, preventing malnutrition, and devising practical ways to deal with feeding problems.[74,75] Because these patients have lower body weight and require higher energy intakes than normal elderly persons, they often require high-caloric supplement beverages to help supply added nourishment.[76,77] Studies generally have identified four major factors that promote optimal intake in long-term care[78]:

- Using skillful individual feeding techniques
- Selecting appropriate food consistency
- Providing adequate time in which to feed
- Focusing on the midday meal when peak cognitive abilities occur

To Sum Up

Individuals facing disabling illness and injury confront a myriad of interacting challenges, including social attitudes and financial, physical, and psychologic barriers. The team approach, involving family and friends in addition to health professionals, becomes an essential basis of care.

The basic principles of nutritional care involve the *prevention* of malnutrition and *restoration* of eating ability. To avoid malnutrition the nutritionist must assess individual nutritional needs to meet basal energy expenditure needs, added metabolic activity factors from any underlying disease process, and requirements to meet physical therapy and other activities. Nutrient intake must be sufficient to meet a variety of needs: protein and fat (linoleic acid) to promote tissue and organ integrity; carbohydrates to counteract impaired after-injury metabolism; and optimal intake of vitamins and minerals, which sometimes requires the use of supplements to guard against deficiencies. To restore eating ability the occupational therapist and nurse play significant roles in promoting adequate swallowing, chewing, and hand and utensil usage skills. To meet the individual's nutritional needs the nutritionist must assess eating skills, estimate eating desire (sensory stimuli, "comfort foods") and help the client develop new ways of eating with various self-help devices.

Disabling conditions that require special nutritional support and modifications to treat underlying disease effects include the following: (1) *musculoskeletal disease* such as various forms of arthritis; (2) *neuromuscular disease* caused by a sudden brain or spinal cord injury or a stroke or by developmental disabilities from cerebral palsy, epilepsy, or spina bifida; and (3) *progressive neurologic disorders* such as Parkinson's and Huntington's diseases, ALS, multiple sclerosis, or dementia as seen in Alzheimer's disease.

QUESTIONS FOR REVIEW

1. What are the two major goals of rehabilitative therapy for disabling conditions? How do the basic principles of nutritional care help meet these goals?
2. Describe the functions of major nutrients in preventing or retarding the catabolic process that often occurs in long-term disabling illness or injury.
3. Select six of the different disease processes or injuries discussed that result in eating disabilities. Describe the nature of the disease or injury and relate it to the disability involved. Outline the medical and nutritional therapy used in each case, giving the rationale for the nutritional management.

REFERENCES

1. Gines DJ: Introduction to nutrition and rehabilitation. In Gines DJ, ed: *Nutrition management in rehabilitation,* Rockville, Md, 1990, Aspen.
2. Institute of Medicine: *The second fifty years: promoting health and preventing disability,* Washington, DC, 1991, National Academy Press.

3. Breslow RA et al: Malnutrition in tubefed nursing home patients with pressure sores, *J Parenteral Enteral Nutr* 15(6):663, 1991.
4. Cassell JA: Interview: Fred Sammons, ORT, *Top Clin Nutr* 3(3):71, 1988.
5. Harris ED: Rheumatoid arthritis: pathophysiology and implications for therapy, *N Engl J Med* 322(18):1277, 1990.
6. Tonger-Decker R: Nutritional considerations in rheumatoid arthritis, *J Am Diet Assoc* 88(3):327, 1985.
7. Wolman PG: Arthritis. In Gines DJ, ed: *Nutrition management in rehabilitation,* Rockville, Md, 1990, Aspen.
8. Mody GM et al: Nutrition assessment in rheumatoid arthritis, *S Afr Med J* 76:255, 1989.
9. Antonelli MAS et al: Herpes zoster in patients with rheumatoid arthritis treated with weekly, low-dose methotrexate, *Am J Med* 90:295, 1991.
10. Endres S et al: The effect of dietary supplementation with n-3 polyunsaturated fatty acids on the synthesis of interleukin-1 and tumor necrosis factor by mononuclear cells, *N Engl J Med* 320(5):265, 1989.
11. Kremer JM et al: Dietary fish oil and olive oil supplementation in patients with rheumatoid arthritis: clinical and immunologic effects, *Arthritis Rheum* 33(6):810, 1990.
12. Pike MC: Antiinflammatory effects of dietary lipid modification, *J Rheumatol* 16:6, 1989.
13. Panush RS: Food induced ("allergic") arthritis: clinical and serologic studies, *J Rheumatol* 17:291, 1990.
14. Price ME, Dilorio C: Swallowing: a practice guide, *Am J Nurs* 90(7):42, 1990.
15. Ostrov BE: Nutrition and pediatric rheumatic disease. Hypothesis: cytokines modulate nutritional abnormalities in rheumatic diseases, *J Rheumatol* 19(suppl 33):49, 1992.
16. Henderson CJ, Gregg DJ: A nutritional screening test for use with children and adolescents with juvenile rheumatoid arthritis, *J Rheumatol* 19:1276, 1992.
17. White-O'Connor B et al: Dietary habits, weight history, and vitamin supplement use in elderly osteoarthritis patients, *J Am Diet Assoc* 89(3):378, 1989.
18. Wolman PG: Management of patients using unproven regimens for arthritis, *J Am Diet Assoc* 87(9):1211, 1987.
19. Tolstoi LG, Levin RM: Osteoporosis—the treatment controversy, *Nutr Today* 27(4):6, 1992.
20. Chesnut CH: Osteoporosis and its treatment, *N Engl J Med* 326:406, 1992.
21. US Department of Health and Human Services, Public Health Service: *Healthy people 2000: national health promotion and disease prevention objectives,* Pub No 91-50212, Washington, DC, 1990, US Government Printing Office.
22. Kearns P: Nutrition in neurological injury, *Nutr Clin Prac* 6(6):211, 1991.
23. National Center for Health Statistics: *Health, United States, 1989 and prevention profile,* Pub No 90-1232, Hyattsville, Md, 1990, US Department of Health and Human Services.
24. Hubert C: Trauma care crisis, *The Sacramento Bee* 273:1, 1993.
25. Stover SL, Fine PR, eds: Spinal cord injury: the facts and figures, Birmingham, Ala, 1986, University of Alabama Press.
26. Konvolinka CW, Morell VO: Nutrition in head trauma, *Nutr Clin Prac* 6(6):251, 1991.
27. Ott L, Young B: Nutrition in the neurologically injured patient, *Nutr Clin Prac* 6(6):223, 1991.
28. Varella L: Barbiturate therapy and nutritional support in head-injured patients, *Nutr Clin Prac* 6(6):239, 1991.
29. Kirby DF et al: Early enteral nutrition after brain injury by percutaneous endoscopic gastrojejunostomy, *J Parenter Enteral Nutr* 15(3):298, 1991.
30. Annis K et al: Nutritional support of the severe head-injured patient, *Nutr Clin Prac* 6(6):245, 1991.
31. Yankelson S: Traumatic brain injury. In Gines DJ, ed: *Nutrition management in rehabilitation,* Rockville, Md, 1990, Aspen.
32. Roye WP Jr et al: Vertical spinal cord injury—a public catastrophe, *J Trauma* 28:1260, 1988.
33. Chin DE, Kearns P: Nutrition in the spinal-injured patient, *Nutr Clin Prac* 6(6):213, 1991.
34. Rice DP et al: *Cost of injury in the United States: a report to Congress, 1989,* San Francisco, 1989, Institute on Health and Aging, University of California, and Injury Prevention Center, The Johns Hopkins University.
35. Cox SAR et al: Energy expenditure after spinal cord injury: evaluation of stable rehabilitating patients, *J Trauma* 25:419, 1985.
36. O'Brien RY: Spinal cord injury. In Gines DJ, ed: *Nutrition management in rehabilitation,* Rockville, Md, 1990, Aspen.
37. Peiffer SC et al: Nutritional assessment during rehabilitation of the spinal cord injury patient, *J Am Diet Assoc* 78:501, 1981.
38. Doolittle ND: Advances in the neurosciences and implications for nursing care, *J Neurosci Nurs* 23(4):207, 1991.
39. Kozlowski BW: Cerebral palsy. In Gines DJ, ed: *Nutrition management in rehabilitation,* Rockville, Md, 1990, Aspen.
40. Thommessen M et al: The impact of feeding problems on growth and energy intake in children with cerebral palsy, *Eur J Clin Health,* 45:479, 1991.
41. Thommessen M et al: Energy and nutrient intakes of disabled children: do feeding problems make a difference? *J Am Diet Assoc* 91(12):1522, 1991.
42. Ross Laboratories: Estimating stature from the knee height. In *Directions for the Ross Knee Height Caliper,* Columbus, Ohio, 1990, Ross Laboratories.
43. Johnson RK, Ferrara MS: Estimating stature from knee height for persons with cerebral palsy: an evaluation of estimation equations, *J Am Diet Assoc* 91(10):1283, 1991.
44. Ferrang TM et al: Dietary and anthropomorphic assessment of adults with cerebral palsy, *J Am Diet Assoc* 92(9):1083, 1992.

45. Gasch AT: Use of the traditional ketogenic diet for treatment of intractable epilepsy, *J Am Diet Assoc* 90(10):1433, 1990.
46. Schwartz RM et al: Ketogenic diets in the treatment of epilepsy: short-term clinical effects, *Dev Med Child Neurol* 31:145, 1989.
47. Pemberton CM et al: *Mayo Clinic diet manual,* ed 6, Philadelphia, 1988, BC Decker.
48. Dustrude A, Prince A: Provision of optimal nutrition care in myelomeningocele, *Top Clin Nutr* 5(2):34, 1990.
49. Atencio PL et al: Effect of level of lesion and quality of ambulation on growth chart measurements in children with myelomeningocele, *J Am Diet Assoc* 92(7):858, 1992.
50. Unonu JN, Johnson AA: Feeding patterns, food energy, nutrient intakes, and anthropometric measurements of selected black preschool children with Down syndrome, *J Am Diet Assoc* 92(7):856, 1992.
51. Rajput AH: Frequency and cause of Parkinson's disease, *Can J Neurol Sci* 19:103, 1992.
52. Guyton AC: *Textbook of medical physiology,* ed 8, Philadelphia, 1991, WB Saunders.
53. Clayman CB, ed: *The American Medical Association guide to prescription and over-the-counter drugs,* New York, 1988, Random House.
54. Tsui JKC: Future treatment of Parkinson's disease, *Can J Neurol Sci* 19:160, 1992.
55. Lindvall O et al: Grafts of fetal dopamine neurons survive and improve motor function in Parkinson's disease, *Science* 247:574, 1990.
56. Paré S et al: Effect of daytime protein restriction on nutrient intakes of free-living Parkinson's disease patients, *Am J Clin Nutr* 55:701, 1992.
57. Gusella J et al: Discovery of Huntington's disease gene, *Cell,* March 22, 1993.
58. Wexler NS et al: Huntington's disease in Venezuela and gene linkage, *Cytogenet Cell Genet* 37:605, 1984.
59. Morales LM et al: Nutritional evaluation of Huntington's disease patients, *Am J Clin Nutr* 50:145, 1989.
60. Honavar M et al: A clinicopathological study of the Guillain-Barré syndrome, *Brain* 114(3):1245, 1991.
61. Hughes RAC, Swan AV: Double-blind trial of intravenous methylprednisolone in Guillain-Barré syndrome, *Lancet* 341:586, March 6, 1993.
62. McNamara JO, Fridovich I: Did radicals strike Lou Gehrig? *Nature* 362(6415):20, 1993.
63. Rosen DR et al: Mutations in Cu/Zn superoxide dismutase gene are associated with familial amyotrophic lateral sclerosis, *Nature* 362(6415):59, 1993.
64. Marx J: Gene linked to Lou Gehrig's disease, *Science* 259(5100):1393, 1993.
65. Pennisi E: Free-radical scavenger gene tied to ALS, *Science News* 143(10):148, 1993.
66. Miller CA: Nutritional needs and care in amyotrophic lateral sclerosis, *Top Clin Nutr* 4(1):15, 1989.
67. Marx J: Testing of autoimmune therapy begins, *Science* 252(5002):27, 1991.
68. Hoffman M: On the trail of the errant T cells of multiple sclerosis, *Science* 254(5031):521, 1991.
69. Lowis GW: The social epidemiology of multiple sclerosis, *Sci Total Environ* 90:163, 1990.
70. Alzheimer A: Uber eine eigenartige Erkrankung der Hirnrinde, *Algemeine Zeitschrift fur Psychiatrie* 64:146, 1907.
71. Yankner BA, Mesulam M: β-Amyloid and the pathogenesis of Alzheimer's disease, *N Engl J Med* 325(26):1849, 1991.
72. Harrell LE: Alzheimer's disease, *South Med J* 84(suppl 1):32, 1991.
73. Schmechel DE: New approaches to therapy for neurodegenerative diseases, *South Med J* 84(suppl 1):11, 1991.
74. Gray GE: Nutrition and dementia, *J Am Diet Assoc* 89(12):1795, 1989.
75. Claggett MS: Nutritional factors relevant to Alzheimer's disease, *J Am Diet Assoc* 89(3):392, 1989.
76. Renvall NJ et al: Body composition of patients with Alzheimer's disease, *JAMA* 93(1):47, 1993.
77. Riley ME, Volicer L: Evaluation of a new nutritional supplement for patients with Alzheimer's disease, *J Am Diet Assoc* 90(3):433, 1990.
78. Suski NS, Nielsen CC: Factors affecting food intake of women with Alzheimer's type dementia in long-term care, *J Am Diet Assoc* 89(12):1770, 1989.

FURTHER READING

Annis K et al: Nutritional support of the severe head-injured patient, *Nutr Clin Prac* 6(6):245, 1991.

Chin DE, Kearns P: Nutrition in the spinal-injured patient, *Nutr Clin Prac* 6(6):213, 1991.

These two articles in the same issue of this helpful journal provide a case study of a 17-year-old boy who suffered severe head injury when the car he was driving left the road and hit a tree, and they provide a full review of care for persons with spinal injuries. Nutritional support plays an essential role in each case.

Breslow RA et al: Malnutrition in tubefed nursing home patients with pressure sores, *J Parenter Enteral Nutr* 15(6):663, 1991.

Price ME, Diloria C: Swallowing: a practice guide, *Am J Nurs* 90(7):42, 1990.

These two articles discuss two basic problems encountered with disabled persons: the problem of pressure sores in bedridden patients and swallowing problems in a variety of neuromuscular and progressive neurologic disorders, both of which often compromise nutritional status.

Gines DJ: *Nutrition management in rehabilitation,* Rockville, Md, 1990, Aspen.

This small reference manual provides a wealth of material for nutritional care of many conditions requiring rehabilitation following injury or during chronic phases of disabling illnesses.

Evers S et al: Nutritional rehabilitation of developmentally disabled residents in a long-term facility, *J Am Diet Assoc* 91(4):471, 1991.
Ferrang TM et al: Dietary and anthropometric assessment of adults with cerebral palsy, *J Am Diet Assoc* 92(9):1083, 1992.

Cerebral palsy is the most common cause of physical disability in children and adults. These two articles provide practical information concerning the nutritional status and needs of children and adults with cerebral palsy and the extent of malnutrition and eating problems.

CASE STUDY

Patient with a Cerebrovascular Accident

James Braddock is a tall (182 cm, or 6 ft 1 in) 57-year-old black man residing until 6 weeks ago at a rehabilitation center to recover from the results of a CVA (stroke) that occurred 6 months ago. At that time he was brought to the local hospital emergency room, accompanied by his wife, who found him unconscious on the bathroom floor after hearing a fall. He had flaccid paralysis on the right side. Pinprick response on the left side was normal, but it was questionable on the right.

Within an hour Mr. Braddock began to regain consciousness but appeared to be confused, disoriented, and apprehensive. An examination conducted by his personal physician revealed a weight of 155 kg (345 lb), which was usual for the patient, pulse rate of 140, and a blood pressure of 190/100. The physician's impression was cerebral hemorrhage in the left-middle cerebral artery prefrontal area with massive extension, paralysis on the right side, and aphasia.

Laboratory tests were ordered, including blood urea nitrogen, fasting blood glucose, and serum cholesterol, hemoglobin, hematocrit, sodium, potassium, and chloride levels and carbon dioxide–combining power. The physician also ordered an intravenous infusion composed of 500 ml of 2.5% dextrose in 0.5% saline every 8 hours. The diet order was clear liquids by mouth as tolerated. Later the laboratory reported these results: blood urea nitrogen, 16 mg/dl; blood glucose, 140 mg/dl; cholesterol, 290 mg/dl; hemogloblin (g/100 ml)/hematocrit (ml/100 ml), 14/40; carbon dioxide, 60 vol/dl; sodium/potassium, 135/4.2 mEq/L; and chloride, 98 mEq/L.

The diet was changed to full liquid the following day, and the intravenous infusion was discontinued. Mr. Braddock was advanced to a soft diet 4 days later. Nurses' notes indicated he was being fed by the staff. Two weeks later he was able to tolerate a full diet. The occupational therapist, together with the clinical nutritionist and the nurse, developed eating aids that would help him learn to feed himself.

After 4 weeks Mr. Braddock was transferred to the rehabilitation center for follow-up therapy. At that time a vigorous physical and speech therapy program began. Self-feeding skills helped him gain more independence, and a diet plan of 1500 kcalories with cholesterol limited to 300 mg and sodium restricted to 1000 mg was designed to promote weight loss and help control his hypertension and vascular disease.

Response to therapy was good. In 6 months Mr. Braddock was able to walk with a cane and had regained much of his ability to speak. He was released to home care, following careful instructions regarding his home care needs. Follow-up home visit reports indicate that Mr. Braddock has been losing weight gradually, has stopped smoking, and is practicing prescribed exercises daily. He is now inquiring about future job possibilities.

Questions for Analysis

1. What underlying conditions may have been responsible for the CVA? What factors indicate this possible association?
2. What was the purpose of each laboratory test ordered? Which values were elevated? Which values were inadequate?
3. What members of the rehabilitative support team are identified? Was any member underused? How could this role have been expanded?
4. Outline the instructions you would give Mrs. Braddock to help her plan nutritional care for her husband at home.

Independent Living Versus the Kindness of Strangers

"I have always relied on the kindness of strangers." If Tennessee Williams' famous line in his play *A Streetcar Named Desire* for his lead character Blanche conjures up images of a blithe Southern belle, you're right—but think again. In today's reality you may well think of a once-independent career woman now confined to her wheelchair, much of her financial resources gone to pay for lengthy and highly specialized care. Before 1978 she would have relied heavily on the "kindness of strangers" to meet most of her basic needs, including transportation to keep medical appointments and to purchase food and help in meal preparation and personal care.

In 1978 the Rehabilitation Act of 1973 was amended to allocate federal funds to establish independent living centers for disabled persons. The number of Americans who cannot perform even simple activities of daily living because of a major illness, disabling injury, or chronic health condition rose dramatically by 83.2% in the one decade between 1966 and 1976, for example, and has been gradually rising during the 1980s. In 1980 about 15% of the free-living population was disabled. This rise is caused primarily by new technologies that have virtually wiped out the infectious diseases that used to kill the disabled, as well as those that together with nutrition have extended the general life span. The causes of disability have changed also with rheumatoid arthritis and diabetes replacing heart disease and other causes.

Disabled persons have traditionally been barred from many activities because of limited mobility. Jobs, education, and recreational facilities have often been denied to them because of inadequate physical access or facilities and even fear and prejudice. Promotion of access, as well as independent living and access to employment, has been a strong civil rights issue in many parts of the United States with many positive results.

The passage of legislation establishing independent living centers across the United States enabled disabled persons to meet their basic needs. It also promoted political awareness among local communities. This legislation has opened the door to disabled persons who can and want to be self-reliant individuals capable of enriching their lives and contributing to their communities. Economic realities have meant that federal authorities have been reluctant to issue costly new regulations regarding the needs of disabled persons, although employment access is now guaranteed under the Americans with Disabilities Act of 1990. But the recent record is mixed, since cutbacks have occurred in programs providing income support via the Social Security Administration. Public support for these programs is also lessening, since the proportion of the public being served is relatively small and their needs are highly specialized.

Will the disabled person once again find it necessary to rely on "the kindness of strangers"? How will the loss of contributed income from working disabled persons affect the economy? And will the kind strangers be capable of filling the gap?

REFERENCES

Cross EW: Implementing the Americans with Disabilities Act, *J Am Diet Assoc* 93(3):273, 1993.

DeJong G, Lifchez R: Physical disability and public policy, *Sci Am* 248(6):40, 1983.

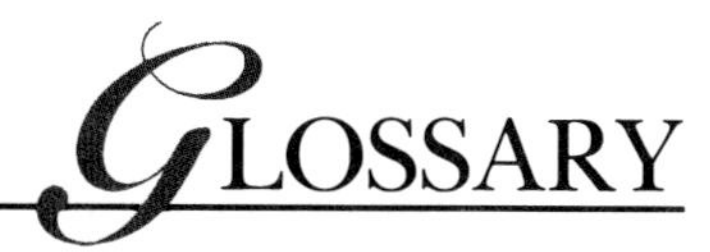

GLOSSARY

25, hydroxycholecalciferol [25,(OH)D_3] Initial product formed in the liver in the process of developing the active vitamin D hormone.

7, dehydrocholesterol A precursor cholesterol compound in the skin that is irradiated by sunlight to produce an initial stage in the process of forming activated vitamin D hormone.

Acetyl (acyl) group (L *acetium,* vinegar; Gr *hyle,* matter) The 2-carbon fragment produced from glucose (acetyl) by process of glycolysis or from fatty acids (acyl) by beta-oxidation, which combines with coenzyme A to fuel the final common energy pathway in the cell's mitochondria—the citric acid cycle.

Acetyl-CoA (L *acetum,* vinegar; Gr *hyle,* matter; *en,* in; *zyme,* leaven) Chief precursor of lipids, an important intermediate in the citric acid cycle; formed by an acetyl group attaching itself to coenzyme A during the oxidation of amino acids, fatty acids, or pyruvate.

Acetylcholine A major neurotransmitter in the body, operating at the myoneural (muscle-nerve) junction; in sympathetic and parasympathetic ganglia and at parasympathetic nerve endings.

Achlasia (Gr *a-,* negative, without; *cholasis,* relaxation) Failure to relax the smooth muscle fibers of the gastrointestinal tract at any point of juncture of its parts; especially failure of the esophagogastric sphincter to relax when swallowing, due to degeneration of ganglion cells in the wall of the organ. The lower esophagus also loses its normal peristaltic activity. Also called cardiospasm.

Acid (L *acidus,* sour) Substance that neutralizes base substances by donating H ions. Acids are essentially ionized hydrogen donors—in solution they provide H ions.

Acidosis Disturbance in acid-base balance in which there is a reduction of the alkali reserve. Acidosis may be caused by an accumulation of acids, as in diabetic acidosis, or by an excess loss of bicarbonate, as in renal disease.

Actin (Gr *aktis,* a radiating activating substance) Myofibril protein whose synchronized meshing action in conjunction with **myosin** causes muscles to contract and relax.

Active transport Movement of solutes in solution (for example, products of digestion such as glucose) across a membrane *against* the usual opposing forces. Such movement requires energy, which is supplied by the cell. Sometimes an additional transporting substance is required, such as sodium, for absorbing glucose.

Acylation Introduction of an acid radical into the molecule of a chemical compound; process of attaching fatty acids to glycerol base to form triglycerides (triacylglycerols).

Adenocarcinoma (Gr *adenos,* gland; *karkinos,* cancer) Tumor arising from glandular tissue or in which tumor cells form glandular structures; usually classified according to type of glandular cell arrangement.

Adenosine triphosphate (ATP) The high energy compound formed in the cell, called the "energy currency" of the cell due to the binding of energy in its high-energy phosphate bonds for release for cell work as these bonds are split. A compound of adenosine (a nucleotide containing adenine and ribose) that has three phosphoric acid groups. ATP is a high-energy phosphate compound important in energy exchange for cellular activity. The splitting off of the terminal phosphate bond (PO_4) of ATP to produce adenosine diphosphate (ADP) releases bound energy and transfers it to free energy available for body work. The reforming of ATP in cell oxidation again stores energy in high-energy phosphate bonds for use as needed. They may be charged and discharged according to conditions in the cell.

ADH mechanism System of body water conservation, controlled by the antidiuretic hormone (ADH) from the pituitary in response to diminished fluid pressure in the kidney nephrons, causing increased water reabsorption.

Adipocyte (L *adipis,* fat; Gr *kytos,* hollow vessel) A fat cell. All cell names end in the suffix *-cyte,* with the type of cell indicated by the root word to which it is added.

Adipose (L *adeps,* fat; *adiposus,* fatty) Fat present in cells of adipose—fatty tissue.

Admixture (L *admixtus,* admixture) A mixture resulting from adding or mingling another ingredient; a combination of two or more substances that are not chemically united or that exist in no fixed proportion to each other.

Adrenocorticotropic hormone (ACTH) Anterior pituitary hormone; stimulates secretion of glucocorticoids from the adrenal cortex; insulin antagonist.

Aerobic (Gr, L *aer,* air or gas) Requiring oxygen to proceed.

Aerobic capacity (Gr *aer,* air or gas) Milliliters of oxygen consumed per kilogram of body weight per minute; influenced by body composition.

Afferent (L *ad,* to, into; *ferre,* to carry, bear) Conveying toward a center, as an afferent nerve.

Agrogenetics (Gr *agros,* field; *gennan,* to produce) The application of the biotechnology of "genetic engineering" to agriculture for the purpose of developing desirable new strains of plants and their produce.

Albinism (L *albus,* white) Congenital absence of pigment in the skin, hair, eyes due to absence or defect of tyrosinase, an enzyme that catalyzes the oxidation of the amino acid tyrosine, a precursor of melanin.

Aldosterone Potent hormone of the cortex of the adrenal glands, which acts on the distal renal tubule to cause reabsorption of sodium in an ion exchange with potassium. The aldosterone mechanism is essentially a sodium-conserving mechanism but indirectly also conserves water since water absorption follows the sodium reabsorption.

Alkalosis Disturbance in acid-base balance in which there is a reduction of the acid partner in the buffer system or an increase in the base. In either case, the necessary 20:1 ratio between base and acid is upset by an increase in the relative amount of base.

Alpha-fetoprotein A fetal antigen in amniotic fluid that provides an early pregnancy test for fetal malformations such as neural tube defect.

alpha-Tocopherol (α-Tocopherol) equivalents Measure of total vitamin E content of the diet, which takes into account the varying vitamin E activity among the different tocopherols making up the group.

Alveolocapillary membrane (L *alveoli,* small sac-like cavity; *membrana,* parchment, membrane) Thin limiting membrane of the pulmonary alveoli (air sacs) and capillaries.

Ameloblasts (Old Fr *amel,* enamel; Gr *blastos,* germ) A cylindrical epithelial cell in the innermost layer of the enamel organ which takes part in developing the tooth enamel.

Amino The monovalent chemical group $-NH_2$.

Amino acid (*Amino,* the monovalent chemical group $-NH_2$) Carriers of the essential element nitrogen; structural units of protein, specific amino acids being linked in specific sequence by peptide chains to form specific proteins.

Amnionic fluid (Gr *amnion,* bowl) The watery fluid within the membrane enveloping the fetus, in which the fetus is suspended.

Amorphous (Gr *amorphos,* shapeless) Lacking definite form; having no specific shape.

Ampullae (L *ampulla,* a jug) A general term for a flasklike wider portions of a tubular structure; spaces under the nipple of the breast for storing milk.

Amyloid (Gr *amylon,* starch; *-oid, eidos,* form, shape) A glycoprotein substance, having a relation to starch-like structure but more a protein compound; an abnormal complex material forming characteristic brain deposits of fibrillary tangles always found in postmortem examinations of patients with Alzheimer's disease, the only means of definitive diagnosis; found in various body tissues which, when advanced, forms lesions that destroy functional cells and injure the organ.

Amylopectin (Gr *amylon,* starch; *pekt,* fixed, congealed) Polysaccharide, the insoluble part of starch, forms paste with hot water and thickens during cooking.

Amylose (Gr *amylon,* starch) Polysaccharide, the soluble part of starch.

Amyotrophic lateral sclerosis (Gr *a-,* negative; *mys,* muscle; *trophē,* nourishment; L *lateralis,* to the side; *sklērōsis,* hardness) A progressive neuromuscular disease characterized by the degeneration of the neurons of the spinal cord and the motor cells of the brain stem, causing a deficit of upper and lower motor neurons; death usually occurs in two to three years.

Anabolism Metabolic process by which body tissues are built.

Ancini Very small units of secretory cells leading into a complex system of transporting channels.

Anemia (Gr *an-,* negative prefix; *haima,* blood) Blood condition characterized by decreased number of circulating red blood cells, hemoglobin, or both.

Anergy (Gr *an-,* negative prefix, *ergon,* work) Diminished immunologic reactivity to specific antigens.

Anion An ion that carries a negative electrical charge.

Anorexia nervosa (Gr "want of appetite") Extreme psychophysiologic aversion to food, resulting in life-threatening weight loss. A psychiatric eating disorder caused by a morbid fear of fatness, in which the person's distorted body-image is reflected as fat when the body is actually malnourished and extremely thin from self-starvation.

Antagonist (Gr *antagonisma,* struggle) Agent that has an opposite, conflicting, or inhibiting action to another substance.

Anthropometry (Gr *anthropos,* man; *metron,* measure) The science of measuring the size, weight, and proportions of the human body.

Antibody Any of numerous protein molecules produced by B cells as a primary immune defense for attaching to specific related **antigens;** animal protein made up of a specific sequence of amino acids that is designed to interact with its specific antigen during an allergic response or to prevent infection.

Antigen (antibody + Gr *gennan,* to produce) Any foreign or "non-self" substances, such as toxins, viruses, bacteria, and foreign proteins, that stimulate the production of **antibodies** specifically designed to interact with them.

Antimetabolite A substance bearing a close structural resemblance to one required for normal physiological functioning, and exerting its effect by interfering with the utilization of the essential metabolite.

Antioxidant (Gr *anti,* against; *oxys* keen) A substance that inhibits oxidation of polyunsaturated fatty acids and formation of free radicals in the cells.

Antiplatelet (Gr *anti-,* against; *platelet,* small plate or disk) Anticoagulation effect; platelet is a blood factor, small disk-shaped structure found in clusters in the blood, chiefly known for its role in blood coagulation; lacks a nucleus and DNA but contains active enzymes and mitochondria.

Antrum (Gr *antron,* cave) The lower part of the stomach opening through the pyloric valve into the duodenum.

Apo- (prefix-protein binder or carrier) (Gr *apo,* from) Prefix implying separation or derivation.

Apoprotein (Gr *apo,* from, separation or derivation from; *prōtos,* first, protein compound) A separate protein compound that attaches to its specific receptor site on a particular lipoprotein and activates certain functions, such as synthesis of a related enzyme. For example, apoprotein C II, an apoprotein of HDL and VLDL that functions to activate the enzyme lipoprotein lipase.

Areola (L *areola,* area, space) A defined space; a circular area of different color surrounding a central point, such as the darkened pigmented ring surrounding the nipple of the breast.

Ariboflavinosis Group of clinical manifestations of riboflavin deficiency.

Arteriole (L *arteriola*) A minute arterial branch, especially one just proximal to a capillary.

Arteriosclerosis (Gr *arteria,* from *ar,* air, and *tērein,* to keep, because of ancient belief that the arteries contained vital air; *sklēros,* hard) Blood vessel disease characterized by thickening and hardening of artery walls, with loss of functional elasticity, mainly affecting the intima (inner lining) of the arteries.

Arthroplasty (Gr *arthron,* joint; *plassein,* to form) Surgical procedure for replacing degenerated joints such as the hip with a mechanical joint of metal or special plastic; formation of moveable joint replacement, developed by team of biomedical engineers and orthopedists.

Ascites (Gr *askites,* from; *askos,* bag) Outflow and accumulation of fluid in the abdominal cavity; also known as *abdominal* or *peritoneal dropsy*.

Asterixis (Gr *a,* negative prefix; *sterixis,* a fixed position) Neuromotor disturbance marked by an inability to hold outstretched hands in a steady position, resulting in an intermittent flapping of the hands, characteristic of hepatic coma.

Atheroma (Gr *athērē,* gruel; *-oma,* a mass or body of tissue) A mass of fatty plaque formed in inner arterial walls in atherosclerosis.

Atherosclerosis (Gr *athere,* gruel; *skleros,* hard) Common form of arteriosclerosis, characterized by the gradual formation, beginning in childhood in genetically predisposed individuals, of yellow cheese-like streaks of cholesterol and fatty material that develop into hardened plaques in the intima or inner lining of major blood vessels such as coronary arteries, eventually in adulthood cutting off blood supply to the tissue served by the vessels; the underlying pathology of coronary heart disease.

Atony (L *atonia,* from a negative; Gr *tonos,* tension) Lack of normal tone or strength, as in lack of muscle tone.

Atrium (L *atrion,* hall) An anatomical chamber; usually used alone to designate one of the pair of smaller upper chambers of the heart, with thin muscular walls, which receives blood from the body's inflowing circulation via the superior and inferior vena cava, and delivers it to the thicker walled ventricles.

Autonomy (Gr *autos,* self; *nomos,* law) The state of functioning independently, without extraneous influence.

Azotemia (Gr *a,* negative; *zoe,* life; *azote,* nitrogen; *haima,* blood) An excess of urea or other nitrogenous substances in the blood.

Basal metabolism (BMR) Amount of energy required to maintain the resting body's internal activities after an overnight fast.

Base Chemical substance that is capable of neutralizing acid by accepting hydrogen ions from the acid. A synonymous term is *alkali.*

Base bicarbonate "Base" in this term refers to *any* base that might be combined with bicarbonate. In the main buffer system of the human body, this base is sodium bicarbonate.

Beikost (Ger) Solid and semisolid baby food.

Benign (L *benignus,* kind, generous) Not malignant or recurrent; favorable for recovery.

Beriberi (Singhalese "I cannot, I cannot") A disease of the peripheral nerves caused by a deficiency of thiamin (vitamin B_1). It is characterized by pain (neuritis) and paralysis of the extremities, cardiovascular changes and edema. Beriberi is common in the Orient, where diets consist largely of milled rice with little protein.

Beta carotene One of the three forms (alpha, beta, and gamma) of carotene, all of which are precursor pro-vitamins and may be converted into vitamin A in the body. Carotene is a yellow or red pigment found in carrots, leafy vegetables, sweet potatoes, mangos, egg yolks, etc.

Beta-oxidation Process of breaking down fatty acids into 2-carbon fragments of acetyl-CoA residues.

Bicarbonate ions (HCO^-_3) Alkaline ions that buffer or neutralize the gastric hydrochloric acid secretions.

Bile (L *bilis,* bile) A fluid secreted by the liver and transported to the gallbladder for concentration and storage; released into duodenum upon entry of fat to facilitate enzymatic fat digestion by acting as an emulsifying agent.

Bilirubin (L *bilis,* bile; *ruber,* red) A reddish bile pigment resulting from the degradation of heme by reticuloendothelial cells in the liver; a high level in the blood produces the yellow-skin symptomatic of jaundice.

Bioavailability Amount of a nutrient ingested in food that is absorbed and thus available to the body for metabolic use.

Bioelectrical impedance analysis A measure of lean body mass by determining how strongly the body prevents a flow of electrical energy through its tissues; resistance readings differentiate between fat and lean tissue.

Bioflavonoids (L *flavus,* yellow) Compounds that are widely distributed in nature as pigments in flowers, fruits, tree barks, vegetables, and grains. They have been found to have little nutritional value, and thus are not considered essential nutrients.

Blastocyst (Gr *blastos,* germ; *kystis,* bladder) Early developmental stage of the embryo, consisting of an inner cell mass, a cavity, and an outer layer, the trophoblast.

Blood urea nitrogen (BUN) The nitrogen component of urea in the blood; a measure of kidney function; elevated levels of BUN indicate a disorder of kidney function.

Body composition The relative sizes of the four basic body compartments that make up the total body: lean body mass (muscle mass), fat, water, and bone.

Body pool The collective quantity of a given substance throughout the body tissues, as in the body's metabolic pool of amino acids.

Bradykinin (Gr *bradys,* slow; *kinein,* to move) A 9-amino acid peptide chain formed from kallidin II by the action of kallikrein; a very powerful vasodilator that causes increased capillary permeability and also constricts smooth muscle.

Brunner's glands John Brunner (1653-1727), Swiss anatomist; mucus-secreting glands in the duodenum that provide mucus to protect the mucosa from irritation and erosion by the strongly acid gastric juices entering from the stomach. Emotional tension and stress inhibit these mucous secretions—a primary factor in duodenal ulcer formation.

Brush border Vast array of microvilli covering each villus on the absorptive surface of the small intestine, holding nutrients ready for absorption within an unstirred layer of water and facilitating their absorption with a greatly expanded surface area. So named because they appear as the bristles of a brush when viewed with an electron microscope.

Buccal (L *bucca,* cheek) Pertaining to or directed toward the cheek.

Buffer Mixture of acidic and alkaline components that, when added to a solution is able to protect the solution against wide variations in its pH, even when strong acids and bases are added to it. If an acid is added, the alkaline partner reacts with it to counteract its acidic effect. If a base is added, the acid partner reacts with it to counteract its alkalizing effect. A solution to which a buffer has been added is called a buffered solution.

Buffered solution A solution to which a buffer has been added.

Bulimia nervosa (L *bous,* ox; *limos,* hunger) A psychiatric eating disorder related to the person's fear of fatness, in which cycles of gorging on large quantities of food are followed by self-induced vomiting and use of diuretics and laxatives to maintain a "normal" body weight.

Cachexia (Gr *kakos,* bad; *hexis,* habit) A specific profound effect caused by malnutrition and a disturbance in glucose metabolism usually seen in patients with terminal cancer or heart failure; general poor health and malnutrition indicated by an emaciated appearance.

Calcitonin (L *calx,* lime, calcium; *tonus,* balance) A polypeptide hormone secreted by the thyroid gland in response to hypercalcemia, which acts to lower both calcium and phosphate in the blood.

Calcitriol Activated hormone form of vitamin D [$1,25(OH)_2D_3$]—1,25, dihydroxycholecalciferol.

Calculus (L *pebble*) Any abnormal accretion within the body of material that forms a "stone." Calculi are usually composed of mineral salts.

Callus (L *callositis,* callus, bone) Unorganized mesh-work of newly grown, woven bone developed on pattern of original fibrin clot (formed after fracture or surgery) and normally replaced in the healing process by hard adult bone.

Calmodulin A calcium-binding protein occurring in many tissues and participating in the regulation of many biochemical and physiological processes.

Calorie (L *calor,* heat) A unit of heat energy. The calorie used in the study of metabolism is the large calorie, or *kilocalorie,* defined as the amount of heat required to raise the temperature of 1 kg of water 1° Celsius (centigrade).

Calorimetry (L *calor,* heat; Gr *metron,* measure) Measurement of amounts of heat absorbed or given out. *Direct method*: measurement of amount of heat produced by a subject enclosed in a small chamber; *indirect method*: measurement of amount of heat produced by a subject by the quantity of nitrogen and carbon dioxide eliminated.

Cancer (L *cancer,* crab) A malignant cellular tumor with properties of tissue invasion and spread to other parts of the body.

Candidiasis (L *candidus,* glowing white) Infection with the fungus of the genus *Candida,* generally caused by *C. albicans,* so-named for the whitish appearance of its small lesions; usually a superficial infection in moist areas of the skin or inner mucous membranes.

Capillary fluid shift mechanism Process that controls the movement of water and small molecules in solution (electrolytes, nutrients) between the blood in the capillary and the surrounding interstitial area. Filtration of water and solutes out of the capillary at the arteriole end and reabsorption at the venule end are accomplished by shifts in balance between the intracapillary hydrostatic blood pressure and the colloidal osmotic pressure exerted by the plasma proteins.

Carbonic acid Acid partner in the carbonic acid-base bicarbonate buffer system in the body.

Carboxyl (COOH) The monovalent radical, -COOH, occurring in those organic acids termed carboxylic acids.

Carboxypeptidase (L *carbo-,* carbon; *oxy,* oxygen) A protein enzyme that splits off the chemical group *carboxyl* (-COOH) at the end of peptide chains, acting on the peptide bond of the terminal amino acidhaving a free-end carboxyl group.

Carcinoma (Gr *karkinos,* crab; *onkoma,* a swelling) A malignant new growth made up of epithelial cells, infiltrating the surrounding tissue and spreading to other parts of the body.

Cardiac output (Gr *kardia,* heart) Total volume of blood propelled from the heart with each contraction; equal to the stroke output multiplied by the number of beats per the time unit used in the calculation.

Cardiac rate Number of heart beats per minute; pulse rate.

Carnitine A naturally occurring amino acid ($C_{17}H_{15}NO_3$) formed from methionine and lysine, required for transport of long-chain fatty acids across the mitochondrial membrane where they are oxidized as fuel substrate for metabolic energy.

Carotinoids Any of a group of red and yellow pigments chemically similar to and including carotene found in dark green and yellow vegetables and fruits.

Cartilage (L *cartilago,* gristle) A specialized fibrous connective tissue, forming most of the temporary skeleton of the embryo, providing a model in which most of the bones develop and constituting an important part of the growth mechanism of the organism.

Casein hydrolysate formula (L *caseus,* cheese) Infant formula with base of hydrolyzed casein, major milk protein, produced by partially breaking down the casein into smaller peptide fragments, making a product that is more easily digested.

Catabolism (Gr *katabole,* a throwing down) The breaking-down phase of metabolism, the opposite of anabolism. Catabolism includes all the processes in which complex substances are progressively broken down into simpler ones. Catabolism usually involves the release of energy. Together, anabolism and catabolism constitute metabolism, which is the coordinated operation of anabolic and catabolic processes into a dynamic balance of energy and substance.

Catalyst (Gr *katalysis,* dissolution) A substance, such as enzymes and their component trace elements, that control specific cell metabolism reactions but are not changed or consumed themselves in the reaction as are their specific substrates on which they work.

Catecholamine (*catechol,* aromatic chemical substance; *amine,* organic compound containing nitrogen) Group of compounds having similar effects to those of the sympathetic nervous system; includes dopamine, norepinephrine, and epinephrine.

Cation (Gr *kata,* down; *ion,* going) An ion having a positive charge owing to the loss of one or more electrons.

Cell differentiation The process of acquiring completely individual characters, as occurs in the progressive specific diversification of all cells, body tissue, and organs of the embryo.

Cellular immunity (L *immunitas,* immunity) Specific acquired immunity in which the role of the T-lymphocytes predominate.

Cellulose (L *cellula,* live cell) An inert carbohydrate $(C_6 10_{10} O_5)_n$; the chief constituent of the cell walls of fibrous plants.

Cerebrospinal (L *cerebrum,* brain) Pertaining to the brain and spinal cord.

Ceruloplasmin Plasma protein containing copper-forming ferroxidase, an enzyme that oxidizes iron in preparation for its absorption.

Cheilosis (Gr *cheilos,* lip) A general symptom of tissue inflammation and breakdown producing swelling and reddening of the lips, a chapped appearance, and fissures at the corners of the mouth; associated with general malnutrition, especially a deficiency of riboflavin.

Chelate (Gr *chele,* claw) Chemical compound capable of grasping and incorporating a metallic ion into its molecular structure. By binding the metal, the chelate removes it from a tissue or from the circulating blood.

Chemical bonding Process of linking the radicals, chemical elements or groups, of a chemical compound.

Chemical reaction (L *re,* again; *agere,* to act) The reciprocal action of chemical agents upon each other; chemical change.

Chemical score A measure of protein quality, based on its amino acid composition.

Chloride-bicarbonate shift Exchange of bicarbonate for chloride. In red blood cells, it provides constant bicarbonate buffering for the rapidly forming carbonic acid from water and carbon dioxide ($H_2O + CO_2$).

Cholecalciferol Chemical name for vitamin D in its inactive dietary form (D_3). When the inactive cholecalciferol is consumed or its counterpart cholesterol compound is developed in the skin, its first stage of activation occurs in the liver and then is completed in the kidney to the active vitamin D hormone form *calcitriol,* 1,25-dihydroxycholecalciferol, or shorter form 1,25 $(OH)_2D_3$.

Cholecystectomy (Gr *cholē,* bile; *kystis,* bladder; *ektomē,* a cutting out) Surgical removal of the gallbladder.

Cholecystokinin (CCK) (Gr *chole,* bile or gall; *kystis,* bladder, *kinein,* to move) A peptide hormone that is secreted by the mucosa of the duodenum in response to the presence of fat. The cholecystokinin causes the gallbladder to contract. This contraction propels bile into the duodenum, where it is needed to emulsify the fat. The fat is thus prepared for digestion and absorption.

Cholesterol A fat-related compound, a sterol ($C_{27}H_{45}OH$). It is a normal constituent of bile and a principal constituent of gallstones. In body metabolism cholesterol is important as a precursor of various steroid hormones such as sex hormones and adrenal corticoids. Cholesterol is synthesized by the liver. It is widely distributed in nature, especially in animal tissue such as glandular meats and egg yolk.

Chorea (L *choreia,* dance) A wide variety of ceaseless involuntary movements that are rapid, complex, and jerky, yet appear to be well coordinated; characteristic movements of Huntington's disease.

Chorion frondosum (Gr *chorion,* outermost trophoblast membrane; L *frondosus,* leafy, bearing fronds or villi) Fetal portion of the placenta. About 2 weeks after implantation occurs, villi develop at the site.

Chorionic gonadotropin (Gr *chorion,* outer trophoblast membrane; L *gonas,* seed; Gr *tropin,* a turning, having an affinity for) A hormone, produced in the initial stage of the placenta of a pregnant woman, that stimulates the production of estrogen and progesterone. Its presence in the blood or urine is an indication of pregnancy.

Chyme (Gr *chymos,* juice) Semifluid food mass in gastrointestinal tract following gastric digestion.

Chymotrypsin (Gr *chymos,* chyme, creamy gruel-like material produced by gastric digestion of food) One of the protein-splitting and milk-curdling pancreatic enzymes, activated in the intestine from precursor chymotrypsinogen; breaks peptide linkages of the amino acids phenylalanine and tyrosine.

Cilia (L *cilium,* hair) Minute hairlike organelles, identical in structure to flagella (long, waving tails of cells such as sperm providing locomotion), that live on the surfaces of certain cells and beat in rhythmic waves, sweeping out debris from external epithelial tissue and moving liquids along internal epithelial tissue.

Cirrhosis (Gr *kirrhos,* orange-yellow) Chronic liver disease, characterized by loss of functional cells, with fibrous and nodular regeneration.

cis (L, on the same side) Having certain atoms or radicals in a chemical structure on the same side. Naturally occurring *cis* fats bend inward at their double bond toward the same side.

Cisterni chyli Cistern or receptacle of the chyle is a dilated sac at the origin of the thoracic duct, which is the common truck that receives all the lymphatic vessels. The cisterna chyli lies in the abdomen between the second lumbar vertebra and the aorta. It receives the lymph from the intestinal trunk, the right and left lumbar lymphatic trunks, and two descending lymphatic trunks. The chyle, after passing through the cisterna chyli, is carried upward into the chest through the thoracic duct and empties into the venous blood at the point where the left subclavian vein joins the left internal jugular vein.

Citric acid A tricarboxylic acid (3 carboxyl -COOH- groups), produced by a turn of the final energy production cycle in the cell mitochondria, then starting the cycle again in a continuous manner.

Citric acid cycle Final energy production pathway in the cell mitochondria that transforms the ultimate fuel acetyl CoA from carbohydrate and fat, capturing this energy in the cell's metabolic enzyme cycle production of high-energy phosphate bonds of ATP.

Clostridial (Gr *kloster,* spindle) Any of several rod-shaped spore-forming, anaerobic bacteria of the genus Clostridium, found in soil and in the intestinal tract of humans and animals.

Coenzyme A (CoA) Central compound in metabolism; catalyzes transfer of acyl (acetyl) groups (acetylation).

Coenzyme factors A major metabolic role of the micronutrients, vitamins and minerals, as essential partners with cell enzymes in a variety of reactions in both energy and protein metabolism.

Cognitive (L *cognoscere,* to know) Pertaining to the mental processes of perceptions, memory, judgment, and reasoning, as contrasted with emotional and volitional processes.

Collagen (Gr *kolla,* glue; *gennan,* to produce) The protein substance of the white fibers (collagenous fibers) of skin, tendon, bone, cartilage, and all other connective tissue; it is converted into gelatin by boiling.

Collagen disease (Gr *kolla,* glue; *gennan,* to produce) Diseases attacking collagen tissues, the protein substance of the white fibers (collagenous fibers) of skin, tendon, bone, cartilage, and other connective tissue; any of a group of diseases that are clinically distinct but have in common widespread pathologic changes in the connective tissue, such as rheumatoid arthritis, lupus erythematosis, scleroderma, and rheumatic fever.

Colloid (Gr *kollōdēs,* glutinous) Glutinous, glue-like; a dispersion of matter throughout a liquid.

Colloidal osmotic pressure (COP) Pressure produced by the protein molecules in the plasma and in the cell. Because proteins are large molecules, they do not pass through the separating membranes of the capillary cells. Thus they remain in their respective compartments, exerting a constant osmotic pull that protects vital plasma and cell fluid volumes in these compartments.

Colostrum (L *colostrum,* pre-milk) Thin yellow fluid first secreted by the mammary gland a few days before and after childbirth, preceding the mature breast milk. It contains up to 20% protein including a large amount of lactalbumin, more minerals and less lactose and fat than does milk, and immunoglobulins representing the antibodies found in maternal blood.

Compartment The collective quantity of material in a given type of space in the body.

Complement (L *complere,* to fill) A complex series of enzymatic proteins occurring in normal serum that interact to combine with and augment (fill out, complete) the antigen-antibody complex of the body's immune system, producing lysis when the antigen is an intact cell; composed of 11 discrete proteins or functioning components, activated by the immunoglobulin factors IgG and IgM.

Complementary proteins A protein that contains the essential amino acids in quantities sufficient for maintenance of the body and for a normal rate of growth. Such proteins are said to have a high biologic value. Egg, milk, cheese, and meat are complete protein foods.

Complete protein food A protein food containing all of the essential amino acids, animal food sources are milk, cheese, meat, eggs. Plant proteins alone are incomplete, but complementary combinations may be planned to make a complete protein mix, as a vegetarian would do.

Compound glands Larger organized glands made up of a number of smaller secretory units whose excretory ducts combine to form ducts of progressively higher order and size.

Cones (L *conus,* cone) One or the cone-shaped cells in the retina of the eye, sensitive to color and intensity of light; a solid figure of body with a circular base tapering to a point.

Conjugated (L *conjugatus,* yoked together) Paired, or equally coupled; working in unison.

Conjunctiva The delicate mucous membrane that lines the exposed portion of the eyeball and inner surface of the eyelids.

Cori cycle Glucose-lactate cycle between muscles and the liver; named for husband-wife team of American biochemists Carl and Getty Cori.

Cornea (L *corneus,* horny) The transparent structure forming the front coating of the eye.

Corticotropin-releasing factor (CRF) (L *cortex,* shell or rind, external layer; Gr *tropikos,* turning, -tropic, suffix indicating turning toward or changing) Hypothalamus factor stimulating release of anterior pituitary hormone ACTH (adrenocorticotropic hormone).

Covalent (L *co,* together; *valentia,* strength) The number of electron pairs that an atom can share with other atoms; the bond formed by sharing of a pair of electrons by two atoms.

Cretinism (F *cretinisine*) A congenital disease due to absence or deficiency of normal thyroid secretion, characterized by physical deformity, dwarfism, and mental retardation, and often by goiters.

Cristae Projections or projecting structure; infolding of inner mitochondrial membrane forming self-like crests or ridges holding in place metabolic cell enzymes.

Cruciferous (L *cruces,* cross; *forma,* form) Bearing a cross; botanical term for plants belonging to the botanical family *Cruciferae* or *Brassicaceae,* the mustard family, so-called because of cross-like, four-petaled flowers; name given to certain vegetables of this family, such as broccoli, cabbage, brussel sprouts, and cauliflower.

Crypts of Lieberkuhn (Gr *kryptein,* to hide) Johann Lieberkuhn (1711-1756) German anatomist; tubular glands of the intestine that secrete intestinal juice. These special secretory organs open between the bases of the villi. Their walls are lined with special cells that secrete digestive enzymes, water, and electrolytes.

Cushing's disease A condition first described by Boston surgeon Harvey Cushing (1869-1939), due to hypersecretion of adrenocorticotropic hormone (ACTH) or excessive intake of glucocorticoids, characterized by rapidly developing fat deposits of face, neck, and trunk, giving an enlarged and rounded "moon-face" or cushingoid appearance.

Cyclosporine An immunosuppressant drug widely used following organ transplants to control the immune system and prevent rejection of the new tissue.

Cystic fibrosis A chronic hereditary disease, primarily affecting infants, children, and young adults, in which there is widespread malfunction of the exocrine glands.

The disease is characterized by the production of thick mucus in the lungs and fibrous tissue formation obstructing the ducts of the pancreas, thus preventing normal secretion of pancreatic enzymes.

Cytokines (Gr *kytos,* hollow vessel, cell; *kinētos,* moveable, changing) Substances produced in tissues that can cause inflammatory changes in tissue cells, e.g., tumor necrosis factor and interleukin-1.

Deamination Removal of amino group (NH_2) from amino acid.

Decarboxylation Key reaction in cell metabolism; the removal of the carboxyl group (-COOH)

Decidua basalis (L *deciduus,* falling off; *basis,* foundation) The base portion of the placenta embedded in the maternal endometrium lining the uterus; the maternal portion of the placenta.

Decubitus ulcer (L *decubitus,* lying down; *ulcus,* ulcer) Pressure sores in long-term bed-bound or immobile patients at points of bony protuberances, where prolonged pressure of body weight in one position cuts off adequate blood circulation to that area, causing tissue death and ulceration.

Dehiscence (L *dehiscere,* to gape) A splitting open; the separation of the layers of a surgical wound, partial or superficial, or complete with total disruption requiring resuturing.

Demographic (Gr *demos,* people; *graphein,* to write) The statistical data of a population, especially those showing average age, income, education, births, deaths, etc.

Deoxyribonucleic acid (DNA) Complex, double-chain protein of high molecular weight, which is the nucleic acid found in the chromosomes of the cell nucleus. It is the chemical basis of heredity and the carrier of genetic information for specific protein synthesis. DNA is composed of four nitrogenous bases (two purines, adenine and guanine, and two pyrimidines, thymine and cytosine), a sugar (deoxyribose), and phosphoric acid. A similar single-chain nucleic acid, ribonucleic acid (RNA), in which the sugar is ribose, also functions with DNA in protein synthesis in the cell.

Depression (L *depressio,* a pressing down) State of general discouragement or despondency, dullness or inactivity; psychiatric syndrome characterized by feelings of dejection or guilt, slowed psychomotor activity, insomnia, weight loss, delusions, etc.

Dextrorotatory (dextro-; R-) (L *dextro-,* right; *rotare,* to turn) Physics term; molecular structure or configuration of a chemical compound that turns the plane of polarized light to the right.

Diabetes insipidus (Gr *dia,* through; *bainein,* to go; *diabetes,* siphon; L *insipidus,* tasteless, not sweet, as compared to diabetes *mellitus,* L honey) A condition of the pituitary gland and insufficiency of one of its hormones, vasopressin or antidiuretic hormone; characterized by a copious output of a nonsweet urine, great thirst and sometimes a large appetite. However, in diabetes insipidus these symptoms result from a specific injury to the pituitary gland, not a collection of metabolic disorders as in diabetes mellitus. The injured pituitary gland produces less vasopressin, a hormone that normally helps the kidneys reabsorb adequate water.

Dialysis (Gr *dia,* through; *lysis,* dissolution) Process of separating crystalloids and colloids in solution by the difference in their rates of diffusion through a semipermeable membrane; crystalloids pass through readily and colloids very slowly or not at all.

Dideoxynucleosides (Chem *di-,* two; *de-,* removal; *oxy-,* oxygen; *nucleoside,* basic type of chemical compound involved) A class of drugs used to treat HIV-infected persons; a nucleoside is a combination of a sugar (a pentose) with a purine or pyrimidine (two types of compounds that provide the cross-linking "ladders" of the double strands of DNA) base.

Dietary fiber Nondigestible form of carbohydrate, of nutritional importance in gastrointestinal disease such as diverticulosis, and in management in serum lipid and glucose levels in risk-reduction related to chronic conditions such as heart disease and diabetes.

Dietetics Management of diet and the use of food; the science concerned with the nutritional planning and preparation of foods.

Diffusion (L *diffundere,* to spread or to pour forth) Processes by which particles in solution spread throughout the solution and across separating membranes from the place of highest solute concentration to all surrounding spaces of lesser solute concentration.

Diglyceride (Gr *di,* two) A glyceride containing two fatty acid molecules in ester linkage.

Dipeptide (Gr *di,* two) A peptide which, on hydrolysis, yields two amino acids.

Disability Mental or physical impairment that prevents an individual from performing one or more gainful activities; not synonymous with *handicap,* which implies serious disadvantage.

Disaccharides (Gr *di,* two; *saccharide,* sugar) Class of compound sugars composed of two molecules of monosaccharide. The three most common are sucrose, lactose, and maltose.

Distal (L *distans,* distant) Remote, farther from any point of reference; opposed to proximal.

Disulfiram White to off-white crystalline antioxidant; inhibits oxidation of the acetaldehyde metabolized from alcohol. It is used in the treatment of alcoholism, producing extremely uncomfortable symptoms when alcohol is ingested following oral administration of the drug.

Diuretic drug (Gr *diouretikos,* promoting urine) An agent that promotes the excretion of urine.

Diverticula (L *divertere,* to turn aside) A blind, tubular sac or process branching off from a canal or cavity, especially an abnormal sac like herniation of the mucosal layer through the muscular wall of the colon.

Diverticulitis (L *divertere,* to turn aside) Inflammation of "pockets" of tissue (diverticuli) in the lining of the mucous membrane of the colon.

Dizygote Two separate fertilized ova developing two different embryos, hence producing different fraternal twins.

Double bond Covalent linking between carbon atoms in a chain, as in fatty acids, where fewer hydrogen atoms occur and the additional bond is taken up by the pair of carbon atoms involved.

Ducts (L *ductus,* from *ducere* to draw or lead) A passage with well-defined walls, especially a tube for the passage of excretions or secretions.

Dynamic (Gr *dynam,* force, power) Characterized by energy and effective action; a force that activates and changes. A dynamic process is one that is constantly changing.

Dysentery (Gr *dys,* painful, bad; *enteron,* intestine) A general term given to a number of disorders marked by inflammation of the intestines, especially of the colon, and attended by abdominal pain and frequent stools containing blood and mucus. The causative agent may be chemical irritants, bacteria, protozoa, or parasites.

Dyspnea (Gr *dysnoia,* difficulty of breathing) Labored, difficult breathing.

Eclampsia (Gr *eklampein,* to shine forth) Advanced pregnancy-induced hypertension (PIH), manifested by convulsions.

Ectoderm (Gr *ektos,* outside; *derma,* skin) Outer layer of embryonic tissue from which the nails, skin glands, nervous system, external sensory organs, and mucous membrane of the mouth are formed.

Edema (Gr *oidema,* swelling) An unusual accumulation of fluid in the intercellular tissue spaces of the body.

Educate (L *e,* from; *ducare,* to lead) To develop and cultivate by systematic instruction.

Eicosanoids (Gr *eikosa,* twenty) Long chain fatty acids composed of 20 carbon atoms.

Elastase A protein enzyme class formed from the inactive proenzyme proelastase, which is secreted by the pancreas. It catalyzes the hydrolysis of peptide bonds. It is so named because it was once thought to attack elastin preferentially.

Electrochemical Chemical changes produced by action of electrical charges in ions.

Electrochemical neutrality A solution that is balanced in terms of chemical changes produced by its electrolyte activity.

Electroencephalogram (EEG) A recording of the electric potentials on the skull generated by currents from nerve cells in the brain.

Electrolytes (Gr *electron,* amber [which emits electricity when rubbed]; *lytos,* soluble) A chemical element or compound, which in solution dissociates as ions carrying a positive or negative charge, for example, H^+, Na^+, K^+, Ca^{++}, Mg^{++}, and Cl^-, HCO^-_3, $HPO^-_4{}^-$, $SO^-_4{}^-$. Electrolytes constitute a major force controlling fluid balances within the body through their concentrations and shifts from one place to another to restore and maintain balance—*homeostasis.*

Electrophoresis (Gr *electron,* amber) The movement of charged particles suspended in a liquid under the influence of an applied electric field. Also, the technique of separating materials that utilizes this phenomenon.

Elemental formula A nutrition support formula composed of simple elemental nutrient components that require no further digestive breakdown and are thus readily absorbed. Infant formula produced with elemental, ready to be absorbed, components of free amino acids and carbohydrate as simple sugars.

Embryo (Gr *embryos,* ingrowing; *bryein,* to swell) The developing organism from about two weeks after fertilization to the end of the seventh or eight week.

Emulsifier An agent that breaks down large fat globules to smaller, uniformly distributed particles. This action is accomplished in the intestine chiefly by the bile acids, which lower surface tension of the fat particles. Emulsification greatly increases the surface area of fat, facilitating contact with fat-digesting enzymes.

Encephalopathy (Gr *enkephalos,* brain; *pathos,* disease) Any degenerative disease of the brain.

Endemic (Gr *endemos,* dwelling in a place) A disease of low morbidity that remains constantly in a human community but is clinically recognizable in only a few.

Endocarditis (Gr *endon,* within; *kardia,* heart) Inflammation of the endocardium, the serous membrane that lines the cavities of the heart.

Endoderm (Gr *endon,* within; *derma,* skin) The inner layer of embryonic tissue from which the epithelium of the respiratory and digestive tract, as well as bladder and urethra, is formed.

Endogenous (Gr *endon,* within; *gennan,* to produce) Developing within an organism.

Endometrium (Gr *endon,* within; *metra,* uterus) The inner mucous membrane of the uterus.

Endoplasmic reticulum (Gr *endon,* within; *plassein,* to form; L *rete,* net) A protoplasmic network in cells of flattened double membrane sheets; important metabolic cell organelles, some with rough surfaces bearing ribosomes for protein synthesis and other smooth surfaces synthesizing fatty acids.

Endothelium (Gr *endo-,* within; *thēlē,* nipple) Layer of epithelial cells that line the cavities of the heart, the blood and lymph vessels, and the serous cavities of the body, originating from the mesoderm.

Enteral (Gr *enteron,* intestine) A mode of feeding that uses the gastrointestinal tract, oral or tube feeding.

Enteric lipase (Gr *enterikos,* intestinal; *lipos,* fat) Fat enzyme in absorbing intestinal wall that completes breakdown of remaining fats, in preparation for resynthesis and transport.

Enteric nervous system (Gr *enterikos,* intestinal) System of nerves, interconnecting nerve centers, and relaying carriers throughout the gastrointestinal wall, controlling neuromuscular and secretory-absorbing actions of the GI system.

Enteritis Inflammation of the intestine.

Enterocyte (Gr *enteron,* intestine) An intestinal epithelial cell.

Enterohepatic circulation (Gr *enteron,* intestine; *hepatikos,* of the liver) Constant circulation of bile between the small intestine, the liver, and the gallbladder, conserving bile for continuous use.

Enterokinase (Gr *enteron,* intestine; *kinesis,* movement) The intestinal peptide hormone that activates the proenzyme trypsinogen to the active protein-splitting enzyme trypsin.

Enzyme (Gr *en,* in; *zyme,* leaven) Various complex proteins produced by living cells that act independently of these cells. Enzymes are capable of producing certain chemical changes in other substances without themselves being changed in the process. Their action is therefore that of a catalyst. Digestive enzymes of the gastrointestinal secretions act on food substances to break them down into simpler compounds and greatly accelerate the speed of these chemical reactions. An enzyme is usually named according to the substance (substrate) on which it acts, with the common suffix *-ase;* for example, sucrase is the specific enzyme for sucrose and breaks it down to glucose and fructose.

Epidemiology (Gr *epidemois,* prevalent; *-ology,* study) The study of factors determining the frequency, distribution, and strength of diseases in population groups.

Epiglottis (Gr *epi,* on; *glottis,* vocal apparatus of the larynx) Lid-like cartilaginous structure overhanging the entrance to the larynx and preventing food from entering the larynx and trachea while swallowing.

Epinephrine (Gr *epi,* on; *nephros,* kidney) A hormone secreted by the inner section (medulla) of the adrenal glands, each of which lies on top of a kidney; secretion stimulated by the central nervous system in response to stress as anger or fear, and acting to increase heart rate, blood pressure, cardiac output, and carbohydrate metabolism.

Episiotomy (Gr *epision,* region of the vulva, the external female genital organ; *tome,* a cutting) A surgical incision into the perineum (the pelvic floor between the vulva and the anus) and the vagina prior to delivery of an infant to enlarge the vaginal opening.

Epithelium (Gr *epi,* on; *thele,* nipple) Tissues lining internal body cavities and making up external skin coverings.

Ergogenic (Gr *ergo,* work; *gennan,* to produce) Tendency to increase work output; various substances that increase work or exercise capacity and output.

Erythema (Gr *erythros,* red; *erythema,* flush upon the skin) Redness of the skin produced by coagulation of the capillaries; results from a variety of causes, e.g., radiant heat or burns.

Erythrocyte (Gr *erythro-,* red; *cyte,* hollow vessel) Red blood cell.

Essential amino acid Any one of nine amino acids that the body cannot synthesize at all or in sufficient amounts to meet body needs, so it must be supplied by the diet, hence a *dietary* essential for these nine specific amino acids: histidine, isoleucine, leucine, lysine, methionine, phenylalanine, threonine, tryptophan, and valine.

Essential hypertension An inherent form of hypertension with no specific discoverable cause, considered to be familial; also called primary hypertension.

Essential nutrient Those nutrients (proteins, minerals, carbohydrates, fat, vitamins) necessary for growth, normal functioning, and maintaining life. They must be supplied by food, since they cannot be synthesized by the body.

Ester A compound produced by the reaction between an acid and an alcohol with elimination of a molecule of water. This process is called esterification. For example, a triglyceride is a glycerol ester. Cholesterol esters are formed in the mucosal cells by combination with fatty acids, largely linoleic acid.

Estrogen (Gr *oistros,* desire, sexual receptivity) Major female sex hormone, produced in the ovaries.

Exogenous (Gr *exo,* outside; *gennan,* to produce) Developing or originating outside a person.

Exponential Rapid, increasingly larger successive number increases by multiples of each preceding value.

Extracellular fluid (ECF) (L *extra,* outside; *cellula,* cell) Alternate term for collective body water or fluids outside of cells.

Exudate (L *exsudare,* to sweat out) Various materials such as cells, cellular debris, and fluids, usually resulting from inflammation, that have escaped from blood vessels and are deposited in or on surface tissues; has a high protein content.

Facilitated diffusion Diffusion across a cell membrane or other biological membrane in which the molecules to be transported form complexes with specific carriers in the membrane, are shuttled across the membrane by the complex, and then released on the other side.

Facultative (L *facultas,* ability) Not obligatory; pertaining to or characterized by the ability to adjust to particular circumstances or to assume a particular role.

FAD (flavin-adenine dinucleotide) A riboflavin enzyme that operates in many reactions affecting amino acids, glucose, and fatty acids.

Fasciculi (L *fascis,* bundle) A general term for a small bundle or cluster of muscle, tendon, or nerve fibers.

Fatty acid The structural components of fats.

Fatty acid synthase System of controlling enzymes for synthesis of new fatty acids.

Feedback mechanism Mechanism that regulates production and secretion by an endocrine gland (A_g) of its hormone (A_h), which stimulates another endocrine gland (T_g; the *target gland*) to produce its hormone (T_h). As sufficient T_h is produced, blood levels of T_h signal A_g to stop secreting A_h.

Femur The bone that extends from the pelvis to the knee, being the longest and largest bone in the body. Thighbone.

Ferritin Protein-iron compound in which iron is stored in tissues; the storage form of iron in the body.

Fetor hepaticas (L *fetor,* stench, offensive odor; *hepaticus,* liver) The peculiar odor of the breath that is characteristic of advanced liver disease.

Fetus (L *fetus,* unborn offspring) The unborn offspring in the post embryonic period, after major structures have been outlined; in humans the growing offspring from seven to eight weeks after fertilization until birth.

Filé In New Orleans Cajun-style cookery, a pungent tasting powder made from the ground leaves of the sassafras tree used as a thickener.

Filtration (L *filtrum,* felt used to strain liquids) Passage of a fluid through a semipermeable membrane (a membrane that permits passage of water and small solutes but not large molecules) as a result of a difference in pressures on the two sides of the membrane. For example, the net filtration pressure in the capillaries is the difference between the outward-pushing hydrostatic force of the blood pressure and the opposing inward-pulling force of the colloidal osmotic pressure exerted by the plasma proteins retained in capillary.

Fistula (L *fistula,* pipe) Abnormal passageway usually between two internal organs, or leading from an internal organ to the surface of the body.

Fluorosis An abnormal condition caused by excessive intake of fluorides, characterized in children by discoloration and pitting of the teeth and in adults by bone changes.

Flushing reaction Short-term reaction resulting in redness of neck and face.

FMN (flavin mononucleotide) A riboflavin phosphate compound that acts as a coenzyme in the deamination of certain amino acids.

Folic acid (Vitamin B_9) The B-vitamin discovered as a factor in the control of pernicious anemia. It functions in metabolism as a coenzyme for transferring single carbon units for attachment in many reactions. In this role, folic acid is a key substance in cell growth and reproduction through aiding in the formation of nucleoproteins and hemoglobin.

Follicle (L *follis,* leather bag) Sac-like secretory cavity surrounding hairs on the skin and nourishing their growth.

Follicular hyperkeratosis Roughed skin area surrounding hair follicles.

Food jags Colloquial expression referring to repeated use of single foods over a brief time.

Fuel factor The kilocalorie value (energy potential) of food nutrients; that is, the number of kilocalories that one gram of the nutrient yields when oxidized. The kilocalorie fuel factor for carbohydrate is 4; for protein, 4; and for fat, 9. The basic figures are used in computing diets and energy values of foods. (For example, 10 grams of fat yields 90 kcal.)

Fulminant (L *fulminare,* to flare up) Sudden, severe; occurring suddenly with great intensity.

Fundus (L *fundus,* bottom) The first part of the stomach at the entering end of the esophagus.

Gadolinium (Gd) A rare earth metallic element, atomic number 64, extracted from the silicate mineral *gadolinate,* named after J. Gadolin (1760-1852), Finnish chemist.

gamma-Carboxyglutamic (γ-Carboxyglutamic) acid (Gla) Activated form of glutamic acid through attachment of a carboxyl (COOH) group.

Ganglia (plural of ganglion) (Gr *ganglion,* knob) Knob or knot-like mass; general term for a group of nerve cell bodies located outside the central nervous system.

Gap junction A narrowed portion (about 3μm) of the intercellular space between absorbing enterocytes which contains channels (about 2μm) linking adjacent cells and through which pass ions, most sugars, amino acids, nucleotides, vitamins, hormones, and cyclic AMP. In electrically excitable tissues, these gap junctions serve to transmit electrical impulses via ionic currents and are known as electronic synapses. They are also present in such tissues as myocardial tissue.

Gastric amylase (Gr *gaster,* stomach; *amylon,* starch) Starch enzyme occurring in the stomach.

Gastric lipase (Gr *gaster,* stomach; *lipos,* fat) Fat enzyme of the gastric secretions, sometimes called *tributyrinase,* which acts on the tributyrin in butterfat.

Gastrin Hormone secreted by mucosal cells in the antrum of the stomach that stimulates the parietal cells to produce hydrochloric acid. Gastrin is released in response to stimulants, especially coffee, alcohol, and meat extractives, into the stomach. When the gastric pH reaches 2.0 to 3.0, a feedback mechanism cuts off gastrin secretion and prevents excess acid formation.

Gastritis (Gr *gaster,* stomach) Inflammation of the stomach.

Gastroenteritis (Gr *gaster,* stomach; *enteron,* intestine) Inflammation of the stomach and intestines.

Gene (Gr *gennan,* to produce) The biologic unit of heredity, self-reproducing and located at a definite position (locus) on a particular chromosome.

Geriatrics (Gr *geras,* old age; *iatrike,* surgery, medicine) Branch of medicine specializing in medical problems associated with old age.

Gerontology (Gr *geronto,* old man; *logy,* work, reason, study) Study of the aging process and its remarkable progressive events.

Gestation (L *gestatio,* from; *gestare,* to bear) The period of embryonic and fetal development from fertilization to birth; pregnancy.

Gingivitis (L *gingiva,* "gum of the mouth") Inflammation of the gum tissue surrounding the base of the teeth.

GIP Glucose-dependent insulinotropic peptide; the most recently established gastrointestinal peptide hormone.

Glomerulosclerosis (L *glomus,* ball, cluster; *sklērōsis,* hardness) Intercapillary degeneration of the nephron glomerulus, a cluster of capillary loops cupped at the head of each nephron, resulting in the degeneration of the entire nephron; a diabetic complication, with symptoms of albuminuria, nephrotic edema, hypertension, and renal insufficiency.

Glossitis (Gr *glossa,* tongue + *itis*) Swollen, reddened tongue; riboflavin deficiency symptom.

Glottis (Gr *glottis,* vocal apparatus of the larynx) Vocal cords and the opening between them.

Glucagon (Gr *glykys,* sweet; *gonē,* seed) A polypeptide hormone secreted by the A cells of the pancreatic islets of Langerhans in response to hypoglycemia; has an opposite balancing effect to that of insulin, raising the blood sugar, thus is used as a quick-acting antidote for the hypoglycemic reaction of insulin. It stimulates the breakdown of glycogen (glycogenolysis) in the liver by activating the liver enzyme phosphorylase, and thus raises blood sugar levels during fasting states to ensure adequate levels for normal nerve and brain function.

Glucocorticoids Group of corticosteroids (adrenocortical hormones) affecting carbohydrate metabolism.

Gluconeogenesis (Gr *gleukos,* sweetness; *neos,* new; *genesis,* production, generation) Production of glucose from keto-acid carbon skeleton from deaminated amino acids and the glycerol portion of fatty acids.

Glucose tolerance factor A biologically active complex of chromium and nicotinic acid that facilitates the reaction of insulin with receptor sites on tissues.

Glutamic acid (Glu) Amino acid base for synthesis of active precursor forms of clotting agents such as prothrombin, a reaction in which vitamin K is an essential coenzyme factor.

Glutathione peroxidase Selenium-containing enzyme system that acts as an antioxidant agent by destroying cell peroxides, preventing their damage to cell membranes.

Glyceride Group name for fats; any of a group of esters obtained from glycerol by the replacement of one, two, or three hydroxyl (OH) groups with a fatty acid. Monoglycerides contain one fatty acid; diglycerides contain two fatty acids; triglycerides contain three fatty acids. Glycerides are the principal constituent of adipose tissue and are found in animal and vegetable fats and oils.

Glycerol A colorless, odorless, syrupy, sweet liquid; a constituent of fats usually obtained by the hydrolysis of fats. Chemically glycerol is an alcohol; it is esterified with fatty acids to produce fats.

Glycogen (Gr *glykys,* sweet; *genes,* born, produced) A polysaccharide, that is, a large compound of many saccharide (i.e., sugar) units. It is the main body storage form of carbohydrate, largely stored (with relatively rapid turnover) in the liver, with lesser amounts stored in muscle tissue.

Glycogenesis Formation of glycogen, the storage form of carbohydrates in animals.

Glycogenolysis (*glycogen* + Gr *lysis,* dissolution) Specific term for conversion of glycogen into glucose in the liver; chemical process of enzymatic hydrolysis or breakdown by which this conversion is accomplished.

Glycolipid (Gr *glykys,* sweet) A lipid containing carbohydrate groups, usually galactose or glucose.

Glycolysis Initial energy production enzyme pathway outside the mitochondria, by which 6-carbon glucose is changed to active 3-carbon fragments of acetyl CoA, the fuel ready for final energy production in the mitochondria to the high-energy phosphate bond compound adenosine triphosphate (ATP).

Glycosuria (Gr *glykys,* sweet; *ouron* urine) Abnormally high concentrations of glucose in the urine.

Goblet cell Special single secretory cells on the mucosal surface that produce mucus. Mucin droplets accumulate in the cell, causing it to swell. The free surface finally ruptures and liberates the mucus. This mucus coats and protects the mucosa.

Goiter (L *guttur,* throat) Enlargement of the thyroid gland caused by lack of sufficient available iodine to produce the thyroid hormone, thyroxine.

Gram (g) (Fr *gramme*) A unit of mass (weight) in the metric system, being the equivalent of 15.432 grains, or 0.035 ounces avoirdupois.

Gravida (L *gravida,* heavy, loaded) A pregnant woman.

Growth acceleration (L *celerare,* to quicken) Period of increased speed of growth at different points of childhood development.

Growth channel The progressive regular growth pattern of children, guided along individual genetically controlled channels, influenced by nutritional and health status.

Growth chart grids Grids comparing stature (length), weight and age of children by percentile. Used for nutritional assessment to determine how their growth is progressing. Most commonly used grids: National Center for Health Statistics (NCHS) by the Fels Research Institute.

Growth deceleration (L *de,* from; *celerare,* to quicken) Period of decreased speed of growth at different points of childhood development.

Growth hormone (GH) A hormone secreted by the anterior pituitary that stimulates growth by exerting direct effects on protein, carbohydrate, and lipid metabolism. Human growth hormone (HGH) is composed of a single chain of 188 amino acids.

Growth velocity (L *velocitas,* speed) Rapidity of motion or movement; rate of childhood growth over normal periods of development, as compared with a population standard.

Guanosine triphosphate (GTP) A high-energy compound similar to adenosine triphosphate (ATP).

Handicap Mental or physical defect that may or may not be congenital that prevents the individual from participating in normal life activities; implies disadvantage.

Heimlich maneuver A first-aid maneuver to relieve a person who is choking from blockage of the breathing passageway by a swallowed foreign object or food particle. Standing behind the person, clasp the victim around the waist, placing one fist just under the sternum (breastbone) and grasping the fist with the other hand. Then make a quick, hard, thrusting movement inward and upward.

Helix (Gr *helix,* snail, coil) A coiled structure, as found in proteins; some are simple chain coils and others may be made of several, as in a triple helix.

Hematuria (Gr *haima,* blood; *ouron,* urine) The abnormal presence of blood in the urine.

Heme iron Dietary iron from animal sources, from heme portion of hemoglobin in red blood cells. More easily absorbed and transported in the body than nonheme iron from plant sources, but supplying the smaller portion of the body's total dietary iron intake.

Hemodialysis (Gr *haima,* blood; *dia,* through; *lysis,* dissolution) Removal of certain elements from the blood according to their rates of diffusion through a semipermeable membrane, e.g., by a hemodialysis machine.

Hemoglobin (Gr *haima,* blood; L *globus,* a ball) Oxygen-carrying pigment in red blood cells; a conjugated protein containing 4 heme groups combined with iron and 4 long polypeptide chains forming the protein globin, named for its ball-like form; made by the developing red blood cells in bone marrow. Carries oxygen in the blood to body cells.

Hemolytic anemia (Gr *haima,* blood; *lysis,* dissolution) An anemia (reduced number of red blood cells) caused by breakdown of red blood cells and loss of their hemoglobin.

Hemophilia (Gr *hemo-,* blood; *philein,* to love) A heredity hemorraghic disease due to deficiency of blood coagulation factor VIII; characterized by spontaneous or traumatic bleeding; transmitted as an X-linked (maternal) recessive trait to male children. This X chromosome-linked deficiency of factor VIII has played a major role in the history of royal families of Europe.

Hemopoiesis (Gr *haima,* blood; *poiein,* to form) The formation of red blood cells.

Hemosiderin (Gr *haima,* blood; *sideros,* iron) Insoluble iron oxide-protein compound in which iron is stored in the liver if the amount of iron in the blood exceeds the storage capacity of ferritin, for example, during rapid destruction of red blood cells (malaria, hemolytic anemia).

Herpes zoster (Gr *herpēs,* herpes; *zoster,* a girdle or encircling structure or pattern) An acute self-limiting viral inflammatory disease of posterior nerve roots causing skin eruptions in a lateral pattern across the back of the torso served by these nerves, accompanied by neuralgic pain; caused by the virus of chicken pox and commonly called *shingles*.

Hexoses (Gr *hex,* six) Class of simple sugars (monosaccharides) that contain 6 carbon atoms ($C_6H_{12}O_6$). The most common are glucose, fructose, and galactose.

Hierarchy (Gr *hieros,* sacred, holy) System of persons or things in a graded order according to held values, functions, or goals.

Hispanic (L *Hispania,* Spain) Spanish, Latin American, American citizen or resident of Spanish or Latin American descent.

Homeostasis (Gr *homoios,* like, unchanging; *stasis,* standing, stable) State of relative dynamic equilibrium within the body's internal environment; a balance achieved through the operation of various interrelated physiologic mechanisms.

Homocystinuria An inborn error of sulfur amino acid (methionine) metabolism due to absence or deficiency of the liver enzyme cystathionine synthase, characterized chemically by elevated levels of methionine and homocystine in the plasma and large amounts of homocystine in the urine. Clinical symptoms of the affected child include cardiovascular and skeletal disorders.

Hormones Various internally secreted substances from the endocrine organs, which are conveyed by the blood to another organ or tissue on which they act to stimulate increased functional activity or secretion. This tissue or substance is called its target organ or substance.

Human diploid fibroblasts (Gr *diploos,* twofold) Having two full sets of chromosomes, as normally found in the body cells of higher organisms. (L *fibro-*, fiber; Gr *blastos,* germ cell) Connective tissue cells forming the fibrous tissues of the body such as skin and tendons, supporting and binding tissues. Skin cells are commonly used in laboratory cultures to study cell replication in its aging process and identify the nature and function of controlling genes.

Humoral immunity (L *humor,* a liquid, a body fluid of semiliquid spongy tissue; *immunitas,* immunity) Specific acquired immunity in which the role of antibodies produced by the B-lymphocytes and plasma cells predominate.

Hydrochloric acid (HCl) Acid secreted by special gastric mucosal oxyntic cells; provides necessary acid medium for enzyme action in the stomach.

Hydrolysis (Gr *hydro,* water; *lysis,* dissolution) Process by which a chemical compound is split into other simpler compounds by taking up the elements of water, as in the manufacture of infant formulas to produce easier-to-digest derivatives of the main protein casein in the cow's milk base; process occurs naturally in digestion.

Hydrophilic (Gr *hydro,* water; *philein,* to love) Readily absorbing water interacting with it; water soluble. Glycerol is hydrophilic.

Hydrophobic (Gr *hydro,* water; *phobein,* to be frightened by) Not readily absorbing water; insoluble in water. Fat is hydrophobic.

Hydrostatic pressure Pressure exerted by a liquid on the surfaces of the walls that contain it. Such pressure is equal in the direction of all containing walls. In body fluid balance hydrostatic pressure usually refers to the blood pressure, which, together with the plasma proteins, maintains fluid circulation and volume in the blood vessels.

Hydroxyapatite The inorganic compound of calcium and phosphorus found in the matrix of bones and teeth, giving rigidity and strength to the structure.

Hygroscopic (Gr *hygros,* moist) Taking up and retaining moisture readily.

Hypercapnia (Gr *hyper,* above; *kapnos,* smoke) Excess carbon dioxide in the blood.

Hyperemesis gravidarum (Gr *hyper,* above, excessive; *emesis,* vomiting; L *gravida,* heavy loaded) Severe vomiting during pregnancy that is potentially fatal.

Hyperkalemia (Gr *hyper,* above; L *Kalium,* potassium; Gr *haima,* blood) Excessive amounts of potassium (K) in the blood plasma.

Hyperkeratosis (Gr *hyper,* super, above; *keras,* horn) Extensive thickening of the horny outer layer of the skin.

Hyperlipoproteinemia (Gr *hyper,* above; *lipoprotein,* fat-protein compound; *—emia,* suffix referring to *haima,* blood) Elevated level of lipoproteins in the blood.

Hypernatremia (Gr *hyper,* above; L *natron,* sodium; *haima,* blood) Excessive levels of sodium in the blood.

Hyperparathyroidism (Gr *hyper,* above; *para,* along side; *thyroidism,* thyroid gland function and, by extension, parathyroid gland function) Abnormally increased activity of the parathyroid gland, resulting in excessive secretion of parathyroid hormone, which normally helps regulate serum calcium levels in balance with vitamin D hormone; excess secretion occurs when the serum calcium level falls below normal, as in chronic renal disease or in vitamin D deficiency.

Hypertension (Gr *hyper,* above) Persistently high arterial blood pressure.

Hypertonic dehydration Loss of water from the cell as a result of hypertonicity (excess solutes, thus greater osmotic pressure) of the surrounding extracellular fluid.

Hyperventilation (Gr *hyper,* above; L *ventilatio,* ventilation) Increased respiration with larger intake and consequent oxygen-carbon dioxide exchange in the lungs above the normal amount.

Hypochloremic alkalosis (Gr *hypo,* under) Excessive loss of gastric secretion (hydrochloric acid).

Hypokalemia Low potassium levels in the blood.

Hypothalamus (Gr *hypo,* under; *thalamus,* inner chamber) A small gland adjacent to the pituitary in the midbasal brain area; serves as a collecting and dispatching center for information about the internal well-being of the body, using much of this neuroendocrine information to stimulate and control many widespread important pituitary hormones.

Hypotonic dehydration Increase of water in the cell (cellular edema) at the expense of extracellular fluid, resulting from hypotonicity (decreased solutes, thus diminished osmotic pressure) of the extracellular fluid surrounding the cell. A dangerous shrinking of the extracellular fluid (especially blood) volume follows.

Hypovolemia (Gr *hypo,* under; *haima,* blood) Abnormally decreased volume of circulating blood in the body.

Hypoxemia (Gr *hypo,* under; *-ox-,* oxygen; *emia (haima),* blood) Deficient oxygenation of the blood, resulting in *hypoxia,* reduced oxygen supply to tissue.

Hypoxic Condition of hypoxia; lack of oxygen in the blood.

Iatrogenic (Gr *iatros,* healer; *genesis,* origin or source) Medical disorder caused by physician diagnosis, manner, or treatment.

Icterus (Gr *ikteros,* jaundice) Alternate term for jaundice. **Nonicteric** indicates absence of jaundice. **Preicteric** indicates a state prior to development of icterus, or jaundice.

Ileum The third and lowest division of the small intestine, extending from the jejunum to the cecum.

Ileus (Gr *eileos,* from *eilein,* to roll up) Obstruction of the intestine, resulting from inhibition of bowel motility, blockage, or persistent spasm or contracture.

Immunocompetence (L *immunis,* free, exempt) The ability or capacity to develop an immune response, that is, antibody production and/or cell-mediated immunity, following exposure to antigen.

Implantation (L *in,* into; *plantare,* to set) The attachment of the early embryo to the lining of the uterus.

Incomplete protein A protein having a ratio of amino acids different from that of the average body protein and therefore less valuable for nutrition than the complete protein.

Indole A compound produced in the intestines by the decomposition of tryptophan; also found in the oil of jasmine and clove.

Infarct (L *infarcire,* to stuff in) An area of tissue necrosis due to local ischemia resulting from obstruction of blood circulation to that area.

Infrared interactance A measure of body fat using infrared light rays, thermal radiation of wavelengths greater than the red end of the visible spectrum, between the red waves and the radio waves.

Insulin (L *insula,* island) Hormone formed in the B cells of the islets of Langerhans in the pancreas. It is secreted when blood glucose and amino acid levels rise and assists their entry into body cells. It also promotes glycogenesis and conversion of glucose into fat and inhibits lipolysis and gluconeogenesis (protein breakdown). Commercial insulin is manufactured from pigs and cows; new "artificial" human insulin products have recently been made available.

Insulin receptor (IR) Special body tissue cell receptor for insulin, necessary for transporting insulin into target tissue cells for work of cell metabolism; if receptors are defective, insulin activity in cells is impaired. The gene controlling IR synthesis was recently discovered.

Insulin-regulatable glucose transporter (GLUT-4) Insulin-controlled glucose transport system in body tissues, necessary for normal insulin availability for cell metabolism; if the transport system is flawed, the glucose available for cell fuel is diminished. The gene controlling GLUT-4 synthesis recently discovered.

Interferon (L *inter,* between; *ferire,* to strike) One of a class of small soluble proteins produced and released by cells invaded by a virus, which induces in non-infected cells the formation of an antiviral protein that interferes with viral multiplication.

Intermittent claudication (L *claudicatio,* limping or lameness) A symptomatic pattern of peripheral vascular disease, characterized by absence of pain or discomfort in a limb, usually the legs, when at rest, followed by pain and weakness when walking, intensifying until walking becomes impossible, then disappears again after a rest period; seen in occlusive arterial disease.

Interstitial fluid (L *inter,* between; *sistere,* to set) The fluid which is situated between parts or in the interspaces of a tissue.

Intervillous spaces (L *inter,* between; *villus,* tuft) Spaces situated between villi, small vascular protrusions.

Intestinal lipase Fat enzyme secreted in the intestine acting upon simple fats to remove fatty acids.

Intima (L *intima,* inner area) General term indicating an innermost part of a structure or vessel; inner layer of the blood vessel wall.

Intracellular fluid (L *intra,* within; *cellula,* cell) The fluid situated or occurring within a cell or cells.

Intrinsic factor (IH) (L *intrinsecus,* on the inside) Substance situated entirely within a part of a body or its secretions; common term for component of the gastric secretions, a mucoprotein, also called Castle's factor, necessary for the absorption of cyanocobalamin (Vitamin B_{12}).

Iodopsin (Gr *iodes,* violet; *opsis* vision) A photosensitive violet retinal pigment found in the retinal cones and important for color vision; called also visual violet.

Ions (Gr *ion,* wanderer) Activated form of certain minerals, such as sodium (Na^+), potassium (K^+), and chloride (Cl^-), that carry an electrical charge and perform a variety of essential metabolic tasks.

Ischemia (Gr *ischein,* to suppress; *haima,* blood) Deficiency of blood to a particular tissue, due to functional blood vessel constriction or actual obstruction.

Islet amyloid polypeptide (IAPP) Precursor of islet *amyloid,* most common pancreatic lesion of the islets of Langerhans in noninsulin-dependent diabetes mellitus (NIDDM); mutant gene controlling synthesis of IAPP recently discovered.

Islets of Langerhans Paul Langerhans (1847-1888), German pathologist; clusters of insulin-secreting cells scattered throughout the pancreas and comprising its endocrine portion.

Isotonicity (Gr *isos,* equal; *tonos,* tone, tension) An isotonic state having the same tension or pressure. Two given solutions are isotonic if they have the same osmotic pressure and therefore balance each other. For example, the law of isotonicity operates between the gastrointestinal fluids and the surrounding extracellular fluid. Shifts of water and electrolytes in and out of the gastrointestinal lumen are controlled to maintain this state of isotonicity.

Isotope (Gr *isos,* equal; *topos,* place) A chemical element having the same atomic number as another element, that is, the same number of nuclear protons, but possessing a different atomic mass, that is, a different number of nuclear neutrons.

Jaundice (Fr *jaune,* yellow) A syndrome characterized by hyperbilirubinemia and deposits of bile pigment in the skin, mucous membranes, and sclera giving a yellow appearance to the patient.

Joule (James Prescott Joule, 1818-1889, English physicist) The international (SI) unit of energy and heat, defined as the work done by the force of 1 newton acting over the distance of 1 meter. A newton (Sir Isaac Newton, 1643-1727, English mathematician, physicist, and astronomer) is the international (SI) unit of force, defined as the amount of force which, when applied in a vacuum to a body having a mass of 1 kg, accelerates it at the rate of 1 meter per second. These are examples of the exactness with which terms and values used by the world's scientific community must be defined, as illustrated in the *Système International d'Unités (SI)*.

Kallikrein (Gr *kallos,* beauty; *kinein,* to change or move) Any of a group of proteolytic enzymes in the blood and various glands that release kinins, e.g. bradykinin, from various globulins.

Keratin A protein which is the principal constituent of skin, hair, nails, horny tissues, and the organizing matrix of the enamel of the teeth. It is a very insoluble protein.

Keratomalacia (Gr *kerato,* horn, cornea; *malakia,* softness) A condition of the eyes associated with vitamin A deficiency. It begins with dry spots on the conjunctiva, while the cornea becomes dry and insensitive; the haze increases until finally the entire cornea becomes soft and tissue breakdown occurs.

Kerckring's folds (valves) Kerckring, Theodorus: Dutch anatomist, 1640-1693. Alternate name for mucosal folds of the small intestine.

Keto acid Amino acid residue after deamination. The glycogenic keto-acids are used to form carbohydrates. The ketogenic keto-acids are used to form fats.

Ketoacidosis Acidosis accompanied by abnormally high concentration of ketone bodies (ketosis) in body tissues and fluids; a complication, for example, of diabetes mellitus and starvation.

Ketones Class of organic compounds, including three keto-acid bases that occur as intermediate products of fat metabolism: acetoacetate, hydroxybutyrate, and acetone; excess production, as in the initial stages of starvation from burning body fat for energy fuel, leads to ketoacidosis, which if continued uncontrolled can bring coma and death.

Kilocalorie (Fr *chilioi,* thousand; L *calor,* heat) The general term *calorie* refers to a unit of heat measure and is used alone to designate the *small calorie*. The calorie used in nutritional science and the study of metabolism is the *large calorie,* 1000 calories, or kilocalorie, to be more accurate and avoid use of very large numbers in calculations.

Kinetic (Gr *kinetikos,* moving) Energy released from body fuels by cell metabolism and now active in moving muscles and energizing all body activities.

Kinin (Gr *kinein,* to change or move) Any of a group of endogenous peptides that cause vasodilation, increase vascular permeability, cause hypotension, and induce contraction of smooth muscle.

Kyphosis (Gr *hyphos,* a hump) Increased, abnormal convexity of the upper part of the spine; hunchback.

Labile (L *labilis,* unstable) A chemically unstable compound.

Lactase Enzyme splitting the disaccharide lactose into its two monosaccharides glucose and galactose.

Lactate (L *lactis,* milk) Produced by anaerobic glycolysis in the muscles during exertion; can be converted to glucose by the liver.

Lactated Ringer's solution Sterile solution of calcium chloride, potassium chloride, sodium chloride, and sodium lactate in water given to replenish fluid and electrolytes; developed by English physiologist Sydney Ringer (1835-1910).

Lactiferous ducts (L *lac,* milk; *ferre,* to bear) Branching channels in the mammary gland that carry breast milk to holding spaces near the nipple ready for the infant's feeding.

Lacuna (L *lacuna,* small pit or cavity) General term for a hollow cavity or space within other body structures; any one of the blood-filled spaces in the trophoblast of the embryo that supplies nutrition.

LCAT (lecithin-cholesterol acyl-transferase) Plasma enzyme necessary for normal transport of cholesterol as cholesterol esters; its deficiency due to a rare genetic defect causes a lipid disorder characterized by high serum levels of free unesterified cholesterol.

Lecithin (Gr *lekithos,* egg yolk) A yellow-brown fatty substance of the group called phospholipids. It occurs in animal and plant tissues and egg yolk. It is composed of units of choline, phosphoric acid, fatty acids, and glycerol. Commercial forms of lecithin, obtained chiefly from soybeans, corn, and egg yolk, are used in candies, foods, cosmetics, and inks. Lecithin plays an important role in the metabolism of fat in the liver. It provides an effective lipotropic factor, choline, which prevents the accumulation of abnormal quantities of fat.

Let-down reflex (L *reflexus,* automatic, involuntary movement or motion) Reflex that stimulates transport of milk from the small storage sacs (alveoli or acini) of the breast to the ducts and into the nipple.

Levorotatory (levo-; L-) (L *levo-,* left; *rotare,* to turn) Physics term; molecular structure or configuration of a chemical compound that turns the plane of polarized light to the left.

Ligand (L *ligare,* to bind, tie) In biochemistry, a molecule, as an antibody, hormone, or drug, that binds to a receptor. In chemistry, a chemical substance that bonds with a central metal or mineral element, making a coordinated compound.

Limiting amino acid The amino acid in foods occurring in the smallest amount, thus limiting its availability for tissue structure.

Linoleic acid The ultimate essential fatty acid for humans.

Lipid bilayer Structure of cell membranes, composed of two layers of phospholipids turned in opposite directions, their fatty acid tails turned inward forming a fat center and their water-soluble phosphoric acid-choline heads turned outward to the interior and exterior sides of the membrane, thus facilitating transport of both fat and water-soluble nutrients.

Lipids (Gr *lipos,* fat) Chemical group name for fats and fat-related compounds such as cholesterol, lipoproteins, and phospholipids; general group name for organic substances of a fatty nature, including fats, oils, waxes, and related compounds.

Lipogenesis (Gr *lipos,* fat; *genesis,* formation) Conversion of carbohydrates and protein into body fat; occurs when excessive amounts of these nutrients are consumed.

Lipolysis (Gr *lipos,* fat; *lysis,* dissolution) The breakdown of fat; fat digestion.

Lipoprotein Noncovalent complexes of fat with protein. The lipoproteins function as major carriers of lipids in the plasma, since most of the plasma fat is associated with them. Such a combination makes possible the transport of fatty substances in a water medium such as plasma.

Lipoprotein lipase Lipid clearing factor in blood circulation; fat enzyme that helps remove the triglycerides from chylomicrons.

Lobule (L *lobus,* a lobe, small defined portion of an organ) General term for a small lobe or one of its divisions; small branching vessels of the mammary gland that make up a lobe of the mammary gland and collect milk while awaiting hormonal stimulus for release.

Logarithm (Gr *logos,* word; *arithmos,* number) The exponent of the power to which a base number must be raised to equal a given number.

Lumen (L *lumen,* light) The cavity or channel within a tube or tubular organ, such as the intestines.

Lymphatic system The system of lymphatic vessels and the lymphoid tissue that drain general tissue fluids and help with initial transport of fats from small intestine into blood circulation.

Lymphocytes (L *lympho-,* water; Gr *kytos,* hollow vessel, suffix for a cell type of the root to which it is designated or attached) Special white cells from lymphoid tissue that participate in humeral and cell-mediated immunity.

Lymphoma (L *lympha,* water; Gr *sōma,* body) General term applied to any neoplastic disorder (cancer) of the lymphoid tissue.

Lysosomes (Gr *lysis,* dissolution; *soma,* body) A cell organelle containing enzymes that digest particles and that disintegrate the cell after its death.

Macrocytic anemia (Gr *makros,* large; *cyte,* hollow vessel, cell) An anemia (deficiency of normal red cells) characterized by abnormally large red cells.

Macronutrients (Gr *makros,* large; L *nutriens,* nourishment) The three large energy-yielding nutrients: carbohydrates, fats, and proteins.

Magnetic resonance imaging Method of producing a series of visual cross sectional images of the body by radio waves within a magnetic field.

Malignant (L *malignare,* to act suspiciously) An abnormal condition such as a tumor, that tends to become progressively worse and results in death.

Malignant melanoma (L *malignans,* acting maliciously; Gr *melos,* black) A tumor tending to become progressively worse, composed of melanin, the dark pigment of the skin and other body tissues, usually arising from the skin and aggravated by excessive sun exposure.

Malonyl coenzyme A Specific coenzyme for synthesizing fatty acids.

Maltase Enzyme acting on the disaccharide maltose, from starch breakdown, into its two component monosaccharides, two units of glucose.

Median (L *medianus,* middle, midpoint) In statistics, the middle number in a sequence of numbers.

Medical foods Specially formulated nutrient mixtures for use under medical supervision for treatment of various metabolic diseases.

Medulla (L *medulla,* marrow, center) General term for the inner or central portion of an organ or structure. The renal medulla is the inner part of the kidney, holding the lower parts (Loop of Henle and collecting tubule) of the nephron, which are organized grossly into pyramids with glomerular heads of the nephrons in the outer portion (cortex) of the kidney.

Megaloblastic anemia (Gr *mega,* great size; *blastos,* embryo, germ) Anemia due to faulty production of abnormally large immature red blood cells, due to a deficiency of vitamin B_{12} and folate.

Melanin (Gr *melas,* black) The dark amorphous pigment of the skin, hair, and various body tissues.

Menaquinone Form of vitamin K synthesized by intestinal bacteria; called also *vitamin* K_2.

Mendel, Gregor Johann (1822-1884) Austrian monk and naturalist; discovered natural laws governing direct inheritance by offspring of certain traits or characters from one or the other parent. The modern study of genetics derives from his work.

Meningitis (Gr *meninx,* membrane) Inflammation of the *meninges,* the three membranes that envelop the brain and spinal cord caused by a bacterial or viral infection and characterized by high fever, severe headache, and stiff neck or back muscles.

Menke's syndrome A hereditary abnormality in copper absorption marked by severe cerebral degeneration and arterial changes resulting in death in infancy and by sparse brittle scalp hair with a twisted appearance microscopically. It is transmitted as an X-linked recessive trait. Also called kinky– or steely–hair syndrome.

Mesentery (Gr *mesos,* little; *enteron,* intestine) A web-like membranous fold attaching the small intestine to the dorsal (rear) body wall.

Mesoderm (Gr *mesos,* middle; *derma,* skin) Central embryonic tissue from which connective tissue, bone, cartilage, muscle, blood, blood vessels, kidney, gonads, lymph, and other organs are derived.

Metabolism (Gr *metaballein,* to change, alter) Sum of all the various biochemical and physiologic processes by which the body grows and maintains itself (anabolism) and breaks down and reshapes tissue (catabolism), transforming energy to do its work. Products of these various reactions are called *metabolites.*

Metabolites Any substance produced by metabolism or by a metabolic process.

Metalloenzyme (L *metallum,* metal) An enzyme containing tightly bound metal atoms as an integral part of its structure, for example, carboxypeptidase and the cytochromes.

Metallothionein Copper-binding protein; plasma transport carrier.

Metastasis (Gr *meta,* after, beyond, over; *stasis,* stand)

Spread or transfer of disease from one organ or part to another not directly connected to the primary site.

Methylmalonic aciduria Excretion of excessive amounts of methylmalonic acid in the urine; a characteristic symptom of the genetic disease in children, methylmalonic acidemia.

Micelle (L *micella,* small body) A microscopic colloid particle of fat and bile formed in the small intestine for initial stage of fat absorption.

Microaneurysm (Gr *mikros,* small; *aneurysma,* a widening) A small sac formed by the widening of the wall of small blood vessels; diabetic aneurysms may form in the basement membrane of capillaries throughout vascular beds, as in the eye.

Microcephaly (Gr *mikros,* small; *kephale,* head) Abnormally small head of a newborn; usually associated with some degree of mental retardation.

Micromole (μmol) (Gr *mikros,* small + mole) One millionth of a mole.

Micronutrients (Gr *mikros,* small; L *nutriens,* nourishment) The two classes of small non-energy-yielding elements and compounds: minerals and vitamins, essential in very small amounts for regulation and control functions in cell metabolism and building certain body structures.

Milliequivalent (mEq) Unit of measure used for electrolytes in a solution. It is based on the number of ions (cations and anions) in solution, as determined by their concentration in a given volume, not the weights of the various particles. The term refers to the chemical combining power of the solution and is expressed as the number of milliequivalents per liter (mEq/L).

Milligram (mg) (L *milli,* thousand; Fr *gramme*) One-thousandth of a gram. A unit of mass (weight) in the metric system, being 10^{-3} gram, or the equivalent of 0.00032 ounces avoirdupois.

Millimole (mmol) or (mM) (L *mille,* thousand; G *mol,* short for molekul) One-thousandth part of a mole.

Mitochondria (Gr *mitos,* thread; *chondrion,* granule) Cell's "powerhouse," small elongated organelles located in the cell cytoplasm; principal site of energy generation (ATP synthesis); contains enzymes of the final energy cycle (citric acid cycle) and cell respiration, as well as ribonucleic acid (RNA) and deoxyribonucleic acid (DNA) for some synthesis of protein.

Mitosis (Gr *mitos,* thread; *osis,* process) The usual method of cell division, characterized typically by the resolving of the chromatin of the nucleus into a threadlike form, which condenses into chromosomes, each of which separates longitudinally into two parts, one part of each chromosome being retained in each of the two new cells resulting from the original cell.

Mole (M) (G *mol,* short for molekul) The molecular weight of a substance expressed in grams; gram molecule.

Monoglyceride (Gr *mono,* single) A compound consisting of one molecule of fatty acid esterified to glycerol.

Monosaccharide (Gr *mono,* single; *sakcharon,* sugar) Simple single sugar; a carbohydrate containing a single saccharide (sugar) unit.

Monounsaturated An unsaturated fatty acid with only one double bond. An example is oleic acid, one of the more abundant unsaturated fatty acids in food fats. Some of these foods include olives and olive oil, peanuts, and peanut oil, almonds, pecans, and avocado.

Monozygote (Gr *zygote,* yolked together) One fertilized ovum developing two identical embryos, hence producing identical twins.

Morula (L *morus,* mulberry) The solid mass of blastocyst cells formed by cleavage of a fertilized ovum.

Motivation Forces that affect individual goal-directed behavior toward satisfying needs or achieving personal goals.

Mucosa (L *mucus*) The mucous membrane comprising the inner surface layer of gastrointestinal tract tissues, providing extensive nutrient absorption and transport functions.

Mucus Viscid fluid secreted by mucous membranes and glands, consisting mainly of mucin (a glycoprotein), inorganic salts, and water. Mucus serves to lubricate and protect the gastrointestinal mucosa and to help move the food mass along the digestive tract.

Myasthenia gravis (Gr *mys,* muscle; *asthenia,* weakness; L *gravis,* heavy, weighty, grave) A progressive neuromuscular disease caused by faulty nerve conduction due to presence of antibodies to acetylcholine receptors at the neuromuscular junction.

Myelin (Gr *myelos,* marrow) High lipid-to-protein substance forming fatty sheath to insulate and protect neuron axons and facilitate their neuromuscular impulses.

Myelin sheath (Gr *myelos,* marrow; *thēkē,* sheath) Covering of myelin, a lipid-protein substance, with a high fat proportion to protein, surrounding nerve axons that serves as electrical insulator and speeds the conduction of nerve impulses, interrupted at intervals along the length of the axon by gaps known as Ranvier's nodes.

Myenteric plexus (Gr *mys,* muscle; *enterikos,* intestine; L *plexuses,* braid) The part of the enteric plexus that is within the intestinal wall; a network of autonomic nerve fibers made up of the submucosal, myenteric, and subserosal plexuses.

Myoclonus (Gr *mys,* muscle; *klonos,* turmoil) Shock-like contractions of muscles restricted to one area of the body.

Myofibril (Gr *mys,* muscle; L *fibrilla,* very small fiber) Slender thread of muscle; runs parallel to the muscle fiber's long axis.

Myofilaments (Gr *mys,* muscle; (L *filare,* to wind thread, spin) Thread-like filaments of actin or myosin which are components of myofibrils.

Myoglobin Muscle protein (globin) that contains iron (also called myohemoglobin).

Myosin (Gr *mys,* muscle) Myofibril protein whose synchronized meshing action in conjunction with **actin** causes muscles to contract and relax.

Na^-,K-ATPase Special cell membrane transport system involving a Na-K pump and energized by ATP (adenine triphosphate).

NAD (Nicotinamide-adenine dinucleotide) A niacin compound that functions in tissue oxidation to release controlled energy.

NADP (Nicotinamide-adenine dinucleotide phosphate) A niacin compound with three high-energy phosphate bonds, which acts as a vital coenzyme in the "respiratory chains" of tissue oxidation within the cell; controlled energy is made available by this reaction.

Necrosis (Gr *nekrosis,* deadness) Cell death caused by progressive enzyme breakdown.

Neoplasm (Gr *neos,* new; *plasma,* formation) Any new or abnormal cellular growth, specifically one that is uncontrolled and progressive.

Nephron (Gr *nephros,* kidney) Microscopic anatomical and functional unit of the kidney which selectively filters and reabsorbs essential blood factors, secretes hydrogen ions as needed for maintaining acid-base balance, then reabsorbs water to protect body fluids, and forms and excretes a concentrated urine for elimination of wastes. The nephron includes the renal corpuscle (glomerulus), the proximal convoluted tubule, the loop of Henle, the distal convoluted tubule, and the collecting tubule, which empties the urine into the renal medulla. The urine passes into the papilla and then to the pelvis of the kidney. Urine is formed by filtration of blood in the glomerulus and by the selective reabsorption and secretion of solutes by cells that comprise the walls of the renal tubules. There are approximately 1 million nephrons in each kidney.

Nephropathy (Gr *nephros,* kidney; *pathos,* disease) Disease of the kidneys; in diabetes, renal damage associated with functional and pathologic changes in the nephrons, which can lead to glomerulosclerosis and chronic renal failure.

Nephrosis (Gr *nephros,* kidney) Nephrotic syndrome caused by degenerative epithelial lesions of the renal tubules of the nephrons, especially the *mesangium,* the thin basement membrane that helps support the capillary loops in a renal glomerulus; marked by edema, albuminuria, and decreased serum albumin.

Neuron Any of the conducting cells of the nervous system.

Neuropathy (Gr *neuron,* nerve; *pathos,* disease) General term for functional and pathologic changes in the peripheral nervous system; in diabetes, a chronic sensory condition affecting mainly the nerves of the legs, marked by numbness from sensory impairment, loss of tendon reflexes, severe pain, weakness, and wasting of muscles involved.

Neurotransmitter (Gr *neuron,* nerve; L *trans,* through, across; *missio,* sending) Large group of some 40 different chemical substances, including compounds as diverse as acetylcholine, various hormones, and several amino acids, which function as essential synaptic transmitters, chemical messengers for sending (or inhibiting) nerve impulses across synapses of connecting nerve endings.

Neutron (L *neutralis,* neutral) A particle of matter that is electrically neutral or uncharged and exists along with protons in the atoms of all elements except the mass 1 isotope of hydrogen.

Niacin equivalent (NE) A measure of the total dietary sources of niacin equivalent to 1 mg of niacin. Thus an NE is 1 mg of niacin or 60 mg of tryptophan.

Night blindness A vitamin A deficiency condition, in which the retina cannot adjust to low levels of light.

Nitrogen balance The metabolic balance between nitrogen intake in dietary protein and output in urinary nitrogen compounds such as urea and creatinine. For every 6.25 g dietary protein consumed, 1 g nitrogen is excreted.

Nonheme iron The larger portion of dietary iron, including all the plant food sources and 60% of the animal food sources, which lacks the more easily absorbed and bioavailable heme iron in the remaining 40% of the animal food sources that contain hemoglobin residues of iron-containing heme.

Norepinephrine (*nor-,* prefix, normal or parent form of a compound; Gr *epi-,* on, upon, or over; *nephros,* kidney) One of the catecholamines; a neurohormone, principal neurotransmitter of adrenergic nerves; secreted by inner part of the adrenal glands which lie on top of the kidneys.

Nucleoproteins (L, combining form of *nucleus*) Any of the class of conjugated proteins occurring in cells and consisting of a protein combined with a nucleic acid, essential for cell division and reproduction.

Nulligravida (L *nullus,* none; *gravida,* pregnant) A woman who has never been pregnant.

Nutrients (L *nutriens,* nourishment) Substances in food that are essential for energy, growth, normal functioning of the body, and maintaining life.

Nutrition (L *nutritio,* nourishment) The sum of the processes involved in taking in food nutrients, assimilating and using them to maintain body tissue and provide energy; a foundation for life and health.

Nutritional science The body of scientific knowledge, developed through controlled research, that relates to the processes involved in nutrition—national, international, community, and clinical.

Obligatory (L *obligare,* to bind) Required as a matter of obligation; mandatory.

Occult bleeding (L *occultus,* concealed) Obscure, difficult to detect, concealed from observation; such a small blood loss that it can be detected only by a microscope or chemical test.

Oligopeptide (Gr *oligos,* little) The structure formed by the linkage of a few amino acids.

Oligosaccharides (Gr *oligos,* little; *saccharide,* sugar) Intermediate products of polysaccharide carbohydrate breakdown, containing a small number (from 4 to 10) of single sugar units of the monosaccharide glucose.

Oliguria (Gr *oligos,* little; *ouron,* urine) Secretion of a very small amount of urine in relation to fluid intake.

Omega (ω) The twenty-fourth and final letter of the Greek alphabet; used in numbering system for fatty acids.

Oncogene (Gr *onkos,* mass; *genesis,* generation, production) Any of various genes that, when activated as by radiation or a virus, may cause a normal cell to become cancerous; viral genetic material carrying the potential of cancer and passed from parent to offspring.

Opsin (Gr *opsis,* vision) A protein of the retinal rods (scotopsin) and cones (photopsin) that combines with 11, *cis*-retinal to form visual pigments. The opsins are also named according to the color of pigment: iodopsin (violet), porphyropsin (red), rhodopsin (purple), etc.

Organelle Specific small bodies within the cell, each having special structure and function.

Organic (Gr *organikos,* organ) Carbon-based chemical compounds.

Orthotopic (Gr *ortho,* straight, normal, correct; *topos,* place) Occurring at the normal place in the body; placement of a transplanted organ in the position formerly occupied by tissue of the same kind.

Osmolality (Gr *osmos,* impulse, osmotic force) Property of a solution which depends on the concentration of the solute per unit of the solvent.

Osmoreceptors (Gr *osmos,* impulse; receptor) Any of a group of specialized neurons in the supraoptic nuclei of the hypothalamus that are stimulated by increased osmolality (chiefly, increased sodium concentration) of the extracellular fluid. Excitation of these receptor cells promotes the release of antidiuretic hormone by the posterior pituitary.

Osmosis (Gr *osmos,* a thrusting) Passage of a solution of different concentrations. The water passes through the membrane from the area of lower concentration of solute to that of higher concentration of solute, which tends to equalize the concentrations of the two solutions. The rate of osmosis depends on (1) the difference in osmotic pressures of the two solutions, (2) the permeability of the membrane, and (3) the electric potential across the membrane.

Osteoblasts (Gr *osteon,* bone; *blastos,* germ) A cell which arises from a fibroblast and which as it matures is associated with the production of bone.

Osteocalcin Gla found in bone BGP (bone Gla protein) which binds calcium to form bone; similar protein in bone matrix MGP (matrix Gla protein).

Osteoclasts (Gr *osteon,* bone; *klan,* to break) A large multinuclear cell associated with the absorption and removal of bone.

Osteodystropathy (Gr *osteon,* bone; *dys,* painful, disordered, abnormal; *trephein,* to nourish) Bone disease resulting from defective bone formation. The general term *dystrophy* applies to any disorder arising from faulty nutrition.

Osteodystrophy (Gr *osteon,* bone) Defective bone formation.

Osteomalacia (Gr *osteon,* bone; *malakia,* softness) Condition marked by softening of the bones due to impaired mineralization with excess accumulation of osteoid (immature young bone matrix that has not had mineralization to harden it); results from deficiency of vitamin D and calcium.

Osteoporosis (Gr *osteon,* bone; *poros,* passage, pore) Abnormal thinning of bone, producing a porous, fragile, lattice-like bone tissue of enlarged spaces, prone to fracture or deformity.

Oxaloacetate A salt of oxaloacetic acid; in biochemistry the term is often used interchangeably with oxaloacetic acid. A crystalline organic acid, $C_4H_4O_5$, that is an important intermediate in the citric acid cycle.

Oxidative phosphorylation The formation of high-energy phosphate bonds of ADP and ATP, in which electrons (H^+) are transferred through a series of substances to combine with oxygen, forming the end product H_2O; respiratory chains in cell energy production.

Oxyntic (Gr *oxyno,* to make acid) Secreting acid, as the parietal (oxyntic [ock-sin-tic]) cells of the gastric mucosa.

Oxytocin (Gr *oxy-,* keen, sharp, sour; *tokos,* birth) Hormone formed in the posterior lobe of the pituitary gland that stimulates uterine contractions and milk ejection from the mammary gland lobules.

P/S ratio Ratio of polyunsaturated to saturated fats in the diet.

Palate (L *palatum,* roof of mouth) The roof of the mouth, consisting of an anterior bony portion (hard palate) and a posterior muscular portion (soft palate) that separate the oral cavity from the nasal cavity.

Palliative (L *palliatus,* cloaked) Care affording relief but not cure; useful for comfort when cure is still unknown or obscured.

Palmar grasp (L *palma,* palm) Early grasp of the young infant, clasping an object in the palm and wrapping the whole hand around it.

Pancreatic enzyme preparations Commercial preparations of pancreatic enzymes—protease, lipase, and amylase—that have the same action as do the human enzymes from the pancreas; used in the treatment of pancreatic insufficiency.

Pancreatitis Inflammation of the pancreas (the large, elongated gland behind the stomach which produces both digestive enzymes and insulin), caused by either disease or injury. The inflammation may be chronic or acute; the acute form is characterized by sudden abdominal pain, nausea, and vomiting, due to autodigestion of pancreatic tissue by its own enzymes.

Pandemic (Gr *pan,* all; *dēmos,* people) A widespread epidemic, distributed through a region, continent, or the world.

Pantothenic acid (Gr *pantothen,* "from all sides" or "in every corner") A B vitamin found widely distributed in nature and occurring throughout the body tissues. Pantothenic acid is an essential constituent of the coenzyme A, which has extensive metabolic responsibility as an activating agent of a number of compounds in many tissues.

Paradigm (Gr *para,* side-by-side; *deiknynai,* to show) A pattern or model serving as an example; a standard or ideal for practice or behavior based on a fundamental value or theme.

Parasite (Gr *para,* along side; *sitos,* food, grain; *parasitos,* one who eats at another's table; in ancient Greece, a term for a person who received free meals in return for amusing or flattering conversation) An organism that lives on or in an organism of another species, know as the host, from whom all life-cycle nourishment is obtained.

Parasympathetic (Gr *para,* along side; *sympathetikos,* sympathetic) The part of the autonomic nervous system that consists of nerves and ganglia arising from the cranial and sacral regions and function in opposition to the sympathetic system, as in inhibiting heart beat or contracting the pupil of the eye.

Parathyroid hormone A polypeptide hormone secreted by the parathyroid glands, which promotes release of calcium from bone into the extracellular fluid by activating osteoclasts and promotes increased intestinal absorption and renal tubular reabsorption of calcium, as well as increased renal excretion of phosphates.

Parenchymal cells (Gr *parenchyma,* "anything poured in beside") Functional cells of an organ as distinguished from the cells comprising its structure or framework.

Parenteral (Gr *para,* along side, beyond, accessory; *enteron,* intestine) A mode of feeding that does not use the gastrointestinal tract, but instead provides nutrition by intravenous delivery of nutrient solutions.

Paresthesia (Gr *para,* beyond; *aisthesis,* perception) Abnormal sensations such as prickling, burning, and "crawling" of skin.

Parity (L *parere,* to bring forth, produce) The condition of a woman with respect to having borne viable offspring.

Parotid (Gr *para,* beyond; *ous,* ear) Situated or occurring near the ear, as the parotid gland.

Pellagra (L *pelle,* skin; Gr *agra,* seizure) A deficiency disease caused by a lack of niacin in the diet and an inadequate amount of protein containing the amino acid, tryptophan, a precursor of niacin. Pellagra is characterized by skin lesions that are aggravated by exposure to sunlight and by gastrointestinal, mucosal, neurologic, and mental symptoms. Four *Ds* often associated with pellagra are dermatitis, diarrhea, dementia, and death.

Pelvic nerve Major nerve of the parasympathetic branch of the autonomic nervous system, arising from the lower spinal cord area of the *sacrum,* the triangular bone just below the lumbar vertebrae, wedged between the two hip bones.

Pepsin The main gastric enzyme specific for proteins. Pepsin begins breaking large protein molecules into shorter chain polypeptides, proteoses, and peptones. Gastric hydrochloric acid is necessary to activate pepsin.

Pepsinogen (Gr *pepsis,* digestion; *gennan,* to produce) An inactive proenzyme secreted by chief cells, mucous neck cells, and pyloric gland cells, which is converted into pepsin in the presence of gastric acid or of pepsin itself.

Peptic (chief) cells Epithelial cells of the stomach, shaped either in columns or cubes, that line the lower portions of the gastric glands and secrete pepsinogen.

Peptidase Protein enzymes that catalyze the final hydrolysis of peptide linkages.

Peptide (Gr *peptos,* digested) Any member of a class of compounds of low molecular weight which yield two or more amino acids on hydrolysis.

Peptide bond The characteristic joining of amino acids to form proteins. Such a chain of amino acids is termed a peptide. Depending on its size, it may be a dipeptide fragment of protein digestion or a large polypeptide.

Peptones (Gr *pepton,* digesting) A derived protein, or a mixture of cleavage products produced by the partial hydrolysis of a native protein either by an acid or by an enzyme.

Percentile (L *per,* throughout, in space or time; *centrum,* a hundred) One of 100 equal parts of a measured series of values; rate or proportion per hundred.

Peristalsis (Gr *peri,* around; *stalsis,* contraction) A wavelike progression of alternate contraction and relaxation of the muscle fibers of the gastrointestinal tract.

Peritoneal dialysis Dialysis through the peritoneum into and out of the peritoneal cavity.

Peritoneum (Gr *per,* around; *teinein,* to stretch) A strong smooth surface, a serous membrane, lining the abdominal/pelvic walls and the undersurface of the diaphragm, forming a sac enclosing the body's vital visceral organs within the peritoneal cavity.

Pernicious anemia A chronic macrocytic anemia occurring most commonly after age 40; caused by absence of the intrinsic factor normally present in the gastric juices and necessary for the absorption of cobalamin (B_{12}); controlled by intramuscular injections of vitamin B_{12}.

pH Power of the hydrogen ion (H^+), a measure indicating degree of acidity or alkalinity of solutions. A pH of 7.0 indicates neutrality, with numbers above it indicating increasing alkalinity and those below, increasing acidity.

Phagocytes (Gr *phagein,* to eat; *kytos,* hollow vessel, cell) Cells that ingest microorganisms, other cells, or foreign particles; macrophages.

Pharynx (Gr *pharynx,* throat) The muscular membranous passage between the mouth and the posterior nasal passages and the larynx and esophagus.

Phospholipid Any of a class of fat-related substances that contain phosphorus, fatty acids, and a nitrogenous base. The phospholipids are essential elements in every cell.

Phosphorylation Combining of glucose with a phosphoric acid radical to produce glucose-6-phosphate as a first step in the cellular oxidation of glucose to produce energy. This reaction is catalyzed by the enzyme glucokinase, the specific hexokinase for this purpose.

Photon (Gr *photos,* light) A particle (quantum) of radiant energy.

Photopsin The protein in the cones of the retina that combines with retinal to form photochemical pigments.

Photosynthesis (Gr *photos,* light; *synthesis,* putting together) Process by which plants containing chlorophyll are able to manufacture carbohydrate by combining CO_2 from air and water from soil. Sunlight is used as energy; chlorophyll is a catalyst. The $6CO_2 + 6H_2O$ + Energy $\rightarrow$ Chlorophyll $\rightarrow C_6H_{12}O_6 + 6O_2$

Phylloquinone A fat-soluble vitamin of the K group, $C_3{,}H_{46}O_2$, found in green plants or prepared synthetically.

Physiologic age (Gr *physis,* nature; *logikos,* or speech or reason) Rate of biologic maturation in individual adolescents that varies widely and accounts for more than does chronological age for wide and changing differences in their metabolic rates, nutritional needs, and food requirements.

Pigment Any substance whose presence in the tissues or cells of animals or plants colors them.

Pincer grasp Later digital grasp of the older infant, usually picking up smaller objects with a precise grip between thumb and forefinger.

Pinocytosis (Gr *pinein,* to drink; *kytos,* cell) The uptake of fluid nutrient material by a living cell by means of incupping and invagination of the cell membrane, which closes off and forms free cell vacuoles.

Placenta (L *placenta,* a flat cake) Special organ developed in early pregnancy that provides nutrients to the fetus and removes metabolic waste.

Plaque (Fr *plaque,* patch or flat area) Thickened deposits of fatty material, largely cholesterol, within the arterial wall that eventually may fill the lumen and cut off blood supply to the tissue served by the damaged vessel.

Plasma protein (Gr *plasma,* molded or formed; *protos,* first) All proteins present in the blood including albumin, fibrinogen, and globulin. In addition to their other functions, all serve to provide colloid osmotic pressure which prevents plasma loss from the capillaries.

Plicae (valvulae) conniventes (L *plica,* a fold; *conniventes,* circular) Circular folds; permanent transverse folds of the luminal surface of the small intestine, involving both the mucosa and submucosa.

Polycyclic alcohols (Gr *poly,* many; *kyklos,* ring) Containing more than one ring or cycle in structure, for example, the four-ring structure of cholesterol.

Polypeptides (Gr *poly,* many; *peptos,* digested) A peptide which on hydrolysis yields more than two amino acids; called tripeptides, tetrapeptides, etc. according to the number of amino acids contained.

Polysaccharides (Gr *poly,* many; *saccharide,* sugar) Class of complex carbohydrates composed of many monosaccharide units. Common members are starch, dextrins, dietary fiber, and glycogen.

Polyunsaturated Carbon chain containing more than one double bond.

Portal An entryway, usually referring to the portal circulation of blood through the liver. Blood is brought into the liver by the portal vein and out by the hepatic vein.

Postprandial (L *post* after; *prandium,* breakfast, a meal) Occurring after a meal.

Potential (L *potentia,* power) Energy existing in stored fuels and ready for action, but not yet released and active.

Prader-Willi syndrome A congenital disease attributed to a chromosome 15 deletion. It is characterized by rounded face, almond-shaped eyes, low forehead, hypogonadism, and mental retardation. The appetite and hunger control centers in the brain's hypothalamus are greatly disordered, resulting in an insatiable voracious appetite and eating of large quantities of food. The resulting obesity in turn leads to respiratory and cardiovascular problems. One of the major goals in caring for these children as they grow older is to help retrain appetites and food habits to control the obesity.

Prealbumin (PAB) Plasma protein with short life used as a biochemical measure for assessing current nutritional status.

Preganglionic (Gr *pre,* before; *ganglions,* knot) Neuron pathways preceding a central or transmitting ganglion of nerves.

Primigravida (L *prima,* first; *gravida,* pregnant) A woman pregnant for the first time.

Proctocolectomy (Gr *prōktos,* anus; *-col-,* colon; *ektomē,* excision) Surgical removal of the rectum and colon.

Proenzyme An inactive precursor converted to the active enzyme by the action of an acid, another enzyme, or other means. Also called zymogen.

Progeria (Gr *pro-,* before; *geras,* old age) Rare condition of premature old age in a child; marked by small stature, absence of normal sexual development, wrinkled skin, gray hair, with facial appearance, attitude, and manner of old age.

Prohormone A precursor of a hormone; larger molecular size than the active hormone.

Prolactin (Gr *pro-,* before; L *lac,* milk) Anterior pituitary hormone that stimulates and sustains lactation in postpartum mothers. The mammary glands are prepared during gestation by other hormones including estrogen, progesterone, growth hormone, and corticosteroids.

Proteinuria (Gr *protos,* first, protein; *ouron,* urine) The presence of an excess of serum proteins such as albumin in the urine.

Proteoses (Gr *protos,* first) A secondary protein derivative or a mixture of split products formed by a hydrolytic cleavage of the protein molecule more complete than that which occurs with the primary protein derivatives, but not so complete as that which forms amino-acids.

Prothrombin (Gr *pro,* before; *thrombos,* clot) Blood-clotting factor (number II), synthesized in the liver from glutamic acid and CO_2, catalyzed by vitamin K.

Protoporphyrin (Gr *protos,* first; *porphyra,* purple) A chemical compound forming the basis for respiratory pigments, such as hemoglobin in humans and in animals, and chlorophyll in plants. Combines with iron to form heme portion of hemoglobin. (See margin flow chart.)

Proximal First portion or front part of a body organ.

Ptyalin (Gr *ptyalon,* spittle) Starch enzyme (amylase) occurring in saliva.

Public health nutritionist A professional nutritionist, accredited by academic degree course of university and special graduate study (MPH, DrPH) in schools of public health accredited by the American Association of Public Health, responsible for nutrition components of public health programs in varied community settings—county, state, national, international.

Puerperium (L *puer,* child; *parere,* to bring forth) The period of time immediately following childbirth.

Pulmonary edema Accumulation of fluid in tissues of the lung.

Pyloric (Gr *phloros,* from *pyle,* gate; *ouros,* guard) The lower opening of the stomach into the duodenum, first section of the small intestine; a valve controlling food mass passage made of a strong band of circular muscle, through which the stomach contents are emptied into the duodenum.

Pyridoxalphosphate (PLP) A major coenzyme involved in amino acid metabolism.

Pyrosis (Gr *pyro,* fire, burning) Heartburn.

Pyruvate Metabolic end product of glycolysis, which may then be converted to lactate or acetyl CoA.

Radiation A form of cancer therapy using electromagnetic rays having both wave and particle functions; radio waves may span the entire spectrum from low-frequency, through white light, to high-frequency gamma rays.

Radical A group of atoms which enters into and goes out of chemical combination without change and which forms one of the fundamental constituents of a molecule.

Radioactive (L *radius,* ray) Used with a chemical element to indicate the quality of electromagnetic radiations related to its nuclear disintegration.

Radiotracers A radioactive chemical element used in medical research and clinical practice to study various body functions to which it is related. For example, radioactive iodine may be used to study the function or malfunction of the thyroid gland.

Raffinose (Fr *raffin,* to refine) A colorless crystalline trisaccharide component of legumes, composed of galactose and sucrose connected by bonds that human enzymes cannot break, thus it remains whole in the intestines and produces gas as bacteria attack it.

Receptor (L *receptor,* receiver) Any one of various specific protein molecules in surface membranes of cells and cell organelles, to which complementary molecules, such as hormones, neurotransmitters, drugs, viruses, or other antigens or antibodies, may become bound.

Recommended Dietary Allowances (RDAs) Recommended daily allowances of nutrients and energy intake for population groups according to age and sex, with defined weight and height. Established and reviewed periodically by a representative group of nutritional scientists, in response to current research. These standards vary very little among the developed countries.

Reducing agent A substance capable of donating electrons to another substance, thereby reducing the second substance and itself becoming oxidized.

Reesterified To combine with an alcohol with elimination of a molecule of water, forming an ester. An ester is any compound formed from an alcohol and an acid by the removal of water. The esters are named as if they were salts of the acid.

Registered Dietitian (RD) A professional dietitian, accredited by academic degree course of university and graduate study (MS, PhD), clinical and administration training, and having passed required registration examinations administered by the American Dietetic Association.

Renal solute load (L *ren,* kidney) Collective number and concentration of solute particles in a solution, carried by the blood to the kidney nephrons for excretion in the urine, usually nitrogenous products from protein metabolism, and the electrolytes Na^+, K^+, Cl^-, and HPO_4^-.

Renal threshold The concentration of a substance in plasma at which it begins to be excreted in the urine.

Renin-angiotensin-aldosterone mechanism Three-stage system of sodium conservation, hence control of water loss, in response to diminished filtration pressure in the kidney nephrons: (1) Pressure loss causes kidney to secret the enzyme renin which combines with and activates angiotensinogen from the liver; (2) active angiotensin stimulates of the adjacent adrenal gland to release the hormone aldosterone; (3) the hormone causes reabsorption of sodium from the kidney nephrons and water follows.

Replicate (L *replicare,* to fold back) To make an exact copy; to repeat, duplicate, or reproduce. In genetics, replication is the process by which double-stranded DNA makes copies of itself, each separating strand synthesizing a complimentary strand. Cell replication is the process by which living cells, under gene control, make exact copies of themselves a programmed number of times during the life span of the organism. The process can be reproduced in the laboratory with cultured cell lines for special studies in cell biology.

Respiratory chains Sequence of special substrate compounds making up the final cell energy production process of oxidative phosphorylation; process of electron (H^+) transfer through a series of substrate compounds, forming high-energy compound ATP, with end product H_2O.

Reticular formation (L *rete,* net) Network of cells in the brain stem controlling the swallowing reflex.

Reticuloendothelial cells A functional rather than anatomical system that serves as an important bodily defense mechanism, composed of highly phagocytic cells such as macrophages of the lymph, liver, spleen, and bone marrow.

Retina (L *retina*) The innermost coat of the posterior part of the eyeball that receives the image produced by the lens; is continuous with the optic nerve, and consists of several layers, one of which contains the rods and cones that are sensitive to light.

Retinal Organic compound that is the aldehyde form of retinol, derived by the enzymatic splitting of absorbed carotene. It performs vitamin A activity. In the retina of the eye, retinal combines with opsins to form visual pigments. In the rods it combines with scotopsin to form rhodopsin (visual purple). In the cones it combines with photopsin to form the three pigments responsible for color vision.

Retinoid Any of the derivatives of retinol, whether naturally occurring or synthetically produced.

Retinol Chemical name for vitamin A derived from its function relating to the retina of the eye and light-dark adaptation. Daily RDA standards are stated in retinol equivalents (RE) to account for sources of the preformed vitamin A and its precursor provitamin A, beta-carotene.

Retinol Equivalent (RE) Unit of measure for dietary sources of vitamin A, both preformed vitamin, retinol, and the precursor provitamin, beta-carotene. 1 RE = 1 μg retinol or 6 μg beta-carotene.

Retinol-binding protein A protein compound that binds and transports retinol.

Retinopathy (L *rete,* net, network; *retina,* innermost layer covering the eyeball; *pathos,* disease) Noninflammatory disease of the retina, visual tissue of the eye, characterized by microaneurysms, intraretinal hemorrhages, waxy yellow exudates, "cotton wool" patches, and macular edema; a complication of diabetes that may lead to proliferation of fibrous tissue, retinal detachment, and blindness.

Retrovirus (L *retro-,* backward) Any of a family of single-strand RNA viruses having an envelope and containing a reverse coding enzyme that allows for a reversal of genetic transcription from RNA to DNA rather than the usual DNA to RNA, the newly transcribed viral DNA then being incorporated into the host cell's DNA strand for the production of new RNA retroviruses.

Rhodopsin (Gr *rhodo,* purple-red; *opsis,* vision) Visual purple: a photosensitive purple-red chromoprotein in the retinal rods which is bleached to visual yellow (all-*trans* retinal) by light, producing stimulation of the retinal sensory endings. It is a conjugated protein, the prosthetic group of which is 11, *cis*-retinal.

Rickets (Gr *rhachitis,* a spinal complaint) A disease of childhood characterized by softening of the bones as a result of inadequate intake of vitamin D and insufficient exposure to sunlight; also associated with impaired calcium and phosphorus metabolism.

RNA (Ribonucleic acid) Vital substance copied from DNA in all living cells, participant in protein synthesis.

Rods One of the rodlike cells in the retina of the eye, sensitive to the low intensities of light; a straight, slim mass of substance.

Rooting reflex A reflex in a newborn in which stimulation of the side of the cheek or the upper or lower lip causes the infant to turn their mouth and face to the stimulus.

Sarcoma (Gr *sarkos,* flesh; *onkoma,* a swelling) Tumors, usually malignant, arising from connective tissue.

Satiety (L *satis,* sufficient; *-ety,* state or condition) A feeling of fullness or satisfaction as after a meal or quenching one's thirst.

Saturated (L *saturare,* to fill) To cause to unite with the greatest possible amount of another substance through solution, chemical combination, or the like. A saturated fat, for example, is one in which the component fatty acids are filled with hydrogen atoms. A fatty acid is said to be saturated if all available chemical bonds of its carbon chain are filled with hydrogen. If one bond remains unfilled, it is a monounsaturated fatty acid. If two or more bonds remain unfilled, it is a polyunsaturated fatty acid. Fats of animal sources are more saturated. Fats of plant sources are unsaturated.

Scoliosis (Gr *skoliosis,* curvature) Lateral curvature of the spine; an appreciable deviation of the normally straight vertical line of the spine.

Scotopsin The protein in the rods of the retina that combines with retinal (11, *cis-* retinal) to form rhodopsin.

Scurvy A hemorrhagic disease caused by lack of vitamin C. Diffuse tissue bleeding occurs, limbs and joints are painful and swollen, bones thicken due to subperiosteal hemorrhage, ecchymoses (large irregular discolored skin areas due to tissue hemorrhages) form, bones fracture easily, wounds do not heal well, gums are swollen and bleeding, and teeth loosen.

Sebaceous (L *sebum,* suet) Secreting the fatty lubricating substance *sebum.*

Secretin Hormone produced in the mucous membrane of the duodenum in response to the entrance of the acid contents of the stomach into the duodenum. Secretin in turn stimulates the flow of pancreatic juice, providing needed enzymes and the proper alkalinity for their action.

Selenium An essential trace element, necessary constituent of the enzyme system glutathione peroxidase, which is closely associated with vitamin E in its antioxidant functions.

Senescence (L *senescere,* to grow old) The process of growing old, consequence of advancing age or of premature aging process from disease.

Sepsis (Gr *sēpsis,* decay) Presence in the blood or other tissues of pathogenic microorganisms or their toxins; conditions associated with such pathogens.

Serosa Outer surface layer of the intestines interfacing with the blood vessels of the portal system going to the liver.

Serotoninergic agent Chemical substance or neuron that activates the secretion of *serotonin,* a neurotransmitter that effectively suppresses appetite and heavy eating.

Serum Ca/P ratio Inverse ratio affecting the absorption rate of each mineral. The *dietary ratio* of 1:1.5 is ideal for periods of rapid growth in children, and 1:1 for normal adult functions. The normal *serum ratio* for adults is 40 (10 mg/dL calcium x 4 mg/dL phosphorus), and for children is 50 (10 mg/dL calcium x 5 mg/dL phosphorus.

SI units Any of the units of the Système International d'Unités, or International System of Units, adopted in 1960. SI units comprise the basic units such as meter (length), kilogram (mass), second (time), watt (power), etc.

Slough Shed or cast off, as sloughing off dead cells from outer edges of epithelial tissue.

Smooth muscle Nonstriated, involuntary muscle, structural component of the gastrointestinal tract walls, providing essential movements and motility for digestion, absorption, and passage of food and it nutrients through the system.

Solutes (Gr *solvere,* to solve) Particles of a substance in solution; a solution consists of solutes and a dissolving medium (solvent), usually a liquid.

Solvent (L *solvens,* to loosen) A liquid that dissolves or that is capable of dissolving.

Somatostatin (Gr *soma,* body; *stasis,* standing still, maintaining a constant level) A hormone formed in the D cells of the pancreatic islets of Langerhans and the hypothalamus. It is a balancing factor in maintaining normal blood glucose levels by inhibiting insulin and glucagon production in the pancreas as needed.

Sphingomyelin A general designation of a group of phospholipids which on hydrolysis yield phosphoric acid, choline, sphingosine, and a fatty acid. They occur primarily in nervous tissue and generally in membranes.

Spina bifida (L *spina,* spine; *bifidus,* cleft into two parts or branches) Congenital defect in the fetal closing of the neural tube to form a portion of the lower spine, leaving the spine unclosed and the spinal cord open in various degrees of exposure and damage.

Splanchnic (Gr *splanchnikos,* viscera) Pertaining to the large interior organs of the body, especially those located in the abdomen.

Sprue Alternate term for adult celiac disease, a malabsorption syndrome.

Staphyloccal (Gr *staphyl,* grapes; *kokkus,* berry) Any of several spherical bacteria of the genus staphylococcus, occurring in irregular clusters resembling bunches of grapes. Certain species such as S. aureus are pathogenic for humans.

Steatorrhea (Gr *steatos,* fat; *rhoia,* flow) Excessive fat amounts in the feces; often caused by malabsorption syndromes.

Stenosis (Gr *stenos,* narrow) A narrowing or obstruction of a body duct, valve, or canal such as a blood vessel.

Sterol (Gr *stereos,* solid; L *oleum,* oil) Steroids with long (8-10 carbons) side-chains and at least one alcohol hydroxyl group. They have lipid-like solubility. Examples are cholesterol and ergosterol.

Stoma (Gr *stoma,* mouth, opening) The opening established in the abdominal wall, connecting with the ileum or colon, for elimination of intestinal wastes after surgical removal of diseased portions of the intestinal tract.

Stomatitis (Gr *stoma,* mouth; *-itis,* inflammation) Inflammation of the oral mucosa, especially the buccal tissue lining the inside of the cheeks, but also may involve the tongue, palate, floor of the mouth, and the gums.

Strategy (Gr *strategia,* generalship; *agein,* to lead) Skillful plan, method or series of actions for achieving a specific goal or result; long-range planning and development.

Striated (L *striatus,* furrowed) Striped; marked by striae or streaks.

Stroke volume (Gr *streich,* to strike or stretch) The amount of blood pumped from a ventricle (chamber of the heart releasing blood to body circulations) with each beat of the heart.

Sublingual (L *sub,* under; *lingualis,* tongue) Located beneath the tongue.

Submandibular (L *sub,* under; *mandibula,* mandible) Below the mandible, the bone of the lower jaw.

Submucosal plexus (L *sub,* under; L *mucosus* slimy; *plexuses,* braid) The part of the enteric plexus that is situated beneath the mucous membrane.

Substrate (L *sub,* under; *stratum,* layer) The specific organic substance on which a particular enzyme acts to produce new metabolic products.

Sucrase Enzyme splitting the disaccharide sucrose into its two monosaccharides of glucose and fructose.

Surfactant A surface-active agent, such as soap or a synthetic detergent. In pulmonary physiology, a mixture of phospholipids secreted by the alveolar type II cells into alveoli and respiratory air passages.

Sympathetic (Gr *sympathetikos,* sympathetic) The part of the autonomic nervous system consisting of nerves that arise from the thoracic and lumbar regions of the spinal cord and functioning in opposition to the parasympathetic system, as in stimulating heartbeat, dilating the pupil of the eye, etc.

Syncytium Mass of protoplasm that results when cells merge, resulting in common actions of the whole.

Synergism (Gr *syn,* with or together; *ergon,* work) The joint action of separate agents in which the total effect of their combined action is greater than the sum of their separate actions.

Synosheath (Gr *syno-,* with, together; *thēkē,* sheath) Protective pliable connective tissue surrounding the bony-collagen mesh and fluid that come together in the synovial area between major bone heads in joints, which allows normal padded and lubricated joint movement and motion.

Tachycardia (Gr *tachys,* swift; *kardia,* heart) Excessively rapid action of the heart; usually applied to a heart rate above 100 beats per minute.

Tactile (L *tactus,* touch) Pertaining to the touch.

Taurine A sulfur-containing amino acid, $NH_2(CH_2)_2SO_2OH$, formed from the essential amino acid methionine. It is found in various body tissues such as lungs and muscles, and in bile and breast milk.

Tetany (Gr *teinein,* to stretch) Condition caused by decrease in ionized serum calcium, marked by intermittent spastic muscle contractions and muscular pain.

Thiamin pyrophosphate (TPP) Activating coenzyme form of thiamin; plays a key role in carbohydrate metabolism.

Thyroxine The iodine-containing hormone produced by the thyroid gland.

Tocopherol (Gr *tokos,* childbirth; *pherein,* to carry) Chemical name for vitamin E, so named by early investigators because their initial work with rats indicated a reproductive function, which did not turn out later to be the case with humans, in whom it functions as a strong antioxidant to preserve structural membranes such as cell walls.

Tomography (Gr *tomē,* a cutting; *graphein,* to write) The recording of internal body images at a particular plane of the body, moving an x-ray source in one direction as the film is moved in the opposite direction, thus showing in detail the desired tissue while blurring or eliminating detail in the other parts. Electronic impulses are processed by a computer for displaying the body cross-section recorded.

Tonicoclonus (Gr *tonos,* tension; *klonos,* turmoil) Spasm of convulsive muscle twitching.

Total body electroconductivity (TOBEC) A method of measuring lean body mass based on the ability of the large water content in muscles to conduct electrical energy.

Trachea (Gr *tracheia,* windpipe) The tube in humans and other air-breathing vertebrates extending from the larynx to the bronchi, serving as the principal passage for conveying air to and from the lungs; the windpipe.

trans (L, through) Having certain atoms or radicals in a chemical structure on opposite sides. Partial hydrogenation of vegetable oil used to make fat spreads such as margarine changes the natural *cis* form of the fatty acid chain to *trans* form, straightening it and bending it in opposite directions.

Transamination Transfer of the amino group (NH_2) from an amino acid to a carbon residue to form another amino acid. The newly formed compound is classed a nonessential amino acid, since the body can synthesize it and does not depend on the diet to supply it.

Transketolation Transfer of the first unit two-carbon group from one sugar to another in glucose oxidation.

Transmangamin Manganese transport carrier, a compound with a plasma protein beta-globulin.

Transmural (L *trans-,* through; *murrus,* wall) Through the wall of an organ; extending through or affecting the entire thickness of the wall of an organ or cavity.

Transthyretin A protein compound that binds and transports both thyroid hormone and retinol.

Triacylglycerol Term used to designate the nature of fat: three fatty acids on a 3-carbon glycerol base. However, the current standardized terminology of the International Union of Pure and Applied Chemistry (IUPAC) and the International Union of Biochemistry (IUB) designates the term *triacylglycerol,* using the more current term *acyl* for the fatty acid units and actually making a more understandable term. Most texts still use these terms interchangeably.

Tricarboxylic acid (TCA) cycle (Gr *kyklos,* circle) The cyclic metabolic mechanism by which the complete oxidation of the acetyl group of acetyl-coenzyme A is accomplished; also called Krebs' cycle and citric acid cycle. A cycle of enzyme-catalyzed reactions in living cells that is the final series of reactions of aerobic metabolism of carbohydrates, proteins, and fatty acids, and by which carbon dioxide is produced, oxygen is reduced and ATP is formed.

Triglyceride (Gr *tri,* three) Chemical name for fat, indicating structure: attachment of three fatty acids to a glycerol base. A neutral fat, synthesized from carbohydrate, stored in adipose tissue. It releases free fatty acids into the blood when hydrolyzed by enzymes.

Tripeptide (Gr *tri,* three) A peptide which on hydrolysis, yields three amino acids.

Trophoblast (Gr *tropho,* nutrition; *blastos,* germ) The outer layer of embryonic ectoderm that chiefly nourishes the embryo or develops into fetal membranes with nutritive functions.

Trypsin (Gr *trypein,* to rub; *pepsis,* digestion) A protein-splitting enzyme formed in the intestine by action of enterokinase on the inactive precursor trypsinogen.

Trypsin inhibitor An initial protective secretion of the pancreas that prevents pancreatic tissues digestion by the activated enzymes. Also occurs naturally in raw soybeans and is responsible for toxin in the beans. Fortunately this substance is destroyed by heat and rendered inactive in the cooked beans.

Tubular glands Any gland made up of or containing a tubule (a small tube) or a number of tubules.

Turgor (L *turgere,* to swell) The natural distention of cells and tissues with fluids that gives form and shape to the body.

Ultrasonography The visualization of deep body structures by recording the echo reflection pulses of ultrasonic waves directed at the body tissues. This diagnostic technique is used, for example, to study heart and brain function as reflections are amplified and processed into visual displays on a television video-scan converted screen.

Unsaturated (L *un,* not; *saturatus,* to fill) A carbon chain, as in fatty acids, having one or more double bonds unfilled with hydrogen atoms.

Urea cycle Special enzyme cycle in the liver for disposing of the nitrogenous compound ammonia by forming urea for excretion in the urine.

Vacuole (L *vacuus,* empty) Any small space or cavity formed in the protoplasm of a cell.

Vagus nerve Either one of the tenth pair of cranial nerves, consisting of motor fibers that innervate the muscles and secretion of the gastrointestinal tract, pharynx, larynx, heart, etc.

Valence (L *valens,* powerful) Power of an element or a radical to combine with or to replace other elements or radicals. Atoms of various elements combine in definite proportions. The valence number of an element is the number of atoms of hydrogen with which one atom of the element can combine.

Varices (plural) (L *varix* (singular), enlarged vein) Varicose veins; enlarged and tortuous veins, full of twists, turns, curves, or windings.

Vasoactive (L *vas,* vessel) Having an effect on the diameter of blood vessels.

Vasopressin (ADH) Hormone formed in the hypothalamus and stored in the posterior pituitary gland. Stimulates muscle contraction of capillaries and arterioles to maintain blood pressure, and acts on the epithelial cells of the distal tubule of the nephron to cause water reabsorption, producing a concentrated urine and preventing water loss. Thus it is also called the antidiuretic hormone (ADH).

Vegan An extreme vegetarian who excludes all animal protein from his diet. Requires careful food combinations of incomplete plant proteins to complement one another and achieve an overall adequacy of essential amino acids for growth needs.

Vena cava (L *vena cava,* hollow vein) Either of two large veins discharging blood into the right atrium of the heart, one (superior vena cava) conveying blood from the head, chest, and upper extremities and the other (inferior vena cava) conveying blood from all parts below the diaphragm.

Ventricle (L *venter,* belly, abdomen; *ventriculus,* diminutive form indicating relation to front aspect of the body) A small cavity; one of the pair of lower chambers of the heart, with thick muscular walls, that make up the bulk of the heart. The ventricles receive blood from the atria and in turn force blood out into body circulation to the lungs for oxygenation and then into systemic body circulation to service the cells.

Venule (L *venulae,* dim. of vena [vein]) Any of the small vessels that collect blood from the capillaries and join to form veins.

Villi (L *villus,* "tuft of hair") Small protrusions from the surface of a membrane; finger-like projections covering mucosal surfaces of the small intestine.

Villous adenoma (L *villus,* tuft of hair, finger-like projection; Gr *adenos,* gland) Epithelial tumor of glandular structure forming soft large protrusion on the mucosa of the large intestine.

Virus (L *virus,* poison; *virion,* individual virus particle) Minute infectious agent, characterized by lack of independent metabolism and by the ability to reproduce with genetic continuity only within living host cells. They range in decreasing size from about 200 nanometers (nm) down to only 15 nanometers (nm). (A nanometer is a linear measure equal to one-billionth of a meter; it is also called a millimicron.) Each particle (virion) consists basically of nucleic acids (genetic material) and a protein shell which protects and contains the genetic material and any enzymes present.

Viscera Abdominal organs associated with the gastrointestinal tract and its accessory secretory organs.

Viscid (L *viscidus*) Glutinous or thick and sticky.

Viscous (viscid) (L *viscidus,* glutinous or sticky) Physical property of a substance dependent on the friction of its component molecules as they slide by one another; viscosity.

VO_2max Maximum uptake volume of oxygen during exercise; used to measure the intensity and duration of exercise a person can perform.

Volition (L *volitio, velle,* to want or wish) The act of willing, choosing, or resolving; a deliberate action.

Werner's syndrome Premature senility of young adults in their 20s, characterized by graying and loss of hair, cataracts, excessive roughing and hardening of the skin from hyperkeratosis, hardened skin changes on the legs leading to chronic ulceration and tissue breakdown.

Wilson's disease Rare hereditary disease in which large amounts of copper are absorbed by and accumulate in the liver, brain, kidneys, and cornea. Produces degenerative changes in brain and liver tissue.

X-ray The name originally given to specially sensitized radiograph films made by electromagnetic radiation capable of penetrating solids. This process was discovered in 1895 by the German physicist Wilhelm Konrad Roentgen, for which he received the Nobel Prize in 1901. He named his discovery *x-ray* to indicate its then unknown nature, little dreaming of how widespread its use would become, and the name has stuck despite our current knowledge.

Xanthoma (Gr *xanthos,* yellow; *-oma,* mass or body of material) A plaque of yellow lipid deposits in the skin, fatty streaks or nodules.

Xerophthalmia (Gr *xeros,* dry; *ophthalmos,* eye) Dryness of the conjunctiva and cornea due to vitamin A deficiency. The condition begins with night blindness and conjunctival xerosis and progresses to corneal xerosis and in late stages to keratomalacia.

Xerosis (Gr *xerosis,* dry) Abnormal dryness, as of the eye, skin, or mouth.

Xerostomia (Gr *xeros,* dry; *stoma,* mouth) Dryness of the mouth from lack of normal secretions.

Zollinger-Ellison syndrome An intractable, sometimes fulminating atypical peptic ulcer disease, characterized by extreme gastric hyperacidity.

Zygote (Gr *zygotos,* yoked together) The cell resulting from union of a male and female gamete (sperm and ovum), until it divides; the fertilized ovum.

ILLUSTRATION CREDITS

Chapter 1: Chapter opener from Potter/Perry: Basic nursing, ed. 2, Mosby, 1991; Figure 1-1, Tom Tracy, Medichrome; Figure 1-2, R. Brady, Medichrome.
Chapter 2: Chapter opener, CLG Photographics, Inc.
Chapter 3: Chapter opener from Potter/Perry: Basic nursing, ed. 2, Mosby, 1991.
Chapter 4: Chapter opener, Photo Researchers.
Chapter 5: Chapter opener from Potter/Perry: Basic nursing, ed. 2, Mosby, 1991.
Chapter 6: Chapter opener, Jack Van Antwerp, The Stock Market; Figure 6-1 from Guthrie: Introductory nutrition, ed. 7, Mosby, 1989.
Chapter 7: Chapter opener, CLG Photographics, Inc.; Figure 7-1, Medical and Scientific Illustration; Figure 7-2, Medical and Scientific Illustration.
Chapter 8: Chapter opener, Walter Iooss, The Image Bank; Figure 8-1, Christine Oleksyk from Seeley/Stephens/Tate: Anatomy and physiology, ed. 2, Mosby, 1992; Figure 8-2, Medical and Scientific Illustration; Figure 8-4, Medical and Scientific Illustration; Figure 8-6, Medical and Scientific Illustration; Figure 8-7, Medical and Scientific Illustration.
Chapter 9: Chapter opener, CLG Photographics, Inc.
Chapter 10: Chapter opener, Howard Sochurek, The Stock Market.
Chapter 11: Chapter opener, CLG Photographics, Inc.
Chapter 12: Chapter opener, P. Forden, SYGMA.
Chapter 13: Chapter opener, Bruce Berman, The Stock Market.
Chapter 14: Chapter opener, CLG Photographics, Inc.

Appendices

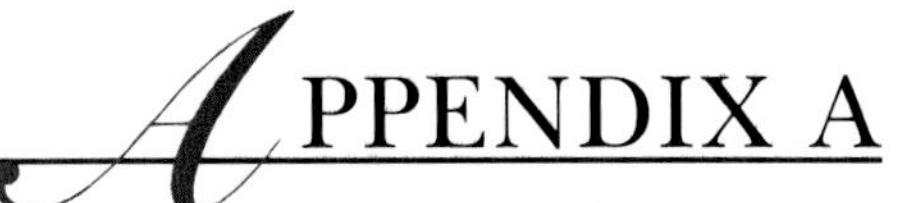

PPENDIX A

Nutritive Values of the Edible Part of Food

Key to Abbreviations

Kcal, Kcalories; *Prot,* protein; *Carb,* carbohydrate; *Fat,* fat; *Chol,* cholesterol; *Safa,* saturated fat; *Mufa,* monounsaturated fat; *Pufa,* polyunsaturated fat; *Sod,* sodium; *Pot,* potassium; *Mag,* magnesium; *Iron,* iron; *Zinc,* zinc; *VA,* vitamin A; *VC,* vitamin C; *Thia,* thiamin; *Ribo,* riboflavin; *Niac,* niacin; *VB_6,* vitamin B_6; *Fol,* folate; *VB_{12},* vitamin B_{12}; *Calc,* calcium; *Phos,* phosphorus; *Sel,* selenium; *Fibd,* dietary fiber; and *VE,* vitamin E

Food name	Portion	Wt (g)	Kcal	Prot (g)	Carb (g)	Fat (g)	Chol (mg)	Safa (g)	Mufa (g)	Pufa (g)	Sod (mg)	Pot (mg)
Baby foods												
Apple Betty	oz	28.4	20	0.1	5.6	0	0	0	0	0	3	14
Apple blueberry	oz	28.4	17	0.1	4.6	0.1	0	—	—	—	0	20
Apple juice	Fl oz	31	14	0	3.6	0	0	0	0	0	1	28
Apple peach juice	Fl oz	31	13	0	3.2	0	0	0	0	0	—	30
Applesauce	oz	28.4	12	0.1	3.1	0	0	0	0	0	1	20
Beans-green	oz	28.4	7	0.4	1.7	0	0	0	0	0	1	45
Beans-green-buttered	oz	28.4	9	0.3	1.9	0.2	—	—	—	—	1	45
Beef	oz	28.4	30	3.9	0	1.5	—	0.73	0.62	0.06	23	62
Beef & egg noodles	oz	28.4	15	0.6	2	0.5	—	—	—	—	8	13
Beef lasagna	oz	28.4	22	1.2	2.8	0.6	—	—	—	—	129	35
Beef stew	oz	28.4	14	1.4	1.5	0.3	3.55	0.16	0.12	0.01	98	40
Beets	oz	28.4	10	0.4	2.2	0	0	0	0	0	24	52
Carrots	oz	28.4	8	0.2	1.7	0	0	0	0	0	11	56
Cereal & egg yolks	oz	28.4	15	0.5	2	0.5	18	0.17	0.22	0.04	9	11
Chicken	oz	28.4	37	3.9	0	2.2	—	0.58	1.01	0.54	13	40
Cookie-arrowroot	Item	6	24	0.4	4.3	0.9	0	0.2	0.52	0.02	22	9
Corn-creamed	oz	28.4	16	0.4	4	0.1	0	0	0	0	12	26
Egg yolks	Serving	28.4	58	2.8	0.3	4.9	223	1.47	1.8	0.54	11	22
Garden vegetables	oz	28.4	11	0.7	1.9	0.1	0	0	0	0	10	48
Ham	oz	28.4	32	3.9	0	1.6	—	0.55	0.78	0.22	12	58
Lamb	oz	28.4	29	4	0	1.3	0	0.66	0.53	0.06	18	58
Liver	oz	28.4	29	4.1	0.4	1.1	52	0.39	0.22	0.02	21	64
Mixed cereal/mix	oz	28.4	32	1.3	4.5	1	0	—	—	—	13	56
Mixed vegetables	oz	28.4	11	0.3	2.7	0	0	0	0	0	2	34
Oatmeal cereal/milk	oz	28.4	33	1.4	4.3	1.2	0	—	—	—	13	58
Orange juice	Fl oz	31	14	0.2	3.2	0.1	0	—	—	—	0	57
Peaches	oz	28.4	20	0.1	5.4	0	0	0	0	0	2	46
Pears	oz	28.4	12	0.1	3.1	0	0	0	0	0	1	37
Peas	oz	28.4	11	1	2.3	0.1	0	0	0	0	1	32
Peas-creamed	oz	28.4	15	0.6	2.5	0.5	0	—	—	—	4	25
Pork	oz	28.4	35	4	0	2	—	0.68	1.02	0.22	12	63
Pretzels	Item	6	24	0.7	4.9	0.1	—	0	0	0	16	8
Rice cereal/milk	oz	28.4	33	1.1	4.7	1	0	—	—	—	13	54
Spinach-creamed	oz	28.4	11	0.7	1.6	0.4	0	—	—	—	14	54
Squash	oz	28.4	7	0.2	1.6	0.1	0	0	0	0	1	51
Sweet potatoes	oz	28.4	16	0.3	3.7	0	0	0	0	0	6	75
Teething biscuits	Item	11	43	1.2	8.4	0.5	0	—	—	—	40	35
Turkey	oz	28.4	32	4	0	1.7	—	0.54	0.62	0.41	15	65
Turkey & rice	oz	28.4	14	0.5	2.1	0.4	2.84	0.12	0.15	0.04	5	12
Veal & vegetables	oz	28.4	20	1.7	1.7	0.8	—	—	—	—	7	43
Zwieback	Piece	7	30	0.7	5.2	0.7	1.46	0.28	0.24	0.05	16	21

Mag (mg)	Iron (mg)	Zinc (mg)	VA (RE)	VC (mg)	Thia (mg)	Ribo (mg)	Niac (mg)	VB_6 (mg)	Fol (µg)	VB_{12} (µg)	Calc (mg)	Phos (mg)	Sel (mg)	Fibd (g)	VE (mg)
—	0.05	—	0	9.8	0.004	0.01	0.013	—	0.1	—	5	—	—	0	0.065
—	0.06	—	1	7.9	0.005	0.01	0.034	0.01	1	—	1	2	0	0.1	0.165
1	0.18	0.009	1	18	0.002	0.005	0.026	0.009	0	—	1	2	0	0.25	0.18
1	0.17	0.008	2	18.1	0.002	0.003	0.066	0.007	0.04	—	1	1	0	0.25	0.18
1	0.06	0.007	0	10.9	0.003	0.008	0.017	0.009	0.5	—	1	2	0	0.7	0.165
7	0.21	0.058	13	1.5	0.007	0.024	0.098	0.011	9.8	—	11	6	0	0.39	0.128
—	0.36	—	13	2.3	0.005	0.03	0.096	—	8.1	—	18	—	0.17	0.7	0.128
5	0.42	0.696	16	0.6	0.003	0.04	0.808	0.04	1.6	0.403	2	24	0.003	0	0.111
2	0.12	0.106	31	0.3	0.01	0.012	0.205	0.014	1.4	0.026	3	8	0.003	0.1	0.062
3	0.25	0.198	100	0.5	0.02	0.025	0.384	0.02	—	—	5	11	—	0.1	0.062
3	0.2	0.247	95	0.9	0.004	0.018	0.372	0.021	—	—	3	12	0.003	0.34	0.062
4	0.09	0.034	1	0.7	0.003	0.012	0.037	0.007	8.7	—	4	4	—	0.4	0.128
3	0.1	0.043	325	1.6	0.007	0.011	0.131	0.021	4.2	—	6	6	0	0.7	0.128
1	0.13	0.081	11	0.2	0.003	0.012	0.014	0.006	0.9	0.02	7	11	—	0	0.071
4	0.4	0.343	11	0.5	0.004	0.043	0.923	0.057	2.9	—	18	27	0.003	0	0.111
1	0.18	0.032	—	0.3	0.03	0.026	0.344	0.002	—	0.004	2	7	—	0	0.014
2	0.08	0.054	2	0.6	0.004	0.013	0.145	0.012	3.2	0.005	6	9	—	0.9	0.128
2	0.78	0.543	107	0.4	0.02	0.075	0.007	0.045	26.1	0.437	22	81	0.005	0	0.17
6	0.24	0.074	172	1.6	0.017	0.02	0.221	0.028	11.4	—	8	8	0	0.7	0.128
4	0.29	0.637	3	0.6	0.039	0.044	0.746	0.071	0.6	—	2	23	0.003	0	0.111
4	0.42	0.781	7	0.3	0.005	0.057	0.829	0.043	0.6	0.621	2	27	0.004	0	0.111
4	1.5	0.844	3247	5.5	0.014	0.514	2.36	0.097	95.7	0.612	1	58	0.007	0	0.111
8	2.96	0.202	6	0.3	0.122	0.165	1.64	0.019	3.2	—	62	40	—	0.25	0.045
—	0.09	—	77	0.8	0.004	0.009	0.142	—	2.3	—	6	—	0	0.25	0.128
10	3.44	0.262	6	0.4	0.143	0.16	1.7	0.017	2.8	—	62	45	0.001	0.7	0.054
3	0.05	0.017	2	19.4	0.014	0.009	0.074	0.017	8.2	—	4	3	0	0.25	0.18
2	0.07	0.024	5	8.9	0.003	0.009	0.173	0.004	1.1	—	2	3	0	0.7	0.165
2	0.07	0.021	1	7	0.004	0.008	0.054	0.002	1	—	2	3	0	0.25	0.165
4	0.27	0.099	16	1.9	0.023	0.017	0.289	0.02	7.4	—	6	12	0	0.7	0.128
—	0.16	0.11	2	0.5	0.025	0.016	0.23	0.013	6.4	0.023	4	9	—	0.7	0.128
3	0.28	0.644	3	0.5	0.041	0.058	0.643	0.058	0.5	0.281	1	27	0.004	0	0.111
2	0.23	0.047	0	0.2	0.028	0.021	0.214	0.005	—	—	1	7	—	0	0.009
13	3.46	0.182	6	0.3	0.132	0.142	1.48	0.032	2.3	—	68	50	0.001	0.25	0.074
16	0.18	0.088	118	2.5	0.004	0.029	0.061	0.021	17.2	—	25	15	—	1.12	0.128
3	0.08	0.04	57	2.2	0.003	0.016	0.1	0.018	4.4	—	7	4	0	0.7	0.128
4	0.1	0.058	183	2.8	0.008	0.009	0.101	0.026	2.8	—	4	7	0	0.7	0.128
4	0.39	0.102	1	1	0.026	0.059	0.476	0.012	—	0.008	29	18	—	0.1	—
4	0.34	0.519	48	0.6	0.005	0.059	1.04	0.051	3.2	0.284	7	36	0.003	0	0.111
—	0.07	—	27	0.3	0.001	0.006	0.087	0.009	0.9	—	6	6	—	0	0.062
2	0.17	0.284	21	0.5	0.006	0.021	0.457	0.024	—	0.128	3	15	—	0.1	0.062
1	0.04	0.038	0	0.4	0.015	0.017	0.092	0.006	—	—	1	4	—	0	—

Continued.

Key to Abbreviations
Kcal, Kcalories; *Prot,* protein; *Carb,* carbohydrate; *Fat,* fat; *Chol,* cholesterol; *Safa,* saturated fat; *Mufa,* monounsaturated fat; *Pufa,* polyunsaturated fat; *Sod,* sodium; *Pot,* potassium; *Mag,* magnesium; *Iron,* iron; *Zinc,* zinc; *VA,* vitamin A; *VC,* vitamin C; *Thia,* thiamin; *Ribo,* riboflavin; *Niac,* niacin; *VB_6,* vitamin B_6; *Fol,* folate; *VB_{12},* vitamin B_{12}; *Calc,* calcium; *Phos,* phosphorus; *Sel,* selenium; *Fibd,* dietary fiber; and *VE,* vitamin E.

Food name	Portion	Wt (g)	Kcal	Prot (g)	Carb (g)	Fat (g)	Chol (mg)	Safa (g)	Mufa (g)	Pufa (g)	Sod (mg)	Pot (mg)
Beverages												
Beer-light	Fl oz	29.5	8	0.1	0.4	0	0	0	0	0	1	5
Beer-regular	Fl oz	29.7	12	0.1	1.1	0	0	0	0	0	2	7
Brandy/cognac-pony	Item	30	73	—	—	0	0	0	0	0	—	—
Carn inst break-choc(env)	Item	36	130	7	23	1	—	—	—	—	136	422
Champagne-domestic-glass	Item	120	84	0.2	3	0	0	0	0	0	—	—
Choc bev drink-no milk-dry	oz	28.4	97.7	0.924	25.3	0.868	0	0.513	0.283	0.025	58.8	165
Cider-fermeted	Fl oz	30	11.8	—	0.3	0	0	0+	0	0	0	—
Club soda	Fl oz	29.6	0	0	0	0	0	0	0	0	6	0
Coffee substitute-prep	Fl oz	30.3	1.52	0.03	0.192	0	0	0	0	0	1.21	7.27
Coffee-brewed	Fl oz	30	1	0	0.1	0	0	0	0	0	1	16
Coffee instant-prep	Fl oz	30.3	0.61	0	0.121	0	0	0	0	0	0.91	10.9
Cordials/liqueur-54-proof	Fl oz	34	97	—	11.5	0	0	0	0	0	1	1
Cream soda	Fl oz	30.9	16	0	4.1	0	0	0	0	0	4	0
Gatorade-thirst quencher	Fl oz	30.1	7	0	1.9	0	0	0	0	0	12	3
Grape drink-can	Cup	253	154	1.42	37.8	0.202	0	0.063	0.008	0.056	7.59	334
Hot cocoa-prep/milk-home	Cup	250	218	9.1	25.8	9.05	33	5.61	2.65	0.33	123	480
Lemon lime soda-7UP	Fl oz	30.7	12	0	3.2	0	0	0	0	0	3	0
Ovaltine-choc-prep/milk	Cup	265	227	9.53	29.2	8.79	—	—	—	—	228	600
Perrier-mineral water	Cup	237	0	0	0	0	0	0	0	0	3	0
Postum-inst grain bev-dry	oz	28.4	103	1.93	24.1	0.028	0	0	0	0	28.4	896
Soda-cola type-carbonated	Cup	246.4	100.8	0	25.6	0	0	0.016	0	0	9.84	2.464
Soda-diet cola-carbonated	Cup	236.8	2.368	0.24	0.24	0	0	0	0	0	14.24	0
Tang-inst drink-orange-dry	oz	28.4	104	0	26.1	0	0	0	0	0	12.8	80.9
Tea-brewed	Fl oz	29.6	0	0	0.1	0	0	0	0	0	1	11
Tea-herb-brewed	Fl oz	29.6	0.17	0.017	0.05	0	0	0	0	0	0	3
Tea-instant-prep-sweet	Cup	259	87	0.1	22.1	0.1	0	0.008	0.003	0.021	—	50
Tea-instant-prep-unsweet	Cup	237	2	0.1	0.4	0	0	0	0	0	8	47
Tonic water-quinine soda	Fl oz	30.5	10	0	2.7	0	0	0	0	0	1	0
Water	Cup	237	0	0	0	0	0	0	0	0	7	1
Whis/gin/rum/vod-100 proof	Fl oz	27.8	82	0	0	0	0	0	0	0	0	0
Whis/gin/rum/vod-80 proof	Fl oz	27.8	64	0	0	0	0	0	0	0	0	1
Whis/gin/rum/vod-86 proof	Fl oz	27.8	69	0	0	0	0	0	0	0	0	1
Whis/gin/rum/vod-90 proof	Fl oz	27.7	73	0	0	0	0	0	0	0	1	0
Whis/gin/rum/vod-94 proof	Fl oz	27.8	76.5	0	0	0	0	0	0	0	0	0
Wine cooler-white wine/7UP	Serving	102	54.9	0.05	5.72	0	0	0	0	0	7.48	41
Wine-dessert	Fl oz	30	46	0.1	3.5	0	0	0	0	0	3	28
Wine-red table	Fl oz	29.5	21	0.1	0.5	0	0	0	0	0	19	40.7
Wine-rose table	Fl oz	29.5	21	0	0.4	0	0	0	0	0	1	29
Wine-vermouth-dry-glass	Item	100	105	0	1	0	0	0	0	0	4	75
Wine-vermouth-sweet-glass	Item	100	167	0	12	0	0	0	0	0	—	—
Wine-white table	Fl oz	29.5	20	0	0.2	0	0	0	0	0	18	33.3
Breads												
Bagel-egg	Item	55	163	6.02	30.9	1.41	8	—	—	—	198	40.7
Bagel-water	Item	55	163	6.02	30.9	1.41	0	0.2	0.4	0.6	198	40.7
Biscuits-prep/mix	Item	28.4	104	1.63	13	5.05	1.4	3.31	1.29	0.196	221	32.8
Bread stick-vienna type	Item	35	106	3.3	20.3	1.1	0	—	—	—	548	33
Corn-home rec	Slice	45	108	2.21	15.6	3.94	0	—	—	—	126	42.3
Cracked wheat	Slice	25	65.5	2.32	12.5	0.868	0	0.1	0.2	0.2	108	33.3
French-enr	Slice	35	98	3.33	17.7	1.36	0	0.2	0.4	0.4	193	30.1
Mixed grain	Slice	25	64.3	2.49	11.7	0.93	0	—	—	—	103	54.5
Pita	Item	38	105	3.95	20.6	0.57	0	—	—	—	215	44.8
Pumpernickel	Slice	32	81.6	2.93	15.4	1.1	0	—	—	—	173	139
Raisin-enr	Slice	25	69.5	2.05	13.2	0.99	0	0.2	0.3	0.2	94	60
Rye-american-light	Slice	25	65.5	2.12	12	0.913	0	—	—	—	174	51
Wheat-firm-toast	Slice	21	59	2.31	10.9	1.05	0	0.1	0.2	0.3	153	42.4
White-firm	Slice	23	61.4	1.9	11.2	0.902	0	0.2	0.3	0.3	118	25.8

Mag (mg)	Iron (mg)	Zinc (mg)	VA (RE)	VC (mg)	Thia (mg)	Ribo (mg)	Niac (mg)	VB_6 (mg)	Fol (μg)	VB_{12} (μg)	Calc (mg)	Phos (mg)	Sel (mg)	Fibd (g)	VE (mg)
1	0.01	0.01	0	0	0.003	0.009	0.116	0.01	1.2	0	1	4	0	0	—
2	0.01	0	0	0	0.002	0.008	0.135	0.015	1.8	0.01	1	4	—	0.07	—
—	—	—	—	—	—	—	—	—	—	—	—	—	—	0	—
80	4.5	3	525	27	0.3	0.07	5	0.4	0	0.6	100	150	—	—	—
—	—	—	—	—	—	—	—	—	—	—	—	—	—	0	—
27.4	0.879	0.434	1.68	0.196	0.01	0.041	0.143	0.003	—	0	10.4	35.8	—	—	0.056
—	—	—	—	—	—	—	—	—	—	—	—	—	—	0	—
0	—	0.03	0	0	0	0	0	0	0	0	1	0	—	0	—
1.21	0.018	0.009	—	—	—	0	0.065	—	—	0	0.91	2.12	—	0	—
2	0.12	0	0	0	0	0	0.066	0	0	0	1	0	0	0	—
1.21	0.015	0.009	0	0	0	0	0.088	0	0	0	0.91	0.91	0	0	0
0	0.02	0.02	—	0	—	—	—	—	—	—	0	0	—	0	—
0	0.02	0.022	0	0	0	0	0	0	0	0	2	0	—	0	—
0	0.02	0.01	0	0	0.002	0	0	0	0	0	0	3	—	0	0
25.3	0.607	0.127	2.02	0.253	0.066	0.094	0.663	0.164	6.58	0	22.8	27.8	—	0	—
56	0.78	1.22	95.5	2.4	0.102	0.435	0.365	0.107	12	0.87	298	270	—	3	—
0	0.02	0.02	0	0	0	0	0.005	0	0	0	1	0	—	0	0
52	4.77	1.13	700	29	0.63	0.97	12.7	0.766	29	0.871	392	302	—	—	—
1	0	0	0	0	0	0	0	0	0	0	32	0	—	0	—
—	1.87	—	0	0	0.165	0.076	6.76	—	—	—	76.7	189	—	0	—
2.464	0.072	0.024	0	0	0	0	0	0	0	0	7.392	29.6	—	0	0
2.368	0.072	0.192	0	0	0.008	0.056	0	0	0	0	9.44	21.28	—	0	—
—	0.028	—	535	107	0	0	0	—	—	—	71	75.8	—	—	—
1	0.01	0.01	0	0	0	0.004	0	0	1.5	0	0	0	0	0	—
0	0.02	0.01	0	0	0.003	0.001	0	0	0.2	0	1	0	—	0	0
5	0.05	0.08	0	0	0	0.047	0.093	—	9.6	0	6	3	0	0	—
5	0.04	0.08	0	0	0	0.005	0.088	0.005	0.7	0	5	3	0	0	—
0	—	—	0	0	0	0	0	0	0	0	0	0	—	0	0
2	0.01	0.06	0	0	0	0	0	0	0	0	5	0	—	0	—
0	0.01	0.01	0	0	0.002	0.001	0.004	0	0	0	0	1	—	0	—
0	0.03	0.02	0	0	0.002	0	0	0	0	0	0	1	0	0	0
0	0.01	0.01	0	0	0.002	0	0.014	0	0	0	0	2	0	0	0
0	0	0	0	0	0	0	0	0	0	0	0	0	0	0	0
0	0.01	0.01	0	0	0.002	0.001	0.004	0	0	0	0	1	—	0	—
5	0.193	0.063	—	—	0.002	0.003	0.043	0.007	0.1	0	6.11	6.95	—	0	—
3	0.07	0.02	—	0	0.005	0.005	0.064	0	0.1	0	2	3	—	0	—
4	0.13	0.03	0	0	0.001	0.008	0.024	0.01	0.6	0	2	4	—	0	—
3	0.11	0.02	—	0	0.001	0.005	0.022	0.007	0.3	0	2	4	—	0	—
—	—	—	—	—	0.01	0.01	0.2	—	—	—	8	—	0.005	0	—
—	—	—	—	—	—	—	—	—	—	—	—	—	—	0	—
3	0.09	0.02	0	0	0.001	0.001	0.02	0.004	0.1	0	3	4	—	0	—
11	1.46	0.286	23.5	0	0.209	0.16	1.94	0.024	13.2	0.052	23.1	36.9	—	1.16	—
11	1.46	0.286	0	0	0.209	0.16	1.94	0.024	13.2	0	23.1	36.9	0.018	1.16	—
3.36	0.616	0.109	37	0	0.101	0.067	1.75	0.011	2.24	0.036	33.9	98.6	0.005	0.504	—
—	0.3	—	0	0	0.02	0.03	0.3	—	—	—	16	31	—	1.02	—
8.1	0.671	0.212	7.25	0	0.081	0.081	0.675	0.032	4.5	0.077	48.6	43.7	0.005	1.17	—
8.75	0.665	—	0	0	0.095	0.095	0.84	0.023	—	0	16.3	31.8	0.011	1.33	0.025
7	1.08	0.221	0	0	0.161	0.123	1.4	0.019	13	0	38.5	28.4	0.01	0.805	0.042
12.3	0.815	0.3	0	0	0.098	0.095	1.04	0.026	16.3	0	26	53	0.011	1.58	0.025
—	0.916	—	0	0	0.171	0.076	1.4	—	—	—	30.8	38	—	0.608	—
21.8	0.877	0.365	0	0	0.109	0.166	1.06	0.049	—	0	22.7	69.8	0.014	1.89	—
6.25	0.775	0.155	0	0	0.083	0.155	1.02	0.009	8.75	0	25.5	22.5	—	0.55	—
6	0.68	0.318	0	0	0.103	0.08	0.828	0.023	9.75	0	20	36.3	0.009	1.55	—
22.5	0.823	0.403	0	0	0.067	0.05	0.92	0.045	13.2	0	17.2	63	0.011	2.38	0.025
4.83	0.653	0.143	0	0	0.108	0.071	0.863	0.008	8.05	0	29	24.8	0.006	0.437	0.028

Continued.

Key to Abbreviations
Kcal, Kcalories; *Prot,* protein; *Carb,* carbohydrate; *Fat,* fat; *Chol,* cholesterol; *Safa,* saturated fat; *Mufa,* monounsaturated fat; *Pufa,* polyunsaturated fat; *Sod,* sodium; *Pot,* potassium; *Mag,* magnesium; *Iron,* iron; *Zinc,* zinc; *VA,* vitamin A; *VC,* vitamin C; *Thia,* thiamin; *Ribo,* riboflavin; *Niac,* niacin; *VB₆,* vitamin B₆; *Fol,* folate; *VB₁₂,* vitamin B₁₂; *Calc,* calcium; *Phos,* phosphorus; *Sel,* selenium; *Fibd,* dietary fiber; and *VE,* vitamin E.

Food name	Portion	Wt (g)	Kcal	Prot (g)	Carb (g)	Fat (g)	Chol (mg)	Safa (g)	Mufa (g)	Pufa (g)	Sod (mg)	Pot (mg)
Breads—cont'd												
White-firm-toast	Slice	20	65	2	12	1	0	0.2	0.3	0.3	117	28
Whole wheat-firm	Slice	25	61.3	2.41	11.3	1.09	0	0.1	0.2	0.3	159	44
Whole wheat-home rec	Slice	25	66.5	2.25	11.6	1.61	0	—	—	—	89	85
Breadcrumbs-dry-grated	Cup	100	390	13	73	5	0	1	1.6	1.4	736	152
Crackers												
Animal	Item	1.9	8.67	0.127	1.47	0.2	0	—	—	—	7.53	1.67
Cheddar snacks	Item	1.6	7.22	0.144	1.11	0.261	—	—	—	—	14.3	2.17
Cheese	Item	1	5.38	0.091	0.52	0.327	—	0.09	0.09	0.03	12	1.86
Graham-plain	Item	7	27.5	0.5	5	0.5	0	0.1	0.25	0.15	33	27.5
Graham-sug/honey	Item	7	30.1	0.519	5.4	0.732	0	0.1	0.4	0.1	32.9	11.7
Ritz	Item	3.33	18	0.233	2.13	0.967	0	—	—	—	32.3	2.67
Rye Krisp-natural	Item	2.1	7.5	0.25	1.67	0.033	0	0	0	0	18.5	10.2
Rye Wafers	Item	6.5	22.5	1	5	0	0	0	0	0	57	39
Saltines	Item	2.75	12.5	0.25	2	0.25	0.75	0.1	0.1	0.05	36.8	3.25
Triscuits	Item	4.5	21	0.4	3.1	0.75	0	—	—	—	—	—
Wheat Thins	Item	1.8	9	0.125	1.25	0.35	0	—	—	—	—	—
Croissant-roll-Sara Lee	Item	26	109	2.3	11.2	6.1	—	—	—	—	140	40
French toast-home rec	Slice	65	153	5.67	17.2	6.73	—	—	—	—	257	85.8
Muffins												
Blueberry-home rec	Item	40	110	3	17	4	21	1.1	1.4	0.7	252	46
Bran-home rec	Item	40	112	2.96	16.7	5.08	21	1.2	1.4	0.8	168	98.8
Corn-home rec	Item	40	125	3	19	4	21	1.2	1.6	0.9	192	54
English-plain	Item	56	133	4.43	25.7	1.09	0	—	—	—	358	314
English-plain-toast	Item	53	154	5.13	29.8	1.26	0	—	—	—	414	364
Plain-home rec	Item	40	120	3	17	4	21	1	1.7	1	176	50
Soy	Item	40	119	3.9	16.7	4.4	0	—	—	—	—	—
Others												
Pancakes-buckwheat-mix	Item	27	55	2	6	2	20	0.8	0.9	0.4	160	66
Pancakes-plain-home rec	Item	27	60	2	9	2	20	0.5	0.8	0.5	160	33
Pancakes-plain-mix	Item	27	58.9	1.85	7.87	2.17	20	0.7	0.7	0.3	160	43.2
Roll-Brown & Serve-enr	Item	26	85	2	14	2	0	0.4	0.7	0.5	144	25
Roll-hamburger/hotdog	Item	40	114	3.43	20.1	2.09	0	0.5	0.8	0.6	241	36.8
Roll-hard-enriched	Item	50	155	5	30	2	0	0.4	0.6	0.5	312	49
Roll-submarine/hoagie-enr	Item	135	390	12	75	4	0	0.9	1.4	1.4	761	122
Roll-whole wheat-homemade	Item	35	90	3.5	18.3	1	0	—	—	—	197	102
Waffles-enr-home rec	Item	75	245	6.93	25.7	12.6	45	2.3	2.8	1.4	445	129
Waffles-froz	Item	37	103	2.15	15.9	3.52	0	—	—	—	265	77.7
Breakfast cereals												
100% Bran	Cup	66	178	8.3	48.1	3.3	0	0.59	0.57	1.87	457	824
All Bran	Cup	85.2	212	12.2	63.4	1.53	0	—	—	—	961	1051
Alpha Bits	Cup	28.4	111	2.2	24.6	0.6	0	—	—	—	219	110
Bran Buds	Cup	85.2	220	11.8	64.8	2.04	0	—	—	—	523	1425
Bran Chex	Cup	49	156	5.1	39	1.4	0	—	—	—	455	394
Bran Flakes-Kellogg's	Cup	39	127	4.9	30.5	0.7	0	0	0	0	363	248
C.W. Post-plain	Cup	97	432	8.7	69.4	15.2	0	11.3	1.72	1.42	167	198
Cheerios	Cup	22.7	88.8	3.42	15.7	1.45	0	0.27	0.515	0.597	246	81
Corn Bran	Cup	36	124	2.5	30.4	1.3	0	—	—	—	310	70
Corn Chex	Cup	28.4	111	2	24.9	0.1	0	0	0	0	271	23
Corn Flakes-Kellogg's	Cup	22.7	88.3	1.84	19.5	0.068	0	0	0	0	281	20.9
Corn Grits-enr	Cup	242	146	3.5	31.4	0.5	0	0.06	0.11	0.2	0	54
Corn-shredded-sugar	Cup	25	95	2	22	0	0	0	0	0	247	—
Cracklin Bran	Cup	60	229	5.5	41.1	8.8	0	—	—	—	487	355
Cream/wheat-instant	Cup	241	53	4.4	31.6	0.6	0	0	0	0	6	48
Cream/wheat-packet	Item	150	132	2.5	28.9	0.4	0	0	0	0	241	55

Mag (mg)	Iron (mg)	Zinc (mg)	VA (RE)	VC (mg)	Thia (mg)	Ribo (mg)	Niac (mg)	VB_6 (mg)	Fol (μg)	VB_{12} (μg)	Calc (mg)	Phos (mg)	Sel (mg)	Fibd (g)	VE (mg)
4.8	0.6	0.142	0	0	0.07	0.06	0.8	0.008	8	0	22	23	0.006	0.5	0.024
23.3	0.855	0.42	0	0	0.088	0.053	0.958	0.047	13.8	0	18	65	0.011	2.83	0.03
23.3	0.67	0.562	10.8	0	0.068	0.038	0.798	0.05	12.3	0.027	19.8	63.3	0.011	2.83	0.025
32	3.6	—	0	0	0.35	0.35	4.8	—	—	—	122	141	0.02	3.65	—
0.267	0.059	0.009	0	0	0.005	0.009	0.073	0	0.2	0.001	0.2	1.2	0	0.027	0.007
0.278	0.068	0.012	0.18	0	0.009	0.007	0.067	0.001	0.222	0.009	1.22	1.89	0.001	0.056	0.006
0.22	0.035	0.01	—	0	0.004	0.004	0.082	—	—	—	1.05	2.1	0	0.025	0.003
3.57	0.25	0.053	0	0	0.01	0.04	0.25	0.006	0.91	0	3	10.5	0.001	0.224	0.026
2.31	0.183	0.053	0	0	0.024	0.019	0.218	0.006	0.91	0	2.66	8.26	0.001	0.119	0.026
—	0.1	—	—	—	0.013	0.013	0.1	—	—	—	5	8	—	0.107	0.012
2.5	0.092	0.057	—	—	0.006	0.005	0.033	0.007	0.833	—	0.833	6.83	0.001	0.34	0.008
—	0.25	—	0	0	0.02	0.015	0.1	—	—	—	3.5	25	0.001	1.05	0.024
0.77	0.125	0.017	0	0	0.125	0.013	0.1	0.001	0.495	0	0.5	2.5	0.004	0.072	0.01
—	—	—	—	—	—	—	—	—	—	—	—	—	0.001	0.155	0.017
—	—	—	—	—	—	—	—	—	—	—	—	—	0	0.099	0.007
7	1.04	—	8.2	0	0.28	0.1	1.2	—	—	—	12	32	—	0.56	—
11.7	1.34	0.553	22.2	0	0.124	0.163	1.01	0.038	17.6	0.291	72.2	84.5	—	2.02	—
10	0.6	—	18	0	0.09	0.1	0.7	—	—	—	34	53	—	0.85	—
35.2	1.26	1.08	40	2.48	0.1	0.112	1.26	0.111	16.8	0.092	53.6	111	—	2.52	—
18.4	0.7	—	25	0	0.1	0.1	0.7	—	—	—	42	68	—	0.95	—
10.6	1.58	0.403	0	0	0.258	0.179	2.1	0.022	17.9	0	90.7	62.7	0.015	1.29	—
12.2	1.83	0.466	0	0	0.239	0.207	2.43	0.026	20.7	0	105	72.6	0.015	1.49	—
10.8	0.6	—	8	0	0.09	0.12	0.9	—	—	—	42	60	—	0.85	—
52	0.9	—	40	0	0.08	0.1	0.5	—	—	—	35	56	—	0.835	—
5.13	0.4	0.192	12	0	0.04	0.05	0.2	0.057	2.97	0.355	59	91	0.002	0.621	—
5.13	0.4	0.192	6	0	0.06	0.07	0.5	0.057	2.97	0.355	27	38	0.002	0.45	—
5.13	0.265	0.192	7.66	0	0.038	0.059	0.254	0.057	2.97	0.355	35.6	70.7	0.003	0.394	—
5.46	0.8	0.19	0	0	0.1	0.06	0.9	0.016	9.88	—	20	23	0.008	0.988	0.203
7.6	1.19	0.248	0	0	0.196	0.132	1.58	0.014	14.8	—	53.6	32.8	0.012	1.01	0.016
11.5	1.2	0.3	0	0	0.2	0.12	1.7	0.018	29.5	0	24	46	0.015	1.5	0.02
—	3	—	0	0	0.54	0.32	4.5	0.047	—	—	58	115	0.041	3.75	0.054
40	0.8	—	0	0	0.12	0.05	1.1	—	—	—	34	98	0.016	1.83	0.035
16.5	1.48	0.653	28	0	0.18	0.24	1.46	0.054	14.3	0.365	154	135	0.011	1.05	—
7.77	1.8	0.303	95	0	0.167	0.2	1.93	0.098	0.74	—	30	141	—	0.888	—
312	8.12	5.74	—	63	1.6	1.8	20.9	2.1	—	6.3	46	801	0.02	19.5	—
318	13.5	11.2	1125	45.2	1.11	1.28	15	1.53	301	—	69	794	0.025	25.5	1.27
17	1.8	1.5	375	—	0.4	0.4	5	0.5	100	1.5	8	51	0.01	0.3	—
271	13.5	11.2	1125	45.2	1.11	1.28	15	1.53	301	—	57.1	740	0.025	23.6	0.903
126	7.8	2.14	11	26	0.6	0.26	8.6	0.9	173	2.6	29	327	0.01	7.9	—
71	11.2	5.1	516	—	0.5	0.6	6.9	0.7	138	2.1	19	192	0.004	5.5	0.164
67	15.4	1.64	1284	—	1.3	1.5	17.1	1.7	342	5.1	47	224	—	2.2	—
31.3	3.61	0.629	300	12	0.295	0.341	4	0.409	4.99	1.2	38.8	107	0.01	0.863	—
18	12.2	4	—	—	0.38	0.7	10.9	0.858	232	1.39	41	52	0.002	6.84	—
4	1.8	0.1	14	15	0.4	0.07	5	0.5	100	1.5	3	11	0.002	0.5	—
2.72	1.43	0.064	300	12	0.295	0.341	4	0.409	80.1	—	0.681	14.3	0.001	0.454	0.023
11	1.55	0.17	—	—	0.24	0.15	1.96	0.058	1	—	1	29	0.024	0.6	0.29
3.5	0.6	0.088	0	13	0.33	0.05	4.4	0.45	88.3	1.33	1	10	0.002	1.54	0.09
116	3.8	3.2	794	32	0.8	0.9	10.6	1.1	212	—	40	241	0.01	9.1	—
14	12	0.41	—	—	0.2	0.1	1.8	—	11	—	59	43	—	2.21	—
9	8.1	0.23	1250	—	0.4	0.2	5	0.5	100	—	40	20	—	2.02	—

Continued.

Key to Abbreviations
Kcal, Kcalories; *Prot,* protein; *Carb,* carbohydrate; *Fat,* fat; *Chol,* cholesterol; *Safa,* saturated fat; *Mufa,* monounsaturated fat; *Pufa,* polyunsaturated fat; *Sod,* sodium; *Pot,* potassium; *Mag,* magnesium; *Iron,* iron; *Zinc,* zinc; *VA,* vitamin A; *VC,* vitamin C; *Thia,* thiamin; *Ribo,* riboflavin; *Niac,* niacin; *VB₆*, vitamin B₆; *Fol,* folate; *VB₁₂*, vitamin B₁₂; *Calc,* calcium; *Phos,* phosphorus; *Sel,* selenium; *Fibd,* dietary fiber; and *VE,* vitamin E.

Food name	Portion	Wt (g)	Kcal	Prot (g)	Carb (g)	Fat (g)	Chol (mg)	Safa (g)	Mufa (g)	Pufa (g)	Sod (mg)	Pot (mg)
Breakfast cereals—cont'd												
Cream/wheat-reg-hot	Cup	251	134	3.8	27.7	0.5	0	0	0	0	2	43
Crispy Rice	Cup	28.4	111	1.8	24.8	0.1	0	0	0	0	205	27
Farina-ckd-enr	Cup	233	116	3.4	24.6	0.2	0	0.02	0.02	0.07	1	30
Fortified Oat Flakes	Cup	48	177	9	34.7	0.7	0	0	0	0	429	343
Frosted Flakes-Kellogg's	Cup	35	133	1.8	31.7	0.1	0	0	0	0	284	22
Frosted Mini Wheats	Item	7.1	25.5	0.731	5.86	0.071	0	0	0	0	2.06	34.2
Granola-homemade	Cup	122	595	15	67.3	33.1	0	5.84	9.37	17.2	12	612
Granola-Nature Val	Cup	113	503	11.5	75.5	19.6	0	13	2.93	2.75	232	389
Grape Nuts	Cup	114	407	13.3	93.5	0.456	0	0	0	0	792	381
Grape Nuts Flakes	Cup	32.5	116	3.48	26.6	0.358	0	0	0	0	250	113
Heartland Natural	Cup	115	499	11.6	78.6	17.7	0	—	—	—	294	385
Honey Bran	Cup	35	119	3.1	28.6	0.7	0	0	0	0	202	151
Honey Nut Cheerios	Cup	33	125	3.6	26.5	0.8	0	0.13	0.31	0.3	299	115
Life-plain/cinnamon	Cup	44	162	8.1	31.5	0.8	0	0	0	0	229	197
Lucky Charms	Cup	32	125	2.9	26.1	1.2	0	0.22	0.43	0.49	227	66
Malt O Meal-ckd	Cup	240	122	3.5	25.8	0.3	0	0	0	0	2	—
Maypo-cook-hot	Cup	240	170	5.8	31.8	2.4	0	—	—	—	9	211
Nutri Grain-barley	Cup	41	153	4.5	33.9	0.3	0	0	0	0	277	108
Nutri Grain-corn	Cup	42	160	3.4	35.5	1	0	—	—	—	276	98
Nutri Grain-rye	Cup	40	144	3.5	33.9	0.3	0	0	0	0	272	72
Nutri Grain-wheat	Cup	44	158	3.8	37.2	0.5	0	0	0	0	299	120
Oatmeal-inst-packet	Item	177	104	4.4	18.1	1.7	0	0.289	0.597	0.697	286	100
Oatmeal-raw	Cup	81	311	13	54.2	5.1	0	0.94	1.8	2.08	3	284
Oats-puffed-sugar	Cup	25	100	3	19	1	0	0.185	0.075	0.465	294	—
Product 19	Cup	33	126	3.2	27.4	0.2	0	0	0	0	378	51
Raisin Bran-Kellogg's	Cup	49.2	154	5.3	37.1	0.984	0	—	—	—	359	256
Ralston-ckd	Cup	253	134	5.5	28.2	0.8	0	0	0	0	4	153
Rice Chex	Cup	25.2	99.5	1.34	22.5	0.101	0	0	0	0	211	29.2
Rice Krispies	Cup	28.4	112	1.9	24.8	0.2	0	0	0	0	340	30
Rice-puffed-plain	Cup	14	56	0.9	12.6	0.1	0	0	0	0	0	16
Rice-puffed-sugar	Cup	28.4	115	1	26	0	0	0	0	0	21	43
Roman meal-ckd	Cup	241	147	6.6	33	1	0	—	—	—	3	302
Special K	Cup	21.3	83.1	4.2	16	0.085	0	0	0	0	199	36.8
Sugar Corn Pops	Cup	28.4	108	1.4	25.6	0.1	0	0	0	0	103	17
Sugar Smacks	Cup	37.9	141	2.65	33	0.72	0	0	0	0	100	56.1
Team	Cup	42	164	2.7	36	0.7	0	0	0	0	259	71
Toasties	Cup	22.7	87.8	1.84	19.5	0.045	0	0	0	0	238	26.3
Total	Cup	33	116	3.3	26	0.7	0	0.1	0.07	0.34	409	123
Trix	Cup	28.4	108	1.5	24.9	0.4	0	0	0	0	179	26
Wheat Chex	Cup	46	169	4.5	37.8	1.1	0	—	—	—	308	174
Wheat Flakes-sugar	Cup	30	105	3	24	0	0	0	0	0	368	81
Wheat Germ-sugar	Cup	113	426	24.7	68.7	9.1	0	1.57	1.32	5.5	3	803
Wheat germ-toasted	Cup	113	431	32.9	56.1	12.1	0	2.07	1.7	7.48	4	1070
Wheat-puffed-plain	Cup	12	44	1.8	9.5	0.1	0	0	0	0	0.48	42
Wheat-puffed-sugar	Serving	38	138	5.59	30.2	0.456	0	—	0.122	0.141	1.52	132
Wheat-rolled-ckd	Cup	240	180	5	41	1	0	0.182	0.07	0.475	535	202
Wheat-shred-biscuit	Item	23.6	83	2.6	18.8	0.3	0	0	0	0	0.472	77
Wheat-whole meal	Cup	245	110	4	23	1	0	0.182	0.07	0.475	535	118
Wheatena-ckd	Cup	243	135	5	28.7	1.1	0	—	—	—	5	187
Wheaties	Cup	29	101	2.8	23.1	0.5	0	0.07	0.05	0.24	363	108
Whole Wheat Natural	Cup	242	151	4.9	33.2	0.9	0	—	—	—	1	171
Combination foods												
Beans/pork/frankfurter-can	Cup	257	366	17.3	39.6	16.9	15	6.05	7.27	2.15	1105	604
Beans/pork/sweet sauce-can	Cup	253	282	13.4	53.1	3.69	17	1.42	1.6	0.473	849	673
Beans/pork/tom sauce-can	Cup	253	247	13	49	2.6	17	1	1.12	0.331	1113	759
Beef & vegetable stew	Cup	245	220	16	15	11	72	4.9	4.5	0.5	1006	613

Mag (mg)	Iron (mg)	Zinc (mg)	VA (RE)	VC (mg)	Thia (mg)	Ribo (mg)	Niac (mg)	VB_6 (mg)	Fol (μg)	VB_{12} (μg)	Calc (mg)	Phos (mg)	Sel (mg)	Fibd (g)	VE (mg)
10	10.3	0.33	—	—	0.2	0.1	1.5	—	9	—	51	42	—	1.94	—
12	0.7	0.46	—	1	0.1	0	2	0.044	3	0.082	5	31	0.004	1	—
4	1.16	0.16	—	—	0.19	0.12	1.28	0.023	6	—	4	28	—	3.26	—
58	13.7	1.5	636	—	0.6	0.7	8.4	0.9	169	2.5	68	176	0.01	1.2	—
3	2.2	0.05	463	19	0.5	0.5	6.2	0.6	124	—	1	26	—	0.77	—
55.8	0.447	0.376	94	3.76	0.092	0.107	1.25	0.128	25.1	—	2.34	18.5	—	0.54	0.026
141	4.84	4.47	10	1	0.73	0.31	2.14	0.428	99	—	76	494	0.023	12.8	—
116	3.78	2.19	—	—	0.39	0.19	0.83	—	85	—	71	354	0.037	4.2	—
76.3	4.95	2.51	1500	—	1.48	1.71	20.1	2.05	402	6.04	43.3	286	0.034	5.47	—
35.8	5.17	0.65	430	—	0.423	0.488	5.72	0.585	115	1.72	13	96.9	0.01	2.08	0.137
147	4.33	3.04	—	—	0.36	0.16	1.61	—	64	—	75	416	—	5.4	—
46	5.6	0.9	463	19	0.5	0.5	6.2	0.6	23	1.9	16	132	—	3.9	—
39	5.2	0.87	437	17	0.4	0.5	5.8	0.6	—	1.7	23	122	—	1.3	—
14	11.6	1.45	—	—	0.95	1	11.6	—	37	—	154	238	—	1.4	—
27	5.1	0.56	424	17	0.4	0.5	5.6	0.6	—	1.7	36	88	—	0.6	—
—	9.5	0.17	—	—	0.4	0.3	5.9	0.019	6	—	5	23	—	0.6	—
51	8.4	1.49	702	28	0.7	0.8	9.4	0.9	9	2.8	125	248	—	1.2	—
32	1.45	5.4	543	22	0.5	0.6	7.2	0.7	145	2.2	11	126	0.027	2.4	—
27	0.89	5.5	556	22	0.5	0.6	7.4	0.8	148	2.2	1	120	0.003	2.6	0.042
31	1.13	5.3	530	21	0.5	0.6	7	0.7	141	2.1	8	104	—	2.56	0.04
34	1.24	5.8	583	23	0.6	0.7	7.7	0.8	155	2.3	12	164	0.007	2.8	0.044
—	6.32	—	455	—	0.53	0.29	5.49	0.742	150	—	163	133	0.015	1.62	1.06
120	3.41	2.48	10	—	0.59	0.11	0.63	0.097	26	—	42	384	0.022	4.6	0.203
28	4	0.693	275	13	0.33	0.38	4.4	0.45	5.5	1.33	44	102	0.006	2.65	0.168
12	21	0.5	1748	70	1.7	2	23.3	2.3	466	7	4	47	—	0.4	—
63.5	6	5.02	500	—	0.492	0.59	6.69	0.689	133	2.02	17.2	183	0.005	5.31	—
59	1.64	1.42	—	—	0.2	0.18	2.05	0.114	18	0.109	14	148	—	4.2	—
6.3	1.59	0.348	1.85	13.4	0.328	—	4.44	0.454	89	1.34	3.53	24.7	0.004	0.151	0.01
10	1.8	0.48	375	15	0.4	0.4	5	0.5	100	—	4	34	0.004	0.1	0.011
3	0.15	0.14	0	0	0.02	0.01	0.42	0.011	3	—	1	14	0.001	0.1	0.094
7.56	0	1.48	300	15	0	0	0	0.504	98.8	1.48	3	14	0.002	0.2	0.188
109	2.12	1.78	—	—	0.24	0.12	3.08	0.113	24	—	30	215	—	2.31	—
11.7	3.39	2.81	280	11.3	0.277	0.32	3.75	0.383	75.2	—	6.18	41.3	0.013	0.17	—
2	1.8	1.5	375	15	0.4	0.4	5	0.5	100	—	1	28	—	0.2	0.026
18.2	2.39	0.379	500	20.1	0.493	0.569	6.67	0.682	134	—	4.17	41.3	—	0.531	—
19	2.57	0.58	556	22	0.5	0.6	7.4	0.8	—	2.2	6	65	0.007	0.4	—
3.41	0.597	0.066	300	—	0.295	0.341	4	0.409	80.1	1.2	0.908	10	—	0.386	—
37	21	0.78	1748	70	1.7	2	23.3	2.3	466	7	56	137	—	2.4	—
6	4.5	0.13	371	15	0.4	0.4	4.9	0.5	—	1.5	6	19	—	0.1	—
58	7.3	1.23	—	24	0.6	0.17	8.1	0.8	162	2.4	18	182	—	3.4	0.193
32.7	4.8	0.669	330	16	0.4	0.45	5.3	0.54	9	1.59	12	83	0.003	2.7	0.126
272	7.71	14.1	—	—	1.41	0.7	4.73	0.829	298	—	38	971	—	5.7	—
362	10.3	18.8	50	7	1.89	0.93	6.31	1.11	398	—	50	1294	—	14.6	15.9
17	0.57	0.28	0	0	0.02	0.03	1.3	0.02	4	—	3	43	—	0.4	0.08
55.1	1.8	0.897	0	0	0.076	0.087	4.1	0.065	12.2	0	10.6	135	—	2.11	—
52.8	1.7	1.15	0	0	0.17	0.07	2.2	—	26.4	—	19	182	—	2.87	2.54
40	0.74	0.59	0	0	0.07	0.06	1.08	0.06	12	—	10	86	—	2.2	0.085
53.9	1.2	1.18	0	0	0.15	0.05	1.5	—	27	—	17	127	—	1.61	2.6
49	1.36	1.68	—	—	0.02	0.05	1.34	0.046	17	—	11	146	0.058	2.6	—
32	4.6	0.65	384	15	0.4	0.4	5.1	0.5	9	1.5	44	100	0.003	2	0.122
54	1.5	1.16	—	—	0.17	0.12	2.15	—	26	—	17	167	0.058	2.7	2.57
71	4.45	4.79	80	5.9	0.149	0.144	2.32	0.118	77.1	0.87	123	267	—	12.8	0.561
87	4.2	3.8	35	7.7	0.119	0.154	0.888	0.215	94.5	0.06	155	266	—	14	0.561
88	8.3	14.8	62	7.8	0.132	0.116	1.26	0.175	56.8	0.03	141	297	—	13.8	0.561
—	2.9	—	480	17	0.15	0.17	4.7	—	—	0.002	29	184	—	3.19	0.515

Continued.

Key to Abbreviations
Kcal, Kcalories; *Prot,* protein; *Carb,* carbohydrate; *Fat,* fat; *Chol,* cholesterol; *Safa,* saturated fat; *Mufa,* monounsaturated fat; *Pufa,* polyunsaturated fat; *Sod,* sodium; *Pot,* potassium; *Mag,* magnesium; *Iron,* iron; *Zinc,* zinc; *VA,* vitamin A; *VC,* vitamin C; *Thia,* thiamin; *Ribo,* riboflavin; *Niac,* niacin; *VB$_6$*, vitamin B$_6$; *Fol,* folate; *VB$_{12}$*, vitamin B$_{12}$; *Calc,* calcium; *Phos,* phosphorus; *Sel,* selenium; *Fibd,* dietary fiber; and *VE,* vitamin E.

Food name	Portion	Wt (g)	Kcal	Prot (g)	Carb (g)	Fat (g)	Chol (mg)	Safa (g)	Mufa (g)	Pufa (g)	Sod (mg)	Pot (mg)
Combination foods—cont'd												
Beef potpie-home rec	Slice	210	515	21	39	30	44	7.9	12.9	7.4	596	334
Beef raviolios-can	oz	28.4	27.5	1.14	4.26	0.568	—	0.11	0.16	0.254	131	45.7
Chicken A La King-home rec	Cup	245	470	27	12	34	186	12.9	13.4	6.2	759	404
Chicken Chow Mein-can	Cup	250	95	7	18	0	98	0	0	0	722	418
Chicken potpie-baked-home rec	Slice	232	545	23	42	31	72	11	13.5	5.5	593	343
Chili Con Carne/beans-can	Cup	255	340	19	31	16	38	7.5	7.2	1	1354	594
Chili with beans-can	Cup	255	286	14.6	30.4	14	43	6	5.95	0.923	1330	932
Macaroni & cheese-enr-can	Cup	240	230	9	26	10	42	4.2	3.1	1.4	729	139
Macaroni & cheese-enr-hom	Cup	200	430	17	40	22	42	8.9	8.8	2.9	1086	240
Meat loaf-celery/onions	Serving	87.6	213	15.8	5.23	13.9	107	5.29	5.9	0.613	103	182
Pizza-cheese-baked	Slice	49	109	5.97	15.9	2.5	7	1.2	0.77	0.382	261	85
Pizza-pepperoni-baked	Slice	53	135	7.56	14.8	5.19	11	1.67	2.34	0.87	199	114
Salads												
Carrot raisin-home	Cup	268	306	3.8	55.8	11.6	—	—	—	—	—	—
Chef ham/cheese	Serving	200	196	13.4	7.42	12.7	46	6.98	4.09	0.739	567	415
Chicken	Cup	205	502	26	17.4	36.2	—	—	—	—	1395	521
Coleslaw	Tbsp	8	6	0.1	0.99	0.21	1	0.031	0.057	0.108	2	14
Fruit-can/juice	Cup	249	125	1.28	32.5	0.06	0	0.01	0.012	0.027	13	288
Green tossed	Serving	207	32	2.6	6.67	0.16	0	0.021	0.008	0.07	53	356
Macaroni	Serving	28.4	50.7	0.7	5.3	3	—	—	—	—	148	21
Mandarin orange gelatin	Serving	28.4	22.7	0.4	5.7	0	—	0	0	0	14	9
Potato	Cup	250	358	6.7	27.9	20.5	171	3.57	6.2	9.3	1323	635
Three bean-Del Monte	oz	28.4	22.4	0.71	5.06	0.056	0	0	0	0	101	38.3
Tuna	Cup	205	350 '	30	7	22	68	4.3	6.3	6.7	434	—
Others												
Sandwich-blt/mayo	Item	148	282	6.8	28.8	15.6	—	—	—	—	—	—
Sandwich-club	Item	315	590	35.6	41.7	20.8	—	—	—	—	—	—
Spaghetti/tom/cheese-can	Cup	250	190	6	39	2	4	0.5	0.3	0.4	955	303
Spaghetti/tom/che-home rec	Cup	250	260	9	37	9	4	2	5.4	0.7	955	408
Spaghetti/tom/meat-can	Cup	250	260	12	29	10	39	2.2	3.3	3.9	1220	245
Spaghetti/tom/meat-home rec	Cup	248	330	19	39	12	75	3.3	6.3	0.9	1009	665
Taco	Item	171	370	20.7	26.7	20.6	57	11.4	6.58	0.959	802	473
Dairy products												
Cheese food-American-proc	oz	28.4	93	5.56	2.07	6.97	18	4.38	2.04	0.2	337	79
Cheese spread-proc	oz	28.4	82	4.65	2.48	6.02	16	3.78	1.76	0.18	381	69
Cheeses												
American-proc	oz	28.4	106	6.28	0.45	8.86	27	5.58	2.54	0.28	406	46
Blue	oz	28.4	100	6.06	0.659	8.14	21	5.29	2.21	0.23	395	72.9
Camembert-wedge	Item	38	114	7.52	0.18	9.22	27	5.8	2.67	0.28	320	71
Cheddar-shred	Cup	113	455	28.1	1.45	37.5	119	23.8	10.6	1.06	701	111
Cottage, 4%-large curd	Cup	225	232	28.1	6.03	10.1	33.8	6.41	2.88	0.315	911	189
Cream	oz	28.4	100	2.17	0.759	10	31.4	6.31	2.82	0.365	85.1	34.4
Feta	oz	28.4	75	4.03	1.16	6.03	25	4.24	1.31	0.17	316	18
Gouda	oz	28.4	101	7.07	0.63	7.78	32	4.99	2.2	0.19	232	34
Limburger	oz	28.4	93	5.68	0.14	7.72	26	4.75	2.44	0.14	227	36
Monterey	oz	28.4	106	6.94	0.19	8.58	—	—	—	—	152	23
Mozzarella-skim milk	oz	28.4	72	6.88	0.78	4.51	16	2.87	1.28	0.13	132	24
Parmesan-grated	Cup	100	456	41.6	3.74	30	79	19.1	8.73	0.66	1862	107
Provolone	oz	28.4	100	7.25	0.61	7.55	20	4.84	2.1	0.22	248	39
Ricotta-skim milk	Cup	246	340	28	12.6	19.5	76	12.1	5.69	0.64	307	308
Romano	oz	28.4	110	9.02	1.03	7.64	29	—	—	—	340	—
Roquefort	oz	28.4	105	6.11	0.57	8.69	26	5.46	2.4	0.37	513	26
Swiss	oz	28.4	107	8.06	0.96	7.78	26	5.04	2.06	0.28	74	31
Swiss-proc	oz	28.4	95	7.01	0.6	7.09	24	4.55	2	0.18	388	61

Mag (mg)	Iron (mg)	Zinc (mg)	VA (RE)	VC (mg)	Thia (mg)	Ribo (mg)	Niac (mg)	VB_6 (mg)	Fol (μg)	VB_{12} (μg)	Calc (mg)	Phos (mg)	Sel (mg)	Fibd (g)	VE (mg)
—	3.8	—	344	6	0.3	0.3	5.5	—	—	—	29	149	—	3.9	1.18
—	0.312	—	50	0.426	0.026	0.023	0.398	—	—	—	4.54	—	—	0.23	0.045
—	2.5	—	226	12	0.1	0.42	5.4	—	—	—	127	358	—	1.2	0.931
—	1.3	—	30	13	0.05	0.1	1	—	—	—	45	85	—	0.9	0
—	3	—	618	5	0.34	0.31	5.5	—	—	—	70	232	0.032	4.2	0.882
—	4.3	—	30	—	0.08	0.18	3.3	0.263	—	—	82	321	—	5	—
115	8.75	5.1	86	4.3	0.122	0.268	0.913	0.337	—	0.03	119	393	—	6.93	—
—	1	—	52	0	0.12	0.24	1	—	—	—	199	182	—	1.44	0.384
52	1.8	—	172	0	0.2	0.4	1.8	—	—	—	362	322	0.028	1.2	0.32
13.6	1.91	3.08	12.3	0.725	0.052	0.148	3.16	0.162	10.9	1.52	22.8	112	0.001	0.11	0.068
12	0.45	0.63	57	1	0.14	0.13	1.93	0.03	46	0.26	90	88	—	1.59	—
6	0.7	0.39	41	1.2	0.1	0.17	2.28	0.04	39	0.14	48	56	—	1.48	—
—	3	—	1100	12	0.16	0.16	1	—	—	—	96	130	—	16.7	—
28.4	1.17	1.73	740	24	0.337	0.24	2.21	0.206	46	0.474	227	251	0.019	2.39	0.719
—	—	—	—	—	—	—	—	—	—	—	—	—	—	—	—
1	0.05	0.02	7	2.6	0.005	0.005	0.022	0.01	2.1	0.002	4	3	—	0.297	—
21	0.62	0.36	149	8.3	0.027	0.035	0.886	—	—	0	28	36	0.001	1.64	—
22	1.3	0.43	235	48	0.06	0.1	1.15	0.16	77	0	26	80	0.001	2.11	0.483
—	—	—	—	—	—	—	—	—	—	—	—	—	—	0.29	—
—	—	—	—	—	—	—	—	—	—	—	—	—	—	0.57	—
39	1.63	0.78	82	24.9	0.193	0.15	2.23	0.353	16.8	0.385	48	130	—	5.25	—
6.25	0.284	0.093	8	0.852	0.014	0.014	0.085	—	—	—	9.66	16.2	—	1.52	—
—	2.7	—	118	2	0.08	0.23	10.3	—	—	—	41	291	—	1.03	0
—	1.5	—	174	13	0.16	0.14	1.6	—	—	—	53	89	—	2.88	—
—	4.3	—	350	27	0.38	0.41	10.2	—	—	—	103	394	—	4.17	—
28	2.8	—	186	10	0.35	0.28	4.5	—	—	—	40	88	0.025	2.5	—
—	2.3	—	216	13	0.25	0.18	2.3	—	—	—	80	135	—	2.5	—
28	3.3	—	200	5	0.15	0.18	2.3	—	—	—	53	113	—	2.75	—
—	3.7	—	—	22	0.25	0.3	4	—	—	—	124	236	0.022	2.73	—
71	2.42	3.93	147	2.2	0.15	0.45	3.22	0.24	23	1.04	221	203	—	2.67	—
9	0.24	0.85	77.8	0	0.008	0.125	0.04	—	—	0.317	163	130	0.006	0	0.179
8	0.09	0.73	67	0	0.014	0.122	0.037	0.033	2	0.113	159	202	0.006	0	0.179
6	0.11	0.85	103	0	0.008	0.1	0.02	0.02	2	0.197	174	211	0.003	0	0.179
6.99	0.09	0.749	61.2	0	0.008	0.108	0.287	0.047	9.98	0.344	150	110	0.006	0	0.179
8	0.12	0.9	105	0	0.011	0.185	0.239	0.086	24	0.492	147	132	0.008	0	0.243
31	0.77	3.51	359	0	0.031	0.424	0.09	0.084	21	0.935	815	579	0.018	0	0.723
11.3	0.315	0.833	110	0	0.047	0.367	0.284	0.151	27	1.4	135	297	0.052	0	1.44
2.03	0.344	0.152	122	0	0.005	0.057	0.029	0.013	4.05	0.122	23.3	30.4	0.001	0	0.181
5	0.18	0.82	—	0	—	—	—	—	—	—	140	96	—	0	0.179
8	0.07	1.11	55	0	0.009	0.095	0.018	0.023	6	—	198	155	0	0	0.179
6	0.04	0.6	109	0	0.023	0.143	0.045	0.024	16	0.295	141	111	—	0	0.179
8	0.2	0.85	80.8	0	—	0.111	—	—	—	—	212	126	0.013	0	0.179
7	0.06	0.78	49.8	0	0.005	0.086	0.03	0.02	2	0.232	183	131	0.003	0	0.179
51	0.95	3.19	211	0	0.045	0.386	0.315	0.105	8	—	1376	807	0.024	0	0.64
8	0.15	0.92	69.4	0	0.005	0.091	0.044	0.021	3	0.415	214	141	—	0	0.179
36	1.08	3.3	319	0	0.052	0.455	0.192	0.049	—	0.716	669	449	—	0	1.57
—	—	—	48.6	0	—	0.105	0.022	—	2	—	302	215	—	0	0.179
8	0.16	0.59	89.2	0	0.011	0.166	0.208	0.035	14	0.182	188	111	—	0	0.179
10.1	0.05	1.11	72.1	0	0.006	0.103	0.026	0.024	2	0.475	272	171	0.002	0	0.179
8	0.17	1.02	68.8	0	0.004	0.078	0.011	0.01	—	0.348	219	216	0.002	0	0.179

Continued.

Key to Abbreviations
Kcal, Kcalories; *Prot*, protein; *Carb*, carbohydrate; *Fat*, fat; *Chol*, cholesterol; *Safa*, saturated fat; *Mufa*, monounsaturated fat; *Pufa*, polyunsaturated fat; *Sod*, sodium; *Pot*, potassium; *Mag*, magnesium; *Iron*, iron; *Zinc*, zinc; *VA*, vitamin A; *VC*, vitamin C; *Thia*, thiamin; *Ribo*, riboflavin; *Niac*, niacin; *VB$_6$*, vitamin B$_6$; *Fol*, folate; *VB$_{12}$*, vitamin B$_{12}$; *Calc*, calcium; *Phos*, phosphorus; *Sel*, selenium; *Fibd*, dietary fiber; and *VE*, vitamin E.

Food name	Portion	Wt (g)	Kcal	Prot (g)	Carb (g)	Fat (g)	Chol (mg)	Safa (g)	Mufa (g)	Pufa (g)	Sod (mg)	Pot (mg)
Creams												
Coffee-table-light	Cup	240	469	6.48	8.78	46.3	159	28.9	13.4	1.72	95	292
Half & Half-fluid	Cup	242	315	7.16	10.4	27.8	89	17.3	8.04	1.03	98	314
Non dairy-powdered	Cup	94	514	4.5	51.6	33.4	0	30.6	0.91	0.01	170	763
Non dairy-coffeemate	Tbsp	15	16	0	2	1	0	0	—	0	5	20
Sour-cultured	Cup	230	493	7.27	9.82	48.2	102	30	13.9	1.79	123	331
Sour-Half & Half	Tbsp	15	20	0.44	0.64	1.8	6	1.12	0.52	0.07	6	19
Sour-imitation	oz	28.4	59	0.68	1.88	5.53	0	5.04	0.17	0.02	29	46
Whip-imit-froz	Cup	75	239	0.94	17.3	19	0	16.3	1.21	0.39	19	14
Whip-imit-pressurized	Cup	70	184	0.69	11.3	15.6	0	13.2	1.35	0.17	43	13
Whip-pressurized	Cup	60	154	1.92	7.49	13.3	46	8.3	3.85	0.5	78	88
Whipping-heavy	Cup	238	821	4.88	6.64	88.1	326	54.8	25.4	3.27	89	179
Milk												
1% Fat-lowfat-fluid	Cup	244	102	8.03	11.7	2.59	10	1.61	0.75	0.1	123	381
2% Fat-lowfat-fluid	Cup	244	121	8.12	11.7	4.68	18	2.92	1.35	0.17	122	377
2% Milk solids add	Cup	245	125	8.53	12.2	4.7	18	2.93	1.36	0.18	128	397
Buttermilk-fluid	Cup	245	99	8.11	11.7	2.16	9	1.34	0.62	0.08	257	371
Chocolate-whole	Cup	250	208	7.92	25.9	8.48	30	5.26	2.48	0.31	149	417
Condensed-sweet-can	Cup	306	982	24.2	166	26.6	104	16.8	7.43	1.03	389	1136
Eggnog-commercial	Cup	254	342	9.68	34.4	19	149	11.3	5.67	0.86	138	420
Evaporated-skim-can	Cup	255	199	19.3	28.9	0.51	10.2	0.309	0.158	0.015	293	847
Evaporated-whole-can	Cup	252	338	17.2	25.3	19.1	73.1	11.6	5.9	0.605	267	764
Human-whole-mature	Cup	246	171	2.53	17	10.8	34	4.94	4.08	1.22	42	126
Nonfat/skim-fluid	Cup	245	86	8.35	11.9	0.44	4	0.287	0.116	0.016	126	406
Whole-3.3% Fat-fluid	Cup	244	150	8.03	11.4	8.15	33	5.07	2.35	0.3	120	370
Whole-low sodium	Cup	244	149	7.56	10.9	8.44	33	5.26	2.44	0.31	6	617
Others												
Milkshake-choc-thick	Item	300	356	9.15	63.5	8.1	32	5.04	2.34	0.3	333	672
Milkshake-vanilla-thick	Item	313	350	12.1	55.6	9.48	37	5.9	2.74	0.35	299	572
Yogurt-fruit flavor-lowfat	Cup	227	231	9.92	43.2	2.45	10	1.58	0.67	0.07	133	442
Yogurt-plain-lowfat	Cup	227	144	11.9	16	3.52	14	2.27	0.97	0.1	159	531
Yogurt-plain-nonfat	Cup	227	127	13	17.4	0.41	4	0.264	0.112	0.012	174	579
Yogurt-plain-whole	Cup	227	139	7.88	10.6	7.38	29	4.76	2.03	0.21	105	351
Desserts												
Angelfood-mix/prep	Slice	53	142	4.2	31.5	0.122	0	—	—	—	142	51.9
Cheesecake-commercial	Slice	85	257	4.61	24.3	16.3	—	—	—	—	189	83.3
Fruitcake-dark-home rec	Slice	15	56.9	0.72	8.96	2.3	6.75	0.48	1.31	0.47	23.7	74.4
Gingerbread-mix/prep	Slice	63	175	2	32	4	1	1.1	1.8	1.1	90	173
Pound-home recipe	Slice	33	160	2	16	10	68	5.9	3	0.6	58	20
Sheet-no icing-home rec	Slice	86	315	4	48	12	1	3.3	4.9	2.6	382	68
Sponge-home recipe	Slice	66	188	4.82	35.7	3.14	162	1.1	1.3	0.5	164	59.4
Strawberry shortcake	Serving	175	344	4.8	61.2	8.9	—	—	—	—	—	—
Yellow/icing-home rec	Slice	69	268	2.9	40.3	11.4	36	3	3	1.4	191	72.5
Cookies												
Choc chip-home rec	Item	10	46.3	0.5	6.41	2.68	5.25	0.6	1.15	0.8	20.6	20.5
Choc chip-mix	Item	10.5	50	0.5	6.96	2.42	5.52	0.7	0.9	0.6	37.8	13.5
Macaroon	Item	19	90	1	12.5	4.5	0	—	—	—	6	88
Oatmeal/raisin-mix	Item	13	61.5	0.732	8.93	2.6	0	0.5	0.825	0.5	37.1	22.6
Peanut butter-mix	Item	10	50	0.8	5.87	2.64	—	—	—	—	56.6	19.4
Sandwich-choc/van	Item	10	50	0.5	7	2.25	0	0.55	0.975	0.55	63	3.75
Sugar-mix	Item	20	98.8	0.908	13.1	4.79	—	—	—	—	109	13.6
Vanilla wafer	Item	4	18.5	0.2	3	0.6	2.5	0.1	0.2	0.1	10	2.9

Mag (mg)	Iron (mg)	Zinc (mg)	VA (RE)	VC (mg)	Thia (mg)	Ribo (mg)	Niac (mg)	VB_6 (mg)	Fol (μg)	VB_{12} (μg)	Calc (mg)	Phos (mg)	Sel (mg)	Fibd (g)	VE (mg)
21	0.1	0.65	519	1.82	0.077	0.355	0.137	0.077	6	0.528	231	192	0.001	0	—
25	0.17	1.23	315	2.08	0.085	0.361	0.189	0.094	6	0.796	254	230	0.001	0	—
4	1.08	0.48	57.4	0	0	0.155	0	0	0	0	21	397	—	0	—
—	—	—	—	—	—	—	—	—	—	—	—	18	—	—	—
26	0.14	0.62	546	1.98	0.081	0.343	0.154	0.037	25	0.69	268	195	—	0	—
2	0.01	0.08	20.4	0.13	0.005	0.022	0.01	0.002	2	0.045	16	14	—	0	—
—	—	—	0	0	0	0	0	0	0	0	1	13	—	0	—
1	0.09	0.02	194	0	0	0	0	0	0	0	5	6	—	0	—
1	0.01	0.01	99.4	0	0	0	0	0	0	0	4	13	—	0	—
6	0.03	0.22	165	0	0.022	0.039	0.042	0.025	—	0.175	61	54	—	0	—
17	0.07	0.55	1051	1.38	0.052	0.262	0.093	0.062	9	0.428	154	149	—	0	—
34	0.12	0.95	150	2.37	0.095	0.407	0.212	0.105	12	0.898	300	235	0.003	0	0.146
33	0.12	0.95	150	2.32	0.095	0.403	0.21	0.105	12	0.888	297	232	0.007	0	0.146
35	0.12	0.98	150	2.45	0.098	0.424	0.22	0.11	13	0.936	313	245	0.007	0	0.147
27	0.12	1.03	24.3	2.4	0.083	0.377	0.142	0.083	—	0.537	285	219	0.003	0	—
33	0.6	1.02	90.7	2.28	0.092	0.405	0.313	0.1	12	0.835	280	251	0.003	0.15	0.225
78	0.58	2.88	302	7.96	0.275	1.27	0.643	0.156	34	1.36	868	775	0.003	0	—
47	0.51	1.17	268	3.81	0.086	0.483	0.267	0.127	2	1.14	330	278	0.003	0	—
68.9	0.74	2.3	300	3.16	0.115	0.788	0.444	0.14	23	0.609	740	497	0.003	0	—
60.5	0.479	1.94	184	4.74	0.118	0.796	0.489	0.126	20.2	0.411	658	509	0.003	0	—
8	0.07	0.42	178	12.3	0.034	0.089	0.435	0.027	13	0.111	79	34	0.004	0	2.16
28	0.1	0.98	150	2.4	0.088	0.343	0.216	0.098	13	0.926	302	247	0.007	0	0.147
33	0.12	0.93	92.2	2.29	0.093	0.395	0.205	0.102	12	0.871	291	228	0.003	0	0.146
12	—	—	95.2	—	0.049	0.256	0.105	0.083	—	0.876	246	209	0.003	0	0.146
48	0.93	1.44	77.5	0	0.141	0.666	0.372	0.075	15	0.945	396	378	0.005	0.75	—
37	0.31	1.22	107	0	0.094	0.61	0.457	0.131	21	1.63	457	361	0.005	0.2	—
33	0.16	1.68	31.2	1.5	0.084	0.404	0.216	0.091	21	1.06	345	271	0.011	0.8	—
40	0.18	2.02	45	1.82	0.1	0.486	0.259	0.111	25	1.28	415	326	0.011	0	—
43	0.2	2.2	4.8	1.98	0.109	0.531	0.281	0.12	28	1.39	452	355	0.011	0	—
26	0.11	1.34	83.8	1.2	0.066	0.322	0.17	0.073	17	0.844	274	215	0.011	0	—
5.83	0.451	0.106	0	0	0.064	0.122	0.594	0.007	4.77	0.015	50	63	0.003	0.037	1.43
8.5	0.408	0.357	43	4.25	0.026	0.111	0.391	0.054	15.3	0.421	47.6	74.8	—	1.79	—
—	0.42	—	3.6	0.06	0.024	0.024	0.165	—	—	—	10.8	17	—	0.313	—
14	0.9	0.284	0	0	0.09	0.11	0.8	0.048	5	0.066	57	63	0.004	1.83	—
—	0.5	—	16	0	0.05	0.06	0.4	—	1.98	—	6	24	0.002	0.08	0.888
12	0.9	0.301	30	0	0.13	0.15	1.1	0.024	6.02	0.087	55	88	0.006	0.96	2.31
7.26	1.11	0.799	25	0	0.092	0.132	0.726	0.037	14.5	0.332	25.1	65.3	0.004	0	1.78
—	2	—	86	89	0.17	0.21	1.3	—	—	—	73	84	—	2.14	—
13.1	0.787	0.338	9.5	0	0.076	0.097	0.656	0.023	5.52	0.123	57.3	60.7	0.004	0.552	1.86
3.5	0.249	0.044	1	0	0.015	0.015	0.146	0.002	0.9	0.01	3.3	8.4	0.001	0.27	0.267
2.52	0.228	0.053	6.09	0	0.014	0.022	0.195	0.002	0.945	—	2.94	7.46	0.001	0.284	0.28
—	0.15	—	0	0	0.01	0.03	0.1	—	—	—	5	16	0.001	0.437	0.507
3.64	0.285	0.085	2.08	0	0.022	0.021	0.241	0.006	1.56	—	4.42	14.4	0.001	0.351	0.347
3.9	0.19	0.75	3.04	0	0.019	0.016	0.381	0.008	2.4	—	11.5	23.5	—	0.18	0.257
5.1	0.175	0.086	0	0	0.015	0.025	0.175	0.004	0.3	0	2.5	24	0.001	0.15	0.257
1.6	0.386	0.054	2.96	0	0.036	0.024	0.466	0.011	1.8	—	20.8	37.8	0.001	0.262	0.514
0.68	0.06	—	1	0	0.01	0.009	0.08	—	—	—	1.6	2.5	0	0.01	0.103

Continued.

Key to Abbreviations

Kcal, Kcalories; *Prot,* protein; *Carb,* carbohydrate; *Fat,* fat; *Chol,* cholesterol; *Safa,* saturated fat; *Mufa,* monounsaturated fat; *Pufa,* polyunsaturated fat; *Sod,* sodium; *Pot,* potassium; *Mag,* magnesium; *Iron,* iron; *Zinc,* zinc; *VA,* vitamin A; *VC,* vitamin C; *Thia,* thiamin; *Ribo,* riboflavin; *Niac,* niacin; *VB$_6$,* vitamin B$_6$; *Fol,* folate; *VB$_{12}$,* vitamin B$_{12}$; *Calc,* calcium; *Phos,* phosphorus; *Sel,* selenium; *Fibd,* dietary fiber; and *VE,* vitamin E.

Food name	Portion	Wt (g)	Kcal	Prot (g)	Carb (g)	Fat (g)	Chol (mg)	Safa (g)	Mufa (g)	Pufa (g)	Sod (mg)	Pot (mg)
Others												
Cupcake/choc icing	Item	36	130	2	21	5	15	2	1.7	0.7	120	42
Custard-baked	Cup	265	305	14	29	15	278	6.8	5.4	0.7	209	387
Danish pastry-plain	Item	65	250	4.06	29.1	13.6	0	4.7	6.1	3.2	249	60.5
Doughnuts-cake-plain	Item	25	104	1.28	12.2	5.77	10	1.2	1.2	2	139	27.3
Doughnuts-yeast-glazed	Item	50	205	3	22	11.2	13	3	5.8	3.3	117	34
Gel-D Zerta-low cal, prep	Cup	240	16	4	0	0	0	0	0	0	—	—
Frozen yogurt-choc	Cup	144	230	5.8	35.8	8.6	6	5.24	2.52	0.32	142	376
Frozen yogurt-fruit variety	Cup	226	216	7	41.8	2	—	—	—	—	—	—
Frozen yogurt-vanilla	Cup	144	28	5.6	34.8	8	4	4.92	2.28	0.3	126	304
Gelatin dessert-prep	Cup	240	140	4	34	0	0	0	0	0	0	—
Gelatin-dry-envelope	Item	7	25	6	0	0	0	0	0	0	8	180
Granola bar	Item	24	109	2.35	16	4.23	—	—	—	—	66.7	78.2
Ice cream-van-hard-10% fat	Cup	133	269	4.8	31.7	14.3	59	8.92	3.6	0.32	116	257
Ice cream-van-soft serve	Cup	173	377	7.04	38.3	22.5	153	13.5	5.85	0.65	153	338
Ice milk-van-soft-2.6% fat	Cup	175	223	8.03	38.4	4.62	13	2.88	1.16	0.1	163	412
Ice cream sundae-hot fudge	Item	165	297	5.89	49.8	9.01	21.5	5.25	2.43	0.843	190	413
Jello-gel-sugar free-prep	Cup	240	16	2	0	0	0	0	0	0	120	—
Pie												
Apple-home rec	Slice	135	323	2.75	49.1	13.6	0	3.9	6.4	3.6	207	115
Banana cream-home rec	Slice	130	285	6	40	12	40	3.8	4.7	2.3	252	264
Cherry-home rec	Slice	135	350	4	52	15	0	4	6.4	3.6	410	142
Crust-mix/prep-baked	Item	160	743	10	70.5	46.5	0	11.4	19.9	11.7	1300	89.5
Custard-home rec	Slice	130	285	8	30	14	—	4.8	5.5	2.5	373	178
Lemon meringue-home	Slice	120	300	3.86	47.3	11.2	0	3.7	4.8	2.3	223	52.8
Mince-home rec	Slice	135	365	3	56	16	0	4	6.6	3.6	604	240
Peach-home rec	Slice	135	345	3	52	14	0	3.5	6.2	3.6	361	21
Pecan-home rec	Slice	118	495	6	61	27	0	4	14.4	6.3	260	145
Pumpkin-home rec	Slice	130	275	5	32	15	0	5.4	5.4	2.4	278	208
Pudding												
Choc-ckd-mix/milk	Cup	260	320	9	59	8	32	4.3	2.6	2	335	354
Choc inst-mix/milk	Cup	260	325	8	63	7	28	3.6	2.2	0.3	322	335
Rice/raisins	Cup	265	387	9.5	70.8	8.2	—	—	—	—	188	469
Tapioca cream-home rec	Cup	165	220	8	28	8	80	4.1	2.5	0.5	257	223
Sherbet-orange-2% fat	Cup	193	270	2.16	58.7	3.82	14	2.38	0.96	0.09	88	198
Turnover-apple	oz	28.4	85.2	0.738	10.5	4.71	1.42	—	—	—	109	13.9
Twinkie-Hostess	Item	42	143	1.25	25.6	4.2	21	—	—	—	189	—
Eggs												
Hard-large-no shell	Item	50	75	6.25	0.61	5.01	213	1.55	1.91	0.682	63	60
Poached-whole-large	Item	50	75	6.25	0.61	5.01	213	1.55	1.91	0.682	63	60
Substitute-liquid	Cup	251	211	30.1	1.61	8.31	2.51	1.65	2.25	4.02	444	828
White-raw-large	Item	33.4	17	3.52	0.34	0	0	0	0	0	55	48
Whole-raw-large	Item	50	75	6.25	0.61	5.01	213	1.55	1.91	0.682	63	60
Yolk-raw-large	Item	16.6	59	2.78	0.3	5.12	213	1.59	1.95	0.698	7	16
Fast foods												
Arthur Treacher-chick sand	Item	156	413	16.2	44	19.2	—	—	—	6.7	708	279
Burger King-Whop hamburger	Item	261	630	26	50	36	104	16.5	13.8	2.22	990	520
Churchs Chick-white meat	Item	100	327	21	10	23	—	—	—	—	498	186
Dairy Queen-banana split	Item	383	540	10	91	15	30	—	—	—	—	—
Dairy Queen-cone, regular	Item	142	226	5.37	33.2	8.43	38.3	4.87	2.5	0.494	126	233
Dairy Queen-dip cone, reg	Item	156	300	7	40	13	20	—	—	—	—	—
Dairy Queen-float	Item	397	330	6	59	8	20	—	—	—	—	—
Dairy Queen-malt-regular	Item	418	600	15	89	20	50	—	—	—	—	—
Dairy Queen-sundae-regular	Item	177	319	6.31	53.4	9.66	23	5.63	2.61	0.904	204	443

Mag (mg)	Iron (mg)	Zinc (mg)	VA (RE)	VC (mg)	Thia (mg)	Ribo (mg)	Niac (mg)	VB_6 (mg)	Fol (μg)	VB_{12} (μg)	Calc (mg)	Phos (mg)	Sel (mg)	Fibd (g)	VE (mg)
—	0.4	—	12	0	0.05	0.06	0.4	—	—	—	47	71	0.003	0.42	0.05
—	1.1	—	87	1	0.11	0.5	0.3	—	—	—	297	310	0.003	1.02	—
9.75	1.2	0.546	11	0	0.156	0.15	1.47	—	—	—	68.9	66.3	—	0.582	—
5.75	0.365	0.128	2.2	0	0.06	0.05	0.428	0.009	2	—	11	55	0.002	0.325	0.18
9.5	0.6	—	5	0	0.1	0.1	0.8	—	11	—	16	33	0.004	1.1	0.36
—	—	—	—	—	—	—	—	—	—	—	—	—	—	0	—
38	0.086	0.72	30.2	0.4	0.052	0.304	0.44	0.108	16	0.42	212	200	—	0	0.078
24	0	—	0	0	0.01	0.26	0	—	—	—	200	200	—	—	—
20	0.44	0.62	82	1.2	0.054	0.322	0.412	0.116	8	0.42	206	186	—	—	—
—	—	—	—	—	—	—	—	—	—	—	—	—	0.016	0	—
—	0.4	—	—	4	0	0	0	0	—	—	0	0	0.002	0	—
—	0.763	—	—	—	0.067	0.026	—	—	—	0	14.4	66.5	—	0.96	—
18	0.12	1.41	133	0.7	0.052	0.329	0.134	0.061	3	0.625	176	134	0.002	0	0.08
25	0.43	1.99	199	0.92	0.08	0.448	0.178	0.095	9	0.996	236	199	0.002	0	0.104
29	0.28	0.86	44	1.17	0.117	0.541	0.184	0.133	5	1.37	274	202	0.003	0	—
34.7	0.611	0.99	46.2	2.48	0.066	0.314	1.12	0.132	9.9	0.677	216	238	—	—	0.693
—	—	—	—	—	—	—	—	—	—	—	—	—	—	0	—
10.8	1.22	0.23	5.1	2	0.149	0.108	1.24	0.035	6.75	0	12.2	31.1	0.015	2.16	2.15
—	1	—	66	1	0.11	0.22	1	—	—	—	86	107	0.015	1.4	—
9.45	0.9	—	118	0	0.16	0.12	1.4	—	—	0	19	34	0.015	1.08	2.15
—	3.05	—	0	0	0.535	0.395	4.95	—	—	—	65.5	136	—	4.23	0.784
—	1.2	—	60	0	0.11	0.27	0.8	—	—	—	125	147	0.015	2.08	2.07
7.2	0.9	0.336	33.4	3.66	0.096	0.12	0.72	0.029	10.8	0.191	15.6	48	0.013	1.44	1.91
24.3	1.9	—	0	1	0.14	0.12	1.4	—	—	—	38	51	0.015	1.96	2.15
9.45	1.2	—	198	4	0.15	0.14	2	—	—	0	14	39	0.015	1.82	2.15
—	3.7	—	40	0	0.26	0.14	1	—	—	—	55	122	0.012	4.13	—
16.9	1	—	320	0	0.11	0.18	1	—	—	—	66	90	0.015	3.51	2.07
—	0.8	—	68	2	0.05	0.39	0.3	—	—	—	265	247	—	0	—
—	1.3	—	68	2	0.08	0.39	0.3	—	—	—	374	237	—	0	—
—	1.1	—	35	0	0.08	0.37	0.5	—	—	—	260	249	—	1.42	—
—	0.7	—	60	2	0.07	0.3	0.2	—	—	—	173	180	—	0.56	—
15	0.31	1.33	39	3.86	0.033	0.089	0.131	0.025	14	0.158	103	74	—	0	—
2.56	0.312	0.054	2.28	0.284	0.028	0.02	0.332	0.011	1.14	0.028	3.98	11.4	—	0.21	0.452
—	0.545	—	8.1	0	0.055	0.06	0.5	—	—	—	19	—	—	—	—
5	0.72	0.55	95.2	0	0.031	0.254	0.037	0.07	23	0.5	25	89	0.012	0	0.35
5	0.72	0.55	95.2	0	0.031	0.254	0.037	0.07	23	0.5	25	89	0.012	0	0.35
21.9	5.27	3.26	542	0	0.276	0.753	0.276	0.008	37.4	0.748	133	304	—	0	—
4	0.01	0	0	0	0.002	0.151	0.031	0.001	1	0.07	2	4	0.005	0	—
5	0.72	0.55	95.2	0	0.031	0.254	0.037	0.07	23	0.5	25	89	0.022	0	0.35
1	0.59	0.52	—	0	0.028	0.106	0.002	0.065	24	0.52	23	81	0.007	0	0.349
27	1.7	—	36.9	19	0.17	0.24	8.1	—	—	—	59	147	—	—	—
50	6	5.25	192	13	0.02	0.03	5.2	0.312	31.2	2.81	104	312	—	—	—
—	1	—	48	1	0.1	0.18	7.2	—	—	—	94	—	—	—	—
—	1.8	—	225	18	0.6	0.6	0.8	—	—	0.9	350	250	—	—	—
21.3	0.213	0.781	87.4	1.56	0.071	0.355	0.426	0.085	7.1	0.284	212	192	—	—	—
—	0.4	—	90.1	0	0.09	0.34	0	—	—	0.6	200	150	—	—	—
—	0	—	30	0	0.12	0.17	0	—	—	0.6	200	200	—	—	—
—	3.6	—	225	3.6	0.12	0.6	0.8	—	—	1.8	500	400	—	—	—
37.2	0.655	1.06	74.5	2.66	0.071	0.336	1.2	0.142	10.6	0.726	232	255	—	—	—

Continued.

Key to Abbreviations
Kcal, Kcalories; *Prot,* protein; *Carb,* carbohydrate; *Fat,* fat; *Chol,* cholesterol; *Safa,* saturated fat; *Mufa,* monounsaturated fat; *Pufa,* polyunsaturated fat; *Sod,* sodium; *Pot,* potassium; *Mag,* magnesium; *Iron,* iron; *Zinc,* zinc; *VA,* vitamin A; *VC,* vitamin C; *Thia,* thiamin; *Ribo,* riboflavin; *Niac,* niacin; *VB_6,* vitamin B_6; *Fol,* folate; *VB_{12},* vitamin B_{12}; *Calc,* calcium; *Phos,* phosphorus; *Sel,* selenium; *Fibd,* dietary fiber; and *VE,* vitamin E.

Food name	Portion	Wt (g)	Kcal	Prot (g)	Carb (g)	Fat (g)	Chol (mg)	Safa (g)	Mufa (g)	Pufa (g)	Sod (mg)	Pot (mg)
Fast foods—cont'd												
Jack/Box-Break Jack sand	Item	121	301	18	28	13	182	—	—	—	1037	190
Jack/Box-Jumbo Jack hamburger	Item	246	551	28	45	29	80	11.4	12.6	2.42	1134	492
Jack/Box-Jumbo Jack/cheese	Item	272	628	32	45	35	110	15	12.6	2.03	1666	499
Jack/Box-Moby Jack	Item	141	455	17	38	26	56	—	—	—	837	246
Jack/Box-Onion rings-bag	Item	83	275	3.7	31.3	15.5	14	6.95	6.65	0.665	430	129
McDonald-Big Mac hamburger	Item	215	560	25.2	42.5	32.4	103	10.1	20.1	1.5	950	237
McDonald-QP hamburger w/ch	Item	194	520	28.5	35.1	29.2	118	11.2	16.5	1.51	1150	341
McDonalds-cheeseburger	Item	116	310	15	31.2	13.8	53	5.17	7.66	0.93	750	223
McDonalds-Egg McMuffin	Item	138	290	18.2	28.1	11.2	226	3.82	6.1	1.29	740	213
McDonalds-Filet O Fish	Item	142	440	13.8	37.9	26.1	50	5.16	10.2	10.8	1030	150
McDonalds-hamburger	Item	102	260	12.3	30.6	9.5	37	3.63	5.09	0.77	500	215
McDonalds-QP hamburger	Item	166	410	23.1	34	20.7	86	8.09	11.4	1.21	660	322
Taco Bell-Bean Burrito	Item	168	332	16.7	42.6	11.5	79	5.6	4.23	0.633	1030	405
Taco Bell-Beef Burrito	Item	110	262	13.3	29.3	10.4	32.5	5.23	3.7	0.427	746	370
Taco Bell-Beefy Tostada	Item	225	334	16.1	29.7	16.9	75	11.5	3.51	0.538	870	490
Taco Bell-Burrito Supreme	Item	225	457	21	43	22	126	7.7	7.35	1.65	367	350
Taco Bell-Taco-regular	Item	171	370	20.7	26.7	20.6	57	11.4	6.58	0.959	802	473
Taco Bell-Tostada-regular	Item	144	223	9.6	26.5	9.86	30	5.37	3.05	0.749	543	403
Wendys-Double hamburger	Item	226	540	34.3	40.3	26.6	122	10.5	10.3	2.8	791	569
Wendys-Single hamburger	Item	218	511	25.7	40.1	27.4	86	10.4	11.4	2.2	825	479
Wendys-Triple hamburger	Item	259	693	50	28.6	41.5	142	15.9	18.2	2.74	713	785
Fats and oils												
Animal fat-cooking-chicken	Tbsp	12.8	115	0	0	12.8	11	3.8	5.7	2.7	—	—
Butter-regular	Tbsp	14	100	0.119	0.008	11.4	30.7	7.07	3.28	0.421	116	3.64
Butter-whipped	Tbsp	9	64.5	0.077	0.005	7.3	19.7	4.54	2.11	0.271	74.3	2.34
Margarine-corn-reg-hard	Tsp	4.7	33.8	0	0	3.8	0	0.6	2.2	0.8	44.3	1.99
Margarine-corn-reg-soft	Tsp	4.7	33.7	0	0	3.8	0	0.7	1.5	1.5	50.7	1.77
Margarine-diet-mazola	Tbsp	14	50	0	0	5.7	0	1	2.1	2.6	130	—
Margarine-reg-hard-stick	Item	113	815	1	1	91.3	0	17.9	40.6	28.8	1070	48.1
Margarine-veg spray-Mazola	Serving	0.72	6	0	0	0.72	0	0.08	0.17	0.4	0	—
Mayonnaise-imitation-soy	Tbsp	15	34.7	0	2.4	2.9	4	0.5	0.7	1.6	74.6	—
Mayonnaise-light-low cal	Tbsp	14	40	0	1	4	5	—	—	—	—	—
Miracle Whip-light-low cal	Tbsp	14	45	0	2	4	5	—	—	—	95	—
Dressings												
Blue Cheese low cal	Tbsp	16	10	0	1	1	4	0.5	0.3	0	177	5
Blue Cheese	Tbsp	15.3	77.1	0.7	1.1	8	9	1.5	1.9	4.3	167	6.12
Caesar	Tbsp	15	70	0	1	7	—	—	—	—	—	—
French	Tbsp	15.6	67	0.1	2.7	6.4	1.95	1.5	1.2	3.4	214	12.3
French-low cal	Tbsp	16.3	21.9	0	3.5	0.9	1	0.1	0.2	0.5	128	13
Italian	Tbsp	14.7	68.7	0	1.5	7.1	0	1	1.7	4.1	116	2
Italian-low cal	Tbsp	15	15.8	0	0.7	1.5	1	0.2	0.3	0.9	118	2
Mayo-low cal	Tbsp	16	20	0	2	2	2	0.4	0.4	1	44	1
Mayonnaise type	Tbsp	14.7	57.3	0	3.5	4.9	4	0.7	1.3	2.6	104	1
Ranch style	Tbsp	15	54	0.4	0.6	5.7	—	—	—	—	97	—
Russian	Tbsp	15.3	76	0.2	1.6	7.8	0	1.1	1.8	4.5	133	24
Russian-low cal	Tbsp	16.3	23.1	0.1	4.5	0.7	1	0.1	0.2	0.4	141	26
Thou Isl-low cal	Tbsp	15.3	24.3	0.1	2.5	1.6	2	0.2	0.4	1	153	17
Thousand Island	Tbsp	15.6	58.9	0	2.4	5.6	4.9	0.9	1.3	3.1	109	18
Vinegar/oil-home	Tbsp	15.6	71.8	0	0.4	8	0	1.5	2.4	3.9	0.1	1.2
Others												
Sandwich spread-commercial	Tbsp	15.3	59.5	0.1	3.4	5.2	12	0.8	1.1	3.1	—	—
Shortening-vegetable-soy	Cup	205	1812	0	0	205	0	51.2	89	52.2	—	—
Vegetable oil-corn	Cup	218	1927	0	0	218	0	27.7	52.7	128	0	0
Vegetable oil-olive	Cup	216	1909	0	0	216	0	30.7	159	18.2	0.08	0

Mag (mg)	Iron (mg)	Zinc (mg)	VA (RE)	VC (mg)	Thia (mg)	Ribo (mg)	Niac (mg)	VB_6 (mg)	Fol (μg)	VB_{12} (μg)	Calc (mg)	Phos (mg)	Sel (mg)	Fibd (g)	VE (mg)
24	2.5	1.8	133	3	0.41	0.47	5.1	0.14	—	1.1	177	310	—	—	—
44	4.5	4.2	73.9	3.7	0.47	0.34	11.6	0.3	—	2.68	134	261	—	—	—
49	4.6	4.8	220	4.9	0.52	0.38	11.3	0.31	—	3.05	273	411	—	—	—
30	1.7	1.1	72.1	1	0.3	0.21	4.5	0.12	—	1.1	167	263	—	—	—
15	0.85	0.35	2.4	0.6	0.09	0.1	0.92	0.06	11	0.12	73	86	—	—	0.587
38	4	4.7	106	1.68	0.48	0.41	6.81	0.27	21	1.8	256	314	—	—	—
41	3.72	5.7	211	3.24	0.37	0.39	6.73	0.23	23	2.15	295	382	—	—	—
21	2.3	2.09	118	2.15	0.29	0.21	3.86	0.12	18	0.94	199	177	—	—	0.53
33	2.77	1.8	150	1.38	0.47	0.33	3.71	0.16	44	0.8	256	319	—	—	—
27	1.83	0.9	43.8	0.06	0.3	0.15	2.68	0.1	20	0.82	165	229	—	1.11	—
23	2.29	2.05	45.6	2.15	0.28	0.16	3.84	0.12	17	0.84	122	110	—	—	0.428
37	3.68	5.1	67	3.24	0.36	0.29	6.7	0.27	23	1.88	142	249	—	—	—
0.407	3.84	3.04	240	3.3	0.275	0.6	3.86	0.205	73	0.995	144	143	—	—	—
40.5	3.05	2.37	41.7	0.55	0.115	0.46	3.23	0.16	19.5	0.985	42	87.5	—	—	—
68	2.45	3.18	383	3.9	0.09	0.5	2.85	0.26	0.26	1.13	190	173	—	—	—
51.8	3.8	5.85	216	8	0.45	0.923	6.17	0.27	42.8	1.53	146	245	—	—	—
71	2.42	3.93	257	2.2	0.15	0.45	3.22	0.24	23	1.04	221	203	—	—	—
59	1.88	1.9	187	1.3	0.1	0.33	1.33	0.17	75	0.68	211	116	—	—	—
49	5.95	5.68	30.6	1.2	0.36	0.39	7.57	0.54	27	4.07	102	314	—	—	—
43	4.92	4.87	93.4	2.5	0.42	0.38	7.28	0.33	36	2.38	96	233	—	—	—
55	8.33	10.8	47.4	1.4	0.31	0.56	11	0.62	31	4.92	65	393	—	—	—
—	—	—	—	—	—	—	—	—	—	—	—	—	—	0	—
0.28	0.022	0.007	105	0	0.001	0.005	0.006	0	0.42	—	3.36	3.22	0	0	0.221
0.18	0.014	0.005	67.9	0	0	0.003	0.004	0	0.27	—	2.16	2.07	0	0	0.142
0.12	—	—	47	0.008	0	0.002	0.001	0	0.06	0.004	1.41	1.08	0	0	0.606
0.11	—	—	47	0.007	0	0.002	0.001	0	0.05	0.004	1.25	0.95	0	0	0.5
—	0	—	130	0	0	0	0	—	—	—	0	—	0	0	0.112
2.95	0.07	—	338	0.181	0.011	0.042	0.026	0.01	1.34	0.108	33.9	26	0.002	0	13.2
—	0	—	0	0	0	0	0	—	—	—	0	0	—	0	—
—	—	0.02	—	—	—	—	—	—	—	—	—	—	—	0	3.11
—	—	—	—	—	—	—	—	—	—	—	—	—	—	0	2.9
—	—	—	—	—	—	—	—	—	—	—	—	—	—	0	—
—	0	—	9	0	0	0.001	0	—	—	—	10	8	—	0	—
—	0	—	9.5	0.3	0	0.02	0	—	—	—	12.4	11.3	—	0.05	—
—	—	—	—	—	—	—	—	—	—	—	—	—	—	0.04	—
—	0.1	0.01	—	—	—	—	—	—	—	—	1.7	2.2	—	0.1	—
—	0.1	0.03	—	—	—	—	—	—	—	—	2	2	—	0.09	—
—	0	0.02	—	—	0	0	0	—	—	—	1	1	—	0.05	—
—	0	—	—	—	0	0	0	—	—	—	0	1	—	0.09	—
—	0	—	12	—	0	0	0	—	—	—	3	4	—	0	—
0.29	0	—	9.6	—	0	0	0	—	—	—	2	4	—	0	—
—	—	—	—	—	—	—	—	—	—	—	—	—	—	0	—
—	0.1	0.07	31.8	1	0.01	0.01	0.1	—	—	—	3	6	—	0	—
—	0.1	—	—	—	—	—	—	—	—	—	3	6	—	0.2	—
—	0.1	—	14.8	0	0	0	0	—	—	—	2	3	—	0.3	—
—	0.1	0.02	15	0	0	0	0	—	—	—	2	3	—	0.6	—
—	—	—	—	—	—	—	—	—	—	—	—	—	—	0	—
—	—	—	—	—	—	—	—	—	—	—	—	—	—	0.02	—
—	—	—	—	—	—	—	—	—	—	—	—	—	—	0	27.9
0	0	0	—	0	0	0	0	0	0	0	0	0	—	0	31.1
0.02	0.83	0.13	—	0	0	0	0	0	0	0	0.38	2.63	—	0	25.7

Continued.

Key to Abbreviations

Kcal, Kcalories; *Prot,* protein; *Carb,* carbohydrate; *Fat,* fat; *Chol,* cholesterol; *Safa,* saturated fat; *Mufa,* monounsaturated fat; *Pufa,* polyunsaturated fat; *Sod,* sodium; *Pot,* potassium; *Mag,* magnesium; *Iron,* iron; *Zinc,* zinc; *VA,* vitamin A; *VC,* vitamin C; *Thia,* thiamin; *Ribo,* riboflavin; *Niac,* niacin; *VB_6,* vitamin B_6; *Fol,* folate; *VB_{12},* vitamin B_{12}; *Calc,* calcium; *Phos,* phosphorus; *Sel,* selenium; *Fibd,* dietary fiber; and *VE,* vitamin E.

Food name	Portion	Wt (g)	Kcal	Prot (g)	Carb (g)	Fat (g)	Chol (mg)	Safa (g)	Mufa (g)	Pufa (g)	Sod (mg)	Pot (mg)
Fish												
Anchovy-fillet-can	Item	4	8.4	1.16	0	0.388	3.4	0.088	0.151	0.102	147	21.8
Bluefish-baked/butter	Item	155	246	40.6	0	8.1	108	1.83	1.84	3.94	161	—
Carp-cooked-dry heat	Serving	85	138	19.4	0	6.1	72	1.18	2.54	1.56	54	363
Catfish-fried-breaded	Serving	85	194	15.4	6.83	11.3	69	2.8	4.77	2.83	238	289
Clam-can-solid/liquid	oz	28.4	12.8	2.33	0.667	0.333	17.7	0.067	0	0	14.7	39.7
Clams-breaded-fried	Serving	85	171	12.1	8.78	9.48	52	2.28	3.86	2.44	309	277
Clams-ckd-moist heat	Serving	85	126	21.7	4.36	1.65	57	0.16	0.146	0.469	95	534
Clams-raw-meat only	Serving	85	63	10.9	2.18	0.83	29	0.08	0.068	0.24	47	267
Cod-ckd-dry heat	Piece	180	189	41.1	0	1.55	99	0.302	0.223	0.526	141	440
Crab cake	Item	60	93	12.1	0.29	4.51	90	0.89	1.69	1.36	198	195
Crab meat-king-can	Cup	135	135	24	1	3.2	135	0.6	0.6	2	675	149
Crab-imitation-surimi	Serving	85	87	10.2	8.69	1.11	17	—	—	—	715	77
Crab-steamed-pieces	Cup	155	150	30	0	2.39	82.2	0.206	0.287	0.831	1662	406
Crayfish-ckd-moist	Serving	85	97	20.3	0	1.15	151	0.197	0.32	0.281	58	298
Flatfish-ckd-dry heat	Serving	85	99	20.5	0	1.3	58	0.309	0.263	0.35	89	292
Grouper-ckd-dry heat	Serving	85	100	21.1	0	1.11	40	0.254	0.228	0.343	45	403
Haddock-cook-dry heat	Serving	85	95	20.6	0	0.79	63	0.142	0.128	0.263	74	339
Halibut-broiled-dry	Serving	85	119	22.7	0	2.49	35	0.354	0.822	0.799	59	490
Lobster-ckd-moist	oz	28.4	27.8	5.82	0.364	0.168	20.4	0.03	0.045	0.026	108	100
Mackeral-Atlantic-can	Cup	190	296	44	0	12	150	3.39	5.16	0.165	720	369
Mackerel-ckd-dry heat	Serving	85	223	20.3	0	15.1	64	3.55	5.96	3.66	71	341
Mussel-blue-ckd-moist	Serving	85	147	20.2	6.28	3.81	48	0.723	0.862	1.03	313	228
Ocean perch-ckd-dry	Serving	85	103	20.3	0	1.78	46	0.266	0.681	0.465	82	298
Oyster-east-ckd-moist	Serving	85	117	12	6.65	4.21	93	1.07	0.425	1.26	190	389
Oyster-eastern-can	Cup	248	170	17.5	9.7	6.14	136	1.57	0.62	1.83	277	568
Oysters-Pacific-raw	Seving	85	69	8.03	4.21	1.96	—	0.434	0.304	0.76	90	143
Oysters-raw-meat only	Cup	248	171	17.5	9.7	6.14	136	1.57	0.62	1.83	277	568
Perch-breaded-fried	Piece	85	915	16	6	11	32	2.7	4.4	2.3	128	242
Perch-ckd-dry heat	Serving	85	99	21.1	0	1	98	0.201	0.166	0.401	67	293
Pollock-Atlantic-raw	Serving	85	78	16.5	0	0.83	60	0.115	0.095	0.411	73	302
Pollock-ckd-dry heat	Serving	85	96	20	0	0.95	82	0.196	0.148	0.445	98	329
Pompano-ckd-dry heat	Serving	85	179	20.1	0	10.3	54	3.82	2.82	1.24	65	541
Red snapper-ckd-dry	Serving	85	109	22.4	0	1.46	40	0.31	0.274	0.5	48	444
Rockfish-ckd-dry heat	Serving	100	121	24	0	2.01	44	0.474	0.447	0.594	77	520
Roe-raw-eggs	oz	28.4	39	6.25	0.42	1.8	105	0.408	0.465	0.744	—	—
Salmon-ckd-moist heat	Serving	85	157	23.3	0	6.4	42	1.19	2.22	1.87	50	454
Salmon-pink-can	Serving	85	118	16.8	0	5.14	—	1.31	1.54	1.74	471	277
Salmon-smoked	Serving	100	117	18.3	0	4.32	23	0.929	2.02	0.995	784	175
Sardine-can/oil	Item	12	25	2.96	0	1.38	17	0.184	0.465	0.618	60.5	47.5
Scallops-steamed	oz	28.4	31.8	6.59	0.511	0.398	15.1	—	—	—	75.2	135
Sea bass-ckd-dry heat	Serving	85	105	20.1	0	2.18	45	0.557	0.462	0.81	74	279
Shad-bake/marg/bacon	Serving	100	201	23.2	0	11.3	69.4	2.45	2.23	5.9	79	377
Shrimp-ckd-moist heat	Serving	85	84	17.8	0	0.92	166	0.246	0.167	0.374	190	154
Shrimp-French fried	Serving	85	206	18.2	9.75	10.4	150	1.77	3.19	3.83	292	191
Shrimp-meat-can	Cup	128	154	29.6	1.32	2.51	222	0.477	0.375	0.966	216	269
Smelt-ckd-dry heat	Serving	85	106	19.2	0	2.64	76	0.492	0.699	0.965	65	316
Sole/flounder-baked	Serving	127	148	30.7	0	1.94	86	0.461	0.392	0.523	133	436
Squid-ckd-fried	Serving	85	149	15.3	6.62	6.36	221	1.6	2.34	1.82	260	237
Stick-bread-froz-ckd	oz	28.4	76	4.38	6.65	3.42	31	0.882	1.42	0.886	163	73
Surimi	Serving	85	84	12.9	5.82	0.77	25.5	—	—	—	122	95
Swordfish-broil/marg	Serving	100	174	28	0	6	4	—	—	—	—	—
Swordfish-ckd-dry	Serving	85	132	21.6	0	4.37	43	1.2	1.68	1.01	98	314
Trout-brook-ckd	Serving	100	196	23.5	0.4	11.2	—	—	—	—	78.8	—
Trout-rainbow-ckd-dry	Serving	85	129	22.4	0	3.66	62	0.707	1.13	1.31	29	539
Tuna-can/oil-drained	Serving	85	169	24.8	0	6.98	15.3	1.3	2.51	2.45	301	176
Tuna-diet-low sodium	oz	28.4	35.5	7.67	0.011	0.54	9.94	0.09	0.163	0.199	11.4	73.8
Tuna-light-can/water	Serving	85	111	25.1	0	0.43	—	0.136	0.122	0.111	303	267

Mag (mg)	Iron (mg)	Zinc (mg)	VA (RE)	VC (mg)	Thia (mg)	Ribo (mg)	Niac (mg)	VB_6 (mg)	Fol (µg)	VB_{12} (µg)	Calc (mg)	Phos (mg)	Sel (mg)	Fibd (g)	VE (mg)
2.8	0.186	0.098	—	—	0.003	0.015	0.796	0.008	—	0.035	9.2	10	0.002	0	0.012
43.3	1.1	—	24	—	0.17	0.16	2.9	—	—	1.64	44.6	445	0.047	0	—
32	1.35	1.62	8.11	1.4	—	—	—	0.186	—	1.25	44	451	0.026	0	—
23	1.22	0.73	7.21	0	0.062	0.113	1.94	—	—	—	37	183	—	0.8	—
—	1.17	0.347	—	—	0.003	0.03	0.3	—	—	5.4	15.7	38.7	0.046	0	0.629
12	11.8	1.24	77.2	—	—	0.207	1.75	—	—	34.2	54	160	—	0.32	—
16	23.8	2.32	145	—	—	0.362	2.85	—	—	84.1	78	287	—	0	—
8	11.9	1.16	76.6	—	—	0.181	1.5	—	—	42	39	144	0.016	0	0.209
76	0.88	1.04	24.9	1.8	0.158	0.142	4.52	0.509	—	1.89	25	248	0.081	0	—
20	0.65	2.46	—	—	—	—	—	—	—	3.56	63	128	0.013	0.03	—
29	1.1	5.83	—	—	0.11	0.11	2.6	—	—	13.5	61	246	0.03	0	1.65
—	0.33	—	—	—	0.027	0.023	0.153	—	—	—	11	—	0.019	0	—
52.7	1.18	11.8	13.5	—	0.082	0.085	2.08	—	—	—	91.5	434	0.034	0	—
27	2.67	1.42	—	2.8	—	0.065	2.5	—	—	2.94	26	280	—	0	—
50	0.28	0.53	9.61	—	0.068	0.097	1.85	0.204	—	2.13	16	246	—	0	—
32	0.96	0.43	—	—	0.069	0.005	0.324	—	—	0.558	18	121	—	0	—
43	1.14	0.41	16.2	—	0.034	0.038	3.94	0.294	—	1.18	36	205	0.025	0	0.51
91	0.91	0.45	45.6	—	0.059	0.077	6.06	0.337	—	1.16	51	242	0.051	0	—
9.94	0.111	0.829	7.42	—	0.002	0.019	0.304	0.022	3.15	0.883	17.3	52.5	0.023	0	—
70	3.88	1.94	248	1.7	0.076	0.403	11.7	0.399	10.2	13.2	458	572	0.089	0	—
82.5	1.33	0.8	45.9	0.3	0.135	0.35	5.82	0.391	—	16.2	13	236	0.03	0	—
32	5.71	2.27	—	—	—	—	—	—	—	—	28	242	—	0	—
33	1	0.52	11.7	—	—	0.114	2.07	—	—	0.981	117	235	0.03	0	—
92.7	11.4	155	—	—	—	0.282	2.12	0.081	15.2	32.5	76	236	0.051	0	—
135	16.6	226	—	—	—	0.412	3.09	0.236	22.1	47.5	111	344	0.149	0	—
19	4.34	14.1	—	—	0.057	0.198	1.71	—	—	—	7	138	0.056	0	0.723
135	16.6	226	222	—	0.34	0.412	3.25	0.124	24.6	47.5	111	344	0.141	0	2.04
—	1.1	—	—	—	0.1	0.1	1.6	—	—	0.85	28	192	0.02	0.05	1.06
33	0.98	1.21	—	—	—	—	—	—	—	—	87	218	0.03	0	—
57	0.39	0.4	9.01	—	0.04	0.157	2.78	0.244	—	2.71	51	188	—	0	—
—	0.24	0.51	19.5	—	0.063	0.065	1.4	0.059	3	3.57	5	—	—	0	—
27	0.57	0.59	—	—	—	—	—	—	—	—	36	290	—	0	—
31	0.2	0.37	—	—	0.045	0.003	0.294	—	—	—	34	171	—	0	—
34	0.53	0.53	65.8	0.87	0.044	0.084	3.92	—	—	—	12	228	0.039	0	—
—	0.17	—	—	3.98	0.028	0.216	0.398	—	—	—	4.25	98.1	0.014	0	—
—	0.76	0.44	—	0.9	—	—	—	—	—	—	—	—	0.026	0	—
29	0.72	0.78	14.1	0	0.02	0.158	5.56	0.255	13.1	5.85	—	279	0.045	0	1.15
18	0.85	0.31	26.4	—	0.023	0.101	4.72	0.278	1.9	3.26	11	164	0.061	0	—
4.5	0.35	0.155	8.11	—	0.01	0.027	0.63	0.02	1.4	1.07	45.8	58.8	0.006	0	—
—	0.852	—	—	—	—	—	—	—	—	—	32.7	96	0.015	0	—
45	0.32	0.44	54.4	—	—	—	—	—	—	—	11	211	—	0	—
—	0.6	—	9.01	—	0.13	0.26	8.6	—	—	—	24	313	—	0	2
29	2.62	1.33	—	—	0.026	0.027	2.2	0.108	2.9	1.27	33	116	0.054	0	—
34	1.07	1.17	—	—	0.11	0.116	2.61	0.083	6.9	1.59	57	185	0.027	0.48	0.807
53	3.5	1.61	22.6	—	0.035	0.047	3.53	0.142	2.3	1.44	75	299	0.041	0	3.64
33	0.98	1.8	—	—	—	0.124	1.5	—	—	3.37	65	251	0.105	0	—
74	0.43	0.8	14.4	—	0.102	0.145	2.77	0.305	—	3.19	23	368	0.16	0	—
33	0.86	1.48	—	3.5	0.048	0.389	2.21	0.049	—	1.04	33	213	—	0.3	—
7	0.21	0.19	9.01	—	0.036	0.05	0.596	0.017	5.1	0.503	6	51	0.003	0.665	—
—	0.22	—	—	—	0.017	0.018	0.187	—	—	—	7	—	—	0	—
—	1.3	—	616	—	0.04	0.05	10.9	—	—	—	—	275	0.047	0	—
29	0.88	1.25	35.1	0.9	0.037	0.099	10	0.324	—	1.72	5	287	—	0	—
35	1.1	—	95.8	1	0.12	0.06	2.5	—	—	—	218	272	—	0	—
33	2.07	1.18	18.9	3.1	0.072	0.191	—	—	—	—	73	272	—	0	—
26	1.18	0.77	19.8	—	0.032	—	—	0.094	4.5	—	11	265	0.061	0	1.42
9.09	0.341	0.142	6.91	—	0.009	0.014	3.52	0.105	0	0.398	1.42	62.5	0.033	0	—
25	2.72	0.37	—	—	—	—	—	0.321	4	—	10	158	0.061	0	—

Continued.

Key to Abbreviations
Kcal, Kcalories; *Prot,* protein; *Carb,* carbohydrate; *Fat,* fat; *Chol,* cholesterol; *Safa,* saturated fat; *Mufa,* monounsaturated fat; *Pufa,* polyunsaturated fat; *Sod,* sodium; *Pot,* potassium; *Mag,* magnesium; *Iron,* iron; *Zinc,* zinc; *VA,* vitamin A; *VC,* vitamin C; *Thia,* thiamin; *Ribo,* riboflavin; *Niac,* niacin; VB_6, vitamin B_6; *Fol,* folate; VB_{12}, vitamin B_{12}; *Calc,* calcium; *Phos,* phosphorus; *Sel,* selenium; *Fibd,* dietary fiber; and *VE,* vitamin E.

Food name	Portion	Wt (g)	Kcal	Prot (g)	Carb (g)	Fat (g)	Chol (mg)	Safa (g)	Mufa (g)	Pufa (g)	Sod (mg)	Pot (mg)
Fish—cont'd												
Tuna-white-can/water	Serving	85	116	22.7	0	2.09	35	0.556	0.551	0.78	333	241
Tuna-yellowfin-raw	Serving	85	92	19.9	0	0.81	38	0.2	0.131	0.241	31	—
White perch-fried filet	Item	65	108	12.5	0	5.3	—	—	—	—	—	—
Whitefish-bake/stuff	Serving	100	215	15.2	5.8	14	—	—	—	—	195	291
Whiting-ckd-dry heat	Serving	85	98	20	0	1.43	71	0.269	0.309	0.456	113	369
Frozen dinners												
Beef dinner-Swanson	Item	326	320	25	34	9	—	—	—	—	1085	—
Beef sirloin tips-Le Menu	Item	326	400	29	27	19	—	—	—	—	1100	—
Beef/green peppers-Stouffer	Item	220	225	10	18	11	—	—	—	—	960	420
Cabbage roll/tom sauc-Horm	oz	28.4	23	1.1	3.2	0.7	3	0.281	0.226	0.043	127	87
Chicken cacciatore-Stouffer	Item	319	310	25	29	11	—	—	—	—	1135	300
Chicken dinner-Swanson	Item	326	660	26	64	33	—	—	—	—	1610	—
Chicken Kiev-Le Menu	Item	234	500	21	35	30	—	—	—	—	745	—
Chicken parmigiana-Le Menu	Item	333	390	26	28	19	—	—	—	—	900	—
Egg roll-beef/shrimp-froz	Item	12	27	0.9	3.5	1	—	—	—	—	80.5	—
Fettucini Alfredo-Stouffer	Item	142	270	8	19	18	—	—	—	—	1195	240
Fish & chips-Van De Kamps	Item	224	500	16	45	30	—	—	—	—	551	—
Fish Divan-Lean Cuisine	Item	351	270	31	16	10	85	—	—	—	780	850
Ham-froz din-Banquet	Item	284	369	16.8	47.7	12.2	—	—	—	—	1590	125
Lasagna-Stouf	Item	298	385	28	36	14	—	—	—	—	1200	580
Manicotti-cheese-Le Menu	Item	241	310	18	29	13	—	—	—	—	840	—
Meatballs/noodles-Stouffer	Item	312	475	25	33	27	—	—	—	—	1620	395
Meatloaf-froz din-Banquet	Item	312	412	20.9	29	23.7	—	—	—	—	1991	468
Mexican dinner-Swanson	Item	454	590	20	64	29	—	—	—	—	1865	—
Salisbury steak din-Banq	Item	312	390	18.1	24	24.6	—	—	—	—	2059	387
Sole-light-Van De Kamp's	Item	142	293	16	17	18	—	—	—	—	412	—
Turkey dinner-Swanson	Item	326	340	20	42	10	—	—	—	—	1295	—
Turkey pie-Stouffer	Item	284	460	20	35	26	—	—	—	—	1735	270
Veal parmigiana-froz din	Item	213	296	24	17	14	—	—	—	—	973	466
Vegetable lasagna-Le Menu	Item	312	400	15	30	24	—	—	—	—	1135	—
Fruits												
Apple juice-can/bottled	Cup	248	116	0.15	29	0.28	0	0.047	0.012	0.082	7	296
Apple juice-froz-diluted	Cup	239	111	0.34	27.6	0.25	0	0.043	0.005	0.074	17	301
Apples-raw-peeled-boiled	Cup	171	91	0.45	23.3	0.61	0	0.099	0.024	0.178	1	150
Apples-raw-unpeeled	Item	138	81	0.27	21.1	0.49	0	0.08	0.021	0.145	1	159
Applesauce-can-sweet	Cup	255	194	0.47	50.8	0.47	0	0.077	0.018	0.138	8	156
Applesauce-can-unsweet	Cup	244	106	0.4	27.6	0.12	0	0.02	0.005	0.034	5	183
Apricot-raw-without pit	Item	35.3	16.9	0.494	3.93	0.138	0	0.01	0.06	0.027	0.353	104
Apricots-can/juice	Cup	248	119	1.56	30.6	0.09	0	0.007	0.042	0.017	9	409
Apricots-dried-ckd-unsweet	Cup	250	211	3.24	54.8	0.41	0	0.028	0.178	0.08	9	1222
Apricots-dried-unckd	Cup	130	310	4.75	80.3	0.6	0	0.042	0.26	0.117	13	1791
Bananas-raw-peeled	Item	114	105	1.18	26.7	0.55	0	0.211	0.047	0.101	1	451
Blackberries-froz-unsweet	Cup	151	97	1.78	23.7	0.65	0	—	—	—	2	211
Blackberries-raw	Cup	144	74	1.04	18.4	0.56	0	0.07	0.17	0.299	0	282
Blueberries-froz-unsweet	Cup	155	78	0.65	18.9	0.99	0	—	—	—	1	83
Blueberries-raw	Cup	145	82	0.97	20.5	0.55	0	0.07	0.16	0.292	9	129
Boysenberries-froz-unsweet	Cup	132	66	1.46	16.1	0.35	0	—	—	—	2	183
Cherries-sweet-raw	Item	6.8	4.9	0.082	1.13	0.065	0	0.015	0.018	0.02	0	15.2
Cranapple juice-can	Cup	253	170	0.253	43.2	0	0	0	0	0	5.06	68.3
Cranberry sauce-can-sweet	Cup	277	419	0.55	108	0.42	0	0.06	0.14	0.22	80	71
Dates-natural-dried-chop	Cup	178	489	3.5	131	0.8	0	0.05	0.31	0.42	5	1161
Figs-dried-unckd	Cup	199	508	6.06	130	2.32	0	0.466	0.513	1.11	22	1418
Fruit cocktail-can/juice	Cup	248	113	1.13	29.4	0.03	0	0.005	0.007	0.015	9	235
Fruit punch drink-can	Fl oz	31	14	0	3.7	0	0	0	0	0	7	8

Mag (mg)	Iron (mg)	Zinc (mg)	VA (RE)	VC (mg)	Thia (mg)	Ribo (mg)	Niac (mg)	VB_6 (mg)	Fol (μg)	VB_{12} (μg)	Calc (mg)	Phos (mg)	Sel (mg)	Fibd (g)	VE (mg)
—	0.51	—	—	—	0.003	0.039	4.93	—	3.5	—	—	—	0.061	0	—
—	0.62	0.45	15	—	0.369	0.04	8.33	—	—	—	14	163	0.085	0	—
—	0.7	—	0	0	0.04	0.05	2.7	—	—	—	9	113	0.016	0	0.813
—	0.5	—	601	0	0.11	0.11	2.3	—	—	—	—	246	—	0.58	—
23	0.36	0.45	29.1	—	0.058	0.051	1.42	0.153	12.8	2.21	53	242	—	0	—
—	—	—	—	—	—	—	—	—	—	—	—	—	—	—	—
—	—	—	—	—	—	—	—	—	—	—	—	—	—	—	—
—	2.33	—	136	0	0.078	0.155	3.88	—	—	—	0	—	—	—	—
4	0.25	0.19	—	0.18	0.76	0.02	0.29	0.03	2.9	0.1	5.9	15.7	—	—	—
—	—	—	—	—	—	—	—	—	—	—	—	—	—	—	—
—	—	—	—	—	—	—	—	—	—	—	—	—	—	—	—
—	—	—	—	—	—	—	—	—	—	—	—	—	—	—	—
—	—	—	—	—	—	—	—	—	—	—	—	—	—	—	—
—	—	—	—	—	—	—	—	—	—	—	—	—	—	0.12	—
—	—	—	—	—	—	—	—	—	—	—	—	—	—	—	—
—	—	—	—	—	—	—	—	—	—	—	—	—	—	—	—
—	—	—	—	—	—	—	—	—	—	—	—	—	—	—	—
—	2.5	—	1311	57	0.57	0.23	3.4	—	—	—	151	278	—	—	—
—	3.15	—	248	0	0.21	0.42	4.2	—	—	—	410	—	—	—	—
—	—	—	—	—	—	—	—	—	—	—	—	—	—	—	—
—	—	—	—	—	—	—	—	—	—	—	—	—	—	—	—
—	4.3	—	427	8	0.16	0.22	4.2	—	—	—	84	243	—	—	—
—	—	—	—	—	—	—	—	—	—	—	—	—	—	—	—
—	3.5	—	791	7	0.16	0.19	3.6	—	—	—	90	206	—	—	—
—	—	—	—	—	—	—	—	—	—	—	—	—	—	—	—
—	—	—	—	—	—	—	—	—	—	—	—	—	—	—	—
—	—	—	—	—	—	—	—	—	—	—	—	—	—	—	—
—	2.3	—	123	6.4	0.3	0.38	6.8	—	—	—	97	—	—	—	—
—	—	—	—	—	—	—	—	—	—	—	—	—	—	—	—
8	0.92	0.07	0.2	2.3	0.052	0.042	0.248	0.074	0.2	0	16	18	0.002	0.52	0.025
12	0.61	0.09	—	1.4	0.007	0.036	0.091	0.079	0.7	0	14	16	0.002	0	0.024
5	0.32	0.07	7.5	0.3	0.027	0.021	0.162	0.075	1	0	8	13	0.001	4.1	0.086
6	0.25	0.05	7.4	7.8	0.023	0.019	0.106	0.066	3.9	0	10	10	0.001	3.04	0.814
7	0.89	0.1	2.8	4.4	0.033	0.071	0.479	0.066	1.5	0	9	17	0.001	3.06	0.23
7	0.29	0.06	7	2.9	0.032	0.061	0.459	0.063	1.4	0	7	18	0.001	3.66	0.22
2.82	0.191	0.092	92.2	3.53	0.011	0.014	0.212	0.019	3.04	0	4.94	6.71	0	0.67	0.314
24	0.74	0.27	420	12.2	0.045	0.047	0.853	—	—	0	30	50	0.001	2.81	2.21
42	4.17	0.66	591	3.9	0.015	0.075	2.36	0.285	0	—	40	104	—	19.5	—
61	6.11	0.97	941	3.1	0.01	0.196	3.9	0.203	13.4	0	59	152	—	10.1	—
33	0.35	0.19	9.2	10.3	0.051	0.114	0.616	0.659	21.8	0	7	22	0.001	1.82	0.308
33	1.21	0.37	17.2	4.7	0.044	0.069	1.82	0.092	51.3	0	44	46	0.001	7.55	—
29	0.83	0.39	23.7	30.2	0.043	0.058	0.576	0.084	18	0	46	30	0.001	8.93	5.04
8	0.28	0.11	12.6	3.8	0.05	0.057	0.806	0.091	10.4	0	12	18	0.001	4.94	—
7	0.24	0.16	14.5	18.9	0.07	0.073	0.521	0.052	9.3	0	9	15	0.001	3.34	—
21	1.12	0.29	8.9	4.1	0.07	0.049	1.01	0.074	83.6	0	36	36	0.001	5.15	—
0.8	0.026	0.004	1.46	0.48	0.003	0.004	0.027	0.002	0.28	0	1	1.3	0	0.1	0.009
5.06	0.152	0.101	—	81	0.013	0.051	0.152	—	0.5	0	17.7	7.59	0.001	0	—
8	0.61	0.14	5.5	5.5	0.042	0.058	0.277	0.039	—	0	10	16	0.001	3.2	—
63	2.05	0.52	8.9	0	0.16	0.178	3.92	0.342	22.4	0	58	70	—	15.5	—
118	4.45	1	26.4	1.7	0.141	0.175	1.38	0.446	15	0	286	136	—	18.5	—
17	0.53	0.21	75.7	6.8	0.03	0.04	0.999	—	—	0	20	34	0.001	1.51	—
1	0.06	0.04	1.2	9.2	0.007	0.007	0.007	0	0.4	0	2	0	0	0	—

Continued.

Key to Abbreviations

Kcal, Kcalories; *Prot*, protein; *Carb*, carbohydrate; *Fat*, fat; *Chol*, cholesterol; *Safa*, saturated fat; *Mufa*, monounsaturated fat; *Pufa*, polyunsaturated fat; *Sod*, sodium; *Pot*, potassium; *Mag*, magnesium; *Iron*, iron; *Zinc*, zinc; *VA*, vitamin A; *VC*, vitamin C; *Thia*, thiamin; *Ribo*, riboflavin; *Niac*, niacin; *VB$_6$*, vitamin B$_6$; *Fol*, folate; *VB$_{12}$*, vitamin B$_{12}$; *Calc*, calcium; *Phos*, phosphorus; *Sel*, selenium; *Fibd*, dietary fiber; and *VE*, vitamin E.

Food name	Portion	Wt (g)	Kcal	Prot (g)	Carb (g)	Fat (g)	Chol (mg)	Safa (g)	Mufa (g)	Pufa (g)	Sod (mg)	Pot (mg)
Fruits—cont'd												
Fruit roll up-cherry	Item	14.4	50	0	12	1	0	—	—	—	5	45
Grape juice-can/bottle	Cup	253	155	1.41	37.9	0.19	0	0.063	0.008	0.056	7	334
Grape juice-froz-diluted	Cup	250	128	0.47	31.9	0.23	0	0.073	0.01	0.065	5	53
Grapefruit juice-can-sweet	Cup	250	116	1.45	27.8	0.23	0	0.03	0.03	0.053	4	405
Grapefruit juice-can-unsweet	Cup	247	93	1.29	22.1	0.24	0	0.032	0.032	0.057	3	378
Grapefruit juice-froz-diluted	Cup	247	102	1.37	24	0.33	0	0.047	0.044	0.079	2	337
Grapefruit juice-raw	Cup	247	96	1.24	22.7	0.25	0	0.035	0.032	0.059	2	400
Grapefruit-raw-pink/red	Item	246	74	1.36	18.5	0.246	0	0.034	0.032	0.06	0	312
Grapefruit-raw-white	Item	236	78	1.63	19.8	0.24	0	0.034	0.03	0.057	0	350
Kiwifruit-raw	Item	76	46	0.75	11.3	0.34	0	0	0	0	4	252
Lemonade-froz-diluted	Cup	248	105	0	28	0	0	0	0	0	0	40
Lemon juice-can/bottle	Cup	244	52	0.98	15.8	0.7	0	0.093	0.027	0.207	50	248
Lemon juice-raw	Cup	244	60	0.92	21.1	0	0	0	0	0	2	303
Lemons-raw-peeled	Item	58	17	0.64	5.41	0.17	0	0.023	0.006	0.052	1	80
Lime juice-can/bottle	Cup	246	51	0.61	16.5	0.57	0	0.064	0.054	0.157	39	185
Lime juice-raw	Cup	246	66	1.08	22.2	0.25	0	0.027	0.025	0.066	2	268
Limes-raw	Item	67	20	0.47	7.06	0.13	0	0.015	0.013	0.037	1	68
Melons-cantaloupe-raw	Cup	160	57	1.4	13.4	0.44	0	0	0	0	14	494
Melons-casaba-raw	Cup	170	45	1.53	10.5	0.17	0	0	0	0	20	357
Melons-honeydew-raw	Cup	170	60	0.77	15.6	0.17	0	0	0	0	17	461
Nectarines-raw	Item	136	67	1.28	16	0.62	0	—	—	—	0	288
Orange juice-can	Cup	249	104	1.46	24.5	0.36	0	0.045	0.062	0.085	6	436
Orange juice-froz-diluted	Cup	249	112	1.68	26.8	0.14	0	0.017	0.025	0.03	2	474
Orange juice-raw	Cup	248	111	1.74	25.8	0.5	0	0.06	0.089	0.099	2	496
Oranges-raw-all varieties	Item	131	62	1.23	15.4	0.16	0	0.02	0.03	0.033	0	237
Papaya nectar-can	Cup	250	142	0.43	36.3	0.38	0	0.118	0.103	0.088	14	78
Papayas-raw	Cup	140	54	0.86	13.7	0.2	0	0.06	0.053	0.043	4	359
Peaches-can/water pack	Cup	244	58	1.07	14.9	0.14	0	0.015	0.051	0.068	8	241
Peaches-dried-ckd-unsweet	Cup	258	198	2.99	50.8	0.63	0	0.067	0.23	0.304	6	825
Peaches-dried-unckd	Cup	160	383	5.77	98.1	1.22	0	0.131	0.445	0.587	12	1594
Peaches-froz-sliced-sweet	Cup	250	235	1.56	59.9	0.33	0	0.035	0.12	0.16	16	325
Peaches-raw-sliced	Cup	170	73	1.19	18.9	0.16	0	0.017	0.058	0.077	1	334
Peaches-raw-whole	Item	87	37	0.61	9.65	0.08	0	0.009	0.03	0.039	0	171
Pears-can/juice	Cup	248	123	0.85	32.1	0.16	0	0.01	0.035	0.037	10	238
Pears-raw-bartlett-unpeeled	Item	166	98	0.65	25.1	0.66	0	0.037	0.139	0.156	1	208
Pineapple-can/juice	Cup	250	150	1.04	39.2	0.21	0	0.015	0.025	0.073	4	304
Pineapple juice-can	Cup	250	139	0.8	34.4	0.2	0	0.013	0.023	0.07	2	334
Pineapple juice-froz-diluted	Cup	250	129	1	31.9	0.08	0	0.005	0.008	0.025	3	340
Pineapple-raw-diced	Cup	155	77	0.6	19.2	0.66	0	0.05	0.074	0.226	1	175
Plums-raw-prune type	Item	28.4	20	0	6	0	0	0	0	0	0	48
Pomegranates-raw	Item	154	104	1.47	26.4	0.46	0	—	—	—	5	399
Prune juice-can/bottle	Cup	256	181	1.55	44.7	0.08	0	0.008	0.054	0.018	11	706
Prunes-dried-unckd	Cup	161	385	4.2	101	0.83	0	0.066	0.547	0.18	6	1200
Raisins-seedless	Cup	145	434	4.67	115	0.67	0	0.218	0.026	0.196	17	1089
Raisins-seedless-packet	Item	14	42	0.451	11.1	0.064	0	0.021	0.003	0.019	1.68	105
Raspberries-raw	Cup	123	61	1.11	14.2	0.68	0	0.023	0.065	0.385	0	187
Rhubarb-raw-ckd-sugar	Cup	270	380	1	97	0	0	0	0	0	5	548
Strawberries-froz-unsweet	Cup	149	52	0.63	13.6	0.16	0	0.009	0.022	0.08	3	220
Strawberries-raw-whole	Cup	149	45	0.91	10.5	0.55	0	0.03	0.077	0.277	2	247
Tangerines-raw-peeled	Item	84	37	0.53	9.4	0.16	0	0.018	0.029	0.031	1	132
Watermelon-raw	Cup	160	50	0.99	11.5	0.68	0	—	—	—	3	186
Grains												
Bisquick mix-dry	Cup	112	480	8	76	16	—	—	—	—	1400	—
Corn chips	oz	28.4	155	1.7	16.9	9.14	0	1.5	3.39	4.25	164	43.3
Cornmeal-degerm-enr-ckd	Cup	240	125	2.88	26.4	0.56	0	0.076	0.14	0.241	1	55
Croutons-herb seasoned	Cup	30	100	4.29	20	0	0	0	0	0	372	38.6

Mag (mg)	Iron (mg)	Zinc (mg)	VA (RE)	VC (mg)	Thia (mg)	Ribo (mg)	Niac (mg)	VB_6 (mg)	Fol (μg)	VB_{12} (μg)	Calc (mg)	Phos (mg)	Sel (mg)	Fibd (g)	VE (mg)
—	—	—	—	—	—	—	—	—	—	—	—	—	—	—	—
24	0.6	0.13	2	0.2	0.066	0.094	0.663	0.164	6.5	0	22	27	0.001	0	—
11	0.26	0.1	1.9	59.7	0.038	0.065	0.31	0.105	3.1	0	9	11	0.001	0	—
24	0.89	0.15	0	67.3	0.1	0.058	0.798	0.05	25.9	0	20	27	0.001	0	0.1
24	0.5	0.21	1.8	72	0.104	0.049	0.571	0.049	25.6	0	18	27	0.001	0.442	0.099
26	0.34	0.13	2.2	83.4	0.101	0.054	0.536	0.109	8.9	0	19	34	0.001	0	0.099
30	0.49	0.13	2.47	93.9	0.099	0.049	0.494	—	51.2	0	22	37	0.001	0.5	0.098
20	0.3	0.18	63.7	91	0.098	0.05	0.492	0.104	23.1	0	36	22	0.001	3.2	0.615
21.2	0.142	0.165	2.4	78.6	0.088	0.048	0.634	0.102	23.6	0	28	18	0.001	2.5	0.59
23	0.31	—	13.3	74.5	0.015	0.038	0.38	—	—	0	20	31	—	2.58	—
—	0.1	—	1	17	0.01	0.02	0.2	—	12	—	2	3	0.001	0.56	—
20	0.31	0.15	3.7	60.4	0.1	0.022	0.481	0.105	24.6	0	26	21	0.001	0.732	—
16	0.08	0.12	4.9	112	0.073	0.024	0.244	0.124	31.5	0	18	14	0.001	0.732	—
—	0.35	0.04	1.7	30.7	0.023	0.012	0.058	0.046	6.2	0	15	9	0.001	0.58	—
16	0.56	0.15	4	15.7	0.081	0.007	0.401	0.066	19.5	0	30	24	0.001	0	—
14	0.08	0.15	2.5	72.1	0.049	0.025	0.246	0.106	—	0	22	18	—	0	—
—	0.4	0.07	0.7	19.5	0.02	0.013	0.134	—	5.5	0	22	12	0.001	0.353	—
17	0.34	0.25	516	67.5	0.058	0.034	0.918	0.184	27.3	0	17	27	0.001	1.28	0.224
14	0.68	—	5.1	27.2	0.102	0.034	0.68	—	—	0	9	12	0.001	2	0.238
12	0.12	—	6.8	42.1	0.131	0.031	1.02	0.1	—	0	10	17	0.001	1.53	0.238
11	0.21	0.12	100	7.3	0.023	0.056	1.35	0.034	5.1	0	6	22	0.001	2.18	—
27	1.1	0.17	43.7	85.7	0.149	0.07	0.782	0.219	136	0	21	36	0.001	0.26	0.1
24	0.24	0.13	19.4	96.9	0.197	0.045	0.503	0.11	109	0	22	40	0.001	0.498	0.1
27	0.5	0.13	49.6	124	0.223	0.074	0.992	0.099	136	0	27	42	0.001	1.98	0.099
13	0.13	0.09	26.9	69.7	0.114	0.052	0.369	0.079	39.7	0	52	18	0.002	3.14	0.314
8	0.86	0.38	27.7	7.5	0.015	0.01	0.375	0.023	5.2	0	24	1	0.001	0.125	—
14	0.14	0.1	282	86.5	0.038	0.045	0.473	0.027	—	0	33	7	0.001	1.27	—
12	0.77	0.22	130	7	0.022	0.046	1.27	0.046	8.2	0	6	25	0.001	1.08	—
35	3.37	0.47	50.8	9.5	0.013	0.054	3.92	0.098	0.2	0	23	99	0.001	6.7	—
67	6.5	0.92	346	7.7	0.003	0.339	7	0.107	10.6	0	45	191	0.001	14	—
12	0.93	0.13	70.9	235	0.033	0.088	1.63	0.045	—	0	6	28	0.001	5.99	—
11	0.19	0.23	91	11.2	0.029	0.07	1.68	0.031	5.8	0	9	21	0.001	2.72	0.17
6	0.1	0.12	46.5	5.7	0.015	0.036	0.861	0.016	3	0	5	11	0.001	1.39	0.087
17	0.71	0.22	1.4	4	0.027	0.027	0.496	—	—	0	21	29	0.001	4.71	—
9	0.41	0.2	3.3	6.6	0.033	0.066	0.166	0.03	12.1	0	19	18	0.001	4.32	0.82
35	0.7	0.24	9.5	23.8	0.238	0.048	0.71	—	—	0	34	16	0.002	1.88	0.25
34	0.65	0.29	1.2	26.7	0.138	0.055	0.643	0.24	57.7	0	42	20	0.002	0.25	—
23	0.75	0.29	2.5	30	0.175	0.05	0.5	0.185	—	0	28	20	0.002	0.3	—
21	0.57	0.12	3.5	23.9	0.143	0.056	0.651	0.135	16.4	0	11	11	0.001	1.86	0.155
1.96	0.1	0.028	8	1	0.01	0.01	0.1	0.023	0.616	0	3	5	0	0.588	0.196
—	0.46	—	—	9.4	0.046	0.046	0.462	0.162	—	0	5	12	0.001	1.1	—
36	3.03	0.52	0.9	10.6	0.041	0.179	2.01	—	1	0	30	64	0.001	2.56	—
73	3.99	0.85	320	5.4	0.13	0.261	3.16	0.425	5.9	0	82	127	0.001	11	—
48	3.02	0.38	1.1	4.8	0.226	0.128	1.19	0.361	4.8	0	71	140	0.001	7.69	1.02
4.62	0.291	0.039	0.112	0.462	0.022	0.012	0.115	0.035	0.462	0	6.86	13.6	0	0.742	0.098
22	0.7	0.57	16	30.8	0.037	0.111	1.11	0.07	6	0	27	15	0.001	5.5	0.369
32.4	1.6	0.216	22	16	0.05	0.14	0.8	0.054	14.3	0	211	41	0.001	5.4	0.54
16	1.12	0.19	6.6	61.4	0.033	0.055	0.688	0.042	25	0	23	20	0.001	3.9	0.313
16	0.57	0.19	4.1	84.5	0.03	0.098	0.343	0.088	26.4	0	21	28	0.001	3.87	0.179
10	0.09	—	77.3	25.9	0.088	0.018	0.134	0.056	17.1	0	12	8	0.001	1.68	—
17	0.28	0.11	58.5	15.4	0.128	0.032	0.32	0.23	3.4	0	13	14	0.001	0.64	—
—	—	—	—	—	—	—	—	—	—	—	—	—	—	3.02	0.302
21.9	0.376	0.435	—	—	0.048	0.026	0.554	0.054	—	0	37.1	54.6	0.002	1.66	—
14	1.4	0.24	14	0	0.243	0.138	1.71	0.087	16	0	2	29	0.006	0.7	0.192
11.4	1.54	0.3	0	—	0.129	0.2	1.72	0	0	—	—	—	—	1.41	—

Continued.

Key to Abbreviations
Kcal, Kcalories; *Prot,* protein; *Carb,* carbohydrate; *Fat,* fat; *Chol,* cholesterol; *Safa,* saturated fat; *Mufa,* monounsaturated fat; *Pufa,* polyunsaturated fat; *Sod,* sodium; *Pot,* potassium; *Mag,* magnesium; *Iron,* iron; *Zinc,* zinc; *VA,* vitamin A; *VC,* vitamin C; *Thia,* thiamin; *Ribo,* riboflavin; *Niac,* niacin; *VB6,* vitamin B_6; *Fol,* folate; *VB12,* vitamin B_{12}; *Calc,* calcium; *Phos,* phosphorus; *Sel,* selenium; *Fibd,* dietary fiber; and *VE,* vitamin E.

Food name	Portion	Wt (g)	Kcal	Prot (g)	Carb (g)	Fat (g)	Chol (mg)	Safa (g)	Mufa (g)	Pufa (g)	Sod (mg)	Pot (mg)
Grains—cont'd												
Flour-wheat-enr-sifted	Cup	115	419	11.9	87.7	1.12	0	0.178	0.1	0.475	1.84	123
Macaroni-ckd-firm-hot	Cup	130	183	6.2	36.9	0.865	0	0.124	0.102	0.355	0.93	40.9
Noodles-egg-enr-ckd	Cup	160	200	7	37	2	50	—	—	—	3	70
Noodles-ramen-oriental	Cup	227	207	5.9	30.7	8.6	—	—	—	—	829	—
Popcorn-popped-plain	Cup	6	25	1	5	0	0	0	0	0	0	—
Popcorn-popped-sugar coat	Cup	35	135	2	30	1	0	0.5	0.2	0.4	0	—
Potato pancakes-home rec	Item	76	495	4.63	26.4	12.6	93	3.42	5.35	2.54	388	538
Pretzel-thin-stick	Item	0.3	1.19	0.028	0.242	0.011	0	0	0	0	4.83	0.303
Rice cake-regular	Item	9.31	35	0.7	7.6	0.28	0	—	—	—	10.8	27.2
Rice-brown-Uncle Ben's	Cup	146	220	5	46.4	1.82	0	0.462	0.425	0.616	2.4	172
Rice-Spanish-home rec	Cup	245	213	4.4	40.7	4.2	0	—	—	—	774	566
Rice-white-instant-hot	Cup	165	161	3.4	35.1	0.27	0	0.073	0.084	0.072	4	7
Rice-white-long grain-ckd	Cup	205	264	5.51	57.2	0.58	0	0.158	0.181	0.155	4	80
Rice-white-parboil-ckd	Cup	175	199	4.01	43.3	0.47	0	0.128	0.147	0.126	6	66
Shake n Bake	oz	28.4	116	2.44	17.7	4.26	—	—	—	—	984	56.8
Spaghetti-cdk-tender-hot	Cup	140	155	5	32	1	0	—	—	—	1	85
Stuffing-mix-dry form	Cup	30	111	3.9	21.7	1.1	—	—	—	—	399	52
Stuffing-mix-prep	Cup	140	501	9.1	49.8	30.5	—	—	—	—	1254	126
Taco shells	Item	11	49.8	0.967	7.24	2.15	0	—	—	—	—	—
Tortilla chips-Doritos	oz	28.4	139	2	18.6	6.6	0	1.43	3.19	1.77	180	51
Tortilla-corn	Item	30	67.2	2.15	12.8	1.14	0	—	—	—	53.4	52.2
Tortilla-flour	Item	30	95	2.5	17.3	1.8	0	—	—	—	—	—
Meats												
Bacon bits	Tbsp	6	26.6	1.92	1.72	1.55	0	—	—	—	165	—
Bacon-pork-broiled/fried	Slice	6.3	36.3	1.93	0.036	3.12	5.33	1.1	1.5	0.367	101	30.7
Beef-liver-fried/marg	Slice	85	184	22.7	6.68	6.8	410	2.4	1.46	1.53	90	309
Bologna-pork	Slice	23	57	3.52	0.17	4.57	14	1.58	2.25	0.49	272	65
Braunschweiger-saus-pork	Slice	18	65	2.43	0.56	5.78	28	1.96	2.68	0.67	206	36
Canadian bacon-pork-grill	Slice	23.3	43	5.64	0.315	1.96	13.5	0.66	0.94	0.185	360	90.5
Corned beef hash-can	Cup	220	400	19	24	25	50	11.9	10.9	0.5	1188	440
Deviled ham-can	Tbsp	13	45	2	0	4	10	1.5	1.8	0.4	160	—
Frankfurter-hot dog-no bun	Item	57	183	6.43	1.46	16.6	29	6.13	7.79	1.56	639	95
Ham-reg-lunch meat-11% fat	Slice	28.4	52	4.98	0.88	3	16	0.96	1.4	0.34	373	94
Ham-reg-roasted-pork	Cup	140	249	31.7	0	12.6	83	4.36	6.22	1.98	2100	573
Hamburger-ground-reg-baked	Serving	85	244	19.6	0	17.8	74	6.99	7.79	0.66	51	188
Hamburger-ground-reg-fried	Serving	85	260	20.3	0	19.2	75	7.53	8.39	0.71	71	255
Italian sausage-pork-link	Item	67	217	13.4	1.01	17.2	52	6.05	8.01	2.2	618	204
Kielbasa-pork/beef	Slice	26	81	3.45	0.56	7.06	17	2.58	3.36	0.8	280	70
Knockwurst-pork/beef-link	Item	68	209	8.08	1.2	18.9	39	6.94	8.71	1.98	687	136
Lamb-chop-lean/fat-broiled	Item	85	307	18.8	0	25.2	84	10.8	10.3	2.02	64	230
Lamb-chop/rib-lean-broiled	Item	57	134	15.8	0	7.38	51.9	2.65	2.97	0.673	48.5	178
Lamb-leg-lean/fat-roast	Slice	85	219	21.7	0	14	79	5.85	5.92	1.01	56	266
Liverwurst/liver saus-pork	Slice	18	59	2.54	0.4	5.14	28	1.91	2.4	0.47	215	—
Mortadella-pork/beef	Slice	15	47	2.46	0.46	3.81	8	1.43	1.71	0.47	187	24
Polish sausage-pork	Item	227	740	32	3.7	65.2	159	23.4	30.6	6.99	1989	538
Pork-chop-lean-broiled	Item	66	169	18.4	0	10.1	63	3.48	4.53	1.23	49	276
Pork-chop-lean/fat-broiled	Item	82	284	19.3	0	22.3	77	8.06	10.2	2.53	54	287
Pork-loin-lean-roast	Slice	72	180	21.4	0	9.81	68	3.38	4.41	1.19	52	271
Pork-loin-lean/fat-roast	Item	88	268	22.4	0	19.1	80	6.92	8.76	2.18	56	284
Pork-tenderloin-lean-roast	oz	28.4	47	8.16	0	1.36	26.3	0.47	0.613	0.163	19	152
Pot roast-arm-beef-ckd	Slice	100	231	33	0	9.98	101	3.79	4.35	0.4	66	289
Roast beef-rib-lean	Slice	51	122	13.9	0	7.03	41.3	2.96	3.06	0.209	37.7	192
Roast beef-rib-lean/fat	Slice	85	308	18.3	0	25.5	73	10.8	11.4	0.9	52	257
Salami-ckd-beef	Slice	23	58	3.38	0.57	4.62	14	1.94	2.14	0.2	266	52
Salami-dry or hard-pork	Slice	10	41	2.26	0.16	3.37	8	1.19	1.6	0.37	226	—
Sausage-link-pork-ckd	Item	13	48	2.55	0.13	4.05	11	1.4	1.81	0.5	168	47

Mag (mg)	Iron (mg)	Zinc (mg)	VA (RE)	VC (mg)	Thia (mg)	Ribo (mg)	Niac (mg)	VB_6 (mg)	Fol (μg)	VB_{12} (μg)	Calc (mg)	Phos (mg)	Sel (mg)	Fibd (g)	VE (mg)
24.8	5.34	0.81	—	0	0.903	0.569	6.79	0.051	30.4	0	16.6	124	0.005	3.11	0.046
23.3	1.82	0.688	—	0	0.266	0.127	2.18	0.046	0.93	0	0.93	70.7	0.032	2.08	0.026
43.2	1.4	—	11	0	0.22	0.13	1.9	0.141	19.2	0	16	94	0.094	3.52	—
—	—	—	—	—	—	—	—	—	—	—	—	—	—	2.04	—
—	0.2	0.5	—	0	—	0.01	0.1	0.012	—	0	1	17	0.001	0.4	—
—	0.5	—	—	0	—	0.02	0.4	—	—	—	2	47	0.007	1.35	—
24	1.21	0.68	8.9	0.4	0.104	0.095	1.61	0.29	21.5	0.217	21	78	—	—	—
0.072	0.006	0.003	0	0	0.001	0.001	0.013	0	0.048	0	0.078	0.273	—	—	0
—	—	—	—	—	—	—	—	—	—	—	—	—	—	0.158	—
—	0.9	—	0	0	0.18	0.04	4.2	—	—	—	16	222	0.057	2.48	0.993
—	1.5	—	162	37	0.1	0.07	1.7	—	—	—	34	96	—	1.83	—
9	1.04	0.4	—	0	0.124	0.076	1.45	0.016	6	0	13	23	0.033	1.32	0.182
26	2.25	0.94	—	0	0.334	0.027	3.03	0.191	7	0	23	95	0.041	2.13	0.226
20	1.97	0.53	—	0	0.437	0.031	2.45	0.033	6	0	33	73	0.035	0.875	0.193
—	0.71	—	62	0.284	0.162	0.184	2.19	—	—	—	13.9	43.5	—	—	—
23.8	1.3	0.7	0	0	0.2	0.11	1.5	0.09	16.8	0	11	70	0.085	2.24	0.084
—	1	—	0	0	0.07	0.08	1	—	—	—	37	57	—	—	—
—	22	—	91	0	0.13	0.17	2.1	—	—	—	92	136	—	—	—
11.4	0.286	0.142	—	—	0.032	0.017	0.189	—	—	0	15.6	25.4	—	0.88	—
21	0.5	0.24	5.2	0	0.03	0.03	0.04	0.1	4	—	30	59	—	1.85	—
19.5	0.57	0.426	—	0	0.048	0.03	0.384	0.091	5.7	0	42	54.9	0.002	1.56	—
7	1.1	—	0.2	0	0.01	0.08	1	—	—	—	46	25	0.005	0.778	—
—	0.3	—	0	0.18	0.025	0.018	0.138	—	—	—	8.4	18.1	—	—	—
1.67	0.103	0.206	0	2.13	0.044	0.018	0.464	0.017	0.333	0.11	0.667	21.3	0.001	0	0.033
20	5.34	4.63	9216	19.4	0.179	3.52	12.3	1.22	187	95	9	392	0.048	0	0.536
3	0.18	0.47	—	8.1	0.12	0.036	0.897	0.06	1	0.21	3	32	0.004	0	0.014
2	1.68	0.51	759	2	0.045	0.275	1.51	0.06	—	3.62	2	30	0.002	0	0.063
5	0.19	0.395	0	5	0.192	0.046	1.61	0.105	1	0.18	2.5	69	0.003	0	—
—	4.4	—	—	—	0.02	0.2	4.6	—	—	—	29	147	—	—	0.066
1.69	0.3	0.238	0	—	0.2	0.01	0.2	0.042	—	0.091	1	12	0.002	0	—
6	0.66	1.05	—	15	0.113	0.068	1.5	0.08	2	0.74	6	49	0.005	0	0.08
5	0.28	0.61	0	8	0.244	0.071	1.49	0.1	1	0.24	2	70	0.013	0	—
30	1.88	3.46	0	31.7	1.02	0.462	8.61	0.43	—	0.98	12	393	0.066	0	0.392
13	2.05	4.16	—	0	0.026	0.136	4.04	0.2	7	1.99	8	117	—	0	0.315
17	2.08	4.31	—	0	0.026	0.17	4.96	0.2	8	2.3	10	145	—	0	0.315
12	1.01	1.59	—	1.3	0.417	0.156	2.79	0.22	—	0.87	16	114	0.022	0	0.107
4	0.38	0.52	—	6	0.059	0.056	0.749	0.05	—	0.42	11	38	0.004	0	0.042
8	0.62	1.13	—	18	0.233	0.095	1.86	0.11	—	0.8	7	67	0.01	0	—
20	1.6	3.4	—	—	0.08	0.19	5.95	0.09	12	2.16	16	151	0.014	0	0.142
16.5	1.26	3	—	—	0.057	0.143	3.73	0.086	12	1.5	9.12	121	0.01	0	0.091
20	1.69	3.74	—	—	0.09	0.23	5.6	0.13	17	2.2	9	162	0.014	0	0.043
—	1.15	—	—	—	0.049	0.185	—	0.03	5	2.42	5	41	0.003	0	0.063
2	0.21	0.32	—	4	0.018	0.023	0.401	0.019	—	0.22	3	15	0.002	0	0.024
31.8	3.27	4.38	—	2.27	1.14	0.336	7.82	0.431	—	2.22	27.2	309	0.066	0	0.363
19	0.61	1.93	1.5	0.2	0.641	0.278	3.93	0.3	4	0.71	5	184	0.011	0	0.106
20	0.66	2.01	2.1	0.2	0.69	0.294	4.32	0.31	4	0.81	5	193	0.014	0	0.131
16	0.82	1.71	1.8	0.3	0.681	0.196	4.09	0.34	0.72	0.45	4	164	0.023	0	0.114
17	0.87	1.8	2.1	0.3	0.727	0.21	4.44	0.35	1	0.53	5	173	0.028	0	0.139
7	0.437	0.85	0.601	0.1	0.266	0.111	1.33	0.12	1.67	0.157	2.33	81.7	0.009	0	0.113
24	3.79	8.66	0	0	0.081	0.289	3.72	0.33	11	3.4	9	268	0.006	0	0.14
12.8	1.33	3.54	0	0	0.042	0.107	2.1	0.153	4.08	1.49	5.1	109	0.012	0	0.092
17	1.77	4.27	0	0	0.065	0.146	2.65	0.25	5	2.37	10	140	0.02	0	0.119
3	0.46	0.49	—	3	0.029	0.059	0.785	0.05	0.46	1.11	2	23	0.004	0	0.025
2	0.13	0.42	—	—	0.093	0.033	0.56	0.06	—	0.28	1	23	0.002	0	0.011
2	0.16	0.33	—	0	0.096	0.033	0.587	0.04	—	0.22	4	24	0.004	0	0.021

Continued.

Key to Abbreviations
Kcal, Kcalories; *Prot,* protein; *Carb,* carbohydrate; *Fat,* fat; *Chol,* cholesterol; *Safa,* saturated fat; *Mufa,* monounsaturated fat; *Pufa,* polyunsaturated fat; *Sod,* sodium; *Pot,* potassium; *Mag,* magnesium; *Iron,* iron; *Zinc,* zinc; *VA,* vitamin A; *VC,* vitamin C; *Thia,* thiamin; *Ribo,* riboflavin; *Niac,* niacin; *VB6,* vitamin B_6; *Fol,* folate; *VB12,* vitamin B_{12}; *Calc,* calcium; *Phos,* phosphorus; *Sel,* selenium; *Fibd,* dietary fiber; and *VE,* vitamin E.

Food name	Portion	Wt (g)	Kcal	Prot (g)	Carb (g)	Fat (g)	Chol (mg)	Safa (g)	Mufa (g)	Pufa (g)	Sod (mg)	Pot (mg)
Meats—cont'd												
Sausage-patty-pork-ckd	Item	27	100	5.31	0.28	8.41	22	2.92	3.75	1.03	349	97
Spareribs-pork-braised	oz	28.4	113	8.23	0	8.58	34.3	3.33	4.01	0.997	26.3	90.7
Steak-chicken fried	Item	100	389	17.9	12.3	30	—	—	—	—	815	126
Steak-rib-ckd	Item	100	225	28	0	11.6	80	4.93	5.1	0.35	69	394
Steak-round-lean/fat	Slice	85	179	26.2	0	7.49	72	2.8	3.08	0.33	51	365
Steak-sirloin-lean-broiled	Item	56	133	17	0	6.63	50	2.71	2.92	0.28	37	226
Steak-sirloin-lean/fat	Item	85	271	22.7	0	19.4	77	8.07	8.67	0.77	52	297
Miscellaneous												
Baking powder-home use	Tsp	3	3.87	0.003	0.936	0	0	0	0	0	329	4.5
Baking powder-low sodium	Tsp	4.3	7.4	0.004	1.79	0	0	0	—	—	0.258	471
Baking soda	Tsp	3	0	0	0	0	0	0	0	0	821	—
Chewing gum-candy coated	Item	1.7	5	—	1.6	—	0	0	0	0	—	—
Chewing gum-Wrigleys	Item	3	10	0	2.3	—	0	0	0	0	0	0
Pickle relish-sweet	Tbsp	15	20	0	5	0	0	0	0	0	124	—
Pickle/hamburger relish	oz	28.4	30	0	7	0	0	0	0	0	325	—
Pickle/hot dog relish	oz	28.4	35	0	8	0	0	0	0	0	200	—
Vinegar-cider	Tbsp	15	0	0	1	0	0	0	0	0	0.125	15
Vinegar-distilled	Cup	240	29	0	12	0	0	0	0	0	2	36
Yeast-baker-dry-act-packet	Serving	7	20	3	3	0	0	0	0	0	1	140
Yeast-brewers-dry	Tbsp	8	25	3	3	0	0	0	0	0	9	152
Nuts and seeds												
Nut-filbert/hazel-dri-chop	Cup	115	727	15	17.6	72	0	5.3	56.5	6.9	3	512
Nut-walnut-Persian/English	Cup	120	770	17.2	22	74.2	0	6.7	17	47	12	602
Nuts-almond-shelled-sliver	Cup	115	677	22.9	23.5	60	0	5.69	39	12.6	12.7	842
Nuts-brazil-dried-shelled	Cup	140	919	20.1	17.9	92.7	0	22.6	32.2	33.8	2	840
Nuts-cashews-dry roast	Cup	137	787	21	44.8	63.5	0	12.5	37.4	10.7	21	774
Nuts-chestnuts-roast	oz	28.4	68	1.27	14.9	0.34	0	0.05	0.176	0.087	1	135
Nuts-coconut cream-raw	Cup	240	792	8.7	16	83.2	0	73.8	3.54	0.91	10	781
Nuts-coconut-dri-flake-can	Cup	77	341	2.58	31.5	24.4	0	21.6	1.04	0.267	15	249
Nuts-coconut-dried-shred	Cup	93	466	2.68	44.3	33	0	29.3	1.4	0.361	244	313
Nuts-macadamia-dried	Cup	134	940	11.1	18.4	98.8	0	14.8	77.9	1.7	6	493
Nuts-mixed-dry roast	Cup	137	814	23.7	34.7	70.5	0	9.45	43	14.8	16	817
Nuts-mixed-oil roast	Cup	142	876	23.8	30.4	80	0	12.4	45	18.9	16	825
Nuts-peanuts-oil roast	Cup	145	840	38.8	26.7	71.3	0	9.9	35.5	22.6	22	1020
Nuts-peanuts-oil-salted	Cup	145	841	38.8	26.8	71.3	0	9.93	35.5	22.6	626	1020
Nuts-peanuts-Spanish-dried	Cup	146	827	37.5	23.6	71.8	0	9.96	35.6	22.7	23	1047
Nuts-Pecans-dried-halves	Cup	108	721	8.37	19.7	73.1	0	5.85	45.5	18.1	1	423
Nuts-pecans-oil roast	Cup	110	754	7.65	17.7	78.3	0	6.27	48.8	19.4	1	395
Nuts-pistachio-dri	Cup	128	739	26.3	31.8	61.9	0	7.84	41.8	9.36	7	1399
Nuts-pistachio-dry roast	Cup	128	776	19.1	35.2	67.6	0	8.56	45.6	10.2	8	1242
Nuts-walnut-black-dried-chop	Cup	125	759	30.4	15.1	70.7	0	4.54	15.9	46.9	2	655
Peanut butter-chunk style	Tbsp	16.1	95	3.88	3.48	8.07	0	1.54	3.8	2.31	78.5	121
Peanut butter-low sodium	Tbsp	16	95	5	2.5	8.5	0	1.36	3.95	2.46	5	110
Peanut butter-old fashion	Tbsp	16	95	4.2	2.7	8.1	0	1.5	—	2.7	75	110
Peanut butter-smooth type	Tbsp	16	95	4.56	2.53	8.18	0	1.36	3.95	2.46	75	110
Seeds-pumpkin/squash-roast	Cup	64	285	11.9	34.4	12.4	0	2.35	3.86	5.66	12	588
Seeds-sesame-roast-whole	oz	28.4	161	4.82	7.31	13.6	0	1.91	5.15	5.98	3	135
Seeds-sunflower-oil roast	Cup	135	830	28.8	19.9	77.6	0	8.13	14.8	51.2	4	652
Poultry												
Chicken-breast-no skin-roast	Item	172	284	53.4	0	6.14	146	1.74	2.14	1.32	126	440
Chicken-thigh-no skin-roast	Item	52	109	13.5	0	5.66	49	1.57	2.16	1.29	46	124
Chicken roll-light	Slice	28.4	45	5.54	0.695	2.09	14	0.575	0.84	0.455	166	64.5
Chicken spread-can	Tbsp	13	25	2	0.7	1.52	—	—	—	—	—	—
Breast-fried/batter	Item	280	728	69.6	25.2	36.9	238	9.86	15.3	8.62	770	564

Mag (mg)	Iron (mg)	Zinc (mg)	VA (RE)	VC (mg)	Thia (mg)	Ribo (mg)	Niac (mg)	VB_6 (mg)	Fol (μg)	VB_{12} (μg)	Calc (mg)	Phos (mg)	Sel (mg)	Fibd (g)	VE (mg)
5	0.34	0.68	—	0	0.2	0.069	1.22	0.09	—	0.47	9	50	0.003	0	0.043
7	0.527	1.3	0.901	—	0.116	0.108	1.55	0.1	1.33	0.307	13.3	74	0.005	0	0.045
—	2.3	—	7.81	—	0.11	0.14	2.7	—	—	—	11	110	—	0	0.13
27	2.57	6.99	0	0	0.105	0.216	4.8	0.4	8	3.32	13	208	0.006	0	0.092
26	2.39	4.59	0	0	0.097	0.221	4.98	0.46	10	2.08	5	203	0.029	0	0.111
17.9	1.88	3.65	3	0	0.071	0.165	2.4	0.252	5.6	1.6	6.16	137	0.019	0	0.073
23	2.49	4.73	15	0	0.092	0.218	3.21	0.33	7	2.22	9	180	0.029	0	0.111
—	0	—	0	0	0	0	0	—	—	—	58	87.1	—	—	—
—	0	—	0	0	0	0	0	—	—	—	207	314	—	—	—
—	—	—	—	0	0	0	0	0	0	0	—	—	—	0	—
—	—	—	—	0	0	0	0	—	—	—	—	—	—	—	—
0	0	0	0	0	0	0	0	0	0	0	3	0	—	—	—
—	0.1	0.01	—	—	—	—	—	—	—	—	3	2	0	—	—
—	0.189	—	—	—	—	—	—	—	—	—	5.67	3.78	0	—	—
—	0.189	—	—	—	—	—	—	—	—	—	5.6	3.7	0	—	—
—	0.1	0.02	—	—	—	—	—	0	—	—	1	1	0.013	0	—
0	—	—	—	—	—	—	—	—	—	—	—	—	0.074	0	—
3.78	1.1	—	0	0	0.16	0.38	2.6	0.14	286	0	3	90	0	2.21	0.006
18.4	1.4	—	0	0	1.25	0.34	3	0.2	313	0	17	140	0	—	—
328	3.76	2.76	7.7	1.2	0.575	0.127	1.3	0.704	82.6	0	216	359	0.002	9.77	27.3
203	2.93	3.28	14.8	3.9	0.458	0.178	1.25	0.67	79.2	0	113	380	0.023	5.76	3.14
340	4.21	3.36	0	0.69	0.243	0.896	3.87	0.13	67.5	0	306	598	0.005	10.7	27.6
315	4.76	6.42	—	1	1.4	0.171	2.27	0.351	5.6	0	246	840	2.26	10.8	8.97
356	8.22	7.67	0	0	0.274	0.274	1.92	0.351	94.8	0	62	671	0.007	10	0.781
26	0.43	0.26	0.1	—	0.043	0.026	0.426	—	—	0	5	29	0.002	2.19	0.142
—	5.47	2.3	0	6.7	0.072	0	2.14	—	—	0	26	293	—	1.6	—
38	1.42	1.23	0	0	0.023	0.015	0.235	—	—	0	11	79	—	4.4	0.539
47	1.78	1.69	0	0.6	0.029	0.019	0.441	—	—	0	14	99	0.016	3.9	0.651
155	3.23	2.29	0	—	0.469	0.147	2.87	—	—	0	94	183	0.007	12.4	—
308	5.07	5.21	2.1	0.6	0.274	0.274	6.44	0.406	69	0	96	596	0.007	11.6	—
333	4.56	7.22	2.8	0.7	0.707	0.315	7.19	0.341	118	0	153	659	0.007	12.8	—
273	2.78	9.6	0	0	0.425	0.146	21.5	0.576	153	0	125	733	0.055	12.8	9.99
273	2.78	9.6	0	0	0.425	0.146	21.5	0.577	153	0	125	733	0.055	12.8	10.1
262	4.71	4.78	0	0	0.969	0.191	20.7	0.432	147	0	85	560	0.007	11.7	11.4
138	2.3	5.91	13.8	2.1	0.916	0.138	0.958	0.203	42.3	0	39	314	0.003	8.3	3.35
142	2.33	6.05	—	—	—	—	—	—	—	0	37	324	0.006	8.47	1.36
203	8.67	1.71	29.9	—	1.05	0.223	1.38	—	74.2	0	173	644	0.007	13.8	6.67
166	4.06	1.74	—	—	0.541	0.315	1.8	—	—	0	90	609	0.007	13.8	6.67
252	3.84	4.28	37	—	0.271	0.136	0.863	—	—	—	72	580	0.024	8.08	1.05
25.6	0.306	0.448	0	0	0.02	0.018	2.21	0.073	14.8	0	6.56	51.1	0.001	1.06	0.969
28	0.29	0.47	—	0	0.024	0.017	2.15	0.062	13.1	0	5	60	0.002	1.7	1.12
30	0.3	0.5	—	—	0.01	0.01	2.3	—	—	—	5	60	0.002	1.06	0.96
28	0.29	0.47	—	0	0.024	0.017	2.15	0.062	13.1	0	5	60	0.002	0.96	1.12
168	2.12	6.59	—	—	—	—	—	—	—	0	35	59	—	29.4	—
101	4.19	2.03	—	—	—	—	—	—	—	0	281	181	—	5.32	—
171	9.05	7.04	—	1.9	0.432	0.378	5.58	—	316	0	76	1538	0.104	9.18	66.8
50	1.78	1.72	10.8	0	0.12	0.196	23.6	1.02	6	0.58	26	392	0.046	0	0.602
12	0.68	1.34	10.2	0	0.038	0.12	3.39	0.18	4	0.16	6	95	0.021	0	0.182
5	0.275	0.205	—	—	0.019	0.037	1.5	—	—	—	12	44.5	—	0	—
—	0.3	—	—	—	0.001	0.015	0.357	—	—	—	16	—	—	—	0.036
68	3.5	2.66	56.5	0	0.322	0.408	29.5	1.2	16	0.82	56	516	0.03	—	0.98

Continued.

Key to Abbreviations
Kcal, Kcalories; *Prot,* protein; *Carb,* carbohydrate; *Fat,* fat; *Chol,* cholesterol; *Safa,* saturated fat; *Mufa,* monounsaturated fat; *Pufa,* polyunsaturated fat; *Sod,* sodium; *Pot,* potassium; *Mag,* magnesium; *Iron,* iron; *Zinc,* zinc; *VA,* vitamin A; *VC,* vitamin C; *Thia,* thiamin; *Ribo,* riboflavin; *Niac,* niacin; *VB₆*, vitamin B_6; *Fol,* folate; *VB₁₂*, vitamin B_{12}; *Calc,* calcium; *Phos,* phosphorus; *Sel,* selenium; *Fibd,* dietary fiber; and *VE,* vitamin E.

Food name	Portion	Wt (g)	Kcal	Prot (g)	Carb (g)	Fat (g)	Chol (mg)	Safa (g)	Mufa (g)	Pufa (g)	Sod (mg)	Pot (mg)
Poultry—cont'd												
Breast-fried/flour	Item	196	436	62.4	3.22	17.4	176	4.8	6.86	3.84	150	506
Breast-no skin-fried	Item	172	322	57.5	0.88	8.1	156	2.22	2.96	1.84	136	474
Breast-roast	Item	196	386	58.4	0	15.3	166	4.3	5.94	3.26	138	480
Breast-stewed	Item	220	404	60.3	0	16.3	166	4.58	6.38	3.48	136	390
Drumstick-fried	Item	49	120	13.2	0.8	6.72	44	1.79	2.66	1.58	44	112
Frankfurter	Item	45	116	5.82	3.06	8.76	45	2.49	3.81	1.82	617	—
Giblets-fried/flour	Cup	145	402	47.2	6.31	19.5	647	5.5	6.41	4.9	164	478
Giblets-simmered	Cup	145	228	37.5	1.37	6.92	570	2.16	1.73	1.56	85	229
Leg-no skin-roast	Item	95	182	25.7	0	8.01	89	2.18	2.9	1.87	87	230
Leg-no skin-stewed	Item	101	187	26.5	0	8.14	90	2.22	2.95	1.9	78	192
Leg-roast	Item	114	265	29.6	0	15.4	105	4.24	5.97	3.42	99	256
Liver pate-can	Tbsp	13	26	1.75	0.85	1.7	—	—	—	—	—	—
Liver-simmered	Cup	140	219	34.1	1.23	7.63	883	2.58	1.88	1.25	71	196
Thigh-fried/flour	Item	62	162	16.6	1.97	9.29	60	2.54	3.64	2.11	55	147
Wing-fried/flour	Item	32	103	8.36	0.76	7.09	26	1.94	2.84	1.58	25	57
Wing-roast	Item	34	99	9.13	0	6.62	29	1.85	2.6	1.41	28	62
Wing-stewed	Item	40	100	9.11	0	6.73	28	1.88	2.64	1.43	27	56
Duck												
Flesh & skin-roast	Item	764	2574	145	0	217	640	73.9	98.6	27.9	454	1560
No skin-roast	Item	442	890	104	0	49.5	396	18.4	16.4	6.3	286	1114
Turkey												
Ham-cured thigh meat	Slice	28.4	36.5	5.37	0.105	1.44	—	0.485	0.325	0.43	283	92
Breast-no skin-roast	Item	612	826	184	0	4.5	510	1.44	0.78	1.2	318	1784
Loaf-breast	Serving	28.4	31.2	6.38	0	0.447	11.5	0.137	0.127	0.078	406	78.8
Pastrami	Slice	28.4	40	5.21	0.47	2.06	—	1.03	0.58	0.45	297	73.5
Roll-light	oz	28.4	42	5.3	0.15	2.05	12	0.57	0.71	0.49	139	71
Dark meat-no skin	Cup	140	262	40	0	10.1	119	3.4	2.29	3.03	110	406
Light-no skin-roast	Cup	140	219	41.9	0	4.5	97	1.44	0.79	1.2	89	426
Light/dark-no skin	Cup	140	238	41	0	6.95	107	2.29	1.45	2	99	418
Sauces and dips												
Dip-French onion-Kraft	Tbsp	15	30	0.5	1.5	2	0	—	—	—	120	—
Dip-guacamole-Kraft	Tbsp	15	25	0.5	1.5	2	0	—	—	—	108	—
Gravy-beef-can	Cup	233	124	8.73	11.2	5.49	7	2.75	2.3	0.21	117	189
Gravy-chicken-can	Cup	238	189	4.59	12.9	13.6	5	3.36	6.08	3.58	1375	260
Gravy-turkey-can	Cup	238	122	6.2	12.2	5.01	5	1.48	2.15	1.17	—	—
Horseradish-prep	Tbsp	15	6	0.2	1.4	0	0	0	0	0	165	44
Mustard-brown-prep	Cup	250	228	14.8	13.3	15.8	0	—	—	—	3268	325
Mustard-yellow-prep	Tsp	5	5	0.1	0.1	0.1	0	0	0	0	65	7
Sauces												
Barbecue	Cup	250	188	4.5	32	4.5	0	0.67	1.94	1.71	2032	435
Bearnaise-mix/milk	Cup	255	701	8.32	17.5	68.2	189	41.8	19.9	3.03	1265	—
Cheese-mix/milk	Cup	279	307	16	23.2	17.1	53	9.32	5.31	1.58	1566	554
Chili-bottled	Tbsp	15	16	0.4	3.7	0	0	0	0	0	201	56
Curry-mix/milk	Cup	272	270	10.7	25.7	14.7	35	6.05	5.16	2.76	1276	—
Heinz 57	Tbsp	15	15	0.4	2.7	0.2	0	0	0	0	265	—
Marinara-can	Cup	250	171	4	25.5	8.38	0	1.2	4.28	2.3	1572	1061
Mushroom-mix/milk	Cup	267	228	11.3	23.8	10.3	34	5.4	3.27	1.1	1533	—
Picante-can	Fl oz	16	9	0.3	1.9	0.5	0	0	0	0	218	77
Salsa/chilies-can	Fl oz	16	10	0.4	2	0.7	0	0	0	0	111	87
Sour cream-mix/milk	Cup	314	509	19.1	45.4	30.3	91	16.1	9.88	2.76	1007	733
Soy	Tbsp	18	11	1.56	1.5	0	0	0	0	0	1029	64
Spaghetti-can	Cup	249	272	4.53	39.7	11.9	0	1.7	6.07	3.25	1236	957
Sweet/sour-mix/prep	Cup	313	294	0.76	72.7	0.08	0	0.01	0.02	0.04	779	66
Tabasco	Tsp	5	0	0.1	0.1	0	0	0	0	0	22	3

Mag (mg)	Iron (mg)	Zinc (mg)	VA (RE)	VC (mg)	Thia (mg)	Ribo (mg)	Niac (mg)	VB_6 (mg)	Fol (μg)	VB_{12} (μg)	Calc (mg)	Phos (mg)	Sel (mg)	Fibd (g)	VE (mg)
58	2.34	2.14	29.4	0	0.16	0.256	26.9	1.14	8	0.68	32	456	0.021	0.07	0.686
54	1.96	1.86	12	0	0.136	0.216	25.4	1.1	8	0.62	28	424	0.031	0	0.602
54	2.08	2	54.7	0	0.13	0.234	24.9	1.08	6	0.64	28	420	0.053	0	0.686
48	2.02	2.12	54.1	0	0.09	0.254	17.2	0.64	6	0.46	28	344	0.053	0	0.77
11	0.66	1.42	12.3	0	0.04	0.11	2.96	0.17	4	0.16	6	86	0.005	0	0.172
—	0.9	—	—	—	0.03	0.052	1.39	—	—	—	43	—	0.01	0	—
37	15	9.09	5195	12.7	0.141	2.21	15.9	0.88	550	19.3	26	414	0.025	—	—
30	9.34	6.63	3234	11.6	0.126	1.38	5.95	0.49	545	14.7	18	331	0.025	0	—
23	1.24	2.71	18	0	0.071	0.22	6	0.35	8	0.31	12	174	0.013	0	0.333
21	1.41	2.81	18	0	0.06	0.218	4.85	0.22	8	0.23	11	151	0.013	0	0.354
26	1.52	2.96	46.2	0	0.078	0.243	7.06	0.37	8	0.35	14	199	0.016	0	0.399
—	1.19	—	28.2	1.3	0.007	0.182	0.977	—	—	—	1	—	—	0	0.036
29	11.9	6.07	6886	22.2	0.214	2.45	6.23	0.82	1077	27.1	20	437	0.099	0	—
15	0.93	1.56	18.3	0	0.058	0.151	4.31	0.21	5	0.19	8	116	0.011	0.04	0.217
6	0.4	0.56	12	0	0.019	0.044	2.14	0.13	1	0.09	5	48	0.006	0	0.112
7	0.43	0.62	16.2	0	0.014	0.044	2.26	0.14	1	0.1	5	51	0.006	0	0.119
6	0.45	0.65	15.9	0	0.016	0.041	1.85	0.09	1	0.07	5	48	0.006	0	0.14
124	20.6	14.2	483	0	1.33	2.06	36.9	1.4	50	2.26	86	1190	—	0	—
88	11.9	11.5	103	0	1.15	2.08	22.5	1.1	44	1.76	52	898	—	0	—
—	0.785	—	—	—	0.015	0.07	1	—	—	—	2.5	54	—	0	—
178	9.36	10.6	0	0	0.264	0.802	45.9	3.42	38	2.36	76	1370	0.049	0	0.551
5.67	0.113	0.318	0	0	0.011	0.03	2.36	0.1	—	0.572	2	64.8	—	0	—
4	0.47	0.61	—	—	0.016	0.071	1	—	—	—	2.5	56.5	—	0	—
5	0.36	0.44	—	—	0.025	0.064	1.99	—	—	—	11	52	—	0	—
34	3.27	6.25	0	0	0.088	0.347	5.11	0.5	13	0.52	45	286	0.035	0	0.896
39	1.88	2.85	0	0	0.085	0.181	9.57	0.75	8	0.52	27	307	—	0	0.126
37	2.49	4.34	0	0	0.087	0.255	7.62	0.64	10	0.52	35	298	0.035	0	0.896
—	—	—	—	—	—	—	—	—	—	—	—	—	—	—	—
—	—	—	—	—	—	—	—	—	—	—	—	—	—	—	—
—	1.63	2.33	0	0	0.074	0.084	1.54	0.023	—	0.23	14	70	—	0.093	—
—	1.12	1.91	264	0	0.041	0.103	1.06	0.024	—	—	48	69	—	—	—
—	1.67	—	0	0	0.048	0.191	3.1	—	—	0	10	—	—	—	—
—	0.1	—	—	—	—	—	—	—	—	—	9	5	—	—	—
—	4.5	—	—	—	—	—	—	—	—	—	310	335	—	—	4.38
2	0.1	—	—	—	—	—	—	—	—	—	4	4	0	0.06	0.088
—	2.25	—	218	17.5	0.075	0.05	2.25	0.188	—	0	48	50	—	2.3	—
—	—	—	—	—	—	—	—	—	—	—	—	—	—	0.09	—
47	0.27	0.972	—	2.3	0.148	0.564	0.318	—	—	—	570	437	—	0.1	—
—	0.1	—	21	2	0.01	0.01	0.2	—	—	—	3	8	0	—	—
—	—	—	—	—	—	—	—	—	—	—	485	280	—	0.9	—
—	—	—	—	—	—	—	—	—	—	—	—	—	0	—	—
59	2	0.67	240	31.9	0.113	0.148	3.98	—	—	0	44	88	—	—	—
—	—	—	—	—	—	—	—	—	—	—	—	—	—	0.5	—
—	0.25	—	23	8.8	0.02	0.01	0.22	—	—	—	3.8	8	—	—	—
—	0.28	—	39	9.1	0.02	0.01	0.29	—	—	—	4.2	9.3	—	—	—
—	0.61	1.37	—	—	—	0.704	0.556	—	—	—	546	—	—	—	—
8	0.49	0.036	0	0	0.009	0.023	0.605	0.031	1.9	0	3	38	—	—	—
60	1.62	0.53	306	27.9	0.137	0.147	3.75	—	—	0	70	90	—	—	—
—	1.62	0.091	—	—	—	0.097	—	—	—	0	41	—	—	—	—
—	—	—	—	—	0	0.01	0	—	—	—	—	—	—	—	—

Continued.

Key to Abbreviations
Kcal, Kcalories; *Prot*, protein; *Carb*, carbohydrate; *Fat*, fat; *Chol*, cholesterol; *Safa*, saturated fat; *Mufa*, monounsaturated fat; *Pufa*, polyunsaturated fat; *Sod*, sodium; *Pot*, potassium; *Mag*, magnesium; *Iron*, iron; *Zinc*, zinc; *VA*, vitamin A; *VC*, vitamin C; *Thia*, thiamin; *Ribo*, riboflavin; *Niac*, niacin; *VB₆*, vitamin B₆; *Fol*, folate; *VB₁₂*, vitamin B₁₂; *Calc*, calcium; *Phos*, phosphorus; *Sel*, selenium; *Fibd*, dietary fiber; and *VE*, vitamin E.

Food name	Portion	Wt (g)	Kcal	Prot (g)	Carb (g)	Fat (g)	Chol (mg)	Safa (g)	Mufa (g)	Pufa (g)	Sod (mg)	Pot (mg)
Sauces—cont'd												
Taco-can	Fl oz	16	11	0.4	2.2	0.7	0	—	—	—	128	88
Tartar-regular	Tbsp	14	75	0	1	8	9	1.5	1.8	4.1	98	11
Teriyaki-bottled	Tbsp	18	15	1.07	2.87	0	0	0	0	0	690	41
Tomato-can-low sod	Cup	226	90	4	18	0	—	0	0	0	65	—
Tomato-can-salt add	Cup	245	74	3.25	17.6	0.41	0	0.059	0.061	0.164	1481	908
Tomato-Spanish-can	Cup	244	80	3.52	17.7	0.64	0	0.092	0.098	0.264	1152	—
Worcestershire	Tbsp	15	12	0.3	2.7	0	0	0	0	0	147	120
Tomato catsup	Tbsp	15	15	0	4	0	0	0	0	0	156	54
Soups												
Bean/bacon-can-water	Cup	253	173	7.89	22.8	5.94	3	1.53	2.18	1.82	952	403
Beef broth-can-ready	Cup	240	16	2.74	0.1	0.53	0.605	0.26	0.22	0.02	782	130
Beef broth-dehy-cubed	Item	3.6	6	0.62	0.58	0.14	0.144	0.07	0.06	0.01	864	15
Beef-chunky-can	Cup	240	171	11.7	19.6	5.14	14	2.55	2.14	0.2	867	336
Black bean-can-water	Cup	247	116	5.64	19.8	1.51	0	0.4	0.54	0.47	1198	273
Cheese-can-milk	Cup	251	230	9.45	16.2	14.6	48	9.12	4.1	0.44	1020	340
Chick broth-can/water	Cup	244	39	4.93	0.93	1.39	1	0.41	0.63	0.29	776	210
Chicken noodle-can	Cup	241	75	4.04	9.35	2.45	7	0.65	1.11	0.55	1107	55
Chicken-chunky-can	Cup	251	178	12.7	17.3	6.63	30	1.98	2.97	1.39	887	176
Chicken/rice-can	Cup	240	127	12.3	13	3.19	12	0.95	1.43	0.67	888	—
Clam-Manhattan-water	Cup	244	78	4.18	12.2	2.31	2	0.44	0.41	1.32	1808	262
Clam-New England-milk	Cup	248	163	9.46	16.6	6.6	22	2.95	2.26	1.08	992	300
Cream/celery-can-milk	Cup	248	165	5.69	14.5	9.68	32	3.95	2.47	2.65	1010	309
Cream/chick-can-milk	Cup	248	191	7.46	15	11.5	27	4.63	4.45	1.64	1046	273
Cream/mushroom-milk	Cup	248	203	6.05	15	13.6	20	5.12	2.98	4.61	1076	270
Cream/potato-can-milk	Cup	248	148	5.78	17.2	6.45	22	3.76	1.73	0.56	1060	323
Minestrone-can-water	Cup	241	83	4.26	11.2	2.51	2	0.54	0.69	1.11	911	312
Onion-can-water	Cup	241	57	3.75	8.18	1.74	0	0.26	0.75	0.65	1053	69
Onion-dehy-packet	Serving	39	115	4.52	20.9	2.33	2	0.54	1.36	0.27	3493	260
Pea-green-can-water	Cup	250	164	8.59	26.5	2.94	0	1.41	1	0.38	987	190
Pea-split-can-water	Cup	253	189	10.3	28	4.4	8	1.76	1.8	0.63	1008	399
Tomato rice-can-water	Cup	247	120	2.11	21.9	2.72	2	0.52	0.6	1.35	815	330
Tomato-can-milk	Cup	248	160	6.09	22.3	6.01	17	2.91	1.6	1.11	932	450
Tomato-can-water	Cup	244	86	2.06	16.6	1.92	0	0.36	0.43	0.96	872	263
Turkey noodle-can	Cup	244	69	3.9	8.63	1.99	5	0.56	0.81	0.49	815	75
Turkey vegetable-can	Cup	241	74	3.09	8.64	3.02	2	0.9	1.33	0.67	905	175
Turkey-chunky-can	Cup	236	136	10.2	14.1	4.41	9	1.22	1.78	1.08	923	361
Vegetable beef-can	Cup	245	79	5.58	10.2	1.9	5	0.85	0.8	0.11	957	173
Vegetarian-can-water	Cup	241	72	2.1	12	1.93	0	0.29	0.83	0.73	823	209
Spices and herbs												
Chili powder	Tsp	2.6	8	0.32	1.42	0.44	0	—	—	—	26	50
Cinnamon-ground	Tsp	2.3	6	0.09	1.84	0.07	0	0.01	0.01	0.01	0.598	11
Oregano-ground	Tsp	1.5	5	0.17	0.97	0.15	0	0.04	0.01	0.08	0.225	25
Paprika	Tsp	2.1	6	0.31	1.17	0.27	0	0.04	0.03	0.17	0.714	49
Parsley-dried	Tsp	0.3	1	0.07	0.15	0.01	0	0	0	0	1.36	11
Pepper-black	Tsp	2.1	5	0.23	1.36	0.07	0	0.02	0.02	0.02	0.924	26
Salt-table	Tsp	5.5	0	0	0	0	0	0	0	0	2132	0
Sugars and sweets												
Almond Joy	oz	28.4	151	1.7	18.5	7.8	—	1.74	2.47	1.72	—	—
Bit O Honey	oz	28.4	121	0.9	21.2	3.6	—	1.65	1.63	0.188	—	—
Caramels-plain/choc	oz	28.4	115	1	22	3	0	1.6	1.1	0.1	74	54
Choc coated peanuts	oz	28.4	160	5	11	12	0	4	4.7	2.1	16	143
Chocolate-semisweet	Cup	170	860	7	97	61	0	36.2	19.8	1.7	3	553
Fondant-uncoated	oz	28.4	105	0	25	1	0	0.1	0.3	0.1	60	1
Fudge-choc-plain	oz	28.4	115	1	21	3	0	1.3	1.4	0.6	54	42

Mag (mg)	Iron (mg)	Zinc (mg)	VA (RE)	VC (mg)	Thia (mg)	Ribo (mg)	Niac (mg)	VB_6 (mg)	Fol (μg)	VB_{12} (μg)	Calc (mg)	Phos (mg)	Sel (mg)	Fibd (g)	VE (mg)
—	0.3	—	4.4	6.2	0.02	0.01	0.27	—	—	—	5.9	9.8	—	—	—
—	0.1	—	3	0	0	0	0	—	—	—	3	4	—	—	—
11	0.31	0.018	0	0	0.005	0.013	0.229	0.018	3.6	0	4	28	—	—	—
—	—	—	—	—	—	—	—	—	—	—	—	—	0.002	3.39	—
46	1.88	0.6	240	32.1	0.162	0.142	2.82	—	—	0	34	78	—	3.68	—
—	8.5	—	240	21	0.18	0.152	3.15	—	—	0	40	—	—	3.66	—
—	0.9	—	5.1	27	0	0.03	0	—	—	—	15	9	—	—	—
3.6	0.1	0.034	21	2	0.01	0.01	0.2	0.016	0.75	0	3	8	0	—	—
44	2.05	1.03	89	1.6	0.089	0.033	0.567	0.04	31.9	—	81	132	0.008	3.2	—
—	0.41	—	0	0	0.005	0.05	1.87	—	—	—	15	31	0.008	0	—
2	0.08	0.008	—	—	0.007	0.009	0.119	—	—	—	—	8	0	—	—
—	2.32	2.64	261	7	0.058	0.151	2.71	0.132	13.4	0.61	31	120	0.008	—	—
42	2.16	1.41	49	0.8	0.077	0.054	0.534	0.094	24.7	0.02	45	107	0.008	—	—
20	0.81	0.688	147	1.2	0.063	0.334	0.502	0.078	—	0.44	288	250	0.008	—	—
2	0.51	0.249	0	0	0.01	0.071	3.35	0.024	—	0.24	9	73	0.008	0	—
5	0.78	0.395	72	0.2	0.053	0.06	1.39	0.027	2.2	—	17	36	0.008	1.45	—
—	1.73	1	130	1.3	0.085	0.173	4.42	0.05	4.6	0.25	24	113	0.008	—	—
—	1.87	—	586	3.8	0.024	0.098	4.1	—	3.8	—	35	—	0.008	1.44	—
10	1.89	0.927	93	3.2	0.063	0.049	1.34	0.083	9.5	2.19	34	57	0.008	—	—
23	1.48	0.799	40	3.5	0.067	0.236	1.03	0.126	9.7	10.3	187	157	0.008	—	—
22	0.69	0.196	68	1.4	0.074	0.248	0.436	0.064	8.5	—	186	151	0.008	0.77	—
18	0.67	0.675	94	1.3	0.074	0.258	0.923	0.067	7.7	—	180	152	0.008	0.5	—
20	0.59	0.64	38	2.3	0.077	0.28	0.913	0.064	—	—	178	156	0.008	—	—
17	0.54	0.675	67	1.1	0.082	0.236	0.642	0.089	9.2	—	166	160	0.008	—	—
7	0.92	0.735	234	1.1	0.053	0.043	0.942	0.099	16.1	0	34	56	0.008	1.9	—
2	0.67	0.612	0	1.2	0.034	0.024	0.6	0.048	15.2	0	26	11	0.008	—	—
25	0.58	0.231	1	0.9	0.111	0.238	1.99	—	6.3	—	55	126	0	2.2	—
39	1.95	1.71	20	1.7	0.108	0.068	1.24	0.053	1.8	0	27	124	0.008	—	—
48	2.28	1.32	44	1.4	0.147	0.076	1.48	0.068	2.5	0	22	213	0.008	—	—
5	0.79	0.514	76	14.8	0.062	0.049	1.06	0.077	—	0	23	33	0.008	1.7	—
23	1.82	0.29	108	67.7	0.134	0.248	1.52	0.164	20.9	0.44	159	148	0.008	0.8	—
8	1.76	0.244	69	66.5	0.088	0.051	1.42	0.112	14.7	0	13	34	0.008	0.9	—
5	0.94	0.583	29	0.2	0.073	0.063	1.4	0.037	—	—	12	48	0.008	0.7	—
4	0.76	0.612	244	0	0.029	0.039	1.01	0.048	—	0.17	17	40	0.008	0.964	—
—	1.91	2.12	716	6.4	0.035	0.106	3.59	0.307	11.1	2.12	50	104	0.008	2.5	—
6	1.11	1.55	189	2.4	0.037	0.049	1.03	0.076	10.6	0.31	17	40	0.008	0.98	—
7	1.08	0.46	300	1.4	0.053	0.046	0.916	0.055	10.6	0	21	35	0.008	1.21	—
4	0.37	0.07	90.8	1.67	0.009	0.021	0.205	—	—	0	7	8	0.001	0.889	—
1	0.88	0.05	0.6	0.65	0.002	0.003	0.03	—	—	0	28	1	0.001	—	—
4	0.66	0.07	10.4	—	0.005	—	0.093	—	—	0	24	3	—	—	—
4	0.5	0.08	127	1.49	0.014	0.037	0.322	—	—	0	4	7	0	—	—
1	0.29	0.01	7	0.37	0.001	0.004	0.024	0.003	—	0	4	1	—	—	—
4	0.61	0.03	0.4	—	0.002	0.005	0.024	—	—	0	9	4	0	0.525	—
0	0	—	0	0	0	0	0	0	0	0	14	—	—	0	0
—	—	—	—	—	—	—	—	—	—	—	—	—	0.001	—	0.308
—	0.25	—	—	—	0	0.13	1.4	—	—	—	13	—	0.001	—	0.048
1	0.4	—	0	0	0.01	0.05	0.1	—	—	—	42	35	0.001	0.784	0.048
—	0.4	—	0	0	0.1	0.05	2.1	—	—	—	33	84	0.001	—	0.196
—	4.4	—	9	0	0.02	0.14	0.9	—	—	—	51	255	0.006	—	1.19
—	0.3	—	0	0	0	0	0	—	—	—	4	2	0.001	0	—
12.6	0.3	—	0	0	0.01	0.03	0.1	—	—	—	22	24	0.001	—	0.196

Continued.

Key to Abbreviations

Kcal, Kcalories; *Prot,* protein; *Carb,* carbohydrate; *Fat,* fat; *Chol,* cholesterol; *Safa,* saturated fat; *Mufa,* monounsaturated fat; *Pufa,* polyunsaturated fat; *Sod,* sodium; *Pot,* potassium; *Mag,* magnesium; *Iron,* iron; *Zinc,* zinc; *VA,* vitamin A; *VC,* vitamin C; *Thia,* thiamin; *Ribo,* riboflavin; *Niac,* niacin; *VB_6,* vitamin B_6; *Fol,* folate; *VB_{12},* vitamin B_{12}; *Calc,* calcium; *Phos,* phosphorus; *Sel,* selenium; *Fibd,* dietary fiber; and *VE,* vitamin E.

Food name	Portion	Wt (g)	Kcal	Prot (g)	Carb (g)	Fat (g)	Chol (mg)	Safa (g)	Mufa (g)	Pufa (g)	Sod (mg)	Pot (mg)
Sugars and sweets—cont'd												
Gum Drops	oz	28.4	100	0	25	0	0	0	0	0	10	1
Hard	oz	28.4	110	0	28	0	0	0	0	0	9	1
Jelly Beans	Item	2.8	6.6	0	2.64	0	—	0	0	0	0.3	0
Kit Kat bar	Item	43	210	3	25	11	—	5.6	3.77	0.448	38	129
Life Savers	Item	2	7.8	0	1.94	0.02	0	0	0	0	0.6	0
Lollipop	Item	28.4	108	0	28	0	0	0	0	0	—	—
M & M's-package	Item	45	220	3	31	10	—	—	—	—	—	—
Milk choc/almonds	oz	28.4	151	2.6	14.5	10.1	—	4.06	3.92	1.38	23	125
Milk choc/peanuts	oz	28.4	154	4	12.6	10.8	—	5.22	5.04	1.78	19	138
Milk choc-plain	oz	28.4	145	2	16	9	0	5.5	3	0.3	28	109
Milky Way bar	Item	60	260	3	43	9	—	5.05	3.61	0.336	—	—
Peanut Brittle	oz	28.4	123	2.4	20.4	4.4	—	1.85	1.79	0.632	9	43
Peanut Butter Cup	Piece	17	92	2.2	8.7	5.35	2.5	2.8	1.83	0.751	54.5	68
Snickers bar	Item	57	270	6	33	13	—	4.73	5.03	2.04	—	—
Honey-strained/extracted	Tbsp	21	65	0	17	0	0	0	0	0	1	11
Icing-cake-choc-mix/prep	Cup	275	1035	9	185	38	0	23.4	11.7	1	882	536
Icing-cake-fudge-mix/water	Cup	245	830	7	183	16	0	5.1	6.7	3.1	568	238
Icing-cake-white-boiled	Cup	94	295	1	75	0	0	0	0	0	134	17
Icing-cake-white-unckd	Cup	319	1200	2	260	21	0	12.7	5.1	0.5	156	57
Icing-cake-white/coco-boil	Cup	166	605	3	124	13	0	11	0.9	0	195	277
Jams/preserves-regular	Tbsp	20	55	0	14	0	0	0	0	0	2	18
Marshmallows	oz	28.4	90	1	23	0	0	0	0	0	11	2
Molasses-cane-blackstrap	Tbsp	20	45	0	11	—	0	—	—	—	18	585
Molasses-cane-light	Tbsp	20	50	0	13	—	0	—	—	—	3	183
Popsicle	Item	95	70	0	18	0	0	0	0	0	0	—
Sugar-brown-pressed down	Cup	220	820	0	212	0	0	0	0	0	66	757
Sugar-Equal-packet	Item	1	4	0	1	0	0	0	0	0	0	0
Sugar-Sweet & Low-packet	Item	1	4	—	0.9	—	0	—	—	—	4	3
Sugar-white-granulated	Tbsp	12	45	0	12	0	0	0	0	0	0.12	0
Sugar-white-powder-sifted	Cup	100	385	0	100	0	0	0	0	0	0.83	3
Vegetables												
Alfalfa seeds-sprouted-raw	Cup	33	10	1.32	1.25	0.23	0	0.023	0.018	0.135	2	26
Artichokes-boil-drain	Item	120	53	2.76	12.4	0.2	0	0.048	0.006	0.086	79	316
Asparagus-froz-boil-spears	Cup	180	50.4	5.31	8.77	0.756	0	0.171	0.023	0.331	7.2	392
Avocado-raw-California	Item	173	306	3.64	12	30	0	4.48	19.4	3.53	21	1097
Beans-baked beans-can	Cup	254	235	12.2	52.1	1.14	0	0.295	0.099	0.493	1008	752
Beans-garbanzo-can	Serving	28.4	27.8	1.31	4.66	0.511	0	0.07	0.17	0.26	113	54.8
Beans-green-froz-French	Cup	135	36	1.84	8.26	0.18	0	0.041	0.007	0.093	17	151
Beans-lima-can	Cup	248	186	11.3	34.4	0.74	0	0.168	0.043	0.358	618	668
Beans-lima-froz-boil-drain	Cup	170	170	10.3	32	0.58	0	0.13	0.034	0.278	90	694
Beans-mung-sprouted-boil	Cup	125	26	2.52	5.2	0.11	0	0.031	0.015	0.04	12	125
Beans-navy pea-dry-ckd	Cup	190	225	15	40	1	0	—	—	—	13	790
Beans-pinto-froz-boil	oz	28.4	46	2.64	8.77	0.135	0	0.017	0.01	0.078	—	—
Beans-red kidney-can	Cup	255	230	15	42	1	0	—	—	—	833	673
Beans-refried beans	Cup	253	270	15.8	46.8	2.7	—	1.04	—	—	1071	994
Beans-shellie-can	Cup	245	75	4.3	15.2	0.47	0	0.056	0.034	0.27	819	268
Beans-snap-green-can-cuts	Cup	135	27	1.55	6	0.135	0	0.03	0.006	0.07	339	147
Beans-snap-green-raw-boil	Cup	125	44	2.36	9.86	0.36	0	0.08	0.014	0.181	4	373
Beans-snap-wax-raw-boil	Cup	125	44	2.36	9.86	0.36	0	0.08	0.014	0.181	4	373
Beans-snap-yellow/wax-can	Cup	136	26	1.56	6.12	0.14	0	0.03	0.006	0.07	340	148
Beets-can-sliced-drain	Cup	170	54	1.56	12.2	0.24	0	0.04	0.048	0.086	479	284
Broccoli-froz-boil-drain	Cup	185	51	5.71	9.85	0.21	0	0.03	0.015	0.101	44	332
Broccoli-raw	Cup	88	24	2.62	4.62	0.3	0	0.048	0.022	0.148	24	286
Broccoli-raw-boil-drain	Cup	155	46	4.64	8.68	0.44	0	0.068	0.032	0.21	16	254
Cabbage-celery-raw	Cup	76	12	0.91	2.46	0.15	0	0.033	0.017	0.055	7	181
Cabbage-common-boil-drain	Cup	145	30.5	1.39	6.92	0.363	0	0.046	0.026	0.173	27.6	297

Mag (mg)	Iron (mg)	Zinc (mg)	VA (RE)	VC (mg)	Thia (mg)	Ribo (mg)	Niac (mg)	VB_6 (mg)	Fol (µg)	VB_{12} (µg)	Calc (mg)	Phos (mg)	Sel (mg)	Fibd (g)	VE (mg)
—	0.1	—	0	0	0	0	0	—	—	—	2	0	0.001	0	—
—	0.5	—	0	0	0	0	0	—	—	—	6	2	0.001	0	0.048
—	0.03	—	0	0	0	—	—	—	—	—	0.3	0.1	0	0	—
19	0.56	0.43	9	—	0.03	0.11	0.1	—	—	—	65	78	0.002	—	0.301
—	0.04	—	0	0	0	0	0	—	—	—	0.4	0.2	0	0	—
—	0	—	0	0	0	0	0	—	—	—	0	0	0.001	0	—
—	—	—	—	—	—	—	—	—	—	—	—	—	0.002	—	0.495
—	0.5	—	21	0	0.02	0.12	0.2	—	—	—	65	77	0.001	—	0.308
—	0.4	—	15	0	0.07	0.07	1.4	—	—	—	49	83	0.001	—	0.308
16	0.3	—	24	0	0.02	0.1	0.1	—	1.96	—	65	65	0.001	—	0.196
—	—	—	—	—	—	—	—	—	—	—	—	—	0.002	—	0.66
—	0.56	—	2.4	0	0.02	0.01	1.3	—	—	—	11	35	0.001	—	—
14.5	0.24	0.24	1	—	0.05	0.03	0.8	—	—	—	14.5	41	0.001	—	0.187
—	—	—	—	—	—	—	—	—	—	—	—	—	0.002	—	0.627
0.63	0.1	0.02	0	0	0	0.01	0.1	0.004	—	0	1	1	0.001	0.06	—
—	3.3	—	174	1	0.06	0.28	0.6	—	—	—	165	305	0.003	—	—
—	2.7	—	0	0	0.05	0.2	0.7	—	—	—	96	218	0.003	—	—
—	0	—	0	0	0	0.03	0	—	—	—	2	2	0.001	0	—
—	0	—	258	0	0	0.06	0	—	—	—	48	38	0.003	0	—
—	0.8	—	0	0	0.02	0.07	0.3	—	—	—	10	50	0.002	—	—
—	0.2	—	0	0	0	0.01	0	0.004	1.6	0	4	2	0	0.2	0.018
—	0.5	0.01	0	0	0	0	0	—	—	—	5	2	0	0	—
—	3.2	—	—	—	0.02	0.04	0.4	0.04	—	0	137	17	0.013	0	0.082
—	0.9	—	—	—	0.01	0.01	0	0.04	—	0	33	9	0.013	0	0.082
—	0	—	0	0	0	0	0	—	—	—	0	—	—	—	—
—	7.5	—	0	0	0.02	0.07	0.4	—	—	—	187	42	0.003	0	—
0	0	0	0	0	0	0	0	0	0	0	0	0	0	—	—
—	—	—	—	—	—	—	—	—	—	—	—	—	0	—	—
—	0	0.006	0	0	0	0	0	—	—	—	0	0	0	0	—
—	0.1	—	0	0	0	0	0	—	—	—	0	0	0.001	0	—
9	0.32	0.3	5.1	2.7	0.025	0.042	0.159	0.011	12.2	0	10	23	—	0.726	—
47	1.62	0.43	17.2	8.9	0.068	0.059	0.709	0.104	53.4	0	47	72	—	4	0.228
23.4	1.15	1	147	43.9	0.117	0.185	1.87	0.036	242	0	41.4	99	0.007	2.16	2.52
70	2.04	0.73	106	13.7	0.187	0.211	3.32	0.484	113	0	19	73	—	6.13	3.66
82	0.74	3.55	43.4	—	0.389	0.152	1.09	0.34	60.7	0	128	264	—	19.6	—
9.37	0.71	0.264	0.568	1.42	0.003	0.011	0.085	—	—	—	11.1	30.1	—	1.4	—
29	1.11	0.84	71.3	11.1	0.065	0.1	0.563	0.076	44.2	0	61	33	0.001	2.16	0.176
84	3.94	1.58	42.8	21.6	0.072	0.106	1.32	0.154	—	0	70	176	0.004	10.4	—
58	2.32	0.74	32.4	21.8	0.12	0.104	1.8	0.208	111	0	38	153	0.001	8.33	0
18	0.81	0.58	1.7	14.1	0.062	0.126	1.01	—	166	0	15	34	—	2.7	—
—	5.1	1.8	0	0	0.27	0.13	1.3	1.06	66.5	0	95	281	0.021	9.31	0.646
—	0.77	—	0	0.19	0.078	0.031	0.18	—	—	0	14.9	—	—	1.39	—
9.94	4.6	1.91	1	7.65	0.13	0.1	1.5	1.12	35.7	0	74	278	0.009	12.5	—
99	4.47	3.45	—	15.2	0.124	0.139	1.23	—	—	—	118	214	—	11.6	—
—	2.43	—	55.9	7.5	0.078	0.132	0.502	—	—	0	72	—	—	12	—
17.5	1.2	0.39	47.1	6.5	0.02	0.075	0.27	0.054	43	0	35	34	0.001	1.76	0.041
32	1.6	0.45	83.3	12.1	0.093	0.121	0.768	0.07	41.6	0	58	46	0.001	2.25	0.025
32	1.6	0.45	83.3	12.1	0.093	0.121	0.768	0.07	41.6	0	58	48	0.001	2.25	0.363
18	1.22	0.4	47.4	6.4	0.02	0.076	0.274	0.057	43	0	36	26	0.001	1.77	0.394
22.1	3.1	0.36	3	5	0.02	0.05	0.2	0.085	40.8	0	32	31	0.001	3.2	0.051
37	1.13	0.56	348	73.7	0.101	0.15	0.843	0.239	104	0	94	101	0.003	7.3	0.851
22	0.78	0.36	136	82	0.058	0.104	0.562	0.14	62.4	0	42	58	0.001	2.46	0.405
94	1.78	0.24	220	98	0.128	0.322	1.18	0.308	107	0	178	74	0.003	4.03	0.713
10	0.23	0.17	91.2	20.5	0.03	0.038	0.304	0.176	59.8	0	58	22	0.002	1.63	0.09
21.8	0.566	0.232	12.5	35.2	0.083	0.08	0.33	0.093	29.4	0	47.9	36.3	0.003	4	2.42

Continued.

Key to Abbreviations
Kcal, Kcalories; *Prot*, protein; *Carb*, carbohydrate; *Fat*, fat; *Chol*, cholesterol; *Safa*, saturated fat; *Mufa*, monounsaturated fat; *Pufa*, polyunsaturated fat; *Sod*, sodium; *Pot*, potassium; *Mag*, magnesium; *Iron*, iron; *Zinc*, zinc; *VA*, vitamin A; *VC*, vitamin C; *Thia*, thiamin; *Ribo*, riboflavin; *Niac*, niacin; *VB6*, vitamin B_6; *Fol*, folate; *VB12*, vitamin B_{12}; *Calc*, calcium; *Phos*, phosphorus; *Sel*, selenium; *Fibd*, dietary fiber; and *VE*, vitamin E.

Food name	Portion	Wt (g)	Kcal	Prot (g)	Carb (g)	Fat (g)	Chol (mg)	Safa (g)	Mufa (g)	Pufa (g)	Sod (mg)	Pot (mg)
Vegetables—cont'd												
Cabbage-common-raw-shred	Cup	90	21.6	1.09	4.83	0.162	0	0.021	0.012	0.078	16.2	221
Cabbage-red-raw-shred	Cup	70	19	0.97	4.29	0.18	0	0.024	0.013	0.088	7	144
Cabbage-white mustard-boil	Cup	170	20	2.65	3.03	0.27	0	0.036	0.02	0.131	57	630
Cabbage-white mustard-raw	Cup	70	9	1.05	1.53	0.14	0	0.018	0.011	0.067	45	176
Carrot-raw-shred-scraped	Cup	110	48	1.12	11.2	0.2	0	0.034	0.008	0.084	38	356
Carrot-raw-whole-scraped	Item	72	31	0.74	7.3	0.14	0	0.022	0.006	0.055	25	233
Carrots-boil-drain-sliced	Cup	156	70	1.7	16.3	0.28	0	0.054	0.014	0.138	104	354
Carrots-can-sliced-drain	Cup	146	34	0.94	8.08	0.28	0	0.052	0.014	0.134	352	262
Carrots-froz-boil-drain	Cup	146	52	1.73	12	0.16	0	0.031	0.007	0.077	86	230
Cauliflower-froz-boil	Cup	180	34	2.9	6.76	0.39	0	0.06	0.028	0.186	32	250
Cauliflower-raw-boil-drain	Cup	124	30	2.32	5.74	0.22	0	0.046	0.022	0.144	8	400
Cauliflower-raw-chop	Cup	100	24	1.99	4.92	0.18	0	0	0	0	15	355
Celery-Pascal-raw-diced	Cup	120	18	0.8	4.36	0.14	0	0.038	0.028	0.072	106	340
Celery-Pascal-raw-stalk	Item	40	6	0.26	1.45	0.05	0	0.013	0.01	0.024	35	114
Chives-raw-chop	Tbsp	3	1	0.08	0.11	0.02	0	0.003	0.003	0.007	0	8
Collards-froz-boil-drain	Cup	170	61	5.04	12.1	0.69	0	—	—	—	85	427
Collards-raw-boil-drain	Cup	190	27	2.1	5.02	0.29	0	—	—	—	36	177
Corn-froz-boil-kernels	Cup	165	134	4.94	33.7	0.12	0	0.018	0.034	0.056	8	228
Corn-kernels	1 Ear	77	83	2.56	19.3	0.98	0	0.152	0.288	0.464	13	192
Corn-kernels & cob-froz-boil	Item	126	118	3.92	28.1	0.92	0	0.144	0.272	0.438	6	316
Corn-sweet-can-drain	Cup	165	132	4.3	30.5	1.64	0	0.254	0.478	0.772	470	160
Corn-sweet-cream style-can	Cup	256	186	4.46	46.4	1.08	0	0.166	0.314	0.506	730	344
Cowpeas-blackeye-froz-boil	Cup	170	224	14.4	40.4	1.13	0	0.298	0.102	0.476	9	638
Cowpeas-blackeye-raw-boil	Cup	165	179	13.4	29.9	1.32	0	0.345	0.117	0.558	7	693
Cucumber-raw-sliced	Cup	104	14	0.56	3.02	0.14	0	0.034	0.004	0.054	2	156
Eggplant-boil-drain	Cup	96	27	0.8	6.37	0.22	0	0.042	0.019	0.089	3	238
Endive-raw-chop	Cup	50	8	0.62	1.68	0.1	0	0.024	0.002	0.044	12	158
Garlic-raw-clove	Item	3	4	0.19	0.99	0.02	0	0.003	0	0.007	1	12
Leeks-boil-drain	Item	124	38	1.01	9.45	0.25	0	0.033	0.004	0.138	13	108
Lettuce-butterhead-leaves	Slice	15	2	0.19	0.35	0.03	0	0.004	0.001	0.018	1	39
Lettuce-iceberg-raw-chop	Cup	55	7.15	0.556	1.15	0.105	0	0.014	0.003	0.055	4.95	86.9
Lettuce-iceberg-raw-leaves	Piece	20	2.61	0.201	0.418	0.038	0	0.005	0.001	0.02	1.81	31.6
Lettuce-looseleaf-raw	Cup	55	10	0.72	1.96	0.16	0	0.022	0.006	0.09	6	148
Lettuce-Romaine-raw-shred	Cup	56	8	0.9	1.32	0.12	0	0.014	0.004	0.06	4	162
Miso-fermented soybeans	Cup	275	565	32.5	76.9	16.7	0	2.42	3.69	9.43	10030	451
Mushrooms-boil-drain	Item	12	3	0.26	0.62	0.06	0	0.007	0.001	0.022	0	43
Mushrooms-can-drain	Item	12	3	0.22	0.6	0.04	0	0.005	0.001	0.014	—	—
Mushrooms-raw-chop	Cup	70	18	1.46	3.26	0.3	0	0.04	0.004	0.12	2	260
Olives-green-pickled-can	Item	4	3.75	0.1	0.1	0.5	0	0.05	0.35	0.035	80.8	1.75
Olives-mission-rip-can	Item	3	5	0.1	0.1	0.667	0	0.067	0.41	0.034	19.2	0.667
Onions-mature-boil-drain	Cup	210	58	1.9	13.2	0.34	0	0.056	0.048	0.132	16	318
Onions-mature-raw-chop	Cup	160	54	1.88	11.7	0.42	0	0.07	0.06	0.164	4	248
Onion rings-froz-prep-heat	Item	10	40.7	0.534	3.82	2.67	0	0.858	1.09	0.511	37.5	12.9
Onions-young-green	Item	5	1.25	0.087	0.278	0.007	0	0.001	0	0	0.2	12.8
Parsley-raw-chop	Tbsp	4	1.2	0.088	0.276	0.012	0	0	0	0	1.6	21.6
Peas-green-can-drain	Cup	170	118	7.52	21.4	0.58	0	0.106	0.052	0.278	372	294
Peas-green-froz-boil-drain	Cup	160	126	8.24	22.8	0.44	0	0.078	0.038	0.206	140	268
Peas-split-dry-ckd	Cup	200	230	16	42	1	0	—	—	—	8	592
Peppers-hot chili-raw	Cup	150	60	3	14.2	0.3	0	0.032	0.016	0.164	10	510
Peppers-hot-red-dried	Tsp	2	5	0	1	0	0	0	0	0	20	20
Peppers-sweet-green-raw	Cup	226	61.1	2.01	14.6	0.43	0	0.063	0.029	0.231	4.53	401
Peppers-jalapeno-can-chop	Cup	136	33	1.09	6.66	0.82	0	0.084	0.046	0.445	1990	185
Pickle-dill-cucumber-med	Item	65	5	0	1	0	0	0	0	0	928	130
Pickle-fresh pack-cucumber	Item	7.5	5	0	1.5	0	0	0	0	0	50	—
Pickle-sweet/gherkin-small	Item	15	20	0	5	0	0	0	0	0	128	—
Potato chips-salt add	Item	2	10.5	0.128	1.04	0.708	0	0.181	0.125	0.36	9.4	26
Potato skin-baked	Item	58	115	2.49	26.7	0.06	0	0.015	0.001	0.025	12	332

Mag (mg)	Iron (mg)	Zinc (mg)	VA (RE)	VC (mg)	Thia (mg)	Ribo (mg)	Niac (mg)	VB_6 (mg)	Fol (μg)	VB_{12} (μg)	Calc (mg)	Phos (mg)	Sel (mg)	Fibd (g)	VE (mg)
13.5	0.504	0.162	11.3	42.6	0.045	0.027	0.27	0.086	51	0	42.3	20.7	0.002	1.8	1.5
11	0.35	0.15	2.8	39.9	0.035	0.021	0.21	0.147	14.5	0	36	29	0.002	1.7	0.14
18	1.77	—	437	44.2	0.054	0.107	0.728	—	—	0	158	49	0.004	2.1	1.19
13	0.56	—	210	31.5	0.028	0.049	0.35	—	—	0	74	26	0.002	1.3	0.084
16	0.54	0.22	3094	10.2	0.106	0.064	1.02	0.162	15.4	0	30	48	0.002	3.52	0.484
11	0.36	0.14	2025	6.7	0.07	0.042	0.668	0.106	10.1	0	19	32	0.002	2.3	0.317
20	0.96	0.46	3830	3.6	0.054	0.088	0.79	0.384	21.6	0	48	48	0.002	5.77	0.651
12	0.94	0.38	2011	4	0.026	0.044	0.806	0.164	13.4	0	38	34	0.002	2.19	0.613
14	0.69	0.35	2585	4.1	0.039	0.054	0.639	0.188	15.8	0	41	39	0.003	5.4	0.613
16	0.74	0.24	4	56.4	0.066	0.096	0.558	0.158	73.8	0	30	44	0.001	3.24	0.054
14	0.52	0.3	1.8	68.6	0.078	0.064	0.684	0.25	63.4	0	34	44	0.001	2.73	0.038
14	0.58	0.18	1.6	71.5	0.076	0.057	0.633	0.231	66.1	0	29	46	0.001	2.4	0.03
14	0.58	0.2	15.2	7.6	0.036	0.036	0.36	0.036	10.6	0	44	32	0	1.92	0.432
5	0.19	0.07	5.1	2.5	0.012	0.012	0.12	0.012	3.6	0	14	10	0	0.64	0.144
2	0.05	—	19.2	2.4	0.003	0.005	0.021	0.005	—	0	2	2	—	0.096	—
52	1.9	0.46	1017	44.9	0.08	0.196	1.08	0.194	129	0	357	46	0.001	5.2	—
21	0.78	1.22	422	18.6	0.032	0.082	0.448	0.08	12.4	0	148	19	0.001	2.1	—
30	0.5	0.56	40.8	4.2	0.114	0.12	2.1	0.164	33.4	0	4	78	0.001	3.47	0.05
24	0.47	0.37	16.7	4.8	0.166	0.055	1.24	0.046	35.7	0	2	79	0.001	6.6	0.056
36	0.78	0.8	26.6	6	0.22	0.086	1.91	0.282	38.4	0	4	94	0.001	2.65	0.069
28	1.4	0.64	25.6	7	0.05	0.08	1.5	0.33	59.4	0	8	81	0.001	2.15	0.066
44	0.98	1.36	24.8	11.8	0.064	0.136	2.46	0.162	115	0	8	130	0.001	3.07	0.102
85	3.6	2.42	12.8	4.5	0.442	0.109	1.24	0.162	240	0	40	208	—	9.8	0.204
83	2.36	1.3	105	2.6	0.112	0.177	1.77	0.083	173	0	46	197	—	11	0.215
12	0.28	0.24	4.6	4.8	0.032	0.02	0.312	0.054	14.4	0	14	18	0.001	1.04	0.156
13	0.34	0.14	6.1	1.3	0.073	0.019	0.576	0.083	13.8	0	5	22	—	2.69	0.029
8	0.42	0.4	103	3.2	0.04	0.038	0.2	0.01	71	0	26	14	—	—	—
1	0.05	—	0	0.9	0.006	0.003	0.021	—	0.1	0	5	5	0	—	0
18	1.36	—	5.7	5.2	0.032	0.025	0.248	—	30.1	0	37	21	0	3.97	1.14
1.65	0.04	0.03	14.6	1.2	0.01	0.01	0.045	0.008	11	0	5	4	0	0.15	0.06
4.95	0.275	0.121	18.2	2.15	0.025	0.017	0.103	0.022	30.8	0	10.5	11	0	0.55	0.22
1.81	0.1	0.044	6.61	0.781	0.009	0.006	0.037	0.008	11.2	0	3.81	4	0	0.2	0.08
6	0.78	0.121	106	10	0.028	0.044	0.224	0.03	76	0	38	14	0	0.76	0.22
4	0.62	—	146	13.4	0.056	0.056	0.28	—	76	0	20	26	0	0.952	0.224
116	7.52	9.13	24	0	0.267	0.688	2.37	0.591	90.8	0.57	183	420	—	9.9	—
1	0.21	0.1	0	0.5	0.009	0.036	0.535	0.011	2.2	0	1	10	0.001	0.264	0.01
—	0.1	0.09	0	—	—	—	—	—	1.5	0	—	—	0.005	0.216	0.01
8	0.86	0.344	0	2.4	0.072	0.314	2.88	0.068	14.8	0	4	72	0.009	0.91	0.056
—	0.05	—	1	—	—	—	—	—	0.04	0	2	0.5	0	0.104	—
—	0.033	0.01	1	—	0	0	—	0	0.033	0	3	0.333	0	0.09	—
22	0.42	0.38	0	12	0.088	0.016	0.168	0.378	26.6	0	58	48	0.007	1.68	0.252
16	0.58	0.28	0	13.4	0.096	0.016	0.16	0.252	31.8	0	40	46	0.003	2.64	0.496
1.9	0.169	0.042	2.25	0.14	0.028	0.014	0.361	0.008	1.3	0	3.1	8.1	—	0.382	0.069
1	0.095	0.022	25	2.25	0.004	0.007	0.001	—	0.685	0	3	1.65	0	0.12	0.006
1.6	0.248	0.028	20.8	3.6	0.003	0.004	0.028	0.006	7.32	0	5.2	1.6	0	0.176	0.07
30	1.62	1.2	131	16.2	0.206	0.132	1.24	0.108	75.4	0	34	114	0.001	6.97	0.034
46	2.52	1.5	107	15.8	0.452	0.16	2.37	0.18	93.8	0	38	144	0.001	6.08	0.192
—	3.4	2.1	8	—	0.3	0.18	1.8	—	—	—	22	178	0.003	10.5	0.18
38	1.8	0.46	116	364	0.136	0.136	1.43	0.418	35	0	26	68	—	3.55	1.03
3.4	0.3	0.054	130	0	0	0.02	0.2	—	—	0	5	4	0	0.685	—
22.6	1.04	0.272	143	202	0.149	0.068	1.15	0.561	49.8	0	20.4	43	—	4.19	1.56
16	3.81	0.26	231	17.7	0.041	0.068	0.68	—	—	0	35	23	0	—	—
7.8	0.7	0.176	7	4	0	0.01	0	0.005	0.65	0	17	14	0	0.78	—
—	0.15	0.02	1	0.5	0	0	0	0.001	0.075	0	2.5	2	0	0.09	—
0.15	0.2	0.02	1	1	0	0	0	0.001	0.15	0	2	2	0	0.165	—
1.2	0.024	0.021	0	0.83	0.003	0	0.084	0.01	0.9	0	0.5	3.1	0	0.029	0.085
25	4.08	0.28	—	7.8	0.071	0.061	1.78	0.356	12.5	0	20	59	—	3.02	—

Continued.

Key to Abbreviations
Kcal, Kcalories; *Prot*, protein; *Carb*, carbohydrate; *Fat*, fat; *Chol*, cholesterol; *Safa*, saturated fat; *Mufa*, monounsaturated fat; *Pufa*, polyunsaturated fat; *Sod*, sodium; *Pot*, potassium; *Mag*, magnesium; *Iron*, iron; *Zinc*, zinc; *VA*, vitamin A; *VC*, vitamin C; *Thia*, thiamin; *Ribo*, riboflavin; *Niac*, niacin; *VB6*, vitamin B_6; *Fol*, folate; *VB12*, vitamin B_{12}; *Calc*, calcium; *Phos*, phosphorus; *Sel*, selenium; *Fibd*, dietary fiber; and *VE*, vitamin E.

Food name	Portion	Wt (g)	Kcal	Prot (g)	Carb (g)	Fat (g)	Chol (mg)	Safa (g)	Mufa (g)	Pufa (g)	Sod (mg)	Pot (mg)
Vegetables—cont'd												
Potato-Au Gratin-home rec	Cup	245	322	12.4	27.6	18.6	58	11.6	5.27	0.676	1060	970
Potato-french fried-froz	Item	5	11.1	0.173	1.7	0.438	0	0.208	0.178	0.033	1.5	22.9
Potato-french fried-raw	Item	5	13.5	0.2	1.8	0.7	0	0.17	0.178	0.033	11.1	42.7
Potato-hash brown-prep-raw	Cup	156	326	3.77	33.3	21.7	—	8.48	9.69	2.5	38	501
Potato-hash brown-froz	Cup	156	340	4.92	43.8	17.9	0	7.01	8.01	2.07	54	680
Potato-mashed-dehy-prep	Cup	210	166	4.2	27.5	4.62	4	1.43	1.35	1.33	491	704
Potato-mashed-milk/butter	Cup	210	222	3.95	35.1	8.87	4	2.17	3.72	2.54	619	607
Potato-scallop-home rec	Cup	245	210	7.03	26.4	9.02	29	5.53	2.55	0.407	821	925
Potato-scallop-mix-prep	oz	28.4	26.4	0.602	3.63	1.22	—	0.748	0.344	0.055	96.8	57.7
Pumpkin pie mix-can	Cup	270	282	2.93	71.3	0.34	0	0.176	0.043	0.019	561	372
Radishes-raw	Item	4.5	0.7	0.027	0.161	0.024	0	0.001	0.001	0.002	1.1	10.4
Rutabagas-boil-drain	Cup	170	58	1.88	13.2	0.32	0	0.042	0.04	0.142	30	488
Sauerkraut-can	Cup	236	44	2.15	10.1	0.33	0	0.083	0.031	0.144	1561	401
Seaweed-wakame-raw	oz	28.4	12.8	0.86	2.6	0.182	0	0.037	0.016	0.062	248	14.2
Soybean-dry-ckd	Cup	180	234	19.8	19.4	10.3	0	—	—	—	4	972
Spinach-can-solids/liquids	Cup	234	44	4.93	6.84	0.87	0	0.14	0.023	0.363	747	539
Spinach-froz-boil-chop	Cup	205	57.4	6.44	10.9	0.431	0	0.068	0.012	0.176	176	611
Spinach-raw-boil-drain	Cup	180	41	5.35	6.75	0.47	0	0.076	0.013	0.194	126	838
Spinach-raw-chop	Cup	56	12	1.6	1.96	0.2	0	0.032	0.006	0.082	44	312
Squash-acorn-baked	Cup	205	115	2.29	29.9	0.29	0	0.059	0.021	0.121	9	896
Squash-butternut-baked	Cup	205	83	1.84	21.5	0.18	0	0.039	0.014	0.078	7	583
Squash-hubbard-boil-mash	Cup	236	70	3.5	15.2	0.88	0	0.179	0.066	0.368	12	504
Squash-summer-boil-sliced	Cup	180	36	1.63	7.76	0.56	0	0.115	0.041	0.236	2	346
Squash-winter-bake-mashed	Cup	205	79	1.81	17.9	1.29	0	0.267	0.096	0.543	3	895
Squash-zucchini-froz-boil	Cup	223	37	2.56	7.94	0.29	0	0.06	0.022	0.123	5	434
Squash-zucchini-italian-can	Cup	227	65	2.33	15.6	0.25	0	0.052	0.018	0.107	850	622
Squash-zucchini-raw-boil	Cup	180	28	1.14	7.08	0.1	0	0.018	0.008	0.038	4	456
Squash-zucchini-raw-sliced	Cup	130	19	1.5	3.78	0.18	0	0.038	0.014	0.078	3	322
Succotash-boil-drain	Cup	192	222	9.73	46.8	1.53	0	0.284	0.298	0.732	32	787
Sweet potato-bake-peel	Item	114	118	1.96	27.7	0.13	0	0.027	0.005	0.056	12	397
Sweet potato-boil-mashed	Cup	328	344	5.4	79.6	0.97	0	0.21	0.036	0.433	42	602
Sweet potato-can-mashed	Cup	255	258	5.05	59.2	0.51	0	0.11	0.02	0.227	191	536
Sweet potato-candied	Piece	105	144	0.91	29.3	3.41	0	1.42	0.658	0.154	73	198
Tofu-soybean curd	Piece	120	86	9.4	2.9	5	0	—	—	—	8	50
Tomato juice-can	Cup	244	42	1.86	10.3	0.14	0	0.02	0.022	0.058	882	536
Tomato juice-low sodium	Cup	244	42	1.86	10.3	0.14	0	0.01	0.022	0.058	24.4	536
Tomato paste-can-low sodium	Cup	262	220	9.9	49.3	2.33	0	0.332	0.351	0.948	172	2442
Tomato paste-can-salt add	Cup	262	220	9.9	49.3	2.33	0	0.332	0.351	0.948	2070	2442
Tomato powder	oz	28.4	85.8	3.67	21.2	0.125	0	0.018	0.019	0.05	38.1	547
Tomato puree-can-low sodium	Cup	250	102	4.18	25.1	0.29	0	0.04	0.043	0.118	49	1051
Tomato puree-can-salt add	Cup	250	102	4.18	25.1	0.29	0	0.04	0.043	0.118	998	1051
Tomato-can-low sodium-diet	Cup	240	47	2.24	10.3	0.59	0	0.084	0.089	0.238	31.2	529
Tomato-raw-red-rip	Item	123	24	1.09	5.34	0.26	0	0.037	0.039	0.107	10	254
Tomato-red-can-stewed	Cup	255	68	2.37	16.5	0.36	0	0.051	0.054	0.148	647	611
Tomato-red-can-whole	Cup	240	47	2.24	10.3	0.59	0	0.084	0.089	0.238	390	529
Tomato-red-raw-boil	Cup	240	60	2.68	13.5	0.65	0	0.091	0.096	0.262	25	624
Tomato-stew-cook-home rec	Cup	101	59	1.77	10.4	2.21	0	0.4	0.701	0.447	374	170
V-8 veg juice-low sodium	Cup	243	51	0	9.72	0	0	0	0	0	58.3	571
Vegetable juice-can	Cup	242	44	1.52	11	0.22	0	0.032	0.034	0.092	884	468
Vegetables-mixed-froz-boil	Cup	182	108	5.22	23.8	0.28	0	0.056	0.018	0.132	64	308

Mag (mg)	Iron (mg)	Zinc (mg)	VA (RE)	VC (mg)	Thia (mg)	Ribo (mg)	Niac (mg)	VB_6 (mg)	Fol (μg)	VB_{12} (μg)	Calc (mg)	Phos (mg)	Sel (mg)	Fibd (g)	VE (mg)
48	1.56	1.69	64.6	24.3	0.157	0.284	2.43	0.426	19.9	0.492	292	278	—	4.41	—
1.1	0.067	0.021	0	0.55	0.006	0.002	0.115	0.012	0.83	0	0.4	4.3	0	0.16	0.01
—	0.07	—	0	1.1	0.007	0.004	0.16	0.009	1.1	0	0.8	5.6	0	0.16	0.01
32	1.27	0.46	—	8.9	0.115	0.031	3.12	0.434	12	0	13	65	—	3.12	—
26	2.34	0.5	—	9.8	0.174	0.032	3.78	0.196	38.8	0	24	112	0.001	1.5	0.295
—	1.26	—	18.9	6.3	0.063	0.105	1.68	—	—	—	65	92	0.001	1.2	—
37	0.55	0.58	35.5	12.9	0.176	0.084	2.27	0.47	16.7	0	54	97	0.001	3.15	0.084
46	1.41	0.98	33.2	26.1	0.169	0.225	2.58	0.436	21.3	0.348	140	154	—	4.41	—
3.98	0.108	0.071	—	0.937	0.005	0.016	0.292	0.012	0.312	—	10.2	15.9	—	0.54	—
43	2.87	0.72	2241	9.5	0.043	0.319	1.01	—	—	0	99	120	—	—	—
0.4	0.013	0.013	0.03	1.03	0	0.002	0.014	0.003	1.22	0	0.9	0.8	0	0.1	—
36	0.8	0.52	0	37.2	0.122	0.062	1.07	0.154	26.4	0	72	84	—	2.5	0.255
31	3.47	0.44	4.2	34.8	0.05	0.052	0.337	0.307	7.05	0	72	46	0.024	6.06	—
30.4	0.619	0.108	10.2	0.852	0.017	0.065	0.454	—	—	0	42.6	22.7	0.001	1.2	—
—	4.9	—	5	0	0.38	0.16	1.1	—	—	—	131	322	—	—	—
132	3.7	0.99	1505	31.6	0.042	0.248	0.634	0.187	136	0	195	74	0.003	5.08	0.047
141	3.12	1.44	1596	25.2	0.123	0.344	0.859	0.299	220	0	299	98.4	0.002	4.51	3.85
157	6.42	1.37	1474	17.7	0.171	0.425	0.882	0.436	262	0	244	100	0.002	3.96	3.38
44	1.52	0.3	376	15.8	0.044	0.106	0.406	0.11	108	0	56	28	0.001	1.46	1.03
87	1.91	0.35	87.8	22.1	0.342	0.027	1.81	0.398	38.4	0	90	93	0.002	4.3	0.246
59	1.22	0.27	1435	30.9	0.148	0.035	1.99	0.254	39.3	0	84	55	0.002	3.5	0.246
32	0.67	0.22	945	15.4	0.099	0.066	0.788	0.243	23	0	23	33	0.002	4.2	0.283
44	0.64	0.71	51.7	10	0.079	0.074	0.923	0.117	36.2	0	48	69	0.006	2.52	0.216
16	0.67	0.54	729	19.7	0.174	0.049	1.44	0.148	57.4	0	28	41	0.006	5.74	0.246
28	1.08	0.44	96.2	8.2	0.091	0.089	0.861	0.1	17.5	0	38	55	0.007	3.23	0.268
31	1.55	0.58	123	5.2	0.095	0.091	1.2	—	—	0	38	66	—	7.02	—
38	0.64	0.32	43.2	8.4	0.074	0.074	0.77	0.14	30.2	0	24	72	0.006	2.3	0.216
28	0.55	0.26	44.2	11.7	0.091	0.039	0.52	0.116	28.8	0	20	42	0.004	2	0.156
102	2.93	1.22	56.4	15.7	0.323	0.184	2.55	0.223	—	0	32	224	—	14	—
23	0.52	0.33	2488	28	0.083	0.145	0.689	0.275	25.7	0	32	62	0.001	3.42	5.2
32	1.83	0.87	5594	55.9	0.174	0.459	2.1	0.8	36.3	0	70	88	0.022	9.84	15
61	3.39	0.54	3857	13.3	0.069	0.23	2.44	0.168	—	0	76	133	0.002	4.59	—
12	1.19	0.16	440	7	0.019	0.044	0.414	0.043	12	0.032	27	27	0.001	1.1	—
—	2.3	—	0	0	0.07	0.04	0.1	—	—	—	154	151	0.002	1.44	—
28	1.42	0.36	136	44.6	0.114	0.076	1.64	0.27	48.4	0	20	46	0.001	2.9	0.535
28	1.42	0.36	136	44.6	0.114	0.076	1.64	0.27	48.4	0	20	46	0.001	2.8	0.537
134	7.83	2.1	647	111	0.406	0.498	8.44	0.996	—	0	91.7	207	0.003	11.3	—
134	7.83	2.1	647	111	0.406	0.498	8.44	0.996	—	0	91.7	207	0.003	11.3	—
50.6	1.3	0.486	490	33.1	0.259	0.216	2.59	0.13	34.1	0	47.1	83.8	—	—	—
60	2.32	0.54	340	88.2	0.178	0.135	4.29	0.38	—	0	37	99	0.003	5.75	0.55
60	2.32	0.54	340	88.2	0.178	0.135	4.29	0.38	—	0	37	99	0.003	5.75	0.55
29	1.45	0.38	145	36.3	0.108	0.074	1.76	0.216	—	0	63	46	0.002	1.69	0.528
14	0.59	0.13	139	21.6	0.074	0.062	0.738	0.059	11.5	0	8	29	0.001	1.6	0.418
29	1.86	0.42	142	33.8	0.117	0.089	1.82	—	7.4	0	84	51	0.002	2.04	0.561
29	1.45	0.38	145	36.3	0.108	0.074	1.76	0.216	7	0	63	46	0.002	1.93	0.53
33	1.44	0.32	325	50.3	0.17	0.144	1.72	0.086	22.6	0	20	70	0.001	1.92	0.816
13	0.78	0.17	102	14.8	0.067	0.064	0.75	0.031	9.9	0	19	32	0.001	1.04	0.343
—	1.46	—	437	53	0.049	0.073	1.94	—	—	—	38.9	—	0.001	2.7	—
26	1.02	0.48	283	67	0.104	0.068	1.76	0.339	—	0	26	40	0.001	2.7	—
40	1.5	0.9	1360	5.8	0.13	0.218	1.55	0.134	34.6	0	44	92	0.001	4.19	—

Continued.

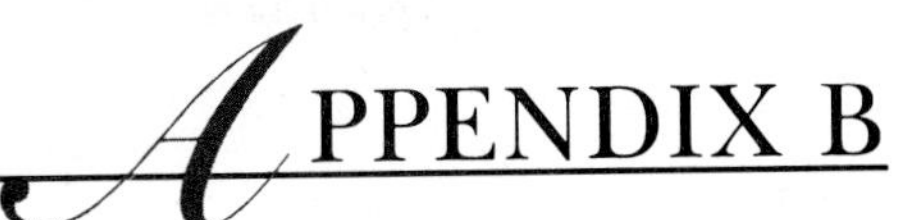

PPENDIX B

Amino Acid Content of Foods, 100 g, Edible Portion

Protein content and nitrogen conversion factor	Trypto-phan (g)	Threo-nine (g)	Iso-leucine (g)	Leucine (g)	Lysine (g)	Methi-onine (g)	Cystine (g)	Phenyl-alanine (g)	Tyro-sine (g)	Valine (g)	Argi-nine (g)	Histi-dine (g)
Milk, milk products												
Milk (protein, N × 6.38)												
Cow												
Fluid, whole and nonfat (3.5% protein)	0.049	0.161	0.223	0.344	0.272	0.086	0.031	0.170	0.178	0.240	0.128	0.092
Canned												
Evaporated, unsweetened (7.0% protein)	0.099	0.323	0.447	0.688	0.545	0.171	0.063	0.340	0.357	0.481	0.256	0.185
Condensed, sweetened (8.1% protein)	0.114	0.374	0.518	0.796	0.631	0.198	0.072	0.393	0.413	0.557	0.296	0.214
Dried												
Whole (25.8% protein)	0.364	1.191	1.648	2.535	2.009	0.632	0.231	1.251	1.316	1.774	0.944	0.680
Nonfat (35.6% protein)	0.502	1.641	2.271	3.493	2.768	0.870	0.318	1.724	1.814	2.444	1.300	0.937
Goat (3.3% protein)	0.039	0.217	0.087	0.278	0.312	0.065	—	0.121	—	0.139	0.174	0.068
Human (1.4% protein)	0.023	0.062	0.075	0.124	0.090	0.028	0.027	0.060	0.071	0.086	0.055	0.030
Indian buffalo (4.2% protein)	0.059	0.212	0.204	0.420	0.331	0.112	0.058	0.177	—	0.255	0.136	0.086
Milk products												
Buttermilk (3.5% protein, N × 6.38)	0.038	0.165	0.219	0.346	0.291	0.082	0.032	0.186	0.137	0.262	0.168	0.099
Casein (100% protein, N × 6.29)	1.335	4.277	6.550	10.048	8.013	3.084	0.382	5.389	5.819	7.393	4.070	3.021
Cheese (protein, N × 6.38)												
Blue mold (21.5% protein)	0.293	0.799	1.449	2.096	1.577	0.559	0.121	1.153	1.028	1.543	0.785	0.701
Camembert (17.5% protein)	0.239	0.650	1.179	1.706	1.284	0.455	0.099	0.938	0.837	1.256	0.639	0.571
Cheddar (25.0% protein)	0.341	0.929	1.685	2.437	1.834	0.650	0.141	1.340	1.195	1.794	0.913	0.815
Cheddar processed (23.2% protein)	0.316	0.862	1.563	2.262	1.702	0.604	0.131	1.244	1.109	1.665	0.847	0.756
Cheese foods, Cheddar (20.5% protein)	0.280	0.761	1.382	1.998	1.504	0.533	0.116	1.099	0.980	1.472	0.749	0.668
Cottage (17.0% protein)	0.179	0.794	0.989	1.826	1.428	0.469	0.147	0.917	0.917	0.978	0.802	0.549
Cream cheese (9.0% protein)	0.080	0.408	0.519	0.923	0.721	0.229	0.085	0.547	0.408	0.538	0.313	0.278
Limburger (21.2% protein)	0.289	0.788	1.429	2.067	1.555	0.552	0.120	1.136	1.014	1.522	0.774	0.691
Parmesan (36.0% protein)	0.491	1.337	2.426	3.510	2.641	0.937	0.203	1.930	1.721	2.584	1.315	1.174
Swiss (27.5% protein)	0.375	1.021	1.853	2.681	2.017	0.715	0.155	1.474	1.315	1.974	1.004	0.896
Swiss processed (26.4% protein)	0.360	0.981	1.779	2.574	1.937	0.687	0.149	1.415	1.262	1.895	0.964	0.861
Lactalbumin (100% protein, N × 6.49)	2.203	5.239	6.209	12.342	9.060	2.250	3.405	4.360	3.806	5.686	3.498	1.911
Whey (protein, N × 6.49)												
Fluid (0.9% protein)	0.010	0.048	0.052	0.074	0.055	0.013	0.018	0.023	0.009	0.045	0.017	0.011
Dried (12.7% protein)	0.147	0.677	0.734	1.043	0.769	0.188	0.250	0.323	0.131	0.640	0.235	0.159
Eggs, chicken (protein, N × 6.25)												
Fresh or stored												
Whole (12.8% protein)	0.211	0.637	0.850	1.126	0.819	0.401	0.299	0.739	0.551	0.950	0.840	0.307
Whites (10.8% protein)	0.164	0.477	0.698	0.950	0.648	0.420	0.263	0.689	0.449	0.842	0.634	0.233
Yolks (16.3% protein)	0.235	0.827	0.996	1.372	1.074	0.417	0.274	0.717	0.756	1.121	1.132	0.368

Courtesy Orr, ML, Watt, BK: *Amino acid content of foods,* Home Economics Research Report No. 4, U.S. Department of Agriculture, 1966. This selected listing reprinted here is taken from the original report of the Agricultural Research Service, which contains data on 18 amino acids in 202 food items.

Protein content and nitrogen conversion factor	Trypto-phan (g)	Threo-nine (g)	Iso-leucine (g)	Leucine (g)	Lysine (g)	Methi-onine (g)	Cystine (g)	Phenyl-alanine (g)	Tyro-sine (g)	Valine (g)	Argi-nine (g)	Histi-dine (g)
Eggs, chicken (protein, N × 6.25)—cont'd												
Dried												
Whole (46.8% protein)	0.771	2.329	3.108	4.118	2.995	1.468	1.093	2.703	2.014	3.474	3.070	1.123
Whites (85.9% protein)	1.306	3.793	5.553	7.559	5.154	3.340	3.089	5.484	3.573	6.693	5.044	1.855
Yolks (31.2% protein)	0.449	1.582	1.907	2.626	2.057	0.799	0.524	1.373	1.448	2.147	2.167	0.704
Meat, poultry, fish and shellfish (their products)												
Meat (protein, N × 6.25)												
Beef carcass or side												
Thin (18.8% protein)	0.220	0.830	0.984	1.540	1.642	0.466	0.238	0.773	0.638	1.044	1.212	0.653
Medium fat (17.5% protein)	0.204	0.773	0.916	1.434	1.529	0.434	0.221	0.720	0.594	0.972	1.128	0.608
Fat (16.3% protein)	0.190	0.720	0.853	1.335	1.424	0.404	0.206	0.670	0.553	0.905	1.051	0.566
Very fat (13.7% protein)	0.160	0.605	0.717	1.122	1.197	0.340	0.173	0.563	0.465	0.761	0.883	0.476
Medium fat, trimmed to retail basis (18.2% protein)	0.213	0.804	0.952	1.491	1.590	0.451	0.230	0.748	0.617	1.010	1.174	0.632
Beef cuts, medium fat												
Chuck (18.6% protein)	0.217	0.821	0.973	1.524	1.625	0.461	0.235	0.765	0.631	1.033	1.199	0.646
Flank (19.9% protein)	0.232	0.879	1.041	1.630	1.738	0.494	0.252	0.818	0.675	1.105	1.283	0.691
Hamburger (16.0% protein)	0.187	0.707	0.837	1.311	1.398	0.397	0.202	0.658	0.543	0.888	1.032	0.556
Porterhouse (16.4% protein)	0.192	0.724	0.858	1.343	1.433	0.407	0.207	0.674	0.556	0.911	1.057	0.569
Rib roast (17.4% protein)	0.203	0.768	0.910	1.425	1.520	0.432	0.220	0.715	0.590	0.966	1.122	0.604
Round (19.5% protein)	0.228	0.861	1.020	1.597	1.704	0.484	0.246	0.802	0.661	1.083	1.257	0.677
Rump (16.2% protein)	0.189	0.715	0.848	1.327	1.415	0.402	0.205	0.666	0.550	0.899	1.045	0.562
Sirloin (17.3% protein)	0.202	0.764	0.905	1.417	1.511	0.429	0.219	0.711	0.587	0.960	1.116	0.601
Beef, canned (25.0% protein)	0.292	1.104	1.308	2.048	2.184	0.620	0.316	1.028	0.848	1.388	1.612	0.868
Beef, dried or chipped (34.3% protein)	0.401	1.515	1.795	2.810	2.996	0.851	0.434	1.410	1.163	1.904	2.212	1.191
Lamb carcass or side												
Thin (17.1% protein)	0.222	0.782	0.886	1.324	1.384	0.410	0.224	0.695	0.594	0.843	1.114	0.476
Medium fat (15.7% protein)	0.203	0.718	0.814	1.216	1.271	0.377	0.206	0.638	0.545	0.774	1.022	0.437
Fat (13.0% protein)	0.168	0.595	0.674	1.007	1.052	0.312	0.171	0.528	0.451	0.641	0.847	0.362
Lamb cuts, medium fat												
Leg (18.0% protein)	0.233	0.824	0.933	1.394	1.457	0.432	0.236	0.732	0.625	0.887	1.172	0.501
Rib (14.9% protein)	0.193	0.682	0.772	1.154	1.206	0.358	0.195	0.606	0.517	0.734	0.970	0.415
Shoulder (15.6% protein)	0.202	0.714	0.809	1.208	1.263	0.374	0.205	0.634	0.542	0.769	1.016	0.434
Pork, packer's carcass or side												
Thin (14.1% protein)	0.183	0.654	0.724	1.038	1.157	0.352	0.165	0.555	0.503	0.733	0.864	0.487
Medium fat (11.9% protein)	0.154	0.552	0.611	0.876	0.977	0.297	0.139	0.468	0.425	0.619	0.729	0.411
Fat (9.8% protein)	0.127	0.455	0.503	0.721	0.804	0.245	0.114	0.386	0.350	0.510	0.601	0.339
Pork cuts, medium fat, fresh												
Ham (15.2% protein)	0.197	0.705	0.781	1.119	1.248	0.379	0.178	0.598	0.542	0.790	0.931	0.525
Loin (16.4% protein)	0.213	0.761	0.842	1.207	1.346	0.409	0.192	0.646	0.585	0.853	1.005	0.567
Miscellaneous lean cuts (14.5% protein)	0.188	0.673	0.745	1.067	1.190	0.362	0.169	0.571	0.517	0.754	0.889	0.501
Pork, cured												
Bacon, medium fat (9.1% protein)	0.095	0.306	0.399	0.728	0.587	0.141	0.106	0.434	0.234	0.434	0.622	0.246
Fat back or salt pork (3.9% protein)	0.006	0.141	0.110	0.367	0.317	0.055	0.043	0.157	0.052	0.168	0.379	0.035
Ham (16.9% protein)	0.162	0.692	0.841	1.306	1.420	0.411	0.273	0.646	0.652	0.879	1.068	0.544
Luncheon meat												
Boiled ham (22.8% protein)	0.219	0.934	1.135	1.762	1.915	0.554	0.368	0.872	0.879	1.186	1.441	0.733
Canned, spiced (14.9% protein)	0.143	0.610	0.741	1.161	1.252	0.362	0.241	0.570	0.575	0.775	0.942	0.479
Rabbit, domesticated, flesh only (21.9% protein)	—	1.021	1.082	1.636	1.818	0.541	—	0.793	—	1.021	1.176	0.474
Veal, carcass or side												
Thin (19.7% protein)	0.258	0.854	1.040	1.444	1.645	0.451	0.233	0.801	0.709	1.018	1.283	0.634
Medium fat (19.1% protein)	0.251	0.828	1.008	1.400	1.595	0.437	0.226	0.776	0.688	0.987	1.244	0.614
Fat (18.5% protein)	0.243	0.802	0.977	1.356	1.545	0.423	0.219	0.752	0.666	0.956	1.205	0.595
Veal cuts, medium fat												
Round (19.5% protein)	0.256	0.846	1.030	1.429	1.629	0.446	0.231	0.792	0.702	1.008	1.270	0.627
Shoulder (19.4% protein)	0.255	0.841	1.024	1.422	1.620	0.444	0.230	0.788	0.698	1.003	1.263	0.624
Stew meat (18.3% protein)	0.240	0.793	0.966	1.341	1.528	0.419	0.217	0.744	0.659	0.946	1.192	0.589

Continued.

Protein content and nitrogen conversion factor	Tryptophan (g)	Threonine (g)	Isoleucine (g)	Leucine (g)	Lysine (g)	Methionine (g)	Cystine (g)	Phenylalanine (g)	Tyrosine (g)	Valine (g)	Arginine (g)	Histidine (g)
Meat, poultry, fish and shellfish (their products)—cont'd												
Poultry (protein, N × 6.25)												
Chicken, fresh only												
Broilers or fryers (20.6% protein)	0.250	0.877	1.088	1.490	1.810	0.537	0.277	0.811	0.725	1.012	1.302	0.593
Hens (21.3% protein)	0.259	0.907	1.125	1.540	1.871	0.556	0.286	0.838	0.750	1.046	1.346	0.613
Ducks, domesticated, flesh only (21.4% protein)	—	0.935	1.109	1.657	1.842	0.531	—	0.842	—	1.027	1.301	0.486
Turkey, flesh only (24.0% protein)	—	1.014	1.260	1.836	2.173	0.664	0.330	0.960	—	1.187	1.513	0.649
Fish and shellfish (protein, N × 6.25)												
Bluefish (20.5% protein)	0.203	0.889	1.040	1.548	1.797	0.597	0.276	0.761	0.554	1.092	1.155	—
Cod												
Fresh (16.5% protein)	0.164	0.715	0.837	1.246	1.447	0.480	0.222	0.612	0.446	0.879	0.929	—
Dried (81.8% protein)	0.811	3.547	4.149	6.178	7.172	2.382	1.099	3.036	2.212	4.358	4.607	—
Croaker (17.8% protein)	0.177	0.772	0.903	1.344	1.561	0.518	0.239	0.661	0.481	0.948	1.002	—
Eel (18.6% protein)	0.185	0.806	0.943	1.405	1.631	0.542	0.250	0.690	0.503	0.991	1.048	—
Flounder (14.9% protein)	0.148	0.646	0.756	1.125	1.306	0.434	0.200	0.553	0.403	0.794	0.839	—
Haddock (18.2% protein)	0.181	0.789	0.923	1.374	1.596	0.530	0.245	0.676	0.492	0.970	1.025	—
Halibut (18.6% protein)	0.185	0.806	0.943	1.405	1.631	0.542	0.250	0.690	0.503	0.991	1.048	—
Herring												
Atlantic (18.3% protein)	0.182	0.793	0.928	1.382	1.605	0.533	0.246	0.679	0.495	0.975	1.031	—
Lake (18.5% protein)	0.184	0.802	0.938	1.397	1.622	0.539	0.249	0.687	0.500	0.986	1.042	—
Pacific (16.6% protein)	0.165	0.720	0.842	1.254	1.455	0.483	0.223	0.616	0.449	0.884	0.935	—
Mackerels												
Raw, common Atlantic (18.7% protein)	0.186	0.811	0.948	1.412	1.640	0.545	0.251	0.694	0.506	0.996	1.053	—
Canned, solids and liquid												
Atlantic (19.3% protein)	0.191	0.837	0.979	1.458	1.692	0.562	0.259	0.716	0.522	1.028	1.087	—
Pacific (21.1% protein)	0.209	0.915	1.070	1.593	1.850	0.614	0.284	0.783	0.571	1.124	1.188	—
Salmon												
Raw, Pacific (Chinook or King) (17.4% protein)	0.173	0.754	0.883	1.314	1.526	0.507	0.234	0.646	0.470	0.927	0.980	—
Canned, solids and liquid (sockeye or red) (20.2% protein)	0.200	0.876	1.025	1.526	1.771	0.588	0.271	0.750	0.546	1.076	1.138	—
Sardines, canned, solids and liquid												
Atlantic type (21.1% protein)	0.209	0.915	1.070	1.593	1.850	0.614	0.284	0.783	0.571	1.124	1.188	—
Pacific type (17.7% protein)	0.176	0.767	0.898	1.337	1.552	0.515	0.238	0.657	0.479	0.943	0.997	—
Shrimp, canned, solids and liquid (18.7% protein)	0.186	0.811	0.948	1.412	1.640	0.545	0.251	0.694	0.506	0.996	1.053	—
Products from meat, poultry, and fish (protein, N × 6.25)												
Brains (10.4% protein)	0.138	0.494	0.504	0.845	0.760	0.220	0.145	0.506	0.433	0.536	0.614	0.278
Chitterlings (8.6% protein)	0.094	0.398	0.308	0.457	0.670	0.193	0.109	0.359	0.228	0.462	1.406	0.169
Fish flour (76.0% protein)	0.754	4.378	4.232	6.189	7.381	2.019	—	2.845	—	3.916	5.204	1.289
Gelatin (85.6% protein, N × 5.55)	0.006	1.912	1.357	2.930	4.226	0.787	0.077	2.036	0.401	2.421	7.866	0.771
Gizzard, chicken (23.1% protein)	0.207	1.072	1.094	1.689	1.567	0.554	0.218	0.968	0.680	1.116	1.741	0.480
Heart												
Beef or pork (16.9% protein)	0.219	0.776	0.857	1.509	1.387	0.403	0.168	0.765	0.627	0.973	1.068	0.433
Chicken (20.5% protein)	0.266	0.941	1.040	1.830	1.683	0.489	0.203	0.928	0.761	1.181	1.296	0.525
Kidney												
Beef (15.0% protein)	0.221	0.665	0.730	1.301	1.087	0.307	0.182	0.706	0.557	0.876	0.934	0.377
Pork (16.3% protein)	0.240	0.722	0.793	1.414	1.181	0.334	0.198	0.767	0.605	0.952	1.015	0.409
Sheep (16.6% protein)	0.244	0.736	0.807	1.440	1.203	0.340	0.202	0.781	0.616	0.969	1.033	0.417
Liver												
Beef or pork (19.7% protein)	0.296	0.936	1.031	1.819	1.475	0.463	0.243	0.993	0.738	1.239	1.201	0.523
Calf (19.0% protein)	0.286	0.903	0.994	1.754	1.423	0.447	0.234	0.958	0.711	1.195	1.158	0.505
Chicken (22.1% protein)	0.332	1.050	1.156	2.040	1.655	0.520	0.272	1.114	0.827	1.390	1.347	0.587
Sheep or lamb (21.0% protein)	0.316	0.998	1.099	1.939	1.572	0.494	0.259	1.058	0.786	1.320	1.280	0.558
Pancreas												
Beef (13.5% protein)	0.175	0.626	0.683	1.054	0.996	0.244	—	0.562	0.590	0.724	0.771	0.266
Pork (14.5% protein)	0.188	0.673	0.733	1.132	1.070	0.262	—	0.603	0.633	0.777	0.828	0.285
Pork or beef, canned (14.3% protein)	0.151	0.618	0.730	1.190	1.345	0.327	0.261	0.579	0.570	0.810	1.050	0.460
Potted meat (16.1% protein)	0.149	0.662	0.641	1.203	1.061	0.361	—	0.641	—	0.943	1.002	0.322

Protein content and nitrogen conversion factor	Tryptophan (g)	Threonine (g)	Isoleucine (g)	Leucine (g)	Lysine (g)	Methionine (g)	Cystine (g)	Phenylalanine (g)	Tyrosine (g)	Valine (g)	Arginine (g)	Histidine (g)
Meat, poultry, fish and shellfish (their products)												
Sausage												
Bologna (14.8% protein)	0.126	0.606	0.718	1.061	1.191	0.313	0.185	0.540	0.481	0.744	1.028	0.398
Braunschweiger (15.4% protein)	0.172	0.668	0.754	1.291	1.200	0.320	0.187	0.700	0.471	0.956	0.954	0.458
Frankfurters (14.2% protein)	0.120	0.582	0.688	1.018	1.143	0.300	0.177	0.518	0.461	0.713	0.986	0.382
Head cheese (15.0 protein)	0.079	0.418	0.509	0.946	0.907	0.250	0.209	0.569	0.569	0.617	1.075	0.278
Liverwurst (16.7% protein)	0.187	0.724	0.818	1.400	1.301	0.347	0.203	0.759	0.510	1.037	1.034	0.497
Pork, links or bulk, raw (10.8% protein)	0.092	0.442	0.524	0.774	0.869	0.228	0.135	0.394	0.351	0.543	0.750	0.290
Pork, bulk, canned (15.4% protein)	0.131	0.631	0.747	1.104	1.239	0.325	0.192	0.562	0.500	0.774	1.069	0.414
Salami (23.9% protein)	0.203	0.979	1.159	1.713	1.923	0.505	0.298	0.872	0.776	1.201	1.660	0.642
Vienna sausage, canned (15.8% protein)	0.134	0.647	0.766	1.133	1.272	0.334	0.197	0.576	0.513	0.794	1.097	0.425
Tongue												
Beef (16.4% protein)	0.197	0.708	0.792	1.286	1.364	0.357	0.207	0.661	0.548	0.840	1.065	0.412
Pork (16.8% protein)	0.202	0.726	0.812	1.317	1.398	0.366	0.212	0.677	0.562	0.860	1.091	0.422
Veal and pork loaf, canned (17.2% protein)	0.198	0.627	0.859	1.236	1.258	0.418	0.209	0.619	0.468	0.958	0.916	0.388
Legumes (dry seed), common nuts, other nuts and dry seeds (their products)												
Legume seeds and their products												
Beans *(Phaseolus vulgaris)* (N × 6.25)												
Pinto and red Mexican (23.0% protein)	0.213	0.997	1.306	1.976	1.708	0.232	0.228	1.270	0.887	1.395	1.384	0.655
Red kidney												
Raw (23.1% protein)	0.214	1.002	1.312	1.985	1.715	0.233	0.229	1.275	0.891	1.401	1.390	0.658
Canned, solids and liquid (5.7% protein)	0.053	0.247	0.324	0.490	0.423	0.057	0.057	0.315	0.220	0.346	0.343	0.162
Other common beans including navy, peabean, white marrow												
Raw (21.4% protein)	0.199	0.928	1.216	1.839	1.589	0.216	0.212	1.181	0.825	1.298	1.287	0.609
Baked with pork, canned (5.8% protein)	0.057	0.274	0.291	0.486	0.354	0.059	0.018	0.333	0.165	0.312	0.251	0.186
Black gram, raw (23.6% protein, N × 6.25)	0.242	0.801	1.390	2.062	1.510	0.332	0.287	1.242	0.551	1.450	1.552	0.559
Broadbeans, raw (25.4% protein, N × 6.25)	0.236	0.829	1.593	2.211	1.426	0.106	0.179	1.057	0.687	1.276	1.780	0.748
Chickpeas (20.8% protein, N × 6.25)	0.170	0.739	1.195	1.538	1.434	0.276	0.296	1.012	0.692	1.025	1.551	0.559
Cowpeas (22.9% protein, N × 6.25)	0.220	0.901	1.110	1.715	1.491	0.352	0.297	1.198	0.678	1.293	1.473	0.692
Dolichos, twinflower (21.6% protein, N × 6.25)	0.221	0.836	1.448	1.707	1.700	0.294	0.480	1.486	0.560	1.286	1.230	0.650
Lentils, whole (25.0% protein, N × 6.25)	0.216	0.896	1.316	1.760	1.528	0.180	0.294	1.104	0.664	1.360	1.908	0.548
Lima beans (20.7% protein, N × 6.25)	0.195	0.980	1.199	1.722	1.378	0.331	0.311	1.222	0.543	1.298	1.315	0.669
Lupine (32.3% protein, N × 6.25)	—	1.101	1.618	1.964	1.447	0.114	—	1.271	—	1.328	2.718	0.811
Moth beans (24.4% protein, N × 6.25)	0.164	—	1.093	1.484	1.202	0.191	0.109	1.003	1.245	0.695	—	0.722
Mung beans (24.4% protein, N × 6.25)	0.180	0.765	1.351	2.202	1.667	0.265	0.152	1.167	0.390	1.444	1.370	0.543
Peanuts (26.9% protein, N × 5.46)	0.340	0.828	1.266	1.872	1.099	0.271	0.463	1.557	1.104	1.532	3.296	0.749
Peanut flour (51.2% protein, N × 5.46)	0.647	1.575	2.410	3.563	2.091	0.516	0.881	2.963	2.100	2.916	6.273	1.425
Peanut butter (26.1% protein, N × 5.46)	0.330	0.803	1.228	1.816	1.066	0.263	0.449	1.510	1.071	1.487	3.198	0.727
Peas *(Pisum sativum)* (N × 6.25)												
Entire seeds (23.8% protein)	0.251	0.918	1.340	1.969	1.744	0.286	0.308	1.200	0.960	1.333	2.102	0.651
Split (24.5% protein)	0.259	0.945	1.380	2.027	1.795	0.294	0.318	1.235	0.988	1.372	2.164	0.670
Pigeonpeas, without seed coat (21.9% protein, N × 6.25)	0.119	0.834	1.346	1.717	1.580	0.256	0.308	1.875	0.725	1.153	1.489	0.617

Continued.

Protein content and nitrogen conversion factor	Tryptophan (g)	Threonine (g)	Isoleucine (g)	Leucine (g)	Lysine (g)	Methionine (g)	Cystine (g)	Phenylalanine (g)	Tyrosine (g)	Valine (g)	Arginine (g)	Histidine (g)
Legumes (dry seed), common nuts, other nuts and dry seeds (their products)—cont'd												
Soybeans, whole (34.9% protein, N × 5.71)	0.526	1.504	2.054	2.946	2.414	0.513	0.678	1.889	1.216	2.005	2.763	0.911
Soybean flour, flakes, and grits (protein, N × 5.71)												
Low fat (44.7% protein)	0.673	1.926	2.630	3.773	3.092	0.658	0.869	2.419	1.558	2.568	3.538	1.166
Medium fat (42.5% protein)	0.640	1.831	2.501	3.588	2.940	0.625	0.826	2.300	1.481	2.441	3.364	1.109
Full fat (35.9% protein)	0.541	1.547	2.112	3.030	2.483	0.528	0.698	1.943	1.251	2.062	2.842	0.937
Soybean curd (7.0% protein, N × 5.71)	—	—	—	—	—	0.081	0.091	—	—	—	—	—
Soybean milk (3.4% protein, N × 5.71)	0.051	0.176	0.175	0.305	0.269	0.054	0.071	0.195	0.193	0.186	0.302	0.121
Vetch (28.8% protein, N × 6.25)	0.203	0.899	2.198	2.290	1.898	0.346	0.336	1.014	0.369	1.442	2.249	0.659
Common nuts and their products												
Almonds (18.6% protein, N × 5.18)	0.176	0.610	0.873	1.454	0.582	0.259	0.377	1.146	0.618	1.124	2.729	0.517
Brazil nuts (14.4% protein, N × 5.46)	0.187	0.422	0.593	1.129	0.443	0.941	0.504	0.617	0.483	0.823	2.247	0.367
Cashews (18.5% protein, N × 5.30)	0.471	0.737	1.222	1.522	0.792	0.353	0.527	0.946	0.712	1.592	2.098	0.415
Coconut (3.4% protein, N × 5.30)	0.033	0.129	0.180	0.269	0.152	0.071	0.062	0.174	0.101	0.212	0.486	0.069
Coconut meal (20.3% protein, N × 5.30)	0.199	0.770	1.076	1.605	0.908	0.421	0.372	1.038	0.605	1.268	2.899	0.414
Filberts (12.7% protein, N × 5.30)	0.211	0.415	0.853	0.939	0.417	0.139	0.165	0.537	0.434	0.934	2.171	0.288
Peanuts, (see Legumes)												
Pecans (9.4% protein, N × 5.30)	0.138	0.389	0.553	0.773	0.435	0.153	0.216	0.564	0.316	0.525	1.185	0.273
Walnuts (English or Persian) (15.0% protein, N × 5.30)	0.175	0.589	0.767	1.228	0.441	0.306	0.320	0.767	0.583	0.974	2.287	0.405
Other nuts and seeds and their products (protein N × 5.30)												
Acorns (10.4% protein)	0.126	0.434	0.561	0.808	0.636	0.139	0.184	0.473	—	0.718	0.722	0.251
Amaranth (14.6% protein)	0.149	0.832	0.882	1.209	1.074	0.372	0.521	1.141	—	0.849	1.747	0.441
Balsam pear seed meal (41.9% protein)	—	—	—	—	1.265	—	0.142	2.609	0.617	—	5.914	0.917
Breadnut tree, Ramon (9.6% protein)	0.261	0.373	0.543	1.041	0.418	0.056	—	0.453	—	0.927	0.884	0.147
Chinese tallow tree-nut flour (57.6% protein)	0.837	2.174	3.510	4.347	1.587	0.924	0.696	2.847	2.011	4.510	10.031	1.587
Chocolate tree, Nicaragua (38.5% protein)	0.588	1.496	2.092	3.952	2.223	0.276	—	2.630	—	2.404	4.220	0.683
Cottonseed flour and meal (42.3% protein)	0.591	1.764	1.884	2.945	2.139	0.686	0.814	2.610	1.365	2.458	5.603	1.325
Earpod tree, Guanacaste (34.1% protein)	0.444	1.165	2.213	4.581	1.930	0.360	—	1.325	—	1.570	2.857	1.004
Lead tree (24.1% protein)	0.191	0.828	1.651	1.787	1.164	0.055	—	0.855	—	0.864	2.410	0.564
Pumpkin seed (30.9% protein)	0.560	0.933	1.737	2.437	1.411	0.577	—	1.749	—	1.679	4.810	0.711
Safflower seed meal (42.1% protein)	0.675	1.462	1.914	2.740	1.525	0.731	—	2.605	—	2.446	4.623	0.985
Sesame												
Seed (19.3% protein)	0.331	0.707	0.951	1.679	0.583	0.637	0.495	1.457	0.951	0.885	1.992	0.441
Meal (33.4% protein)	0.573	1.223	1.645	2.905	1.008	1.103	0.857	2.521	1.645	1.531	3.447	0.763
Sunflower												
Kernel (23.0% protein)	0.343	0.911	1.276	1.736	0.868	0.443	0.464	1.220	0.647	1.354	2.370	0.586
Meal (39.5% protein)	0.589	1.565	2.191	2.981	1.491	0.760	0.797	2.094	1.110	2.325	4.069	1.006
Grains and their products												
Barley (12.8% protein, N × 5.83)	0.160	0.433	0.545	0.889	0.433	0.184	0.257	0.661	0.466	0.643	0.659	0.239
Bread, white (4% nonfat dry milk, flour basis) (8.5% protein, N × 5.70)	0.091	0.282	0.429	0.668	0.225	0.142	0.200	0.465	0.243	0.435	0.340	0.192
Buckwheat flour												
Dark (11.7% protein, N × 6.25)	0.165	0.461	0.440	0.683	0.687	0.206	0.228	0.442	0.240	0.607	0.930	0.256
Light (6.4% protein, N × 6.25)	0.090	0.252	0.241	0.374	0.376	0.113	0.125	0.242	0.131	0.332	0.509	0.140
Canihua (14.7% protein, N × 6.25)	0.118	0.706	1.000	0.851	0.882	0.263	0.162	0.529	0.294	0.677	1.162	0.367

Protein content and nitrogen conversion factor	Trypto-phan (g)	Threo-nine (g)	Iso-leucine (g)	Leucine (g)	Lysine (g)	Methi-onine (g)	Cystine (g)	Phenyl-alanine (g)	Tyro-sine (g)	Valine (g)	Argi-nine (g)	Histi-dine (g)
Grains and their products—cont'd												
Cereal combinations												
Corn and soy grits (18.0% protein, N × 6.25)	0.161	0.792	0.841	1.656	0.772	0.271	0.311	0.832	0.562	1.054	0.982	0.472
Infants food, precooked, mixed cereals with nonfat dry milk and yeast (19.4% protein, N × 6.25)	0.118	—	—	—	0.273	0.310	0.137	0.543	0.447	—	0.447	0.233
Oat-corn-rye mixture, puffed (14.5% protein, N × 5.83)	0.172	0.545	0.841	1.368	0.343	0.388	0.234	0.933	0.622	0.900	0.776	0.326
Corn, field (10.0% protein, N × 6.25)	0.061	0.398	0.462	1.296	0.288	0.186	0.130	0.454	0.611	0.510	0.352	0.206
Corn flour (7.8% protein, N × 6.25)	0.047	0.311	0.361	1.011	0.225	0.145	0.101	0.354	0.477	0.398	0.275	0.161
Corn grits (8.7% protein, N × 6.25)	0.053	0.347	0.402	1.128	0.251	0.161	0.113	0.395	0.532	0.444	0.306	0.180
Cornmeal												
Whole ground (9.2% protein, N × 6.25)	0.056	0.367	0.425	1.192	0.265	0.171	0.119	0.418	0.562	0.470	0.324	0.190
Degermed (7.9% protein, N × 6.25)	0.048	0.315	0.365	1.024	0.228	0.147	0.102	0.359	0.483	0.403	0.278	0.163
Corn products												
Flakes (8.1% protein, N × 6.25)	0.052	0.275	0.306	1.047	0.154	0.135	0.152	0.354	0.283	0.386	0.231	0.226
Germ (14.5% protein, N × 6.25)	0.144	0.622	0.578	1.030	0.791	0.232	0.130	0.483	0.343	0.789	1.134	0.464
Gluten (10.0% protein, N × 6.25)	0.059	0.344	0.443	1.563	0.179	0.282	0.141	0.558	0.582	0.512	0.322	0.200
Hominy (8.7% protein, N × 6.25)	0.084	0.316	0.349	0.810	0.358	0.099	—	0.333	0.331	0.398	0.444	0.203
Masa (2.8% protein, N × 6.25)	0.010	—	—	—	0.103	0.108	0.030	—	—	—	—	—
Pozol (5.9% protein, N × 6.25)	0.042	0.336	0.304	0.591	0.234	0.087	—	0.254	—	0.267	0.197	0.122
Tortilla (5.8% protein, N × 6.25)	0.031	0.235	0.345	0.939	0.145	0.111	—	0.252	—	0.304	0.223	0.128
Zein (16.1% protein, N × 6.25)	0.010	0.495	0.822	3.184	—	0.281	0.162	1.664	0.981	0.654	0.286	0.216
Job's tears (13.8% protein, N × 5.83)	0.066	0.620	1.065	3.506	0.362	0.459	0.265	0.703	—	—	0.518	0.317
Millets												
Foxtail millet (9.7% protein, N × 5.83)	0.103	0.323	0.790	1.737	0.218	0.291	—	0.697	—	0.717	0.374	0.218
Little millet (7.2% protein, N × 5.83)	0.047	0.262	0.517	0.841	0.138	0.178	—	0.370	—	0.471	0.363	0.147
Pearl millet (11.4% protein, N × 5.83)	0.248	0.456	0.635	1.746	0.383	0.270	0.152	0.506	—	0.682	0.524	0.240
Ragimillet (6.2% protein, N × 5.83)	0.085	0.270	0.398	0.620	0.202	0.270	0.187	0.263	—	0.473	0.100	0.079
Oatmeal and rolled oats (14.2% protein, N × 5.83)	0.183	0.470	0.733	1.065	0.521	0.209	0.309	0.758	0.524	0.845	0.935	0.261
Quinoa (11.0% protein, N × 6.25)	0.120	0.523	0.722	0.781	0.729	0.278	0.107	0.394	0.253	0.447	0.820	0.297
Rice												
Brown (7.5% protein, N × 5.95)	0.081	0.294	0.352	0.646	0.296	0.135	0.102	0.377	0.343	0.524	0.432	0.126
White and converted (7.6% protein, N × 5.95)	0.082	0.298	0.356	0.655	0.300	0.137	0.103	0.382	0.347	0.531	0.438	0.128
Rice products												
Flakes or puffed (5.9% protein, N × 5.95)	0.046	—	—	—	0.056	—	0.044	0.286	0.124	—	0.137	0.137
Germ (14.2% protein, N × 5.95)	0.270	2.177	0.630	0.838	1.707	0.420	0.169	0.750	0.929	0.938	1.559	0.430
Rye (12.1% protein, N × 5.83)	0.137	0.448	0.515	0.813	0.494	0.191	0.241	0.571	0.390	0.631	0.591	0.276
Rye flour												
Light (9.4% protein, N × 5.83)	0.106	0.348	0.400	0.632	0.384	0.148	0.187	0.443	0.303	0.490	0.459	0.214
Medium (11.4% protein, N × 5.83)	0.129	0.422	0.485	0.766	0.465	0.180	0.227	0.538	0.368	0.594	0.557	0.260
Sorghum (11.0% protein, N × 6.25)	0.123	0.394	0.598	1.767	0.299	0.190	0.183	0.547	0.303	0.628	0.417	0.211
Teosinte (22.0% protein, N × 6.25)	0.049	—	—	—	0.348	0.496	—	—	—	—	—	—
Wheat, whole grain												
Hard red spring (14.0% protein, N × 5.83)	0.173	0.403	0.607	0.939	0.384	0.214	0.307	0.691	0.523	0.648	0.670	0.286
Hard red winter (12.3% protein, N × 5.83)	0.152	0.354	0.534	0.825	0.338	0.188	0.270	0.608	0.460	0.570	0.589	0.251
Soft red winter (10.2% protein, N × 5.83)	0.126	0.294	0.443	0.684	0.280	0.156	0.224	0.504	0.382	0.472	0.488	0.208
White (9.4% protein, N × 5.83)	0.116	0.271	0.408	0.630	0.258	0.143	0.206	0.464	0.351	0.435	0.450	0.192
Durum (12.7% protein, N × 5.83)	0.157	0.366	0.551	0.852	0.348	0.194	0.279	0.627	0.475	0.588	0.608	0.259
Wheat flour												
Whole grain (13.3% protein, N × 5.83)	0.164	0.383	0.577	0.892	0.365	0.203	0.292	0.657	0.497	0.616	0.636	0.271

Continued.

Protein content and nitrogen conversion factor	Tryptophan (g)	Threonine (g)	Isoleucine (g)	Leucine (g)	Lysine (g)	Methionine (g)	Cystine (g)	Phenylalanine (g)	Tyrosine (g)	Valine (g)	Arginine (g)	Histidine (g)
Grains and their products—cont'd												
Intermediate extraction (12.0% protein, N × 5.70)	—	0.392	0.619	0.924	0.356	0.198	0.320	0.732	0.335	0.583	0.549	0.286
White (10.5% protein, N × 5.70)	0.129	0.302	0.483	0.809	0.239	0.138	0.210	0.577	0.539	0.453	0.466	0.210
Wheat products												
Bran (12.0% protein, N × 6.31)	0.196	0.342	0.485	0.717	0.491	0.145	0.270	0.434	0.259	0.552	0.742	0.280
Bulgar (12.4% protein, N × 5.83)	0.070	—	—	—	0.430	0.300	0.319	—	—	—	—	—
Farina (10.9% protein, N × 5.70)	0.124	—	—	—	0.199	0.143	0.184	0.579	0.447	—	0.424	0.268
Flakes (10.8% protein, N × 5.70)	0.121	0.356	0.496	0.891	0.360	0.127	0.191	0.478	0.311	0.572	0.559	0.231
Germ (25.2% protein, N × 5.80)	0.265	1.343	1.177	1.708	1.534	0.404	0.287	0.908	0.882	1.364	1.825	0.687
Gluten, commercial (80.0% protein, N × 5.70)	0.856	2.119	3.677	5.993	1.530	1.389	1.726	4.351	2.596	3.789	3.481	1.825
Gluten flour (41.4% protein, N × 5.70)	0.443	1.097	1.903	3.101	0.792	0.719	0.893	2.252	1.344	1.961	1.801	0.944
Macaroni or spaghetti (12.8% protein, N × 5.70)	0.150	0.499	0.642	0.849	0.413	0.193	0.243	0.669	0.422	0.728	0.582	0.303
Noodles, containing egg solids (12.6% protein, N × 5.70)	0.133	0.533	0.621	0.834	0.411	0.212	0.245	0.610	0.312	0.745	0.621	0.301
Shredded Wheat (10.1% protein, N × 5.83)	0.085	0.405	0.449	0.684	0.331	0.139	0.204	0.481	0.236	0.577	0.523	0.236
Whole wheat with added germ (12.8% protein, N × 5.83)	0.136	—	—	—	0.466	—	0.246	0.755	0.481	—	0.742	0.371
Fruits (protein, N × 6.25)												
Abiu (1.7% protein)	0.028	—	—	—	0.085	0.013	—	—	—	—	—	—
Avocados (1.3% protein)	0.014	—	—	—	0.074	0.012	—	—	—	—	—	—
Bananas, ripe												
Common (1.2% protein)	0.018	—	—	—	0.055	0.011	—	—	0.031	—	—	—
Dwarf (1.2% protein)	0.012	—	—	—	0.049	0.004	—	—	—	—	—	—
Dates (2.2% protein)	0.061	0.061	0.074	0.077	0.065	0.027	—	0.063	—	0.094	0.049	0.049
Grapefruit (0.5% protein)	0.001	—	—	—	0.006	0.000	—	—	—	—	—	—
Guavas, common (1.0% protein)	0.010	—	—	—	0.030	0.010	—	—	—	—	—	—
Limes (0.8% protein)	0.003	—	—	—	0.015	0.002	—	—	—	—	—	—
Mamey (0.5% protein)	0.006	—	—	—	0.040	0.007	—	—	—	—	—	—
Mangos (0.7% protein)	0.014	—	—	—	0.093	0.008	—	—	—	—	—	—
Muskmelons (0.6% protein)	0.001	—	—	—	0.015	0.002	—	—	—	—	—	—
Oranges, sweet (0.9% protein)	0.003	—	—	—	0.024	0.003	—	—	—	—	—	—
Orange juice (0.8% protein)	0.003	—	—	—	0.021	0.002	—	—	—	—	—	—
Oranges, mandarin, including tangerines (0.8% protein)	0.005	—	—	—	0.028	0.004	—	—	—	—	—	—
Papayas (0.6% protein)	0.012	—	—	—	0.038	0.002	—	—	—	—	—	—
Pineapple (0.4% protein)	0.005	—	—	—	0.009	0.001	—	—	—	—	—	—
Plaintain or baking banana (1.1% protein)	0.010	0.027	0.056	0.059	0.050	0.005	0.016	0.049	—	0.065	0.045	—
Soursop (1.0 protein)	0.011	—	—	—	0.060	0.007	—	—	—	—	—	—
Sugarapple (1.8% protein)	0.009	—	—	—	0.071	0.008	—	—	—	—	—	—
Vegetables												
Immature seeds (protein, N × 6.25)												
Corn, sweet, white or yellow												
Raw (3.7% protein)	0.023	0.151	0.137	0.407	0.137	0.072	0.062	0.207	0.124	0.231	0.174	0.095
Canned, solids and liquid (2.0% protein)	0.012	0.082	0.074	0.220	0.074	0.039	0.033	0.112	0.067	0.125	0.094	0.052
Cowpeas (9.4% protein)	0.099	0.353	0.465	0.653	0.617	0.131	—	0.523	—	0.513	0.615	0.310
Lima beans												
Raw (7.5% protein)	0.097	0.338	0.460	0.605	0.474	0.080	0.083	0.389	0.259	0.485	0.454	0.247
Canned, solids and liquid (3.8% protein)	0.049	0.171	0.233	0.306	0.240	0.041	0.042	0.197	0.131	0.246	0.230	0.125
Peas												
Raw (6.7% protein)	0.056	0.245	0.308	0.418	0.316	0.054	0.073	0.257	0.163	0.274	0.595	0.109
Canned solids and liquid (3.4% protein)	0.028	0.125	0.156	0.212	0.160	0.027	0.037	0.131	0.083	0.139	0.302	0.055

Protein content and nitrogen conversion factor	Trypto- phan (g)	Threo- nine (g)	Iso- leucine (g)	Leucine (g)	Lysine (g)	Methi- onine (g)	Cystine (g)	Phenyl- alanine (g)	Tyro- sine (g)	Valine (g)	Argi- nine (g)	Histi- dine (g)
Vegetables—cont'd												
Leafy vegetables, raw (protein, N × 6.25)												
Amaranth (3.5% protein)	0.038	0.056	0.164	0.206	0.141	0.025	0.024	0.096	0.105	0.136	0.134	0.069
Beet greens (2.0% protein)	0.024	0.076	0.084	0.129	0.108	0.034	—	0.116	—	0.101	0.083	0.026
Brussels sprouts (4.4% protein)	0.044	0.153	0.186	0.194	0.197	0.046	—	0.148	—	0.193	0.279	0.106
Cabbage (1.4% protein)	0.011	0.039	0.040	0.057	0.066	0.013	0.028	0.030	0.030	0.043	0.105	0.025
Chard (1.4% protein)	0.014	0.058	0.060	0.076	0.055	0.004	—	0.046	—	0.055	0.035	0.018
Chicory (1.6% protein)	0.024	—	—	—	0.052	0.016	0.006	—	0.040	—	—	0.024
Collards (3.9% protein)	0.055	0.114	0.121	0.218	0.202	0.046	0.059	0.124	0.151	0.195	0.258	0.087
Kale (3.9% protein)	0.042	0.139	0.133	0.252	0.121	0.035	0.036	0.158	—	0.184	0.202	0.062
Lettuce (1.2% protein)	0.012	—	—	—	0.070	0.004	—	—	—	—	—	—
Mustard greens (2.3% protein)	0.037	0.060	0.075	0.062	0.111	0.024	0.035	0.074	0.121	0.108	0.167	0.041
Parsley, curly garden (2.5% protein)	0.050	—	—	—	0.160	0.012	—	—	—	—	—	—
Spinach (2.3% protein)	0.037	0.102	0.107	0.176	0.142	0.039	0.046	0.099	0.073	0.126	0.116	0.049
Turnip greens (2.9% protein)	0.045	0.125	0.107	0.207	0.129	0.052	0.045	0.146	0.105	0.149	0.167	0.051
Watercress (1.7% protein)	0.028	0.084	0.076	0.131	0.091	0.010	—	0.062	0.036	0.084	0.053	0.034
Starchy roots and tubers (protein, N × 6.25)												
Apio arracacia (1.2% protein)	0.008	—	—	—	0.042	0.003	—	—	—	—	—	—
Cassava												
Flour (1.6% protein)	0.021	0.044	0.045	0.066	0.066	0.010	0.018	0.045	0.030	0.049	0.159	0.025
Root (1.1% protein)	0.014	0.030	0.031	0.045	0.045	0.007	0.012	0.031	0.021	0.033	0.110	0.017
Potatoes												
Raw (2.0% protein)	0.021	0.079	0.088	0.100	0.107	0.025	0.019	0.088	0.036	0.107	0.099	0.029
Canned, solids and liquid (1.7% protein)	0.018	0.067	0.075	0.085	0.091	0.021	0.016	0.075	0.030	0.091	0.084	0.024
Flour (7.1% protein)	0.076	0.279	0.311	0.353	0.378	0.089	0.068	0.314	0.127	0.379	0.350	0.102
Sweet potatoes *(Ipomaea batatas)*												
Raw (1.8% protein)	0.031	0.085	0.087	0.103	0.085	0.033	0.029	0.100	0.081	0.135	0.094	0.036
Dehydrated (5.0% protein)	0.087	0.235	0.241	0.286	0.236	0.093	0.080	0.278	0.225	0.374	0.261	0.099
Taro (1.9% protein)	0.035	0.089	0.099	0.169	0.110	0.021	—	0.099	—	0.114	0.118	0.032
Yam (*Dioscorea* spp.) (2.1% protein)	0.035	—	—	—	0.110	0.034	—	—	—	—	—	—
Yautia malanga (1.7% protein)	0.023	—	—	—	0.067	0.016	—	—	—	—	—	—
Other vegetables (protein, N × 6.25)												
Asparagus												
Raw (2.2% protein)	0.027	0.066	0.080	0.096	0.103	0.032	—	0.069	—	0.106	0.123	0.036
Canned, solids and liquid (1.9% protein)	0.023	0.057	0.069	0.083	0.089	0.027	—	0.060	—	0.092	0.106	0.031
Beans, snap												
Raw (2.4% protein)	0.033	0.091	0.109	0.139	0.126	0.035	0.024	0.057	0.050	0.115	0.101	0.045
Canned, solids and liquid (1.0% protein)	0.014	0.038	0.045	0.058	0.052	0.014	0.010	0.024	0.021	0.048	0.042	0.019
Beets												
Raw (1.6% protein)	0.014	0.034	0.051	0.055	0.086	0.006	—	0.027	—	0.049	0.028	0.022
Canned, solids and liquid (0.9% protein)	0.0008	0.019	0.029	0.031	0.048	0.003	—	0.015	—	0.028	0.016	0.012
Broccoli (3.3% protein)	0.037	0.122	0.126	0.163	0.147	0.050	—	0.119	—	0.170	0.192	0.063
Carrots												
Raw (1.2% protein)	0.010	0.043	0.046	0.065	0.052	0.010	0.029	0.042	0.020	0.056	0.041	0.017
Canned, solids and liquid (0.5% protein)	0.004	0.018	0.019	0.027	0.022	0.004	0.012	0.018	0.008	0.023	0.017	0.007
Cauliflower (2.4% protein)	0.033	0.102	0.104	0.162	0.134	0.047	—	0.075	0.034	0.144	0.110	0.048
Celery (1.3% protein)	0.012	—	—	—	0.021	0.015	0.006	—	0.016	—	—	—
Chayote (0.6% protein)	0.008	—	—	—	0.038	0.001	—	—	—	—	—	—
Cowpeas, yardlong, immature pod (3.4% protein)	0.034	—	—	—	0.203	0.021	—	—	—	—	—	—
Cucumbers (0.7% protein)	0.005	0.019	0.022	0.030	0.031	0.007	—	0.016	—	0.024	0.053	0.001
Cushaw (1.5% protein)	0.014	—	—	—	0.044	0.008	—	—	—	—	—	—
Eggplant (1.1% protein)	0.010	0.038	0.056	0.068	0.030	0.006	—	0.048	—	0.065	0.037	0.019
Mallow (3.7% protein)	0.144	0.155	—	0.259	0.155	0.030	—	0.166	—	0.181	0.189	0.063

Continued.

Protein content and nitrogen conversion factor	Tryptophan (g)	Threonine (g)	Isoleucine (g)	Leucine (g)	Lysine (g)	Methionine (g)	Cystine (g)	Phenylalanine (g)	Tyrosine (g)	Valine (g)	Arginine (g)	Histidine (g)
Vegetables—cont'd												
Mushrooms												
*(Agaricus campestris)**	0.006	—	0.532	0.281	—	0.167	—	—	—	0.378	0.235	—
(*Lactarius* spp.)†	0.006	0.156	0.201	0.139	0.088	0.021	—	0.018	—	0.116	0.021	0.027
Okra (1.8% protein)	0.018	0.066	0.069	0.101	0.076	0.022	0.017	0.065	0.079	0.091	0.093	0.030
Onions, mature (1.4% protein)	0.021	0.022	0.021	0.037	0.064	0.013	—	0.039	0.046	0.031	0.180	0.014
Peppers (1.2% protein)	0.009	0.050	0.046	0.046	0.051	0.016	—	0.055	—	0.033	0.024	0.014
Prickly pears (1.1% protein)	0.009	0.053	0.044	0.057	0.044	0.008	—	0.059	—	0.041	0.032	0.016
Pumpkin (1.2% protein)	0.016	0.028	0.044	0.063	0.058	0.011	—	0.032	0.016	0.045	0.043	0.019
Radishes (1.2% protein)	0.005	0.059	—	—	0.034	0.002	—	—	—	0.030	—	—
Seepweed (2.6% protein)	0.027	0.089	0.113	0.152	0.089	0.013	—	0.116	—	0.091	0.062	0.036
Soybean sprouts (6.2% protein)	—	0.159	0.225	0.265	0.211	0.045	—	0.186	—	0.225	0.225	0.133
Squash, summer (0.6% protein)	0.005	0.014	0.019	0.027	0.023	0.008	—	0.016	—	0.022	0.027	0.009
Tomatoes and cherry tomatoes (1.0% protein)	0.009	0.033	0.029	0.041	0.042	0.007	—	0.028	0.014	0.028	0.029	0.015
Turnips (1.1% protein)	—	—	0.020	—	0.057	0.012	—	0.020	0.029	—	—	—
Waxgourd, Chinese (0.4% protein)	0.002	—	—	—	0.009	0.003	—	—	—	—	—	—
Miscellaneous food items												
Vegetable patty or steak (principally wheat protein) (15% protein, N × 5.70)	0.142	0.411	0.884	1.079	0.321	0.253	—	0.811	—	0.705	0.597	0.321
Yeast												
Baker's, compressed‡ (N × 6.25)	0.122	0.655	0.655	1.151	0.914	0.248	0.120	0.607	0.580	0.840	0.536	0.353
Brewer's dried¶ (N × 6.25)	0.710	2.353	2.398	3.226	3.300	0.836	0.548	1.902	1.902	2.723	2.250	1.251
Primary, dried												
(Saccharomyces cerevisiae) (N × 6.25)	0.636	2.353	2.708	3.300	3.337	0.851	0.444	1.813	2.472	2.553	1.931	1.103
(Torulopsis utilis)¶ (N × 6.25)	0.636	2.331	3.323	3.707	3.648	0.710	0.422	2.361	2.464	2.901	3.337	1.251

*Total nitrogen is 0.58%. This is equivalent to 2.4% protein on the basis that two thirds of the nitrogen is protein nitrogen. If total nitrogen is used for the calculation, the protein content is 3.6%.

†Total nitrogen is 0.69%. This is equivalent to 2.9% protein on the basis that two thirds of the nitrogen is protein nitrogen. If total nitrogen is used for the calculation, the protein content is 4.3%.

‡Total nitrogen is 2.1%. This is equivalent to 10.6% protein on the basis that four fifths of the nitrogen is protein nitrogen. If total nitrogen is used for the calculation, the protein content is 13.1%.

¶Total nitrogen is 7.4%. This is equivalent to 36.9% protein on the basis that four fifths of the nitrogen is protein nitrogen. If total nitrogen is used for the calculation, the protein content is 46.1%.

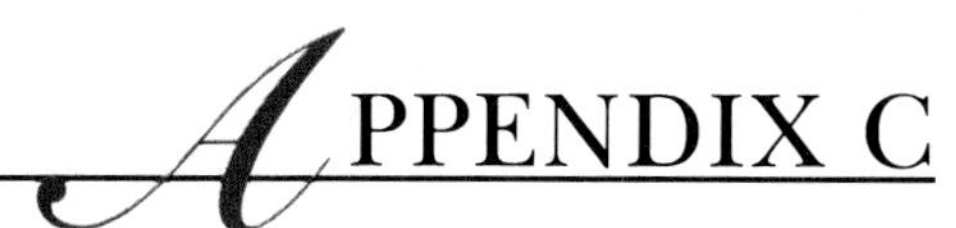

APPENDIX C

Fatty Acid Content of Common Vegetable Oils

Vegetable oil	Polyunsaturated (%)	Monounsaturated (%)	Saturated (%)
Safflower	74	12	9
Walnut	66	15	11
Sunflower	64	21	10
Wheat germ	61	16	17
Corn	58	25	13
Soybean (unhydrogenated)	58	23	15
Cottonseed	51	19	26
Sesame seed	40	40	15
Soybean (partially hydrogenated)	40	47	13
Peanut	30	46	19
Olive	9	72	14
Palm	9	38	48
Coconut	2	6	86

Adapted from Brown, H.B.: Current focus on fat in the diet, ADA White Paper, J. Am. Diet. Assoc. 68:25, 1977. Other substances in the oils that make up total composition (100%) include such materials as sterols, vitamins, phospholipids, and water.

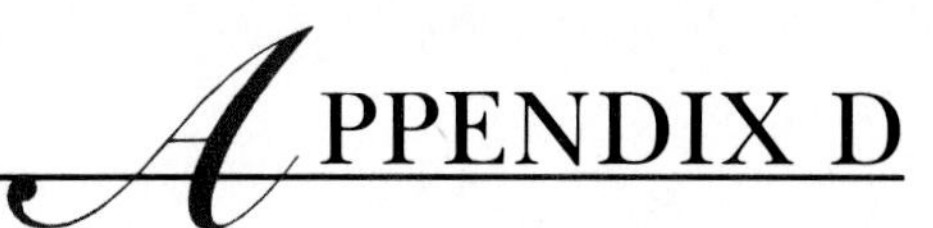

Relative Ratios of Polyunsaturated Fat and Saturated Fat (P/S Ratio) in Representative Foods

P/S ratio	Foods
High	Almonds
>2.5:1	Corn oil
	Cottonseed oil
	Mayonnaise (made with oils in this group)
	Safflower oil
	Sesame oil
	Soft margarines
	Soybean oil
	Sunflower oil
	Walnuts
Medium high	Chicken
2:1	Fish
	Peanut oil
	Semisolid margarines
Medium	Beef heart, liver
1:1	Hydrogenated or hardened vegetable oils (shortenings, special products)
	Peanuts, peanut butter
	Pecans
	Solid margarines
Low	Chicken liver
0.1-0.5:1	Lamb
	Lard
	Olive oil
	Palm oil
	Pork
	Veal
Very low	Beef
<0.1:1	Butter, cream
	Coconut oil
	Egg yolk
	Whole milk, milk products

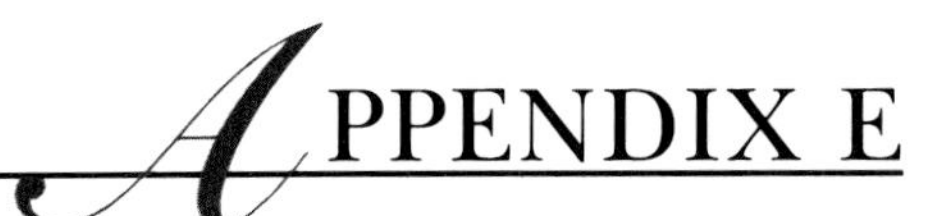

APPENDIX E

Cholesterol Content of Foods

Item	Amount of cholesterol		Refuse from item as purchased (%)
	100 g edible portion* (mg)	Edible portion of 450 g (1 lb) as purchased (mg)	
Beef, raw			
With bone†	70	270	15
Without bone†	70	320	0
Brains, raw	>2000	>9000	0
Butter	250	1135	0
Caviar or fish roe	>300	>1300	0
Cheese			
Cheddar	100	455	0
Cottage, creamed	15	70	0
Cream	120	545	0
Other (25%-30% fat)	85	385	0
Cheese spread	65	295	0
Chicken, flesh only, raw	60	—	0
Crab			
In shell†	125	270	52
Meat only†	125	565	0
Egg, whole	550	2200	12
Egg white	0	0	0
Egg yolk			
Fresh	1500	6800	0
Frozen	1280	5800	0
Dried	2950	13,380	0
Fish			
Steak†	70	265	16
Fillet†	70	320	0
Heart, raw	150	680	0
Ice cream	45	205	0
Kidney, raw	375	1700	0
Lamb, raw			
With bone†	70	265	16
Without bone†	70	320	0
Lard and other animal fat	95	430	0
Liver, raw	300	1360	0
Lobster			
Whole†	200	235	74
Meat only†	200	900	0
Margarine			
All vegetable fat	0	0	0
Two-thirds animal fat, one-third vegetable fat	65	295	0

From Watt, BK, Merrill, AL: *Composition of foods—raw, processed, prepared,* U.S. Department of Agriculture, Agriculture Handbook No 8, Dec 1963.

*Data apply to 100 g of edible portion of the item, although it may be purchased with the refuse indicated and described or implied in the first column.

†Items that have the same chemical composition for the edible portion but differ in the amount of refuse.

Continued.

Item	Amount of cholesterol: 100 g edible portion* (mg)	Amount of cholesterol: Edible portion of 450 g (1 lb) as purchased (mg)	Refuse from item as purchased (%)
Milk			
Fluid, whole	11	50	0
Dried, whole	85	385	0
Fluid, skim	3	15	0
Mutton			
With bone†	65	250	16
Without bone†	65	295	0
Oysters			
In shell†	>200	>90	90
Meat only†	>200	>900	0
Pork			
With bone†	70	260	18
Without bone†	70	320	0
Shrimp			
In shell†	125	390	31
Flesh only†	125	565	0
Sweetbreads (thymus)	250	1135	0
Veal			
With bone†	90	320	21
Without bone†	90	410	0

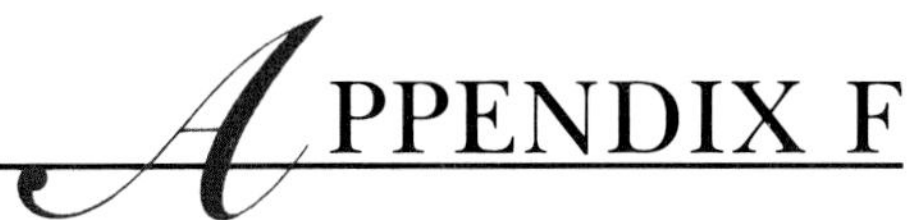

APPENDIX F

Dietary Fiber in Selected Plant Foods

Food	Amount	Weight (g)	Total dietary fiber (g)	Noncellulose polysaccharides (g)	Cellulose (g)	Lignin
Apple	1 med					
Flesh		138	1.96	1.29	0.66	0.01
Skin		100	3.71	2.21	1.01	0.49
Banana	1 small	119	2.08	1.33	0.44	0.31
Beans						
Baked	1 cup	255	18.53	14.45	3.59	0.48
Green, cooked	1 cup	125	4.19	2.31	1.61	0.26
Bread						
White	1 slice	25	0.68	0.50	0.18	Trace
Whole meal	1 slice	25	2.13	1.49	0.33	0.31
Broccoli, cooked	1 cup	155	6.36	4.53	1.78	0.05
Brussels sprouts, cooked	1 cup	155	4.43	3.08	1.24	0.11
Cabbage, cooked	1 cup	145	4.10	2.55	1.00	0.55
Carrots, cooked	1 cup	155	5.74	3.44	2.29	Trace
Cauliflower, cooked	1 cup	125	2.25	0.84	1.41	Trace
Cereals						
All-Bran	1 oz	30	8.01	5.35	1.80	0.86
Corn Flakes	1 cup	25	2.75	1.82	0.61	0.33
Grapenuts	¼ cup	30	2.10	1.54	0.38	0.17
Puffed Wheat	1 cup	15	2.31	1.55	0.39	0.37
Rice Krispies	1 cup	30	1.34	1.04	0.23	0.07
Shredded Wheat	1 biscuit	25	3.07	2.20	0.66	0.21
Special K	1 cup	30	1.64	1.10	0.22	0.32
Cherries	10 cherries	68	0.84	0.63	0.17	0.05
Cookies						
Ginger	4 snaps	28	0.56	0.41	0.08	0.07
Oatmeal	4 cookies	52	2.08	1.64	0.21	0.22
Plain	4 cookies	48	0.80	0.68	0.05	0.06
Corn	1 cup	165	7.82	7.11	0.51	0.20
Canned	1 cup	165	9.39	8.20	1.06	0.13
Flour						
Bran	1 cup	100	44.00	32.70	8.05	3.23
White	1 cup	115	3.62	2.90	0.69	0.03
Whole meal	1 cup	120	11.41	7.50	2.95	0.96
Grapefruit	½ cup	100	0.44	0.34	0.04	0.06
Jam, strawberry	1 tbsp	20	0.22	0.17	0.02	0.03
Lettuce	⅙ head	100	1.53	0.47	1.06	Trace
Marmalade, orange	1 tbsp	20	0.14	0.13	0.01	Trace
Onions, raw, sliced	1 cup	100	2.10	1.55	0.55	Trace
Orange	1 cup	200	0.58	0.44	0.08	0.06
Parsnips, raw, diced	1 cup	100	4.90	3.77	1.13	Trace
Peach, flesh and skin	1 med	100	2.28	1.46	0.20	0.62
Peanuts	1 oz	30	2.79	1.92	0.51	0.36
Peanut butter	1 tbsp	16	1.21	0.90	0.31	Trace

Adapted from Southgate, DAT, et al: A guide to calculating intakes of dietary fiber, *J Hum Nutr* 30:303, 1976.

Continued.

Food	Amount	Weight (g)	Total dietary fiber (g)	Noncellulose polysaccharides (g)	Cellulose (g)	Lignin
Pear	1 med					
Flesh		164	4.00	2.16	1.10	0.74
Skin		100	8.59	3.72	2.18	2.67
Peas, canned	1 cup	170	13.35	8.84	3.91	0.60
Peas, raw or frozen	1 cup	100	7.75	5.48	2.09	0.18
Plums	1 plum	66	1.00	0.65	0.15	0.20
Potato, raw	1 med	135	4.73	3.36	1.38	Trace
Raisins	1 oz	30	1.32	0.72	0.25	0.35
Strawberries	1 cup	149	2.65	1.39	1.04	0.22
Tomato						
Raw	1 med	135	1.89	0.88	0.61	0.41
Canned, drained	1 cup	240	2.04	1.08	0.89	0.07
Turnips, raw	1 med	100	2.20	1.50	0.70	Trace

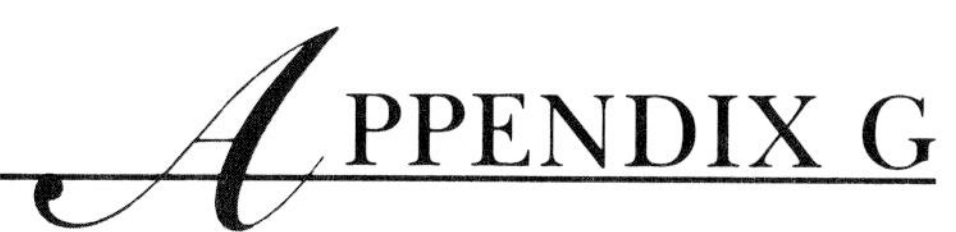

APPENDIX G

Sodium and Potassium Content of Foods, 100 g, Edible Portion

Food and description	Sodium (mg)	Potassium (mg)
Almonds		
Dried	4	773
Roasted and salted	198	773
Apple brown betty	153	100
Apple butter	2	252
Apple juice, canned or bottled	1	101
Apples		
Raw, pared	1	110
Frozen, sliced, sweetened	14	68
Applesauce, canned, sweetened	2	65
Apricot nectar, canned (approx. 40% fruit)	Trace	151
Apricots		
Raw	1	281
Canned, syrup pack, light	1	239
Dried, sulfured, cooked, fruit, and liquid	8	318
Asparagus		
Cooked spears, boiled, drained	1	183
Canned spears, green		
Regular pack, solids and liquid	236[1]	166
Special dietary pack (low sodium), solids and liquid	3	166
Frozen		
Cuts and tips, cooked, boiled, drained	1	220
Spears, cooked, boiled, drained	1	238
Avocados, raw, all commercial varieties	4	604
Bacon, cured, cooked, broiled or fried, drained	1021	236
Bacon, Canadian, cooked, broiled or fried, drained	2555	432
Baking powders		
Home use		
Straight phosphate	8220	170
Special low-sodium preparations	6	10,948
Bananas, raw, common	1	370
Barbecue sauce	815	174
Bass, black sea, raw	68	256
Beans, common, mature seeds, dry		
White		
Cooked	7	416
Canned, solids and liquid, with pork and tomato sauce	463	210
Red, cooked	3	340
Beans, lima		
Immature seeds		
Cooked, boiled, drained	1	422
Canned		
Regular pack, solids and liquid	236[1]	222

Numbers in parentheses denote values inputed, usually from another form of the food or from a similar food. Dashes denote lack of reliable data for a constituent believed to be present in measurable amount. Values are selected from Watt, BK, Merrill, AL: *Composition of foods—raw, processed, prepared,* U.S. Department of Agriculture, Agriculture Handbook No 8, Dec 1963. For notes see p. A-63.

Continued.

Food and description	Sodium (mg)	Potassium (mg)
Special dietary pack (low sodium), solids and liquid	4	222
Frozen, thin-seeded types, commonly called baby limas, cooked, boiled, drained	129	394
Mature seeds, dry, cooked	2	612
Beans, mung, sprouted seeds, cooked, boiled, drained	4	156
Beans, snap		
Green		
Cooked, boiled, drained	4	151
Canned		
Regular pack, solids and liquid	236[1]	95
Special dietary pack (low sodium), solids and liquid	2	95
Frozen, cut, cooked, boiled, drained	1	152
Yellow or wax		
Cooked, boiled, drained	3	151
Canned		
Regular pack, solids and liquid	236[1]	95
Special dietary pack (low sodium), solids and liquid	2	95
Frozen, cut, cooked, boiled, drained	1	164
Beans and frankfurters, canned	539	262
Beef		
Retail cuts, trimmed to retail level		
Round	60	370
Rump	60	370
Hamburger, regular ground, cooked	47	450
Beef and vegetable stew, canned	411	174
Beef, corned, boneless		
Cooked, medium fat	1740	150
Canned corned-beef hash (with potato)	540	200
Beef, dried, cooked, creamed	716	153
Beef potpie, commercial, frozen, unheated	366	93
Beet greens, common, cooked, boiled, drained	76	332
Beets, common, red		
Canned		
Regular pack, solids and liquid	236[1]	167
Special dietary pack (low sodium), solids and liquid	46	167
Beverages, alcoholic		
Beer, alcohol 4.5% by volume (3.6% by weight)	7	25
Gin, rum, vodka, whisky		
80 proof (33.4% alcohol by weight)	1	2
86 proof (36.0% alcohol by weight)	1	2
90 proof (37.9% alcohol by weight)	1	2
94 proof (39.7% alcohol by weight)	1	2
100 proof (42.5% alcohol by weight)	1	2
Wines		
Dessert, alcohol 18.8% by volume (15.3% by weight)	4	75
Table, alcohol 12.2% by volume (9.9% by weight)	5	92
Biscuit dough, commercial, frozen	910	86
Biscuit mix, with enriched flour, and biscuits baked from mix		
Dry form	1300	80
Made with milk	973	116
Biscuits, baking powder, made with enriched flour	626	117
Blackberries, including dewberries, boysenberries, and youngberries, raw	1	170
Blackberries, canned, solids and liquid		
Water pack, with or without artificial sweetener	1	115
Syrup pack, heavy	1	109
Blueberries		
Raw	1	81
Frozen, not thawed, sweetened	1	66
Bluefish, cooked		
Baked or broiled	104	—
Fried	146	—
Boston brown bread	251	292
Bouillon cubes or powder	24,000	100
Boysenberries, frozen, not thawed, sweetened	1	105
Bran, added sugar and malt extract	1060	1070
Bran flakes (40% bran), added thiamine	925	—

For notes, see p. A-63.

Food and description	Sodium (mg)	Potassium (mg)
Bran flakes with raisins, added thiamine	800	—
Brazil nuts	1	715
Bread crumbs, dry, grated	736	152
Bread stuffing mix and stuffings prepared from mix, dry form	1331	172
Breads		
Cracked wheat	529	134
French or Vienna, enriched	580	90
Italian, enriched	585	74
Raisin	365	233
Rye, American (⅓ rye, ⅔ clear flour)	557	145
White enriched, made with 3%-4% nonfat dry milk	507	105
Whole wheat, made with 2% nonfat dry milk	527	273
Broccoli		
Cooked spears, boiled, drained	10	267
Frozen, spears, cooked, boiled, drained	12	220
Brussels sprouts, frozen, cooked, boiled, drained	14	295
Buffalo fish, raw	52	293
Bulgur (parboiled wheat), canned, made from hard red winter wheat		
Unseasoned[2]	599	87
Seasoned[3]	460	112
Butter[4]	987	23
Buttermilk, fluid, cultured (made from skim milk)	130	140
Cabbage		
Common varieties (Danish, domestic, and pointed types)		
Raw	20	233
Cooked, boiled until tender, drained, shredded, cooked in small amount of water	14	163
Red, raw	26	268
Cabbage, Chinese (also called celery cabbage or petsai)	23	253
Cakes		
Baked from home recipes		
Angel food	283	88
Fruit cake, made with enriched flour, dark	158	496
Gingerbread, made with enriched flour	237	454
Plain cake or cupcake, without icing	300	79
Pound, modified	178	78
Frozen, commercial, devil's food, with chocolate icing	420	119
Candy		
Caramels, plain or chocolate	226	192
Chocolate, sweet	33	269
Chocolate coated, chocolate fudge	228	193
Gum drops, starch jelly pieces	35	5
Hard	32	4
Marshmallows	39	6
Peanut bars	10	448
Carp, raw	50	286
Carrots		
Raw	47	341
Canned		
Regular pack, solids and liquid	236[1]	120
Special dietary pack (low sodium), solids and liquid	39	120
Cashew nuts	15[5]	464
Catfish, freshwater, raw	60	330
Cauliflower		
Cooked, boiled, drained	9	206
Frozen, cooked, boiled, drained	10	207
Caviar, sturgeon, granular	2200	180
Celery, all, including green and yellow varieties		
Raw	126	341
Cooked, boiled, drained	88	239
Chard, Swiss, cooked, boiled, drained	86	321
Cheese straws	721	63
Cheeses		
Natural cheeses		
Cheddar (domestic type, commonly called American)	700	82

For notes, see p. A-63.

Continued.

Food and description	Sodium (mg)	Potassium (mg)
Cottage (large or small curd)		
Creamed	229	85
Uncreamed	290	72
Cream	250	74
Parmesan	734	149
Swiss (domestic)	710	104
Pasteurized process cheese, American	1136[6]	80
Pasteurized process cheese spread, American	1625[6]	240
Cherries		
Raw, sweet	2	191
Canned		
Sour, red, solids and liquid, water pack	2	130
Sweet, solids and liquid, syrup pack, light	1	128
Frozen, not thawed, sweetened	2	130
Chicken, all classes		
Light meat without skin, cooked, roasted	64	411
Dark meat without skin, cooked, roasted	86	321
Chicken potpie, commercial, frozen, unheated	411	153
Chicory, Witloof (also called French or Belgian endive), bleached head (forced), raw	7	182
Chili con carne, canned, with beans	531	233
Chocolate, bitter or baking	4	830
Chocolate syrup, fudge type	89	284
Chop suey, with meat, canned	551	138
Chow mein, chicken (without noodles), canned	290	167
Citron, candied	290	120
Clams, raw		
Soft, meat only	36	235
Hard or round, meat only	205	311
Clams, canned, including hard, soft, razor, and unspecified solids and liquid	—	140
Cocoa and chocolate-flavored beverage powders		
Cocoa powder with nonfat dry milk	525	800
Mix for hot chocolate	382	605
Cocoa, dry powder, high-fat or breakfast		
Plain	6	1522
Processed with alkali	717	651
Coconut cream (liquid expressed from grated coconut meat)	4	324
Coconut meat, fresh	23	256
Cod		
Cooked, broiled	110	407
Dehydrated, lightly salted	8100	160
Coffee, instant, water-soluble solids		
Dry powder	72	3256
Beverage	1	36
Coleslaw, made with French dressing (commercial)	268	205
Collards, cooked, boiled, drained, leaves, including stems, cooked in small amount of water	25	234
Cookie dough, plain, chilled in roll, baked	548	48
Cookies		
Assorted, packaged, commercial	365	67
Butter, thin, rich	418	60
Gingersnaps	571	462
Molasses	386	138
Oatmeal with raisins	162	370
Sandwich type	483	38
Vanilla wafer	252	72
Corn, sweet		
Cooked, boiled, drained, white and yellow, kernels, cut off cob before cooking	Trace	165
Canned		
Regular pack, cream style, white and yellow, solids and liquid	236[1]	(97)
Special dietary pack (low sodium), cream style, white and yellow, solids and liquid	2	(97)
Frozen, kernels cut off cob, cooked, boiled, drained	1	184
Corn fritters	477	133
Corn grits, degermed, enriched, dry form	1	80

For notes, see p. A-63.

Food and description	Sodium (mg)	Potassium (mg)
Corn products used mainly as ready-to-eat breakfast cereals		
Corn flakes, added nutrients	1005	120
Corn, puffed, added nutrients	1060	—
Corn, rice, and wheat flakes, mixed, added nutrients	950	—
Cornbread, baked from home recipes, southern style, made with degermed cornmeal, enriched	591	157
Cornbread mix and cornbread baked from mix, cornbread, made with egg, milk	744	127
Cornmeal, white or yellow, degermed, enriched, dry form	1	120
Cornstarch	Trace	Trace
Cowpeas, including blackeye peas		
Immature seeds, canned, solids and liquid	236[1]	352
Young pods, with seeds, cooked, boiled, drained	3	196
Crab, canned	1000	110
Crackers		
Butter	1092	113
Graham, plain	670	384
Saltines	(1100)	(120)
Sandwich type, peanut-cheese	992	226
Soda	1100	120
Cranberries, raw	2	82
Cranberry juice cocktail, bottled (approx. 33% cranberry juice)	1	10
Cranberry sauce, sweetened, canned, strained	1	30
Cream, fluid, light, coffee, or table, 20% fat	43	122
Cream substitutes, dried, containing cream, skim milk (calcium reduced), and lactose	575	—
Cream puffs with custard filling	83	121
Cress, garden, raw	14	606
Croaker, Atlantic, cooked, baked	120	323
Cucumbers, raw, pared	6	160
Custard, baked	79	146
Dates, domestic, natural and dry	1	648
Doughnuts, cake type	501	90
Duck, domesticated, raw, flesh only	74	285
Eggplant, cooked, boiled, drained	1	150
Eggs, chicken		
Raw		
Whole, fresh and frozen	122	129
Whites, fresh and frozen	146	139
Yolks, fresh	52	98
Endive (curly endive and escarole), raw	14	294
Farina		
Enriched		
Regular		
Dry form	2	83
Cooked	144	9
Quick-cooking, cooked	165	10
Instant-cooking, cooked	188	13
Nonenriched, regular, dry form	2	83
Figs, canned, solids and liquid, syrup pack, light	2	152
Flatfishes (flounders, soles, sand dabs), raw	78	342
Fruit cocktail, canned, solids and liquid, water pack, with or without artificial sweetener	5	168
Garlic, cloves, raw	19	529
Ginger root, fresh	6	264
Gizzard, chicken, all classes, cooked, simmered	57	211
Goose, domesticated, flesh only, cooked, roasted	124	605
Gooseberries, canned, solids and liquid, syrup pack, heavy	1	98
Grapefruit		
Raw, pulp, pink, red, white, all varieties	1	135
Canned, juice, sweetened	1	162
Grapefruit juice and orange juice blended, canned, sweetened	1	184
Grapes, raw, American type (slip skin), such as Concord, Delaware, Niagara, Catawba, and Scuppernong	3	158
Grapejuice, canned or bottled	2	116

For notes, see p. A-63.

Continued.

Food and description	Sodium (mg)	Potassium (mg)
Guavas, whole, raw, common	4	289
Haddock, cooked, fried	177	348
Hake, including Pacific hake, squirrel hake, and silver hake or whiting; raw	74	363
Halibut, Atlantic and Pacific, cooked, broiled	134	525
Ham croquette	342	83
Heart, beef, lean, cooked, braised	104	232
Herring		
Raw, Pacific	74	420
Smoked, hard	6231	157
Honey, strained or extracted	5	51
Horseradish, prepared	96	290
Ice cream and frozen custard, regular, approximately 17% fat	63[7]	181
Ice cream cones	232	244
Ice milk	68[7]	195
Jams and preserves	12	88
Kale, cooked, boiled, drained, leaves including stems	43	221
Kingfish; southern, gulf, and northern (whiting); raw	83	250
Lake herring (cisco), raw	47	319
Lamb, retail cuts	70	290
Lemon juice, canned or bottled, unsweetened	1	141
Lettuce, raw crisphead varieties such as Iceberg, New York, and Great Lakes strains	9	175
Lime juice, canned or bottled, unsweetened	1	104
Liver, beef, cooked, fried	184	380
Lobster, northern, canned or cooked	210	180
Loganberries, canned, solids and liquid, syrup pack, light	1	111
Macadamia nuts	—	164
Macaroni, unenriched, dry form	2	197
Macaroni and cheese, canned	304	58
Margarine[8]	987	23
Marmalade, citrus	14	33
Milk, cow		
Fluid (pasteurized and raw)		
Whole, 3.7% fat	50	144
Skim	52	145
Canned, evaporated (unsweetened)	118	303
Dry, skim (nonfat solids), regular	532	1745
Malted		
Dry powder	440	720
Beverage	91	200
Chocolate drink, fluid, commercial		
Made with skim milk	46	142
Made with whole (3.5% fat) milk	47	146
Molasses, cane		
First extraction or light	15	917
Third extraction or blackstrap	96	2927
Muffin mixes, corn, and muffins baked from mixes		
Made with egg, milk	479	110
Made with egg, water	346	104
Mushrooms		
Raw	15	414
Canned, solids and liquid	400	197
Muskmelons, raw, cantaloupes, other netted varieties	12	251
Mussels, Atlantic and Pacific, raw, meat only	289	315
Mustard greens, cooked, boiled, drained	18	220
Mustard, prepared		
Brown	1307	130
Yellow	1252	130
Nectarines, raw	6	294
New Zealand spinach, cooked, boiled, drained	92	463
Noodles, egg noodles, enriched, cooked	2	44
Oat products used mainly as hot breakfast cereals, oatmeal or rolled oats		
Dry form	2	352
Cooked	218	61

For notes, see p. A-63.

Food and description	Sodium (mg)	Potassium (mg)
Oat products used mainly as ready-to-eat breakfast cereals, with or without corn, puffed, added nutrients	1267	—
Ocean perch, Atlantic (redfish)		
Raw	79	269
Cooked, fried	153	284
Ocean perch, Pacific, raw	63	390
Oils, salad or cooking	0	0
Okra		
Raw	3	249
Cooked, boiled, drained	2	174
Olives, pickled; canned or bottled		
Green	2400	55
Ripe, Ascolano (extra large, mammoth, giant jumbo)	813	34
Ripe, salt-cured, oil-coated, Greek style	3288	—
Onions, mature (dry), raw	10	157
Onions, young green (bunching varieties), raw, bulb and entire top	5	231
Oranges, raw, peeled fruit, all commercial varieties	1	200
Orange juice		
Raw, all commercial varieties	1	200
Canned, unsweetened	1	199
Frozen concentrate, unsweetened, diluted with 3 parts water, by volume	1	186
Oysters		
Raw, meat only, Eastern	73	121
Cooked, fried	206	203
Frozen, solids and liquid	380	210
Oyster stew, commercial frozen, prepared with equal volume of milk	366	176
Pancake and waffle mixes and pancakes baked from mixes, plain and buttermilk, made with egg, milk	564	154
Parsnips, cooked, boiled, drained	8	379
Peaches		
Raw	1	202
Canned, solids and liquid, water pack, with or without artificial sweetener	2	137
Frozen, sliced, sweetened, not thawed	2	124
Peanut butters made with small amounts of added fat, salt	607	670
Peanuts		
Roasted with skins	5	701
Roasted and salted	418	674
Pears		
Raw, including skin	2	130
Canned, solids and liquid, syrup pack, light	1	85
Peas, green, immature		
Cooked, boiled, drained	1	196
Canned, Alaska (early or June peas)		
Regular pack, solids and liquid	236[1]	96
Special dietary pack (low sodium), solids and liquid	3	96
Frozen, cooked, boiled, drained	115	135
Peas, mature seeds, dry, whole, raw	35	1005
Peas and carrots, frozen, cooked, boiled, drained	84	157
Pecans	Trace	603
Peppers, hot, chili, mature, red, raw, pods excluding seeds	25	564
Peppers, sweet, garden varieties, immature, green, raw	13	213
Perch, yellow, raw	68	230
Pickles, cucumber, dill	1428	200
Piecrust or plain pastry, made with enriched flour, baked	611	50
Pies, baked, piecrust made with unenriched flour		
Apple	301	80
Cherry	304	105
Mince	448	178
Pumpkin	214	160
Pike, walleye, raw	51	319
Pineapple		
Raw	1	146
Frozen chunks, sweetened, not thawed	2	100

For notes, see p. A-63.

Continued.

Food and description	Sodium (mg)	Potassium (mg)
Pizza, with cheese, from home recipe, baked		
With cheese topping	702	130
With sausage topping	729	168
Plate dinners, frozen, commercial, unheated		
Beef pot roast, whole oven-browned potatoes, peas, corn	259	244
Chicken, fried; mashed potatoes; mixed vegetables (carrots, peas, corn, beans)	344	112
Meat loaf with tomato sauce, mashed potatoes, peas	393	115
Turkey, sliced; mashed potatoes; peas	400	176
Plums		
Raw, Damson	2	299
Canned, solids and liquid, purple (Italian prunes), syrup pack, light	1	145
Popcorn, popped		
Plain	(3)	—
Oil and salt added	1940	—
Pork, fresh, retail cuts, trimmed to retail level, loin	65	390
Pork, lightly cured, commercial, ham, medium-fat class, separable, lean, cooked, roasted	930	326
Pork, cured, canned ham, contents of can	(1100)	(340)
Potatoes		
Cooked, boiled in skin	3[9]	407
Dehydrated mashed, flakes without milk		
Dry form	89	1600
Prepared, water, milk, table fat added	231	286
Pretzels	1680[10]	130
Prunes, dried, "softenized," cooked (fruit and liquid), with added sugar	3	262
Pudding mixes and puddings made from mixes, with starch base		
With milk, cooked	129	136
With milk, without cooking	124	129
Pumpkin, canned	2	240
Radishes, raw, common	18	322
Raisins, natural (unbleached), cooked, fruit and liquid, added sugar	13	355
Raspberries		
Canned, solids and liquid, water pack, with or without artificial sweetener, red	1	114
Frozen, red, sweetened, not thawed	1	100
Rennin products		
Tablet (salts, starch, rennin enzyme)	22,300	—
Dessert mixes and desserts prepared from mixes		
Chocolate, dessert made with milk	52	125
Other flavors (vanilla, caramel, fruit flavorings)		
Mix, dry form	6	—
Dessert, made with milk	46	128
Rhubarb, cooked, added sugar	2	203
Rice		
Brown		
Raw	9	214
Cooked	282	70
White (fully milled or polished), enriched, common commercial varieties, all types		
Raw	5	92
Cooked	374	28
Rice products used mainly as ready-to-eat breakfast cereals		
Rice flakes, added nutrients	987	180
Rice, puffed; added nutrients, without salt	2	100
Rice, puffed or open-popped, presweetened, honey and added nutrients	706	—
Rockfish, including black, canary, yellowtail, rasphead, and bocaccio, cooked, oven-steamed	68	446
Roe, cooked, baked or broiled, cod and shad[11]	73	132
Rolls and buns, commercial, ready-to-serve		
Danish pastry	366	112
Hard rolls, enriched	625	97
Plain (pan rolls), enriched	506	95
Sweet rolls	389	124
Rusk	246	161
Rutabagas, cooked, boiled, drained	4	167
Rye, flour, medium	(1)	203

For notes, see p. A-63.

Food and description	Sodium (mg)	Potassium (mg)
Rye wafers, whole grain	882	600
Salad dressings, commercial[12]		
Blue and Roquefort cheese		
Regular	1094	37
Special dietary (low calorie), low fat (approx. 5 kcal/tsp)	1108	34
French		
Regular	1370	79
Special dietary (low calorie), low fat (approx. 5 kcal/tsp)	787	79
Mayonnaise	597	34
Thousand Island		
Regular	700	113
Special dietary (low calorie, approx. 10 kcal/tsp)	700	113
Salmon, coho (silver)		
Raw	48[13]	421
Canned, solids and liquid	351[14]	339
Salt pork, raw	1212	42
Salt sticks, regular type	1674	92
Sandwich spread (with chopped pickle)		
Regular	626	92
Special dietary (low calorie, approx. 5 kcal/tsp)	626	92
Sardines, Atlantic, canned in oil, drained solids	823	590
Sardines, Pacific, in tomato sauce, solids and liquid	400	320
Sauerkraut, canned, solids and liquid	747[15]	140
Sausage, cold cuts, and luncheon meats		
Bologna, all samples	1300	230
Frankfurters, raw, all samples	1100	220
Luncheon meat, pork, cured ham or shoulder, chopped, spiced or unspiced, canned	1234	222
Pork sausage, links or bulk, cooked	958	269
Scallops, bay and sea, cooked, steamed	265	476
Soups, commercial, canned		
Beef broth, bouillon, and consomme, prepared with equal volume of water	326	54
Chicken noodle, prepared with equal volume of water	408	23
Tomato		
Prepared with equal volume of water	396	94
Prepared with equal volume of milk	422	167
Vegetable beef, prepared with equal volume of water	427	66
Soy sauce	7325	366
Spaghetti, enriched, cooked, tender stage	1	61
Spaghetti, in tomato sauce with cheese, canned	382	121
Spinach		
Cooked, boiled, drained	50	324
Canned		
Regular pack, drained solids	236[1]	250
Special dietary pack (low sodium), solids and liquid	34	250
Frozen, chopped, cooked, boiled, drained	52	333
Squash, summer, all varieties, cooked, boiled, drained	1	141
Squash, frozen		
Summer, yellow crookneck, cooked, boiled, drained	3	167
Winter, heated	1	207
Strawberries		
Raw	1	164
Frozen, sweetened, not thawed, sliced	1	112
Sturgeon, cooked, steamed	108	235
Succotash (corn and lima beans), frozen, cooked, boiled, drained	38	246
Sugars, beet or cane, brown	30	344
Sweet potatoes		
Cooked, all, baked in skin	12	300
Canned, liquid pack, solids and liquid, regular pack in syrup	48	(120)
Dehydrated flakes, prepared with water	45	140
Tangerines, raw (Dancy variety)	2	126
Tapioca, dry	3	18
Tapioca desserts, tapioca cream pudding	156	135
Tartar sauce, regular	707	78

For notes, see p. A-63

Continued.

Food and description	Sodium (mg)	Potassium (mg)
Tea, instant (water-soluble solids), carbohydrate added		
Dry powder	—	4530
Beverage	—	25
Tomato catsup, bottled	1042[16]	363
Tomato juice, canned or bottled		
Regular pack	200	227
Special dietary pack (low sodium)	3	227
Tomato juice cocktail, canned or bottled	200	221
Tomato puree, canned		
Regular pack	399	426
Special dietary pack (low sodium)	6	426
Tomatoes, ripe		
Raw	3	244
Canned, solids and liquid, regular pack	130	217
Tongue, beef, medium fat, cooked, braised	61	164
Tuna, canned		
In oil, solids and liquid	800	301
In water, solids and liquid	41[17]	279[17]
Turkey, all classes		
Light meat, cooked, roasted	82	411
Dark meat, cooked, roasted	99	398
Turkey potpie, commercial, frozen, unheated	369	114
Turnips, cooked, boiled, drained	34	188
Turnip greens, leaves, including stems		
Canned, solids and liquid	236[1]	243
Frozen, cooked, boiled, drained	17	149
Veal, retail cuts, untrimmed	80	500
Vinegar, cider	1	100
Waffles, frozen, made with enriched flour	644	158
Walnuts		
Black	3	460
Persian or English	2	450
Watercress leaves including stems, raw	52	282
Watermelon, raw	1	100

For notes, see p. A-63.

Food and description	Sodium (mg)	Potassium (mg)
Wheat flours		
Whole (from hard wheats)	3	370
Patent		
All-purpose or family flour, enriched	2	95
Self-rising flour, enriched (anhydrous monocalcium phosphate used as a baking acid)[18]	1079	—[19]
Wild rice, raw	7	220
Yeast		
Baker's, compressed	16	610
Brewer's, debittered	121	1894
Yogurt, made from whole milk	47	132
Zweiback	250	150

[1]Estimated average based on addition of salt in the amount of 0.6% of the finished product.
[2]Processed, partially debranned, whole-kernel wheat with salt added.
[3]Processed, partially debranned, whole-kernel wheat with chicken fat, chicken stock base, dehydrated onion flakes, salt, monosodium glutamate, and herbs.
[4]Values apply to salted butter. Unsalted butter contains less than 10 mg of either sodium or potassium per 100 g. Value for vitamin A is the year-round average.
[5]Applies to unsalted nuts. For salted nuts, value is approximately 200 mg per 100 g.
[6]Values for phosphorus and sodium are based on use of 1.5% anhydrous disodium phosphate as the emulsifying agent. If emulsifying agent does not contain either phosphorus (P) or sodium (Na), the content of these two nutrients in milligrams per 100 g is as follows:

	Na	P
American process cheese	650	444
Swiss process cheese	681	540
American cheese food	—	427
American cheese spread	1139	548

[7]Value for product without added salt.
[8]Values apply to salted margarine. Unsalted margarine contains less than 10 mg/100 g of either sodium or potassium. Vitamin A value based on the minimum required to meet federal specifications for margarine with vitamin A added, 15,000 IUA/lb.
[9]Applies to product without added salt. If salt is added, an estimated average value for sodium is 236 mg/100 g.
[10]Sodium content is variable. For example, very thin pretzel sticks contain about twice the average amount listed.
[11]Prepared with butter or margarine, lemon juice or vinegar.
[12]Values apply to products containing salt. For those without salt, sodium content is low, ranging from less than 10 to 50 mg/100 g; the amount usually is indicated on the label.
[13]Sample dipped in brine contained 215 mg sodium/100 g.
[14]For product canned without added salt, value is approximately the same as for raw salmon.
[15]Values for sauerkraut and sauerkraut juice are based on salt content of 1.9% and 2.0%, respectively, in the finished products. The amounts in some samples may vary significantly from this estimate.
[16]Applies to regular pack. For special dietary pack (low sodium), values range from 5-35 mg/100 g.
[17]One sample with salt added contained 875 mg of sodium/100 g and 275 mg of potassium.
[18]The acid ingredient most commonly used in self-rising flour. When sodium acid pyrophosphate in combination with either anhydrous monocalcium phosphate or calcium carbonate is used, the value for calcium is approximately 120 mg/100 g; for phosphorus, 540 mg; for sodium, 1360 mg.
[19]90 mg of potassium/100 g contributed by flour. Small quantities of additional potassium may be provided by other ingredients.

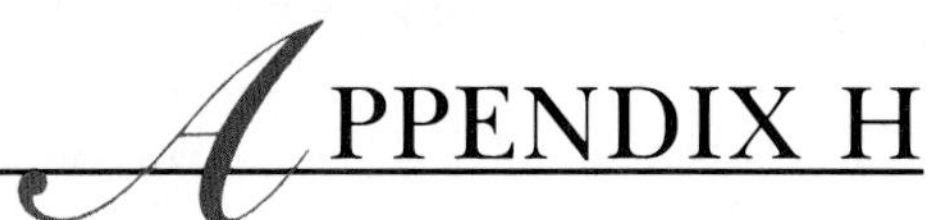

APPENDIX H

Sodium Levels in Mineral Waters and Soft Drinks

Sodium Levels in Mineral Waters

Sodium levels	Beverage (8 fl oz)
Low (less than 5 mg)	Black Mountain spring water
	Bel-Air mineral water
	Perrier
	Poland Springs sparkling water
	Sheffield's O_2 sparkling spring water
Moderate-low (30-60 mg)	Calistoga mineral water
	Canada Dry club soda
	Napa Valley springs mineral water
	Schweppes club soda
Moderate-high (100-110 mg)	Calso water
High (more than 400 mg)	Lady Lee club soda

Adapted from *Sodium in mineral waters—8 fluid ounce servings,* American Heart Association, Alameda County Chapter. Oakland, Calif, Feb 1981.

Sodium Levels in Soft Drinks

Regular beverage	Sugar-free beverage
Less than 20 mg/12 fl oz	
Aspen, Bubble-Up, Canada Dry ginger ale, Canada Dry tonic water, Orange Crush, Pepsi, Schweppes ginger ale, Schweppes tonic water, Shasta cola, Squirt	
20-40 mg/12 fl oz	
Canada Dry collins mix, Coca-Cola, Dr. Pepper, Fanta (orange, grape, root beer), Mountain Dew, Mr. Pibb, Seven-Up, Shasta (all flavors except cola, strawberry, lemon-lime), Sunkist, Teem	Sugar-free Dr. Pepper, Diet Shasta grape, Diet Squirt
40-60 mg/12 fl oz	
Fanta ginger ale, Schweppes bitter lemon, Shasta (lemon-lime, strawberry), Sprite	Fresca, Sugar-free Mr. Pibb, Pepsi Light, Diet Seven-Up, Diet Shasta (all flavors except grape), Tab, Tab-Strawberry
60-80 mg/12 fl oz	
	Diet-Rite Cola, Diet Pepsi, Sugar-free Sprite, Tab (black cherry, ginger ale, grape, lemon-lime, orange, root beer)
80-100 mg/12 fl oz	
	Sugar-free Bubble-Up, Diet Mug Root Beer, Diet Sunkist

Adapted from *Sodium in soft drinks—12 fl oz servings,* American Heart Association, Alameda County Chapter, Oakland, Calif, Feb 1981.

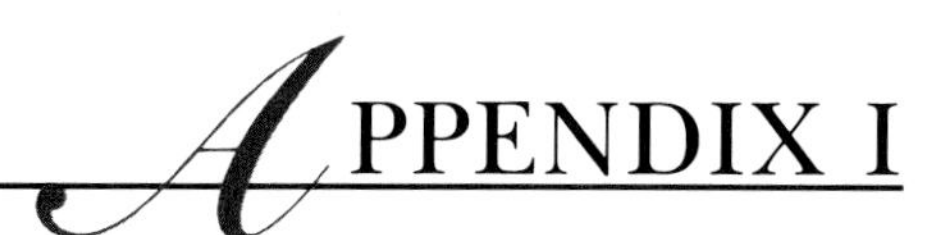

APPENDIX I

Sodium Content of Popular Condiments, Fats, and Oils

Product	Portion size	Sodium (mg)
Salt	1 tsp	1938
Garlic salt	1 tsp	1850
Meat tenderizer (regular)	1 tsp	1750
Onion salt	1 tsp	1620
Soy sauce	1 tbsp	1029
Dill pickle	1 pickle	928
Baking soda	1 tsp	821
Teriyaki sauce	1 tbsp	690
MSG (monosodium glutamate)	1 tsp	492
Baking powder	1 tsp	339
Green olives	4 olives	323
A-1 Steak Sauce	1 tbsp	275
French dressing (dry mix, prepared)	1 tbsp	253
Chili sauce (regular)	1 tbsp	227
French dressing (bottled, store bought)	1 tbsp	214
Worchestershire sauce	1 tbsp	206
Horseradish (prepared)	1 tbsp	198
Tartar sauce	1 tbsp	182
Italian dressing (dry mix, prepared)	1 tbsp	172
Catsup (regular)	1 tbsp	156
Thousand Island dressing (low kcalorie)	1 tbsp	153
Blue cheese dressing	1 tbsp	153
Margarine (regular)	1 tbsp	140
Russian dressing	1 tbsp	133
Barbecue sauce	1 tbsp	130
Pickle, sweet	1 pickle	128
Relish (sweet)	1 tbsp	124
Italian dressing (bottled, store bought)	1 tbsp	116
Butter (regular)	1 tbsp	116
Thousand Island dressing (regular)	1 tbsp	109
Pickles, bread-and-butter	2 slices	101
Mission olives, ripe	3 olives	96
French dressing (home recipe)	1 tbsp	92
Mayonnaise	1 tbsp	78
Butter (whipped)	1 tbsp	74
Mustard (prepared)	1 tsp	65
Chili powder	1 tsp	26
Tabasco sauce	1 tsp	24
Chili sauce (low sodium)	1 tbsp	11
Parsley, dried	1 tbsp	6
Catsup (low sodium)	1 tbsp	3
French dressing (low sodium)	1 tbsp	3
Butter (unsalted)	1 tbsp	2
Meat tenderizer (low sodium)	1 tsp	1
Onion powder	1 tsp	1
Black pepper	1 tsp	1
Vinegar	½ cup	1
Margarine (unsalted)	1 tbsp	1
Oil, vegetable (corn, olive, soybean)	1 tbsp	0

Adapted from *The sodium content of your food,* Home and Garden Bulletin No 233, U.S. Department of Agriculture, Washington, DC, Aug 1980, U.S. Government Printing Office.

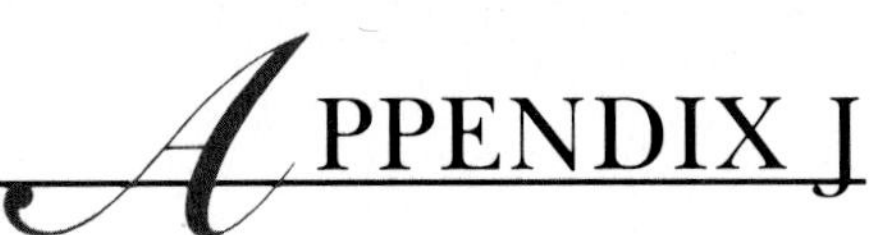

PPENDIX J

Salt-Free Seasoning Guide

Fish

- Breaded, battered fillets
  - Dry mustard, onion; oregano, basil, garlic; thyme
- Broiled steaks or fillets
  - Chili or curry powder; tarragon
- Fillets in butter sauce
  - Thyme, chervil; dill; fennel
- Fish soup
  - Italian seasoning; bay leaf, thyme, tarragon
- Fish cakes
  - Tarragon, savory; dry mustard, white pepper; red pepper, oregano

Beef

- Swiss steak
  - Rosemary, black pepper; bay leaf, thyme; clove
- Roast beef
  - Basil, oregano; bay leaf; nutmeg; tarragon, marjoram
- Beef stew
  - Chili powder; bay leaf, tarragon; caraway; marjoram
- Meatballs
  - Garlic, thyme; basil, oregano, onion; thyme, garlic; black pepper, dry mustard
- Beef stroganoff
  - Red pepper, onion, garlic; nutmeg, onion; curry powder

Poultry and veal

- Fried chicken
  - Basil, oregano, garlic; onion, dill; sesame seed, nutmeg
- Roast chicken or turkey
  - Ginger, garlic; onion, thyme, tarragon
- Chicken croquettes
  - Dill; curry; chili, cumin; tarragon, oregano
- Veal patties
  - Italian seasoning; tarragon; dill, onion, sesame seed
- Barbecue chicken
  - Garlic, dry mustard; clove, allspice, dry mustard; basil, garlic, and oregano

Gravies and sauces

- Barbecue
  - Bay leaf, thyme, red pepper; cinnamon, ginger, allspice, dry mustard, red pepper; chili powder
- Brown
  - Chervil, onion; onion, bay leaf, thyme; onion, nutmeg; tarragon
- Chicken
  - Dry mustard; ginger, garlic; marjoram, thyme, bay leaf
- Cream
  - White pepper, dry mustard; curry powder; dill, onion, paprika; tarragon, thyme

Soups

- Chicken
  - Thyme, savory; ginger; clove, white pepper, allspice
- Clam chowder
  - Basil, oregano; nutmeg, white pepper; thyme, garlic powder
- Mushroom
  - Ginger; oregano; thyme, tarragon; bay leaf, black pepper; chili powder
- Onion
  - Curry, carraway; marjoram, garlic; cloves
- Tomato
  - Bay leaf, thyme; Italian seasoning; oregano, onion; nutmeg
- Vegetable
  - Italian seasoning; paprika, caraway; rosemary, thyme; fennel, thyme

Salads

- Chicken
  - Curry or chili powder; Italian seasoning; thyme, tarragon
- Coleslaw
  - Dill; caraway; poppy; dry mustard, ginger
- Fish or seafood
  - Dill; tarragon, ginger, dry mustard, red pepper; ginger, onion, garlic
- Macaroni
  - Dill; basil, thyme, oregano; dry mustard, garlic
- Potato
  - Chili powder; curry; dry mustard, onion

Pasta, beans, and rice

- Baked beans
  - Dry mustard; chili powder; clove, onion; ginger, dry mustard
- Rice and vegetables
  - Curry; thyme, onion, paprika; rosemary, garlic; ginger, onion, garlic
- Spanish rice
  - Cumin, oregano, basil; Italian seasoning
- Spaghetti
  - Italian seasoning, nutmeg; oregano, basil, nutmeg; red pepper, tarragon
- Rice pilaf
  - Dill; thyme; savory, black pepper

Vegetables

- Asparagus
  - Ginger; sesame seed; basil, onion
- Broccoli
  - Italian seasoning; marjoram, basil; nutmeg, onion; sesame seed
- Cabbage
  - Caraway; onion, nutmeg; allspice, clove
- Carrots
  - Ginger; nutmeg; onion, dill
- Cauliflower
  - Dry mustard; basil; paprika, onion
- Tomatoes
  - Oregano; chili powder; dill, onion
- Spinach
  - Savory, thyme; nutmeg; garlic, onion

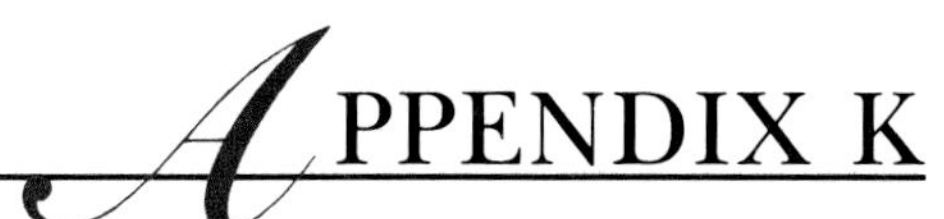

APPENDIX K

Caffeine Content of Common Beverages and Drugs

Source	Caffeine (mg)
Beverages (180 ml cup)	
Brewed coffee	80-140
Instant coffee	60-100
Decaffeinated coffee	1-6
Leaf tea	30-80
Tea bags	25-75
Instant tea	30-60
Cocoa	10-50
Cola drinks (8 oz)	15-50
Candy bar, chocolate (1 oz)	20
Caffeine-containing analgesics	
General	30 (per unit)
Excedrine	60 (per unit)
Cafergot	100 (per unit)

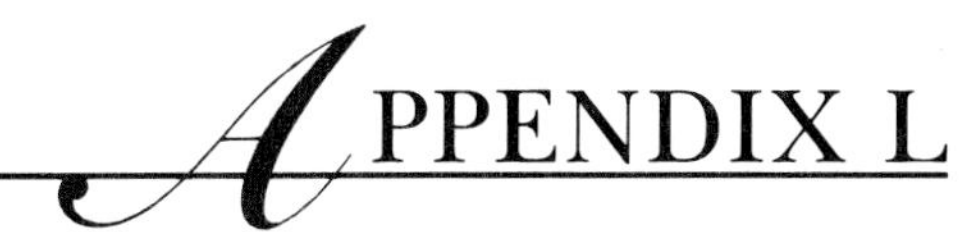

Appendix L

Composition of Beverages: Alcoholic and Carbonated Nonalcoholic (per 100 g)

	Food energy	Protein	Carbo-hydrate	Calcium	Phos-phorus	Iron	Thiamin	Ribo-flavin	Niacin
Alcoholic beverages									
Beer, alcohol 4.5% by volume (3.6% by weight)	42	0.3	3.8	5	30	Trace	Trace	0.03	0.6
Gin, rum, vodka, whisky									
80 proof (33.4% alcohol by weight)	231	—	Trace	—	—	—	—	—	—
86 proof (36.0% alcohol by weight)	249	—	Trace	—	—	—	—	—	—
90 proof (37.9% alcohol by weight)	263	—	Trace	—	—	—	—	—	—
94 proof (39.7% alcohol by weight)	275	—	Trace	—	—	—	—	—	—
100 proof (42.5% alcohol by weight)	295	—	Trace	—	—	—	—	—	—
Wines									
Dessert, alcohol 18.8% by volume (15.3% by weight)	137	0.1	7.7	8	—	—	0.01	0.02	0.2
Table, alcohol 12.2% by volume (9.9% by weight)	85	0.1	4.2	9	10	4	Trace	0.01	0.1
Carbonated nonalcoholic beverages									
Carbonated water									
Sweetened (quinine sodas)	31	—	8	—	—	—	—	—	—
Unsweetened (club sodas)	—	—	—	—	—	—	—	—	—
Cola type	39	—	10	—	—	—	—	—	—
Cream sodas	43	—	11	—	—	—	—	—	—
Fruit-flavored sodas (citrus, cherry, grape, strawberry, Tom Collins mixer, other) (10%-13% sugar)	46	—	12	—	—	—	—	—	—
Ginger ale, pale dry and golden	31	—	8	—	—	—	—	—	—
Root beer	41	—	10.5	—	—	—	—	—	—
Special dietary drinks with artificial sweetener (less than 1 kcal/oz)	—	—	—	—	—	—	—	—	—

From Watt, BK, Merrill, AL: *Composition of foods—raw, processed, prepared.* U.S. Department of Agriculture, Agriculture Handbook No 8, Dec 1963.

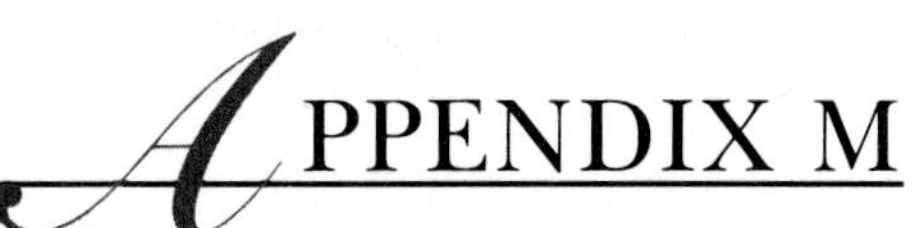

Appendix M

Kilocalorie Values of Some Common Snack Foods

Food	Weight (g)	Approximate measure	Kilocalories
Beverages			
Carbonated, cola type	180	1 bottle, 6 oz	70
Malted milk	405	1 regular (1½ cups)	420
Chocolate milk (made with skim milk)	250	1 cup	190
Cocoa	200	1 cup	235
Soda, vanilla ice cream	242	1 regular	260
Cake			
Angel food	40	2-in sector	110
Cupcake, chocolate, iced	50	1 cake, 2¾-in diameter	185
Fruit cake	30	1 piece, 2 × 2 × ½ in	115
Candy and popcorn			
Butterscotch	15	3 pieces	60
Candy bar, plain	57	1 bar	295
Caramels	30	3 medium	120
Chocolate-coated creams	30	2 average	130
Fudge	28	1 piece	115
Peanut brittle	30	1 oz	125
Popcorn with oil added	14	1 cup	65
Cheese			
Camembert	28	1 oz	85
Cheddar	28	1 oz	105
Cream	28	1 oz	105
Swiss (domestic)	28	1 oz	105
Cookies			
Brownies	30	1 piece, 2 × 2 × ¾ in	140
Cookies, plain and assorted	25	1 cookie, 3-in diameter	120
Crackers			
Cheese	18	5 crackers	85
Graham	14	2 medium	55
Saltines	16	4 crackers	70
Rye	13	2 crackers	45
Dessert-type cream puff and doughnuts			
Cream puff, custard filling	105	1 average	245
Doughnut, cake type, plain	32	1 average	125
Doughnut, jelly	65	1 average	225
Doughnut, raised	30	1 average	120
Miscellaneous			
Hamburger and bun	96	1 average	330
Ice cream, vanilla	62	3½ oz container	130
Sherbet	96	½ cup	120
Jams, jellies, marmalades, preserves	20	1 tbsp	55
Syrup, blended	80	¼ cup	240
Waffles	75	1 waffle, 4½ × 5½ × ½ in	210
Nuts			
Mixed, shelled	15	8-12	95
Peanut butter	16	1 tbsp	95
Peanuts, shelled, roasted	144	1 cup	840

Food	Weight (g)	Approximate measure	Kilocalories
Pie			
Apple	135	4-in sector	345
Cherry	135	4-in sector	355
Custard	130	4-in sector	280
Lemon meringue	120	4-in sector	305
Mince	135	4-in sector	365
Pumpkin	130	4-in sector	275
Potato chips	20	10 chips, 2-in diameter	115
Sandwiches			
Bacon, lettuce, tomato	150	1 sandwich	280
Egg salad	140	1 sandwich	280
Ham	80	1 sandwich	280
Liverwurst	90	1 sandwich	250
Peanut butter	85	1 sandwich	330
Soups, commercial canned			
Bean with pork	250	1 cup	170
Beef noodle	250	1 cup	70
Chicken noodle	250	1 cup	65
Cream (mushroom)	240	1 cup	135
Tomato	245	1 cup	90
Vegetable with beef broth	250	1 cup	80

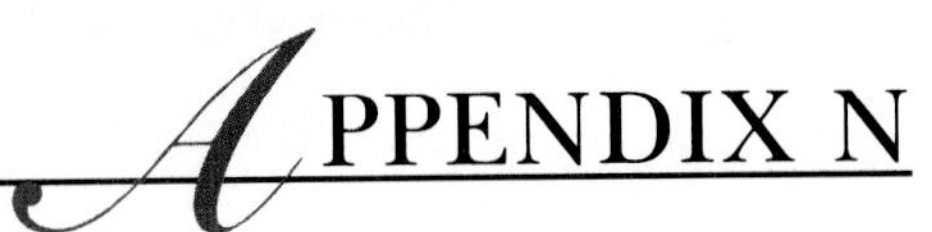

APPENDIX N

Nutritional Analysis of Fast Foods

Food Name	Portion	WT. Gm	KCAL Kc	PROT Gm	CARB Gm	FAT Gm	CHOL Mg	SAFA Gm	MUFA Gm	PUFA Gm	SOD Mg	POT Mg
ARBY'S-BEEF AND CHEESE SANDWICH	ITEM	176	402	32.2	27.1	18	77	9.03	3.66	3.51	1634	345
ARBY'S-CHICKEN BREAST SANDWICH	ITEM	184	493	23	47.9	25	91	5.1	9.6	10.3	1019	330
ARBY'S-CLUB SANDWICH	ITEM	252	560	30	43	30	100	11.6	9.28	8.4	1610	466
ARBY'S-HAM AND CHEESE SANDWICH	ITEM	146	353	20.7	33.4	15.5	58	6.44	6.74	1.38	772	290
ARBY'S-ROAST BEEF SANDWICH	ITEM	139	346	21.5	33.5	13.8	52	3.61	6.8	1.71	792	316
ARBY'S-SUPER ROAST BEEF SANDWICH	ITEM	234	501	25.1	50.4	22.1	40	8.5	8.2	5.4	798	503
ARBY'S-TURKEY DELUXE	ITEM	236	510	28	46	24	70	—	—	—	1220	—
ARBYS-SOUP-BOSTON CLAM CHOWDER	SERVING	227	207	10	18	11	28	4	5	2	1157	319
ARBYS-SOUP-CREAM OF BROCCOLI	SERVING	227	180	9	19	8	3	5	2	1	1113	455
ARBYS-SOUP-FRENCH ONION	SERVING	227	67	2	7	3	0	1	2	1	1248	106
ARBYS-SOUP-LUMBERJACK MIXED VEGETABLE	SERVING	227	89	2	13	4	4	2	1	1	1075	268
ARBYS-SOUP-OLD FASHIONED CHICKEN NOODLE	SERVING	227	99	6	15	2	25	1	1	1	929	78
ARBYS-SOUP-PILGRIM CLAM CHOWDER	SERVING	227	193	10	18	11	28	4	5	2	1157	379
ARBYS-SOUP-ROAST BEEF AND VEGETABLE	SERVING	227	96	5	14	3	10	1	1	1	996	211
ARBYS-SOUP-SPLIT PEA AND HAM	SERVING	227	200	8	21	10	30	5	1	1	1029	272
ARBYS-SOUP-TOMATO FLORENTINE	SERVING	227	84	3	15	2	2	1	1	1	910	221
ARBYS-SOUP-WISCONSIN CHEESE	SERVING	227	287	9	19	19	31	8	8	3	1129	441
BEEF BURGER-FAST FOOD	OUNCE	28.3	72.3	4.99	7.26	2.58	—	—	—	—	54.7	45.9
BUN-HAMBURGER/HOTDOG-FAST FOOD	OUNCE	28.3	97.8	2.66	16.3	2.41	—	—	—	—	22.1	31.2
BURGER KING-BACON DOUBLE CHEESE-DELUXE	SERVING	195	592	33	28	39	111	16	14	6	804	463
BURGER KING-BARBECUE BACON DOUBLE CHEESE	ITEM	174	536	32	31	31	105	14	13	2	795	429
BURGER KING-BK BROILER	ITEM	168	379	24	31	18	53	3	7.96	3.84	764	324
BURGER KING-BK BROILER SAUCE	SERVING	14	90	0	0	10	7	1	2	5	95	—
BURGER KING-CHICKEN TENDERS	PIECE	90	39.3	2.67	2.33	2.17	7.67	0.5	0.833	0.5	90.2	249
BURGER KING-CROISSANT-EGG AND CHEESE	ITEM	127	369	12.8	24.3	24.7	216	14.1	7.54	1.37	551	174
BURGER KING-CROISSANT-EGG/CHEESE/HAM	ITEM	152	475	18.9	24.2	33.6	213	17.5	11.4	2.36	1080	272
BURGER KING-DOUBLE CHEESEBURGER	ITEM	172	483	30	29	27	100	13	11	2	851	344
BURGER KING-FISH TENDERS	SERVING	99	267	12	18	16	28	3	7	4	870	176
BURGER KING-MUSHROOM SWISS DOUBLE CHEESE	ITEM	176	473	31	27	27	95	12	11	2	746	—
BURGER KING-RANCH DIP SAUCE	SERVING	28	171	0	2	18	0	3	4	10	208	—
BURGER KING-SWEET & SOUR SAUCE	SERVING	28	45	0	11	0	0	0	0	0	52	9.14
BURGER KING-TARTAR DIP SAUCE	SERVING	28	174	0	3	18	16	3	4	11	302	13.8
BURGER KING-TATER TENDERS	SERVING	71	213	2	25	12	3	3	6	3	318	—

MAG Mg	IRON Mg	ZINC Mg	V-A RE	V-C Mg	THIA Mg	RIBO Mg	NIAC Mg	V-B6 Mg	FOL Ug	VB12 Ug	CALC Mg	PHOS Mg	SEL Mg	FIBD Gm	V-E Mg
40	5.05	5.37	58	0	0.38	0.46	5.9	0.34	41	2.05	183	401	—	1.06	0.484
45.8	3.45	1.66	15.3	0	0.447	0.388	14.8	0.65	32.3	0.339	111	290	—	1.56	3.1
46.2	3.6	3.13	127	28.3	0.68	0.43	7	0.396	43.6	0.937	200	433	—	2.27	3.92
16	3.25	1.38	95.8	2.7	0.31	0.49	2.69	0.2	71	0.54	130	152	—	1.04	1.36
31	4.23	3.39	63.1	2.1	0.38	0.31	5.86	0.27	40	1.22	54	239	—	0.974	0.257
58.3	6.38	10.7	0	0	0.526	0.601	9.44	0.484	41.1	4.29	115	402	—	1.64	0.432
—	2.7	—	—	—	0.45	0.34	8	—	—	—	80	—	—	—	—
20.4	1.36	0.731	100	3.6	0.061	0.216	0.944	0.116	8.85	9.38	170	143	—	1.36	0.163
54.8	0.792	0.738	50	9	0.113	0.422	0.751	0.175	45.5	0.588	237	193	—	1.75	1.7
2.27	0.636	0.577	10	2.4	0.032	0.023	0.565	0.045	14.3	0	25	11.4	—	0.908	0.326
5.68	1.87	2.72	250	9	0.061	0.102	1.85	0.152	14.2	0.295	40.9	90.8	—	1.25	0.436
4.54	0.726	0.372	200	1.2	0.05	0.057	1.31	0.025	2.04	0.136	15.9	34	—	0.681	0.079
19.2	1.95	1.06	350	3.6	0.061	0.163	1.34	0.148	9.36	9.67	134	126	—	1.92	0.275
4.54	1.04	1.44	300	4.8	0.034	0.045	0.96	0.07	9.76	0.295	15.9	38.6	—	0.454	0.354
36.3	2.02	2.95	300	1.2	0.109	0.089	2.38	0.204	4.31	0.227	31.8	168	—	3.86	0.163
10.2	1.64	0.236	100	12	0.091	0.093	1.34	0.116	15	0.102	44.8	57.9	—	0.454	2.8
6.81	1.32	1.13	90.1	2.4	0.03	0.238	0.704	0.045	6.81	0	252	241	—	1.82	0.436
—	0.255	—	8.22	0.17	0.017	0.037	0.822	—	—	—	3.4	24.9	—	0.028	—
—	0.227	—	0	0.142	0.071	0.023	0.397	—	—	—	9.36	13	—	0	—
37.5	3.95	6.36	71.4	7.59	0.298	0.392	8.12	0.365	31.4	3.24	156	373	—	1.06	1.78
36.1	3.96	6.52	48.7	4.42	0.294	0.393	8.25	0.348	27.1	3.34	158	379	—	0.799	0.758
29.1	3.23	3.17	43.7	6.22	0.274	0.262	5.21	0.242	37.5	1.52	73.7	153	—	1.8	3.1
—	—	—	—	—	—	—	—	—	—	—	—	—	—	0	—
21.6	1.03	0.738	25.2	0	0.135	0.117	6.21	0.315	9	0.297	9	234	—	0.27	0.362
22	2.2	1.76	300	0.2	0.19	0.38	1.51	0.1	36	0.78	244	349	—	2.05	0.83
26	2.13	2.17	135	11.4	0.52	0.3	3.19	0.23	36	1.01	144	336	—	—	—
30.6	2.95	3.95	100	5.84	0.215	0.308	4.94	0.237	31.4	1.81	189	305	—	1.44	2.12
33.1	1.7	0.589	19.6	0.005	0.232	0.167	2.29	0.055	22.7	1.05	60	191	—	1.12	1.55
—	4.14	—	—	—	—	—	—	—	—	—	—	—	—	—	—
—	—	—	—	—	—	—	—	—	—	—	—	—	—	—	—
2.09	0.1	0.013	0	0	0.001	0.003	0.059	0.003	0.301	0	1.02	2.65	—	0.014	—
1.01	0.255	0.053	25.5	0.248	0.002	0.005	0.013	0.076	2.17	0.059	6.99	7.81	—	0.042	4.67
—	—	—	—	—	—	—	—	—	—	—	—	—	—	—	—

Continued.

Food Name	Portion	WT. Gm	KCAL Kc	PROT Gm	CARB Gm	FAT Gm	CHOL Mg	SAFA Gm	MUFA Gm	PUFA Gm	SOD Mg	POT Mg
CHEESE BURGER-FAST FOOD	OUNCE	28.3	78	5.61	6.55	3.26	12.3	1.73	1.65	0.241	198	68
CHICKEN-BREAST AND WING-BREADED-FRIED	SERVING	163	494	35.7	19.6	29.5	149	7.84	12.2	6.79	975	566
CHICKEN-BREAST-FAST FOOD	OUNCE	28.3	73.1	7.65	2.61	3.57	23.6	0.616	0.852	0.467	142	85
CHICKEN-DRUMSTICK & THIGH-BREADED-FRIED	SERVING	148	430	30.1	15.7	26.7	165	7.05	10.9	6.32	756	446
CHICKEN-DRUMSTICK-FAST FOOD	OUNCE	28.3	59	7.03	4.2	1.56	25.6	0.858	1.2	0.703	133	73.7
CHICKEN-FRIED-FAST FOOD-VARIOUS PORTIONS	OUNCE	28.3	82.2	4.71	5.67	4.51	25.4	1.14	1.66	0.958	153	70.9
CHICKEN-MEAT-SHAPED-FRIED-FAST FOOD	OUNCE	28.3	81.6	4.85	4.65	4.85	—	—	—	—	141	39.7
CHICKEN-SHOULDER-FAST FOOD	OUNCE	28.3	92.4	5.33	3.18	6.49	—	—	—	—	150	73.7
CHICKEN-THIGH-FAST FOOD	OUNCE	28.3	104	7.26	2.75	7.14	26.2	1.22	1.73	0.962	139	68
CHICKEN-WING-FAST FOOD	OUNCE	28.3	91.9	7.85	2.78	5.47	—	—	—	—	198	53.9
COLESLAW-FAST FOOD	OUNCE	28.3	23.8	0.68	2.75	1.13	1.07	0.206	0.374	0.759	76.5	45.4
DOUBLE CHEESE BURGER-FAST FOOD	OUNCE	28.3	66.3	4.2	6.63	2.55	16.6	2.2	1.94	0.238	49.9	85.3
FAST FOOD-PIZZA WITH CHEESE	OUNCE	28.4	63.2	3.46	9.23	1.45	4.25	0.693	0.445	0.221	151	49.3
FAST FOOD-PIZZA WITH PEPPERONI	OUNCE	28.4	72.3	4.04	7.93	2.78	5.67	0.893	1.25	0.465	107	61
FISH CAKE-FRIED-WITH BUN-FAST FOOD	OUNCE	28.3	84.5	2.72	7.63	4.79	19.7	0.388	0.761	0.455	167	51.6
FRANKFURTER-CONEY DOG-FAST FOOD	OUNCE	28.3	69.2	3.12	6.95	3.2	14.7	3.09	3.99	0.81	242	48.8
FRANKFURTER-HOT DOG-FAST FOOD	OUNCE	28.3	77.7	3.12	7.37	3.97	14.7	3.09	3.99	0.81	219	48.2
HAMBURGER-DOUBLE PATTY-EVERYTHING ON IT	OUNCE	28.4	67.8	4.3	5.05	3.33	15.3	1.32	1.3	0.351	99.2	71.4
HARDEE-BACON AND EGG BISCUIT	SERVING	124	410	15	35	24	155	5	14	5	990	180
HARDEE-BACON EGG AND CHEESE BISCUIT	SERVING	137	460	17	35	28	165	8	15	5	1220	200
HARDEE-BIG COUNTRY BREAKFAST-COUNTRY HAM	SERVING	254	670	29	52	38	345	9	21	8	2870	710
HARDEE-BIG COUNTRY BREAKFAST-SAUSAGE	SERVING	274	850	33	51	57	340	16	31	11	1980	670
HARDEE-BIG COUNTRY BREAKFAST-WITH BACON	SERVING	217	660	24	51	40	305	10	22	8	1540	530
HARDEE-BIG COUNTRY BREAKFAST-WITH HAM	SERVING	251	620	28	51	33	325	7	19	8	1780	620
HARDEE-BIG ROAST BEEF SANDWICH	SERVING	134	300	18	32	11	45	5	5	2	880	320
HARDEE-BIG TWIN HAMBURGER	SERVING	173	450	23	34	25	55	11	9	5	580	280
HARDEE-BISCUIT N GRAVY	SERVING	221	440	9	45	24	15	6	14	5	1250	210
HARDEE-CHICKEN N PASTA SALAD	SERVING	414	230	27	23	3	55	1	1	1	380	620
HARDEE-CRISPY CURLS	SERVING	85	300	4	36	16	0	3	8	5	840	370
HARDEE-GRILLED CHICKEN SANDWICH	SERVING	192	310	24	34	9	60	1	3	5	890	410
HARDEE-HAM & EGG BISCUIT	SERVING	138	370	15	35	19	160	4	12	4	1050	210
HARDEE-HAM EGG & CHEESE BISCUIT	SERVING	151	420	18	35	23	170	6	13	4	1270	230
HARDEE-MUSHROOM N SWISS HAMBURGER	SERVING	186	490	30	33	27	70	13	12	2	940	370
HARDEE-REGULAR ROAST BEEF SANDWICH	SERVING	114	260	15	31	9	35	4	4	2	730	260
HARDEE-THE LEAN ONE SANDWICH	ITEM	220	420	27	37	18	85	8	8	2	760	510
HARDEE-THREE PANCAKES	SERVING	137	280	8	56	2	15	1	1	1	890	240
KFC-CHICKEN HOT WINGS	PIECE	119	62.6	3.66	2.99	3.99	24.6	0.832	10.3	0.666	113	218
KFC-CHICKEN SANDWICH	SERVING	166	482	21	39	27	47	6	3.91	9	1060	297
KFC-CRISPY CHICKEN-BREAST	PIECE	135	342	33	12	20	114	5	4.7	2	790	347
KFC-CRISPY CHICKEN-DRUMSTICK	PIECE	69	204	14	6	14	71	3	3.72	2	324	157
KFC-CRISPY CHICKEN-THIGH	PIECE	119	406	20	14	30	129	8	6.95	4	688	280
KFC-CRISPY CHICKEN-WING	PIECE	65	254	12	9	19	67	4	5.74	3	422	115
LONG JOHN SILVER-BATTERED SHRIMP-9 PIECE	PIECE	357	95.4	2.66	9.76	4.99	13.9	1.11	3.22	0.555	163	94.3

MAG Mg	IRON Mg	ZINC Mg	V-A RE	V-C Mg	THIA Mg	RIBO Mg	NIAC Mg	V-B6 Mg	FOL Ug	VB12 Ug	CALC Mg	PHOS Mg	SEL Mg	FIBD Gm	V-E Mg
5.88	0.567	0.722	9.36	0.283	0.023	0.048	0.624	0.038	6.79	0.311	25.2	33.2	—	0.057	0.142
38	1.49	1.55	57.7	0	0.14	0.3	12	0.57	9	0.67	60	307	—	0.261	1.18
7.6	0.17	0.287	9.36	0.68	0.02	0.048	1.98	0.158	1.13	0.09	3.97	51.9	—	0	0.089
37	1.6	3.24	66.7	0	0.14	0.43	7.21	0.33	10	0.83	36	240	—	0.237	1.58
6.47	0.312	0.807	6.52	0.425	0.02	0.062	1.42	0.096	2.25	0.09	4.25	41.1	—	0	0.089
7.05	0.283	0.575	6.52	0.454	0.02	0.051	1.62	0.116	1.76	0.087	4.25	38.6	—	0	0.212
—	0.312	—	5.95	0.425	0.009	0.006	0.794	—	—	—	3.97	33.5	—	0	—
—	0.142	—	4.25	0.34	0.02	0.037	1.87	—	—	—	3.69	31.8	—	0	—
6.19	0.085	0.664	6.24	0.283	0.023	0.068	1.42	0.087	1.97	0.082	4.25	36.9	—	0	0.089
—	0.227	—	6.52	0.624	0.017	0.043	1.47	—	—	—	5.1	31.2	—	0	—
3.81	0.51	0.045	7.65	0.425	0.009	0.003	0.028	0.022	8.87	0.008	9.92	9.07	—	0	0.498
5.86	0.624	0.906	7.94	0.057	0.02	0.04	0.765	0.045	5.39	0.422	3.4	30.9	—	0.142	0.139
7.09	0.261	0.366	33.2	0.567	0.082	0.074	1.12	0.02	26.4	0.15	52.4	50.7	—	0.576	0.386
3.4	0.374	0.207	21.8	0.652	0.054	0.094	1.22	0.023	21	0.074	25.8	30.1	—	0.576	—
7.98	0.482	0.682	5.67	0.113	0.017	0.043	1.39	0.033	11.8	0.845	13.9	34.3	—	0	0.389
2.86	0.964	0.554	7.37	0.51	0.065	0.068	1.08	0.031	1.02	0.333	12.2	30.3	—	0	0.08
2.86	0.567	0.554	4.54	0.454	0.011	0.006	0.567	0.031	1.02	0.333	5.67	33.2	—	0	0.08
6.24	0.734	0.712	1.42	0.142	0.045	0.048	0.95	0.068	5.84	0.51	12.8	39.4	—	0.285	0.172
24.8	2.18	1.37	116	2.92	0.331	0.445	3.01	0.136	13.9	0.467	253	358	—	0.625	1.45
27.4	2.41	1.52	129	3.23	0.366	0.492	3.32	0.151	15.4	0.516	279	396	—	0.69	1.61
—	—	—	—	—	—	—	—	—	—	—	—	—	—	—	—
—	—	—	—	—	—	—	—	—	—	—	—	—	—	—	—
23.4	2.46	2.54	333	0	0.312	0.796	1.84	0.343	52.8	1.5	77.5	347	—	0	5.69
—	—	—	—	—	—	—	—	—	—	—	—	—	—	—	—
33.4	3.65	6.14	0	0	0.301	0.344	5.41	0.277	23.5	2.45	66	230	—	0.939	0.247
34.9	4	4.57	16.7	3.26	0.277	0.306	6.72	0.27	33.9	2.27	79.6	197	—	1.74	1.05
—	—	—	—	—	—	—	—	—	—	—	—	—	—	—	—
—	9	—	—	—	—	—	—	—	—	—	—	—	—	—	—
—	—	—	—	—	—	—	—	—	—	—	—	—	—	—	—
44.1	3	2.66	413	0.033	0.43	0.593	4.17	0.1	31	0.472	542	611	—	2.21	4.09
25.5	2.75	1.62	127	8.73	0.56	0.535	3.87	0.207	39.3	0.73	94.9	234	—	1.06	2.33
30.2	2.65	1.67	142	3.56	0.403	0.542	3.66	0.166	16.9	0.569	308	436	—	0.761	1.78
—	—	—	—	—	—	—	—	—	—	—	—	—	—	—	—
28.4	3.11	5.22	0	0	0.257	0.293	4.6	0.236	20	2.09	56.1	196	—	0.799	0.211
—	—	—	—	—	—	—	—	—	—	—	—	—	—	—	—
25.4	1.86	0.914	63.2	0.719	0.215	0.388	1.39	0.099	13.5	0.415	341	411	—	1.35	1.86
22.3	1.48	2.1	63.4	0.206	0.05	0.149	7.65	0.491	3.69	0.333	17.9	175	—	0.061	1.05
41.4	3.11	1.5	13.8	0	0.403	0.35	13.4	0.586	29.1	0.305	99.9	261	—	1.41	2.8
40.2	1.61	1.47	20	0	0.113	0.171	18.4	0.771	5.38	0.459	21.4	312	—	0.08	0.742
16	0.92	1.98	17.4	0	0.057	0.155	4.14	0.238	5.54	0.217	8.42	120	—	0.041	0.637
28.8	1.77	2.97	35.2	0	0.108	0.293	8.22	0.395	9.75	0.362	16	221	—	0.136	0.668
12.4	0.81	1.14	24.5	0	0.038	0.089	4.33	0.265	2.33	0.18	9.87	97.2	—	0.056	0.72
132	10.3	4.23	242	4.89	0.3	0.496	9.86	0.364	33.5	3.4	214	764	—	1.77	16.9

Continued.

Food Name	Portion	WT. Gm	KCAL Kc	PROT Gm	CARB Gm	FAT Gm	CHOL Mg	SAFA Gm	MUFA Gm	PUFA Gm	SOD Mg	POT Mg
LONG JOHN SILVER-BREADED SHRIMP	PIECE	420	51	1.19	6.19	2.43	5.95	0.524	1.57	0.286	85.2	41
LONG JOHN SILVER-CATFISH FILLET	SERVING	373	860	28	90	42	65	10	26	6	990	1180
LONG JOHN SILVER-CHICKEN PLANK-4 PIECE	SERVING	415	940	39	94	44	70	10	29	5	1660	1320
LONG JOHN SILVER-CHICKEN-LIGHT HERB	SERVING	498	630	35	85	17	85	3	5	7	2170	790
LONG JOHN SILVER-CLAM CHOWDER WITH COD	SERVING	198	140	11	10	6	20	2	3	2	590	380
LONG JOHN SILVER-CLAM DINNER	SERVING	363	980	21	122	45	15	10	30	6	1200	870
LONG JOHN SILVER-COLE SLAW	SERVING	98	140	1	20	6	15	1	2	4	260	190
LONG JOHN SILVER-FISH & CHICKEN ENTREE	SERVING	398	870	35	91	40	70	9	26	5	1520	1290
LONG JOHN SILVER-FISH & MORE ENTREE	SERVING	381	800	31	88	37	70	8	23	5	1390	1260
LONG JOHN SILVER-FISH AND FRYES-3 PIECE	SERVING	358	810	42	77	38	85	9	27	2	1630	1340
LONG JOHN SILVER-FISH SAND-WICH PLATTER	SERVING	379	870	26	108	38	55	8	22	7	1110	1050
LONG JOHN SILVER-FRIES	SERVING	85	220	3	30	10	5	3	7	1	60	390
LONG JOHN SILVER-GARDEN SALAD	SERVING	246	170	9	13	9	5	0.846	1	0.777	380	20
LONG JOHN SILVER-GUMBO-COD & SHRIMP BOBS	SERVING	198	120	9	4	8	25	2	3	3	740	310
LONG JOHN SILVER-HOMESTYLE FISH SANDWICH	SERVING	196	510	22	58	22	45	5	13	3	780	470
LONG JOHN SILVER-HOMESTYLE FISH-3 PIECE	SERVING	456	960	43	97	44	100	10	29	5	1890	1540
LONG JOHN SILVER-HOMESTYLE FISH-6 PIECE	SERVING	513	1260	49	124	64	130	14	43	6	1590	1660
LONG JOHN SILVER-HUSH-PUPPIES	PIECE	24	70	2	10	2	5	1	1	1	25	65
LONG JOHN SILVER-LIGHT FISH-LEMON	SERVING	291	320	24	49	4	75	1	1	1	900	470
LONG JOHN SILVER-LIGHT FISH-PAPRIKA	SERVING	284	300	24	45	2	70	1	1	1	650	460
LONG JOHN SILVER-MIXED VEGE-TABLES	SERVING	113	60	2	9	2	0	1	1	1	330	120
LONG JOHN SILVER-OCEAN CHEF SALAD	SERVING	321	250	24	19	9	80	2	2	2	1340	160
LONG JOHN SILVER-RICE PILAF	SERVING	142	210	5	43	2	0	1	1	1	570	140
LONG JOHN SILVER-SEAFOOD PLATTER	SERVING	400	970	30	109	46	70	10	30	6	1540	1100
LONG JOHN SILVER-SEAFOOD SALAD	SERVING	337	270	16	36	7	90	1	2	3	670	100
LONG JOHN SILVER-SEAFOOD SALAD-SCOOP	SERVING	142	210	14	26	5	90	1	2	3	570	100
LONG JOHN SILVER-SHRIMP & FISH DINNER	SERVING	348	770	25	85	37	80	8	23	5	1250	1030
LONG JOHN SILVER-SHRIMP FISH & CHICKEN	SERVING	380	840	31	89	40	80	9	26	5	1450	1170
LONG JOHN SILVER-SHRIMP SCAMPI	SERVING	529	610	25	87	18	220	3	6	7	2120	560
MCDONALDS-APPLE BRAN MUFFIN	SERVING	85	190	5	46	0	0	0	0	0	230	202
MCDONALDS-APPLE DANISH	SLICE	115	390	5.8	51.2	17.9	25.7	3.49	10.8	1.96	370	68.6
MCDONALDS-APPLE PIE	SERVING	83	260	2.2	30	14.8	0	4.83	9.11	0.87	240	49.5
MCDONALDS-BACON AND EGG BISCUIT	SERVING	156	440	17.5	33.3	26.4	253	8.22	16.1	2.01	1230	237
MCDONALDS-BACON BITS	SERVING	3	16	1.3	0.1	1.19	0	0	1.19	0	95	4.35
MCDONALDS-BARBEQUE (BARBE-CUE) SAUCE	SERVING	32	50	0.3	12.1	0.5	0	0.06	0.19	0.22	340	55.7
MCDONALDS-BISCUIT WITH SPREAD	SERVING	75	260	4.6	31.9	12.7	1	3.39	8.64	0.64	730	99.5
MCDONALDS-CHEF SALAD	SERVING	283	230	20.5	7.5	13.3	128	5.91	6.52	0.91	490	—
MCDONALDS-CHICKEN MCNUG-GETS-6 PIECE	SERVING	113	290	19	16.5	16.3	65	4.1	10.4	1.78	520	—

MAG Mg	IRON Mg	ZINC Mg	V-A RE	V-C Mg	THIA Mg	RIBO Mg	NIAC Mg	V-B6 Mg	FOL Ug	VB12 Ug	CALC Mg	PHOS Mg	SEL Mg	FIBD Gm	V-E Mg
156	12.1	4.97	285	5.75	0.353	0.584	11.6	0.428	39.4	3.99	252	899	—	2.08	19.9
121	4.63	3.43	317	11	0.201	0.489	9.69	0.869	67.4	9.41	200	1017	—	0.071	6.85
—	—	—	—	—	—	—	—	—	—	—	—	—	—	—	—
94.6	4.83	3.59	120	0	0.324	0.647	26.3	1.05	9.96	0.747	214	782	—	0	1.58
16.7	1.7	0.923	73.9	4.21	0.053	0.143	1.17	0.129	8.17	8.44	117	110	—	1.67	0.24
40.6	56.7	6.18	365	46.9	0.341	0.911	7.17	0.258	54.1	201	209	572	—	0	5.41
13.1	0.5	0.149	225	29.8	0.039	0.026	0.256	0.127	36.8	0.032	36.1	23.1	—	2.33	5.28
—	—	—	—	—	—	—	—	—	—	—	—	—	—	—	—
131	3.25	2.14	71.2	5	0.392	0.495	12.3	0.724	46.4	5.17	133	769	—	1.69	9.28
—	—	—	—	—	—	—	—	—	—	—	—	—	—	—	—
93.7	6.39	2.25	64.6	2.14	0.872	0.648	11.1	0.421	89.1	2.29	238	488	—	4.06	6.82
28.9	0.646	0.323	0	8.76	0.15	0.024	2.76	0.201	24.6	0	16.1	79.1	—	2.93	0.209
40	1.73	1.1	239	25.6	0.14	0.15	11.4	0.561	65.7	0.268	42	217	—	2.07	1.12
41.1	2.28	0.776	300	21.4	0.117	0.079	1.98	0.168	46.5	0.24	100	105	—	3.02	2.09
48.4	18	1.16	33.4	1.11	0.451	0.335	5.73	0.218	46.1	1.19	123	252	—	2.1	3.53
157	3.89	2.56	85.3	5.99	0.47	0.593	14.7	0.866	55.5	6.19	159	920	—	2.02	11.1
177	4.38	2.88	95.9	6.74	0.528	0.667	16.6	0.975	62.4	6.97	179	1035	—	2.27	12.5
—	—	—	—	—	—	—	—	—	—	—	—	—	—	—	—
56.1	2.29	1.39	79.7	10.2	0.291	0.146	3.38	0.335	46.1	0.576	40.4	238	—	2.43	3.66
97.7	2.43	1.6	53.1	3.73	0.293	0.369	9.18	0.54	34.6	3.86	99	573	—	1.26	6.91
24.1	0.899	0.536	75	3.5	0.078	0.132	0.931	0.081	20.8	0.003	28.5	56.4	—	5.9	0.935
—	—	—	—	—	—	—	—	—	—	—	—	—	—	—	—
16.6	1.77	0.618	59.5	0.565	0.148	0.016	1.51	0.082	5.32	0.006	16.9	44.6	—	0.778	0.936
114	4.13	2.2	59	13.4	0.42	0.368	8.22	0.876	36.9	1.68	109	484	—	5.33	5.2
86	3.22	5.2	129	19.9	0.128	0.158	3.72	0.27	46.7	2.89	148	444	—	1.33	8.9
36.2	1.36	2.19	250	8.38	0.054	0.067	1.57	0.114	19.7	1.22	62.5	187	—	0.562	3.76
81.7	3.45	1.55	27.5	16.5	0.372	0.212	6.64	0.64	35	1.06	54.1	422	—	7.33	5.29
—	—	—	—	—	—	—	—	—	—	—	—	—	—	—	—
203	13.6	6.22	364	11.3	0.132	0.196	13.6	0.55	9.89	5.57	299	1156	—	0	15.5
54.8	0.6	1.23	1	0.7	0.02	0.08	0.4	0.374	76.8	0.784	31	178	—	4.47	0.454
8.09	1.37	0.232	34.5	16.1	0.28	0.2	2.2	0.026	3.42	0	14	30.7	—	1.57	4.51
5.84	0.71	0.168	0	11.4	0.06	0.02	0.32	0.019	2.47	0	10.7	22.1	—	1.13	3.25
31.2	2.56	1.73	160	0	0.36	0.33	2.47	0.172	17.5	0.588	185	451	—	0.786	1.82
2.85	0	0.056	0	0	0	0	0	0.002	3.81	0.036	0	6.51	—	0	0.248
5.76	0.31	0.064	30	2.34	0.01	0.01	0.17	0.024	1.28	0	12.8	6.4	—	1.89	2.1
14.1	1.31	0.704	0	0	0.23	0.11	1.65	0.028	5.95	0.102	75	168	—	0.977	2.14
—	1.51	—	411	13.6	0.31	0.29	3.6	—	—	—	256	—	—	—	—
—	1	—	0	0	0.11	0.12	8.97	—	—	—	12.8	—	—	—	—

Continued.

Food Name	Portion	WT. Gm	KCAL Kc	PROT Gm	CARB Gm	FAT Gm	CHOL Mg	SAFA Gm	MUFA Gm	PUFA Gm	SOD Mg	POT Mg
MCDONALDS-CHOCOLATE MILK-SHAKE-LOWFAT	SERVING	293	320	11.6	66	1.7	10	0.76	0.92	0.05	240	—
MCDONALDS-CHUNKY CHICKEN SALAD	SERVING	250	140	23.1	5.3	3.4	78	0.94	1.99	0.52	230	436
MCDONALDS-CINNAMON AND RAISIN DANISH	ITEM	110	440	6.4	57.5	21	34.7	4.2	13	1.6	430	—
MCDONALDS-COOKIE-CHOCOLATY	SERVING	56	330	4.2	41.9	15.6	4	5.04	10.2	0.39	280	71.7
MCDONALDS-COOKIE-MCDONALD-LAND	SERVING	56	290	4.2	47.1	9.2	0	1.85	6.8	0.52	300	37.5
MCDONALDS-CROUTONS	SERVING	11	50	1.39	6.8	2.17	0	0.45	1.32	0.11	140	19.9
MCDONALDS-ENGLISH MUFFIN	SERVING	59	170	5.4	26.7	4.6	9	2.38	1.68	0.5	270	74.3
MCDONALDS-FRENCH FRIES-LARGE	SERVING	122	400	5.61	45.9	21.6	16	9.06	11.6	0.89	200	866
MCDONALDS-FRENCH FRIES-MEDIUM	SERVING	97	320	4.44	36.3	17.1	12	7.17	9.21	0.7	150	692
MCDONALDS-FRENCH FRIES-REGULAR ORDER	SERVING	68	220	3.13	25.6	12	9	5.05	6.49	0.5	110	484
MCDONALDS-GARDEN SALAD	SERVING	213	110	7.1	6.2	6.6	83	2.9	3.16	0.53	160	450
MCDONALDS-HASHBROWN POTATO	SERVING	55	130	1.4	14.9	7.3	9	3.24	3.66	0.37	330	238
MCDONALDS-HONEY SAUCE	SERVING	14	45	0	11.5	0	0	0	0	0	0	—
MCDONALDS-HOT CAKES WITH SYRUP	SERVING	176	410	8.2	74.4	9.2	21	3.66	3.09	2.46	640	187
MCDONALDS-HOT CARAMEL SUNDAE	SERVING	174	270	6.6	59.3	2.8	13	1.51	1.22	0.09	180	414
MCDONALDS-HOT FUDGE SUNDAE	SERVING	169	240	7.3	50.5	3.2	6	2.35	0.76	0.05	170	274
MCDONALDS-HOT MUSTARD SAUCE	SERVING	30	70	0.5	8.2	3.6	5	0.51	1.23	1.86	250	25.6
MCDONALDS-ICED CHEESE DANISH	SERVING	110	390	7.4	42.3	21.8	47	5.95	12.1	1.77	420	—
MCDONALDS-McCHICKEN SAND-WICH	SERVING	190	490	19.2	39.8	28.6	42.6	5.4	11.5	11.6	780	340
MCDONALDS-McDLT HAMBURGER	ITEM	234	580	26.3	36	36.8	109	11.5	16.7	8.5	990	—
MCDONALDS-MCLEAN DELUXE HAMBURGER	SERVING	206	320	22	35	10	60	4	5	1	670	290
MCDONALDS-MILKSHAKE-CHOCO-LATE-LOWFAT	SERVING	293	320	12	66	2	10	1	1	0	240	—
MCDONALDS-MILKSHAKE-STRAW-BERRY-LOWFAT	SERVING	293	320	11	67	1	10	1	1	0	170	—
MCDONALDS-MILKSHAKE-VA-NILLA-LOWFAT	SERVING	293	290	11	60	1	10	1	1	0	170	643
MCDONALDS-PORK SAUSAGE	SERVING	48	180	8.4	0	16.3	48	5.88	8.51	1.9	350	—
MCDONALDS-RASPBERRY DANISH	ITEM	117	410	6.1	61.5	15.9	26	3.11	10.2	1.1	310	—
MCDONALDS-SALAD DRESSING-PEPPERCORN	OUNCE	28.4	160	0	2	18	14	2	4	10	170	22.4
MCDONALDS-SALAD DRESSING-RED FRENCH	OUNCE	28.4	80	0	10	4	0	0	2	2	220	22.4
MCDONALDS-SAUSAGE AND EGG BISCUIT	ITEM	180	520	19.9	32.6	34.5	275	11.2	20	2.54	1250	319
MCDONALDS-SAUSAGE BISCUIT	ITEM	123	440	13	31.9	29	49	9.27	17.2	2.54	1080	196
MCDONALDS-SAUSAGE MCMUFFIN	ITEM	117	370	16.5	27.3	21.9	64	7.79	11.7	2.43	830	179
MCDONALDS-SAUSAGE MCMUFFIN WITH EGG	ITEM	167	440	22.6	27.9	26.8	263	9.45	14.2	3.15	980	255
MCDONALDS-SCRAMBLED EGGS	SERVING	98	140	12.4	1.2	9.8	399	3.33	5.03	1.44	290	102
MCDONALDS-SIDE SALAD	SERVING	115	60	3.7	3.3	3.3	41	1.45	1.59	0.27	85	219
MCDONALDS-STRAWBERRY MILK-SHAKE-LOWFAT	SERVING	293	320	10.7	67	1.3	10	0.63	0.64	0.05	170	—
MCDONALDS-STRAWBERRY SUNDAE	SERVING	171	210	5.7	49.2	1.1	5	0.63	0.39	0.04	95	263
MCDONALDS-SWEET AND SOUR SAUCE	SERVING	32	60	0.2	13.8	0.2	0	0.03	0.1	0.1	190	10.4
MCDONALDS-VANILLA MILK-SHAKE-LOWFAT	SERVING	293	290	10.8	60	1.3	10	0.63	0.67	0.05	170	—
MCDONALDS-VANILLA-FROZEN YOGURT	SERVING	80	100	4	22	0.75	3	0.41	0.28	0.06	80	—
PIZZA-BEEF/CHICKEN/ONION	OUNCE	28.3	72.6	5.53	7.23	2.38	—	—	—	—	267	49
PIZZA-BEEF/ONION	OUNCE	28.3	72.9	4.34	7.88	2.66	—	—	—	—	132	49.9
PIZZA-CHICKEN CURRY/PEAS	OUNCE	28.3	81.6	3.74	9.41	3.23	—	—	—	—	146	44.5
PIZZA-CHICKEN/MUSHROOM/TOMATO	OUNCE	28.3	60.7	4.9	7.31	1.3	—	—	—	—	167	44.2

MAG Mg	IRON Mg	ZINC Mg	V-A RE	V-C Mg	THIA Mg	RIBO Mg	NIAC Mg	V-B6 Mg	FOL Ug	VB12 Ug	CALC Mg	PHOS Mg	SEL Mg	FIBD Gm	V-E Mg
—	0.84	—	91.9	0	0.13	0.5	0.4	—	—	—	332	—	—	—	—
36.6	1.02	2.94	366	19.9	0.22	0.17	8.5	0.6	26.6	0.63	33.8	257	—	0.955	13
—	1.81	—	33	3.2	0.32	0.24	2.8	—	—	—	35.1	—	—	—	—
20.2	2.18	0.515	0	0	0.18	0.21	2.47	0.028	5.04	0.073	23.9	71.1	—	1.12	1.73
12.9	2.07	0.325	0	0	0.25	0.18	2.54	0.028	3.92	0.067	8.91	91.3	—	0.56	1.73
4.62	0.35	0.103	0	0.14	0.05	0.03	0.42	0.007	3.41	0	6.48	15.4	—	0.517	0.114
12.2	1.61	0.396	36.6	0	0.33	0.14	2.47	0.097	51.1	0.001	151	59.8	—	1.56	0.16
40.1	0.93	0.633	0	14.6	0.24	0	3.29	0.317	40.1	0.147	17.8	162	—	4.21	0.3
32	0.73	0.506	0	11.6	0.19	0	2.6	0.253	32	0.117	14.1	129	—	3.35	0.239
22.4	0.52	0.354	0	8.16	0.14	0	1.84	0.177	22.4	0.082	9.93	90.4	—	—	—
34.7	1.26	0.956	391	13.5	0.1	0.16	0.59	0.486	56.9	0.232	149	188	—	1.8	0.974
9.3	0.27	0.175	0	1.59	0.06	0.02	0.85	0.069	3.55	0	5.58	39.4	—	1.09	0.125
—	0.07	—	0	0.14	0	0.01	0.04	—	—	—	—	—	—	—	—
25	2.08	0.6	52	4.71	0.32	0.33	2.82	0.12	9	0.19	114	501	—	—	—
50.5	0.08	1.1	87.4	0	0.08	0.35	0.26	0.383	19.1	0.661	222	198	—	1.04	1.38
32	0.48	1.29	64.3	0	0.08	0.35	0.3	0.074	7.23	0.597	235	178	—	1.25	1.36
5.47	0.22	0.094	1.6	0.45	0.01	0.01	0.15	0.01	1.27	0	15	7.3	—	0.252	1.45
—	1.42	—	37.6	1.1	0.29	0.23	2.1	—	—	—	32.9	—	—	—	—
47.3	2.61	1.72	31.2	2.42	0.96	0.21	8.92	0.671	33.3	0.35	143	299	—	1.61	3.19
—	3.91	—	226	7.38	0.39	0.36	6.87	—	—	—	225	—	—	—	—
34.8	3.78	3.24	66.6	9.74	0.354	0.311	5.81	0.257	47.7	1.48	92.5	170	—	2.4	3.2
—	—	—	—	—	—	—	—	—	—	—	332	—	—	—	—
—	—	—	—	—	—	—	—	—	—	—	327	—	—	—	—
48.1	0.205	2.43	38.1	2.2	0.123	0.589	0.314	0.132	30.8	1.54	327	394	—	0	0.12
—	0.67	—	0	0	0.27	0.1	2.31	—	—	—	8.24	—	—	0	—
—	1.47	—	35.1	3.2	0.33	0.21	2.1	—	—	—	14.2	—	—	—	—
0	0.114	0.023	5.68	0	0.002	0.005	0.001	0.003	1.19	0.039	3.12	3.98	—	0	2.87
0	0.114	0.023	5.68	0	0.002	0.005	0.001	0.003	1.19	0.039	3.12	3.98	—	0	2.87
25	3.16	2.16	88.3	0.1	0.53	0.35	3.99	0.2	40	1.37	116	490	—	—	—
19.8	1.98	1.54	0	0	0.49	0.21	3.96	0.114	8.73	0.504	83.2	443	—	1.35	3.66
20	2.3	1.67	72.1	1.27	0.6	0.29	4.8	0.133	47.7	0.503	235	273	—	1.1	1.94
28.6	3.34	2.39	150	0	0.64	0.42	4.82	0.19	68.1	0.718	263	390	—	1.56	2.77
10.2	2.08	1.09	156	1.18	0.07	0.26	0.05	0.075	27.2	1.68	57	136	—	0	3.44
12.4	0.67	0.252	217	7.4	0.05	0.08	0.32	0.059	40.3	0	763	25.5	—	1.23	0.469
—	0.09	—	91.9	0	0.13	0.48	0.31	—	—	—	327	—	—	—	—
19	0.16	1.17	64.3	1.3	0.07	0.29	0.25	0.067	8.77	0.54	190	127	—	0.687	0.754
2.38	0.17	0.014	64.8	0.64	0	0.01	0.08	0.004	0.344	0	10.9	3.03	—	0.016	—
—	0.1	—	91.9	0	0.13	0.48	0.31	—	—	—	327	—	—	—	—
—	0.23	—	38.4	0	0.04	0.18	0.37	—	—	—	112	—	—	—	—
—	0.709	—	23.2	1.25	0.026	0.023	1.25	—	—	—	72.9	53	—	0.028	—
—	0.17	—	23.2	0.227	0.011	0.017	0.879	—	—	—	21.3	35.7	—	0.113	—
—	0.17	—	29.8	0.198	0.02	0.026	1.73	—	—	—	19.3	36.6	—	0.198	—
—	0.198	—	22.7	0.312	0.009	0.011	0.765	—	—	—	24.1	36.6	—	0.085	—

Continued.

Food Name	Portion	WT. Gm	KCAL Kc	PROT Gm	CARB Gm	FAT Gm	CHOL Mg	SAFA Gm	MUFA Gm	PUFA Gm	SOD Mg	POT Mg
PIZZA-CHICKEN/PINEAPPLE	OUNCE	28.3	80.5	4.22	6.32	4.25	—	—	—	—	267	37.4
PIZZA-COMBINATION SUPREME	OUNCE	28.3	50.5	4.14	7.09	0.624	5.66	1.33	1.47	0.408	165	45.1
PIZZA-CURRY BEEF/PEAS	OUNCE	28.3	70.6	4.51	7.31	2.58	8.33	0.856	1.62	1.01	130	47.3
PIZZA-ONION/TOMATO/GREEN PEPPER/MUSHROOM	OUNCE	28.3	45.4	3.49	6.58	0.567	—	—	—	—	136	42.8
PIZZA-PEPPERONI/BEEF/SALAMI/ MUSHROOM/ETC	OUNCE	28.3	83.3	5.07	4.56	4.96	—	—	—	—	367	61.2
PIZZA-SHRIMP/CUCUMBER	OUNCE	28.3	68.6	4.45	6.83	2.61	—	—	—	—	143	46.2
PIZZA-SHRIMP/SQUID/MUSH- ROOM	OUNCE	28.3	70.3	4.96	7.43	2.3	—	—	—	—	160	33.2
POTATOES-FRENCH FRIED-FAST FOOD	OUNCE	28.3	91.3	1.08	10.3	5.07	2.76	1.8	1.93	0.755	17	130
POTATOES-MASHED-FAST FOOD	OUNCE	28.3	26.4	0.624	5.44	0.227	0.544	0.284	0.481	0.328	82.2	48.2
RAX-GRILLED CHICKEN SAND- WICH	ITEM	190	440	24	36	19	87.9	2.92	4.48	5.37	1050	340
SALAD-FAST FOOD	OUNCE	28.3	33.5	0.454	3.29	2.04	—	—	—	—	128	39.7
SPAGHETTI-VEGETABLES/ SAUCE/CHEESE	OUNCE	28.3	28.3	3.8	3.01	0.113	—	—	—	—	83.6	52.4
SUBWAY SANDWICH-HAM AND CHEESE-ON WHEAT	ITEM	194	673	39	86	22	73	7	8	4	2508	918
SUBWAY-BMT SANDWICH-ON HONEY WHEAT ROLL	ITEM	220	1011	45	88	57	133	20	25	7	3199	1002
SUBWAY-BMT SANDWICH-ON ITALIAN ROLL	ITEM	213	982	44	83	55	133	20	24	7	3139	917
SUBWAY-CLUB SANDWICH-ON HONEY WHEAT	ITEM	220	722	47	89	23	84	7	9	4	2777	1055
SUBWAY-CLUB SANDWICH-ON ITALIAN ROLL	ITEM	213	693	46	83	22	84	7	8	4	2717	971
SUBWAY-COLD CUT COMBO SAND- WICH-ITALIAN	ITEM	184	853	46	83	40	166	12	15	10	2218	876
SUBWAY-COLD CUT COMBO SAND- WICH-ON WHEAT	ITEM	191	883	48	88	41	166	12	15	10	2278	1010
SUBWAY-HAM & CHEESE SAND- WICH-ON ITALIAN	ITEM	184	643	38	81	18	73	7	8	4	1710	834
SUBWAY-MEATBALL SANDWICH-ON ITALIAN ROLL	ITEM	215	918	42	96	44	88	17	17	4	2022	1210
SUBWAY-MEATBALL-ON HONEY WHEAT ROLL	ITEM	224	947	44	101	45	88	17	18	4	2082	1498
SUBWAY-ROAST BEEF SANDWICH- ITALIAN ROLL	ITEM	184	689	42	84	23	83.3	8	9	4	2288	910
SUBWAY-ROAST BEEF SANDWICH- ON WHEAT ROLL	ITEM	189	717	41	89	24	75	8	9	4	2348	994
SUBWAY-SALAD DRESSING- BUTTERMILK RANCH	SERVING	56.7	348	1	2	37	6	5	7	24	492	17
SUBWAY-SALAD DRESSING-LITE ITALIAN	SERVING	56.7	23	1	4	1	0	3.97	6.35	15.9	952	13
SUBWAY-SEAFOOD/CRAB SAND- WICH-ON ITALIAN	ITEM	210	986	29	94	57	56	11	15	28	1967	557
SUBWAY-SEAFOOD/CRAB SAND- WICH-ON WHEAT	ITEM	219	1015	31	100	58	56	11	16	28	2027	641
SUBWAY-SPICY ITALIAN SAND- WICH-ON ITALIAN	ITEM	213	1043	42	83	63	137	23	28	7	2282	880
SUBWAY-STEAK & CHEESE SAND- WICH-ITALIAN	ITEM	213	765	43	83	32	82	12	12	4	1556	909
SUBWAY-TURKEY BREAST SAND- WICH-WHEAT ROLL	ITEM	192	674	42	88	20	67	6	7	7	2520	605
TACO BELL-DOUBLE BEEF BURRITO SUPREME	ITEM	255	457	23.6	41.7	21.8	56.8	10.1	15.4	2.09	1053	431
TACO BELL-ENCHIRITO	ITEM	213	382	19.8	30.9	19.7	54.2	9.32	—	1.51	1243	—
TACO BELL-MEXICAN PIZZA	SERVING	223	575	21.3	39.7	36.8	52	11.4	8.16	9.74	1031	408
TACO BELL-NACHOS	SERVING	106	346	7.49	37.5	18.5	8.82	5.74	9.96	1.55	399	159
TACO BELL-NACHOS BELL- GRANDE	SERVING	287	649	21.6	60.6	35.3	36.3	12.3	—	2.61	997	674
TACO BELL-PINTOS & CHEESE	SERVING	128	190	8.97	19	8.72	16.2	3.6	4.92	0.814	642	399
TACO BELL-SOFT TACO	ITEM	92.1	228	11.8	17.9	11.8	31.8	5.37	3.71	1.21	516	178
TACO BELL-TACO BELLGRANDE	ITEM	163	355	18.3	17.7	23.1	55.9	10.9	6.57	1.32	472	334
TACO BELL-TACO LIGHT	ITEM	170	410	19	18.1	28.8	55.6	11.6	—	5.36	594	316
TACO BELL-TACO SALAD WITH SALSA/NO SHELL	SERVING	530	520	30.6	30	31.4	79.8	14.4	19.2	1.7	1431	1151

MAG Mg	IRON Mg	ZINC Mg	V-A RE	V-C Mg	THIA Mg	RIBO Mg	NIAC Mg	V-B6 Mg	FOL Ug	VB12 Ug	CALC Mg	PHOS Mg	SEL Mg	FIBD Gm	V-E Mg
—	0.397	—	25.2	0.879	0.026	0.026	2.13	—	—	—	85.9	114	—	0.057	—
6.45	0.227	0.343	9.64	0.624	0.017	0.017	1.81	0.038	6.9	0.084	26.6	39.4	—	0.17	0.348
7.03	0.17	0.725	28.6	0.879	0.02	0.023	3.57	0.058	2.45	0.366	23.8	37.7	—	0.17	0.784
—	0.227	—	9.07	0.425	0.014	0.023	1.64	—	—	—	24.7	32.9	—	0.227	—
—	0.227	—	21.5	0.198	0.02	0.003	3.06	—	—	—	76.3	58.7	—	0.085	—
—	0.198	—	11.9	0.397	0.009	0.011	2.32	—	—	—	24.7	48.2	—	0.142	—
—	0.17	—	13	0.369	0.009	0.014	0.936	—	—	—	22.4	37.7	—	0.142	—
9.62	0.595	0.108	6.24	0.312	0.023	0.011	0.369	0.067	8.21	0	2.27	20.1	—	0	0.07
5.15	0.765	0.077	14.7	0.227	0.017	0.011	0.198	0.063	2.25	0.016	3.12	14.2	—	0	0.208
47.3	3.56	1.72	15.8	0	0.462	0.401	15.3	0.671	33.3	0.35	114	299	—	1.61	3.19
—	0.652	—	4.25	0.85	0.017	0.006	0.028	—	—	—	5.39	14.2	—	0	—
—	0.312	—	3.97	0.085	0.011	0.011	0.227	—	—	—	3.97	9.64	—	0.34	—
—	—	—	—	—	—	—	—	—	—	—	—	—	—	6	—
—	—	—	—	—	—	—	—	—	—	—	—	—	—	6	—
66.1	4.26	6.08	66.5	5.4	0.271	0.341	5.06	0.481	62.6	2.33	63.6	308	—	5	6.1
39.7	3.18	1.39	83	15.1	0.486	0.348	9.3	0.455	43.1	0.44	96.3	247	—	6	5.04
65.6	3.09	2.5	74	20.2	0.477	0.334	12.5	0.581	47	0.946	57.5	384	—	5	1.61
27.5	2.86	2.73	87	17.3	0.359	0.333	3.8	0.201	39	1.23	227	315	—	5	1.08
28.5	2.97	2.83	90.3	18	0.372	0.346	3.94	0.208	40.5	1.28	23.5	327	—	6	1.13
49.6	2.17	2.8	174	16.8	0.528	0.388	3.56	0.335	45.1	0.756	304	527	—	5	4.6
47.1	4.97	6.2	71.9	18.7	0.333	0.391	9.36	0.4	34.9	3.21	77.6	263	—	3.02	1.18
—	—	—	—	—	—	—	—	—	—	—	—	—	—	—	—
57.1	3.68	5.26	57.5	4.67	0.234	0.294	4.37	0.416	54.1	2.01	54.9	266	—	5	5.26
58.6	3.78	5.4	59	4.79	0.24	0.302	4.49	0.427	55.6	2.07	56.4	273	—	6	5.4
1.13	0.113	0.102	47.6	0	0.007	0.014	0.002	0.01	3.56	0.118	7.94	14.7	—	0	2.72
0.363	0.113	0.062	13.6	0	0.006	0.011	0.002	0.007	2.77	0.092	5.67	2.84	—	0	5.86
—	—	—	—	—	—	—	—	—	—	—	—	—	—	—	—
61.7	4.41	5.28	107	5.49	0.51	0.383	6.95	0.258	91.3	6.54	230	336	—	2.49	3.01
—	—	—	—	—	—	—	—	—	—	—	—	—	—	5	—
43.1	4.22	6.78	119	5.82	0.33	0.464	5.06	0.381	36.4	2.54	231	456	—	6	1.01
—	—	—	—	—	—	—	—	—	—	—	—	—	—	7	—
87.2	3.95	5.93	286	8.68	0.427	2.19	3.68	0.354	132	2.18	145	548	—	5.68	2.78
—	2.84	—	290	28.1	0.256	0.418	2.32	—	—	—	269	—	—	—	—
62.9	3.74	2.32	295	30.9	0.319	0.326	2.96	0.274	113	0.198	257	360	—	5.75	3.02
42.8	0.934	2.58	169	1.88	0.006	0.163	0.679	0.122	15.7	0.615	191	439	—	1.39	3.36
—	3.48	—	341	57.8	0.104	0.339	2.17	—	—	—	297	—	—	—	—
49.8	1.42	1.08	132	51.4	0.05	0.146	0.396	0.192	98.1	0.076	156	175	—	4.87	1.68
30.6	2.27	1.36	64	1.22	0.387	0.224	2.74	0.159	40.3	0.31	116	132	—	2.56	1.1
54.1	1.92	2.4	254	5.48	0.107	0.291	2.02	0.282	71.3	0.549	182	234	—	4.54	1.94
—	2.44	—	199	4.7	0.199	0.325	2.51	—	—	—	155	—	—	—	—
111	5.14	9.14	908	76.1	0.264	0.64	3.17	0.779	98.8	4.29	367	567	—	7.04	7.25

Continued.

Food Name	Portion	WT. Gm	KCAL Kc	PROT Gm	CARB Gm	FAT Gm	CHOL Mg	SAFA Gm	MUFA Gm	PUFA Gm	SOD Mg	POT Mg
TACO BELL-TACO SALAD WITH SALSA/SHELL	SERVING	595	941	36	63.1	61.3	80.4	18.7	21.6	12.1	1662	1212
TACO BELL-TACO SALAD-NO SALSA-NO SHELL	SERVING	530	502	29.5	26.3	31.3	79.8	14.4	19.2	1.7	1056	988
WENDYS-BACON AND CHEESE POTATO	SERVING	347	450	15	57	18	10	37.1	38.2	14.1	1125	1580
WENDYS-BIG CLASSIC-QUARTER POUND BURGER	SERVING	277	570	27	46	33	85	15.9	14.8	4.26	1075	590
WENDYS-BROCCOLI AND CHEESE POTATO	SERVING	377	400	9	59	16	0	—	—	—	470	1555
WENDYS-CHEESE POTATO	SERVING	348	470	13	57	21	0	12.1	9.26	4	580	1435
WENDYS-CHEESE SAUCE	SERVING	56	40	1	5	2	0	1.87	1.06	0.319	300	70
WENDYS-CHEESE TORTELLINI/ SPAGHETTI SAUCE	SERVING	112	120	4	24	1	5	2.8	2.15	0.888	280	110
WENDYS-CHICKEN CLUB SAND-WICH	SERVING	231	500	30	42	24	75	5.45	8.46	8.02	950	515
WENDYS-CHICKEN SALAD	SERVING	56	120	7	4	8	0	3	2.81	3	215	60
WENDYS-CHILI	SERVING	255	220	21	23	7	45	3	5.66	1.05	750	495
WENDYS-FRENCH FRIES-REGULAR SIZE	SERVING	134	440	5	53	23	25	8.51	9.13	3.58	265	855
WENDYS-KIDS MEAL HAMBURGER	SERVING	104	260	14	30	9	35	3.5	4.75	0.768	545	205
WENDYS-REFRIED BEANS	SERVING	56	70	4	10	3	0	1	2.21	1	215	210
WENDYS-SEAFOOD SALAD	SERVING	56	110	4	7	7	0	1	4.46	4	455	40
WENDYS-SINGLE CHEESEBURGER/ EVERYTHING	SERVING	252	490	29	35	27	90	10.8	11.2	4.58	1155	495
WENDYS-SINGLE HAMBURGER/ EVERYTHING	SERVING	234	420	25	35	21	70	6.72	9.4	4.43	865	495
WENDYS-SPANISH RICE	SERVING	56	70	2	13	1	0	0.121	0.298	1	440	130
WENDYS-TACO SALAD WITH TACO CHIPS	SERVING	791	660	40	46	37	35	28.8	28.7	15.4	1110	1330
WENDYS-TUNA SALAD	SERVING	56	100	8	4	6	0	1	0.796	3	290	90

MAG Mg	IRON Mg	ZINC Mg	V-A RE	V-C Mg	THIA Mg	RIBO Mg	NIAC Mg	V-B6 Mg	FOL Ug	VB12 Ug	CALC Mg	PHOS Mg	SEL Mg	FIBD Gm	V-E Mg
125	7.1	10.3	888	77	0.508	0.753	4.78	0.875	111	4.82	398	637	—	7.91	8.14
111	4.54	9.14	572	74.3	0.246	0.498	3.17	0.779	98.8	4.29	331	567	—	7.04	7.25
167	15.3	6.99	266	76.5	1.04	0.805	14.5	1.94	75.4	2.26	713	1015	—	9.85	5.83
49.2	4.75	6.36	162	9.41	0.346	0.496	7.95	0.382	50.5	2.92	304	491	—	2.32	3.42
—	—	—	—	—	—	—	—	—	—	—	—	—	—	—	—
71.9	2.25	2.43	288	33.9	0.223	0.425	3.47	0.574	30.6	0.299	417	398	—	3.59	2.75
9.52	0.056	0.195	23.5	0.448	0.03	0.113	0.064	0.028	2.52	0.224	114	87.9	—	0.168	0.08
14.3	1.34	0.643	110	4.24	0.12	0.175	1.21	0.085	12.2	0.17	74.5	92.3	—	1.01	1.14
41.7	14.4	1.46	87.1	15.8	0.511	0.365	16	0.478	45.3	0.462	101	259	—	2.3	5.29
8.2	0.5	0.659	21.5	1.08	0.022	0.077	1.79	0.134	5.96	0.141	12.8	57.5	—	0.214	2.89
53.2	6.3	4.12	146	18.9	0.158	0.258	4.81	0.232	41.3	1.46	55.2	228	—	6	2.11
45.6	1.02	0.509	0	13.8	0.237	0.038	4.36	0.316	38.9	0	25.5	125	—	4.62	0.33
21.6	2.47	2.22	7.3	1.43	0.226	0.198	3.82	0.135	24.9	0.998	62.6	110	—	1.32	0.641
24.7	1.16	0.493	0	1.68	0.082	0.039	0.177	0.087	71.1	0	24.6	72.3	—	3	0.566
14.3	0.535	0.865	21.4	3.3	0.021	0.026	0.619	0.045	7.76	0.481	24.7	73.7	—	0.222	1.48
43.7	4.31	4.27	136	10.9	0.403	0.423	6.52	0.302	55.1	1.8	234	348	—	2.69	3.8
39.5	4.29	3.69	75.6	11.1	0.402	0.353	6.6	0.292	54.2	1.68	105	193	—	2.73	3.64
8.92	0.692	0.196	23.9	9.2	0.046	0.017	0.586	0.057	3.6	0	15.3	17.4	—	0.744	0.36
166	9.23	13.6	1478	67.4	0.396	0.925	15.2	1.16	147	6.41	532	847	—	10.5	10.8
10.3	0.557	0.176	14.9	1.23	0.018	0.041	3.75	0.045	3.9	0.679	9.25	61.9	—	0.312	0.638

APPENDIX O

Water and Electrolyte Balance Problem

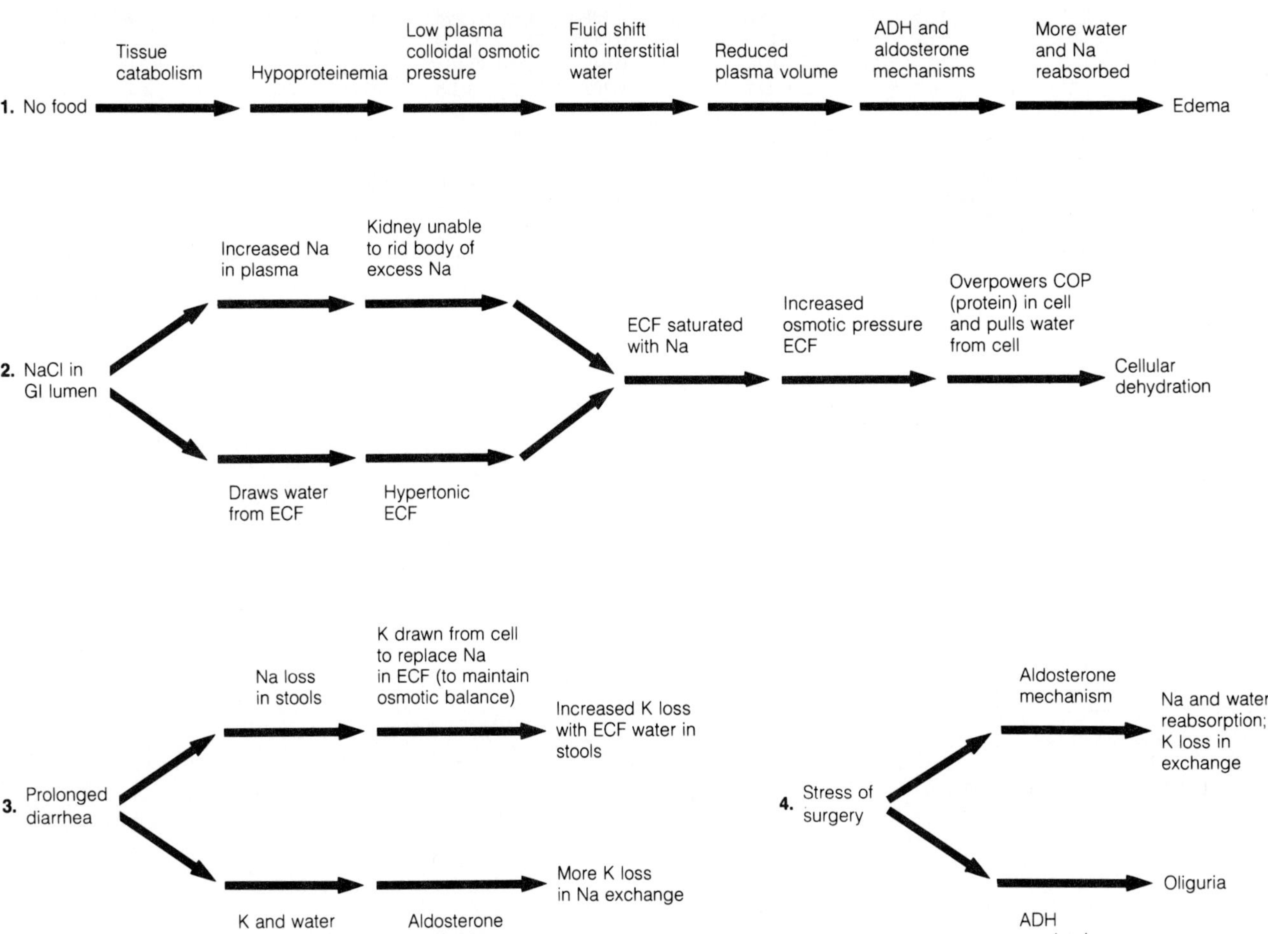

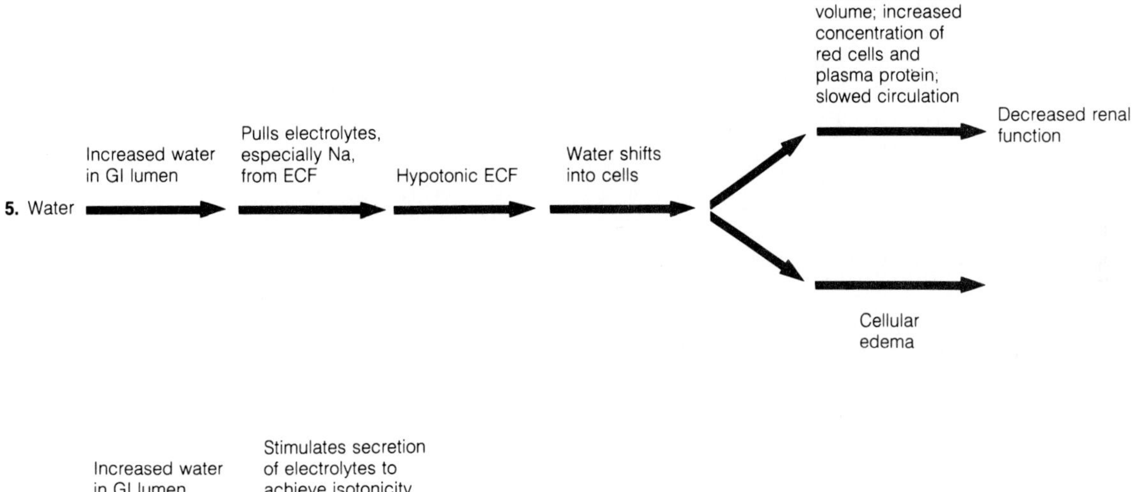

6. Water → Increased water in GI lumen → Stimulates secretion of electrolytes to achieve isotonicity → Water and electrolytes lost in suction

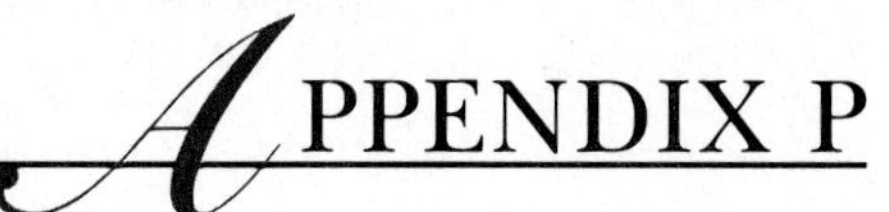

Appendix P

Physical Growth NCHS Percentiles

GIRLS: BIRTH TO 36 MONTHS
PHYSICAL GROWTH
NCHS PERCENTILES*

NAME ______________________ RECORD # __________

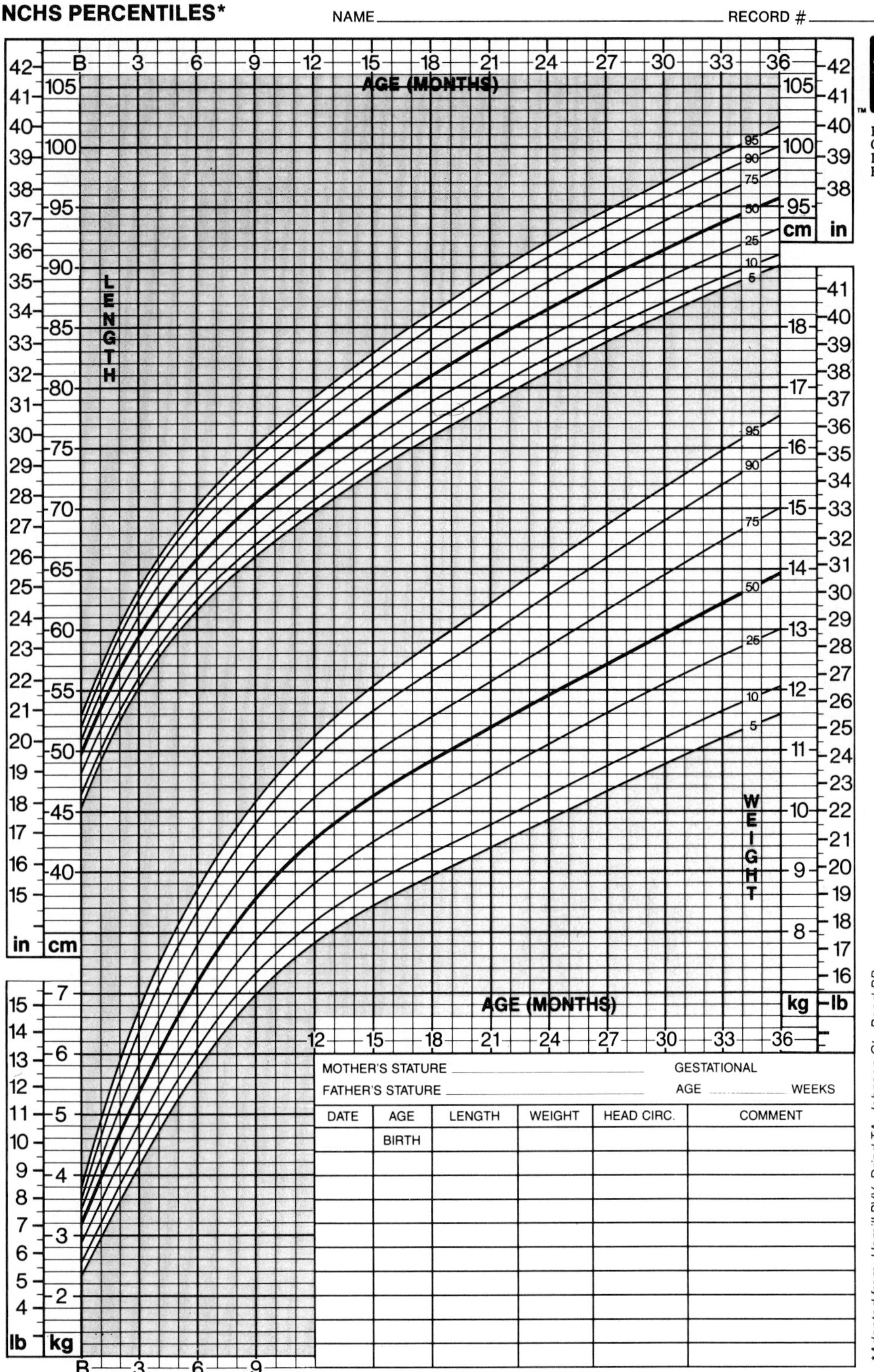

Ross Growth & Development Program

*Adapted from: Hamill PVV, Drizd TA, Johnson CL, Reed RB, Roche AF, Moore WM: Physical growth: National Center for Health Statistics percentiles. AM J CLIN NUTR 32:607-629, 1979. Data from the Fels Research Institute, Wright State University School of Medicine, Yellow Springs, Ohio.

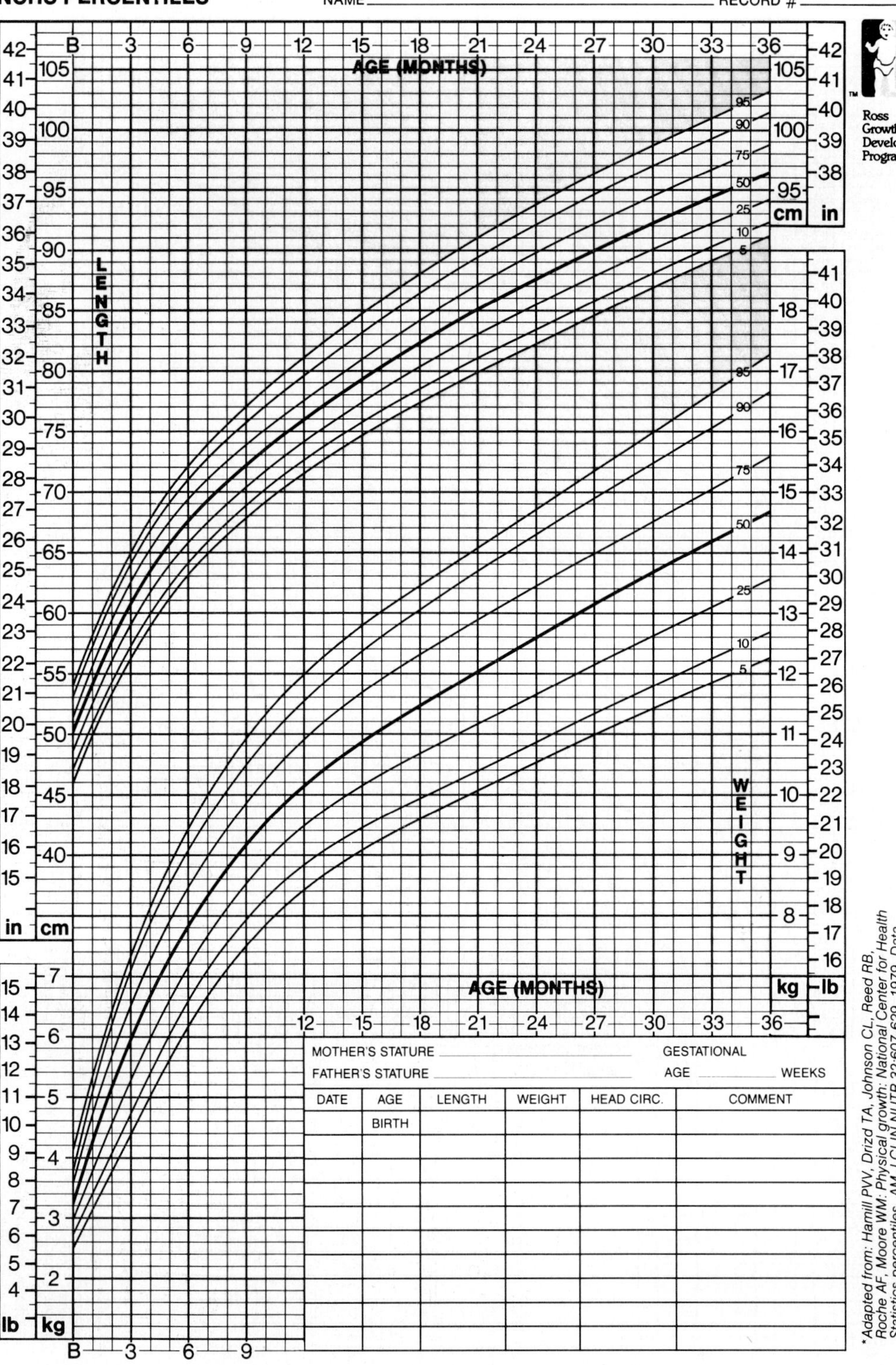

*Adapted from: Hamill PVV, Drizd TA, Johnson CL, Reed RB, Roche AF, Moore WM: Physical growth: National Center for Health Statistics percentiles. AM J CLIN NUTR 32:607-629, 1979. Data from the Fels Research Institute, Wright State University School of Medicine, Yellow Springs, Ohio.

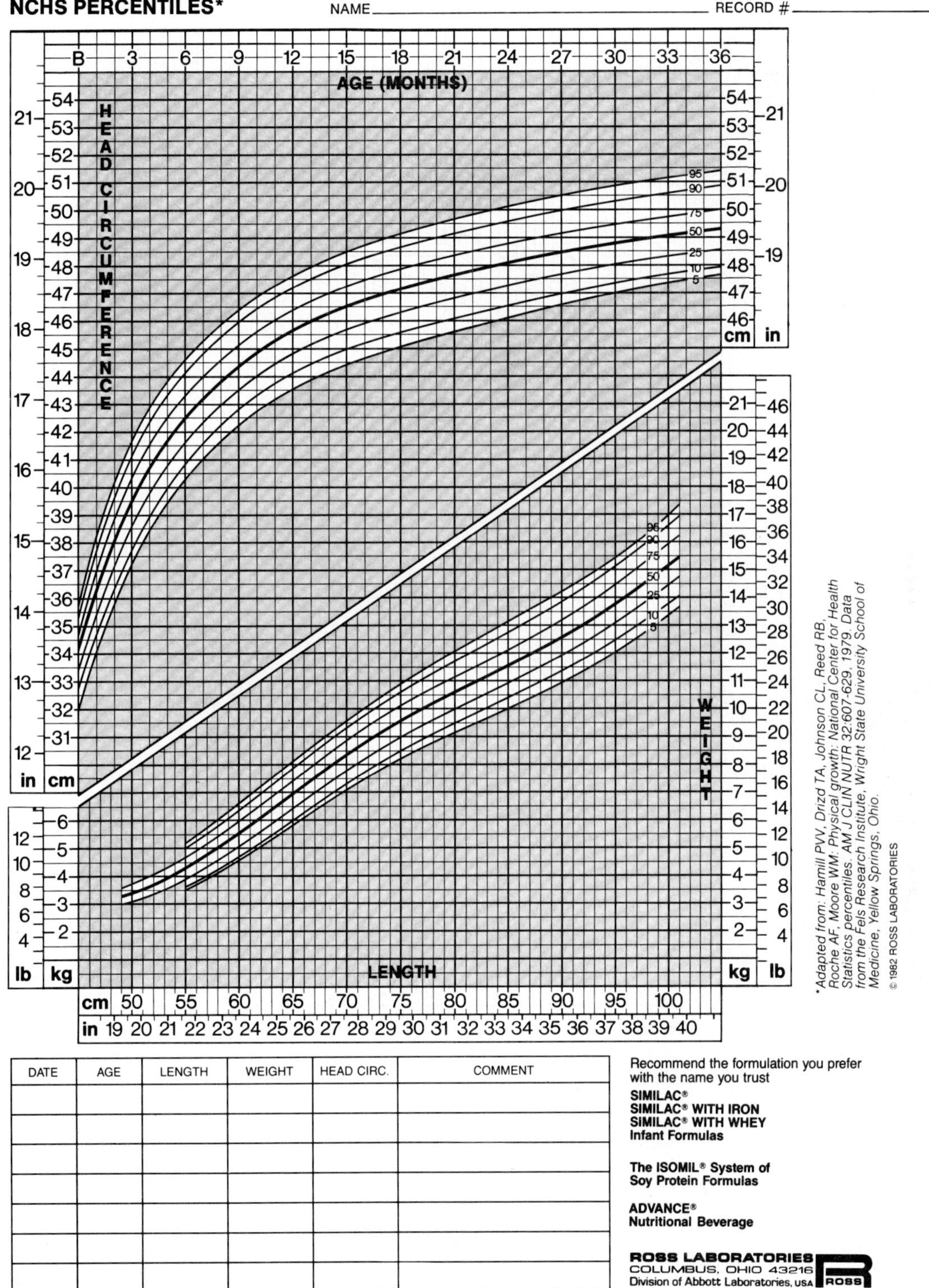
GIRLS: BIRTH TO 36 MONTHS
PHYSICAL GROWTH
NCHS PERCENTILES*
NAME
RECORD #
AGE (MONTHS)
B 3 6 9 12 15 18 21 24 27 30 33 36
HEAD CIRCUMFERENCE
WEIGHT
LENGTH
cm
in
kg
lb
95
90
75
50
25
10
5
cm 50 55 60 65 70 75 80 85 90 95 100
in 19 20 21 22 23 24 25 26 27 28 29 30 31 32 33 34 35 36 37 38 39 40
DATE
AGE
LENGTH
WEIGHT
HEAD CIRC.
COMMENT
*Adapted from: Hamill PVV, Drizd TA, Johnson CL, Reed RB, Roche AF, Moore WM: Physical growth: National Center for Health Statistics percentiles. AM J CLIN NUTR 32:607-629, 1979. Data from the Fels Research Institute, Wright State University School of Medicine, Yellow Springs, Ohio.
© 1982 ROSS LABORATORIES
Recommend the formulation you prefer with the name you trust
SIMILAC®
SIMILAC® WITH IRON
SIMILAC® WITH WHEY
Infant Formulas
The ISOMIL® System of Soy Protein Formulas
ADVANCE®
Nutritional Beverage
ROSS LABORATORIES
COLUMBUS, OHIO 43216
Division of Abbott Laboratories, USA
ROSS
G106/JUNE 1983
LITHO IN USA

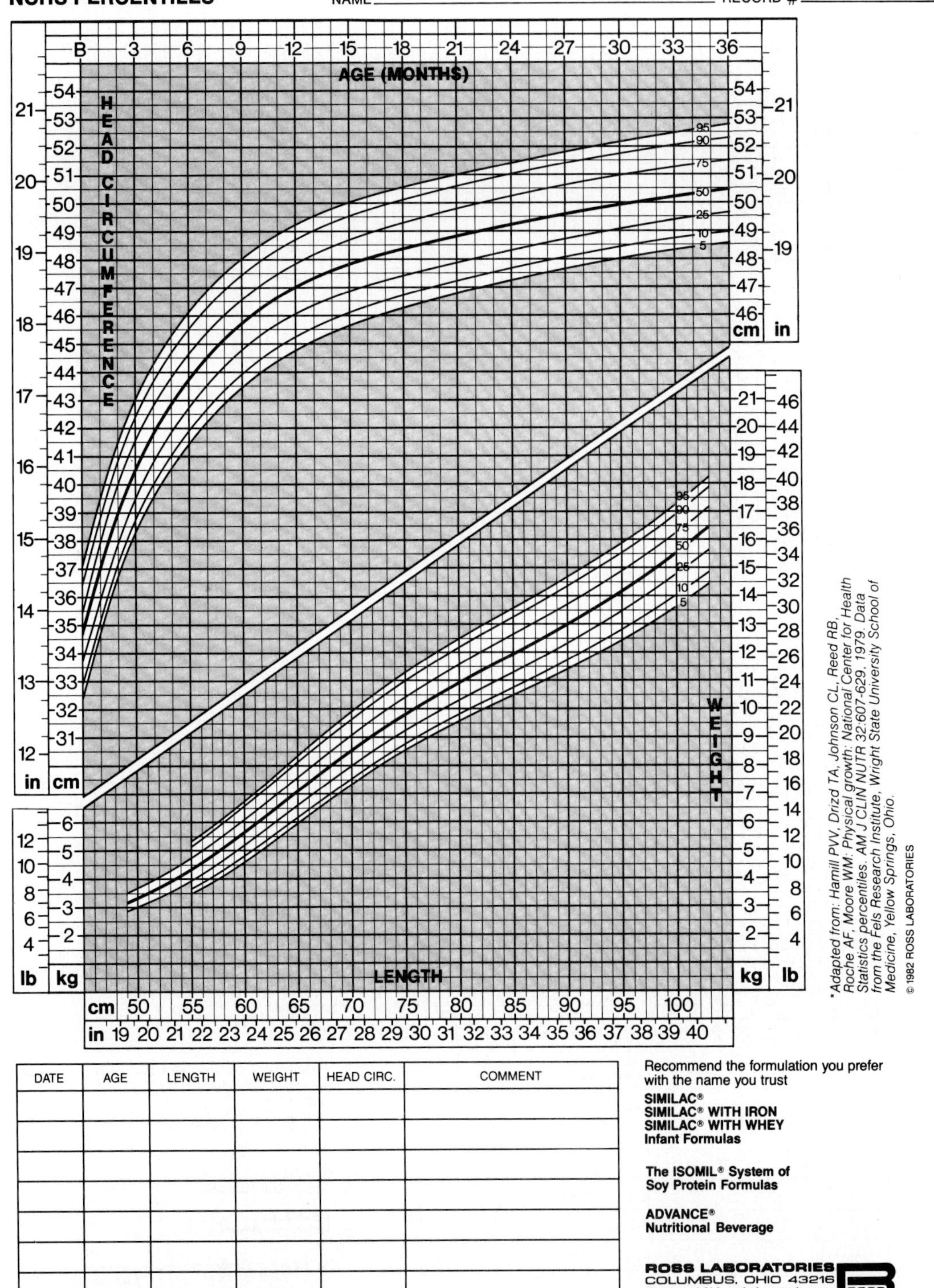

BOYS: BIRTH TO 36 MONTHS
PHYSICAL GROWTH
NCHS PERCENTILES*

NAME ______________ RECORD # ______________

*Adapted from: Hamill PVV, Drizd TA, Johnson CL, Reed RB, Roche AF, Moore WM: Physical growth: National Center for Health Statistics percentiles. AM J CLIN NUTR 32:607-629, 1979. Data from the Fels Research Institute, Wright State University School of Medicine, Yellow Springs, Ohio.

DATE	AGE	LENGTH	WEIGHT	HEAD CIRC.	COMMENT

GIRLS: 2 TO 18 YEARS
PHYSICAL GROWTH
NCHS PERCENTILES*

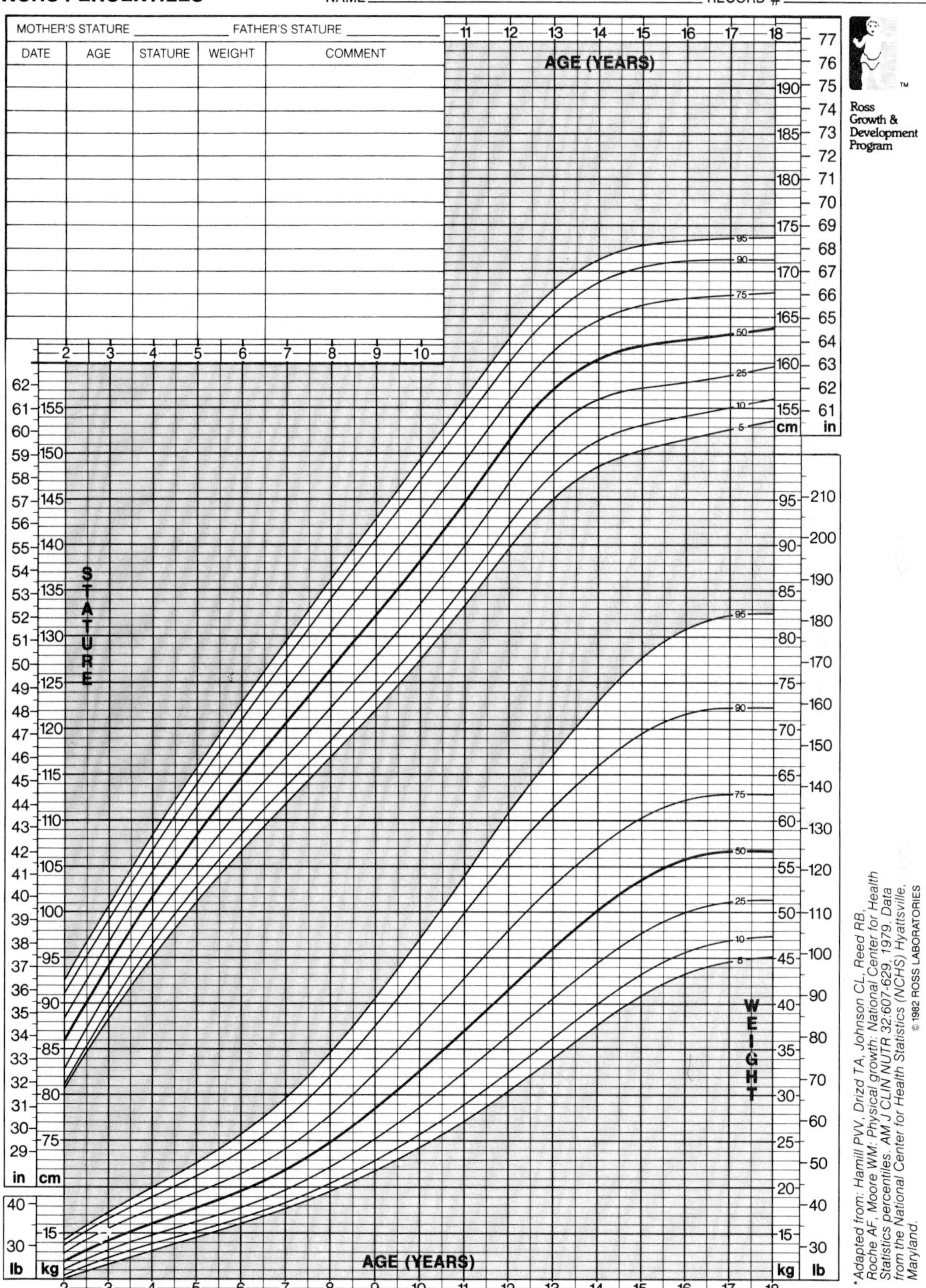

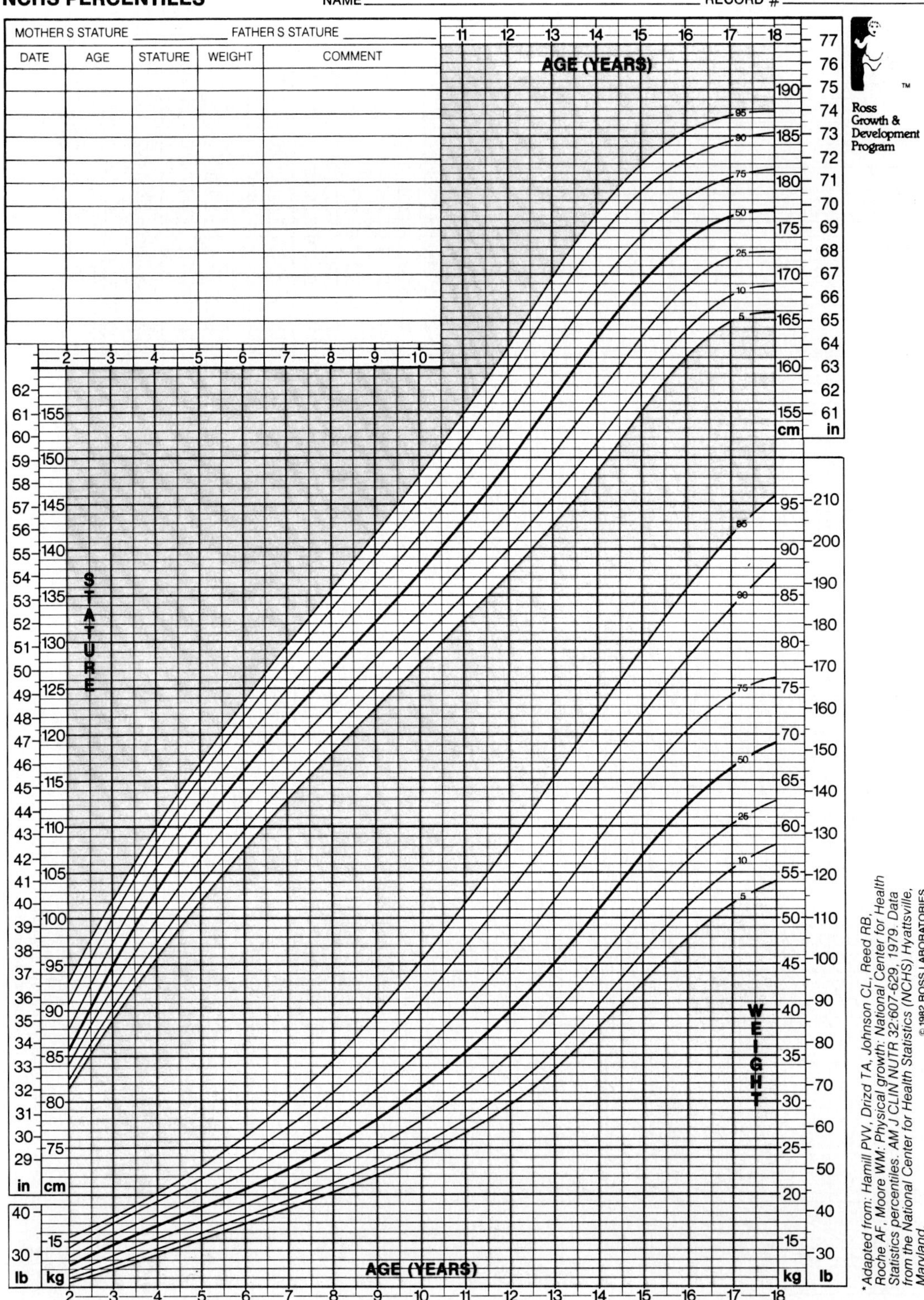

BOYS: 2 TO 18 YEARS
PHYSICAL GROWTH
NCHS PERCENTILES*
NAME
RECORD #
MOTHER'S STATURE
FATHER'S STATURE
DATE
AGE
STATURE
WEIGHT
COMMENT
AGE (YEARS)
STATURE
WEIGHT
in
cm
lb
kg
Ross Growth & Development Program
*Adapted from: Hamill PVV, Drizd TA, Johnson CL, Reed RB, Roche AF, Moore WM: Physical growth: National Center for Health Statistics percentiles. AM J CLIN NUTR 32:607-629, 1979. Data from the National Center for Health Statistics (NCHS) Hyattsville, Maryland.
© 1982 ROSS LABORATORIES

GIRLS: PREPUBESCENT PHYSICAL GROWTH NCHS PERCENTILES*

NAME ______________________ RECORD # ______________

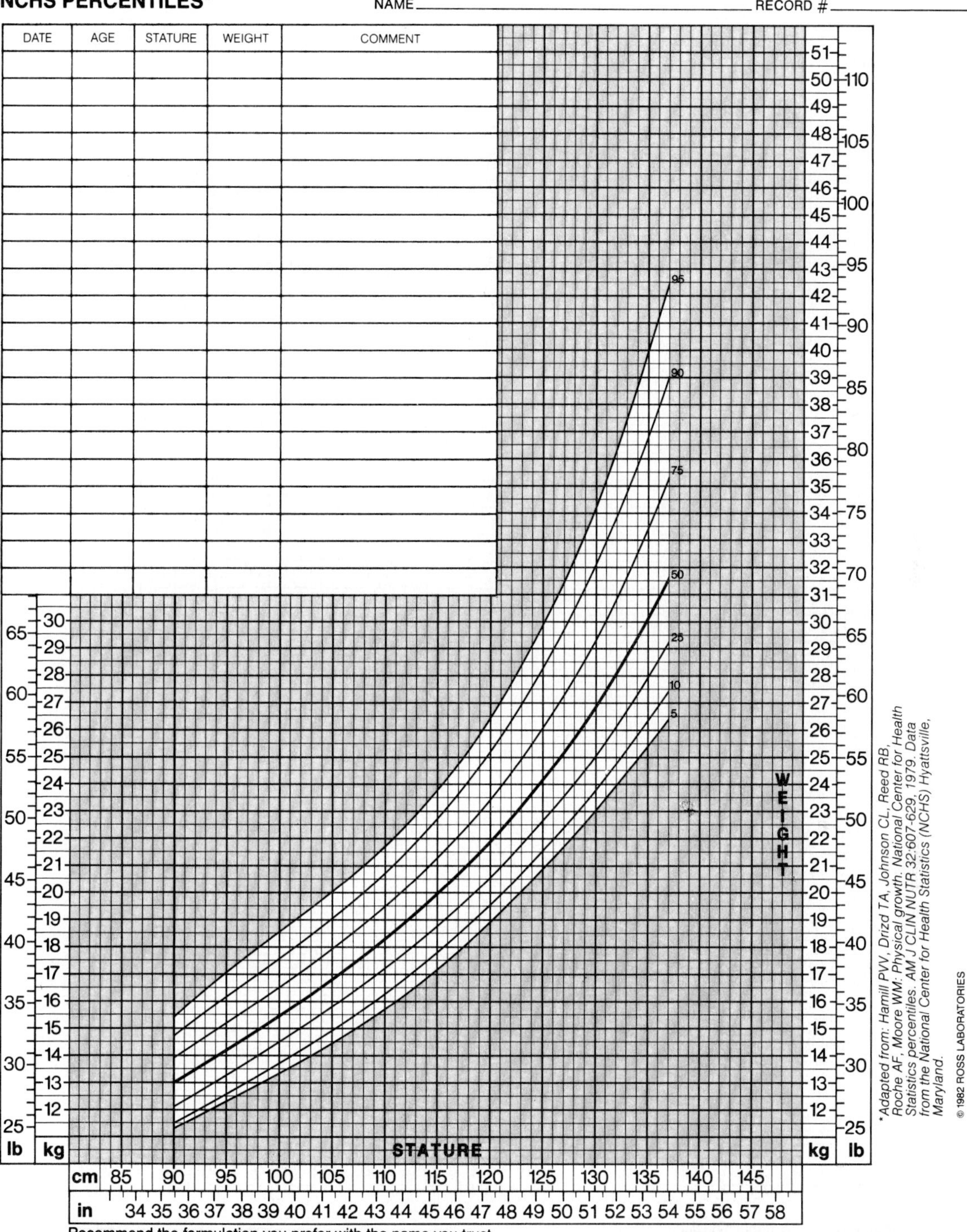

*Adapted from: Hamill PVV, Drizd TA, Johnson CL, Reed RB, Roche AF, Moore WM: Physical growth: National Center for Health Statistics percentiles. AM J CLIN NUTR 32:607-629, 1979. Data from the National Center for Health Statistics (NCHS) Hyattsville, Maryland.

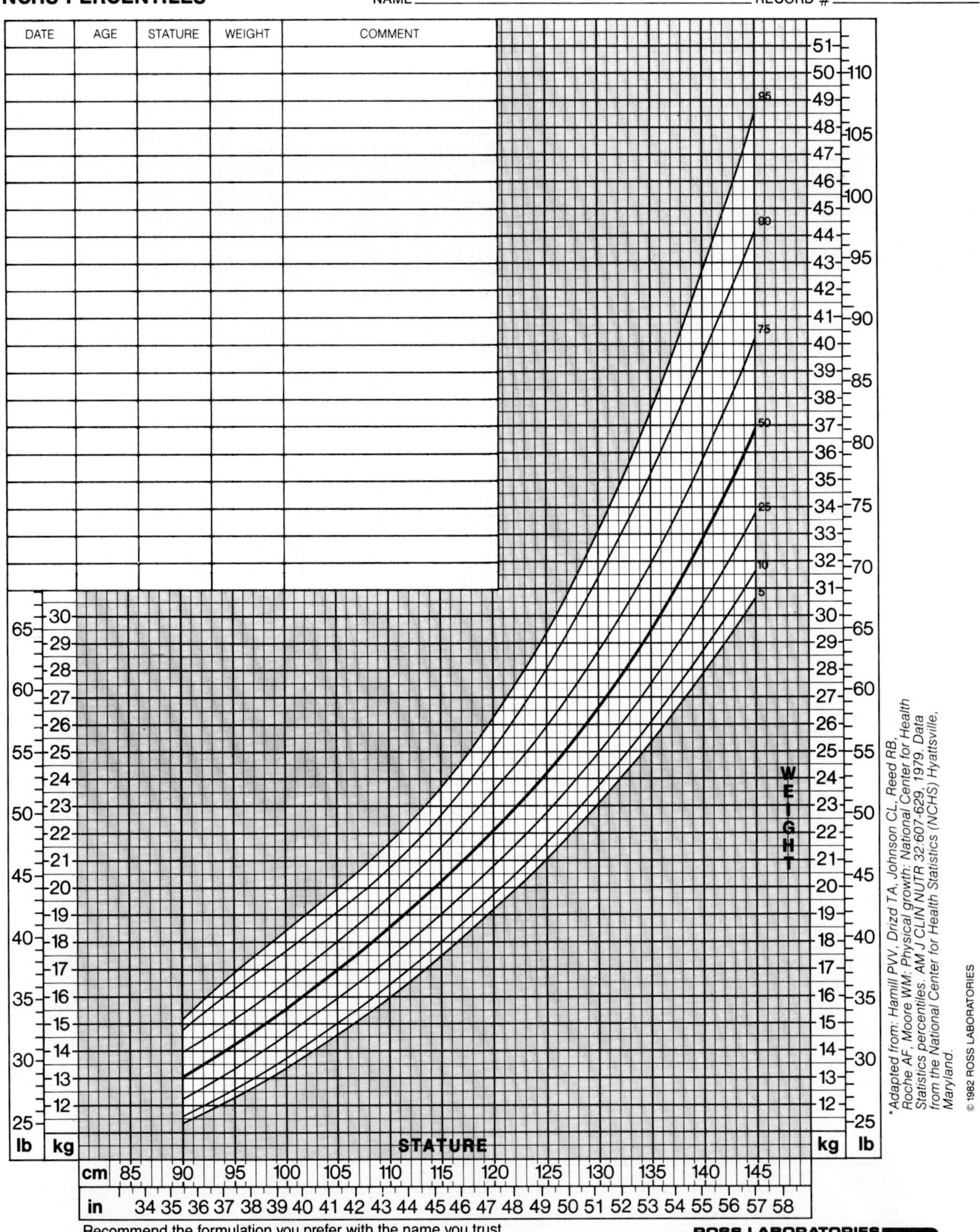
BOYS: PREPUBESCENT
PHYSICAL GROWTH
NCHS PERCENTILES*
NAME
RECORD #
DATE
AGE
STATURE
WEIGHT
COMMENT
95
90
75
50
25
10
5
WEIGHT
STATURE
lb
kg
cm
in
*Adapted from: Hamill PVV, Drizd TA, Johnson CL, Reed RB, Roche AF, Moore WM: Physical growth: National Center for Health Statistics percentiles. AM J CLIN NUTR 32:607-629, 1979. Data from the National Center for Health Statistics (NCHS) Hyattsville, Maryland.
© 1982 ROSS LABORATORIES
Recommend the formulation you prefer with the name you trust
SIMILAC®
SIMILAC® WITH IRON
SIMILAC® WITH WHEY
Infant Formulas
The ISOMIL® System of
Soy Protein Formulas
ADVANCE®
Nutritional Beverage
ROSS LABORATORIES
COLUMBUS, OHIO 43216
Division of Abbott Laboratories, USA
ROSS
G107/JUNE 1983
LITHO IN USA

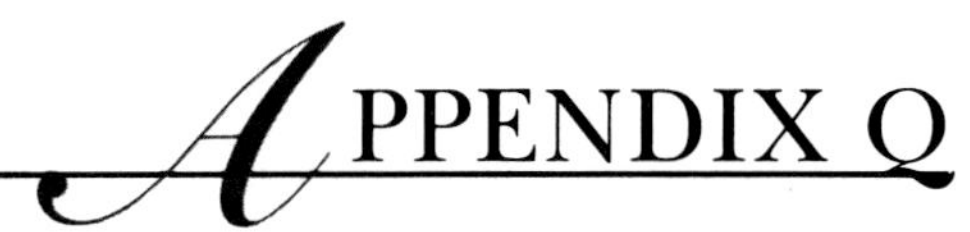

APPENDIX Q

Assessment of Nutritional Status: Percentiles

Mid–Upper-Arm Circumference Percentiles (cm)

	Female percentiles					Male percentiles				
Age (yr)	**5th**	**25th**	**50th**	**75th**	**95th**	**5th**	**25th**	**50th**	**75th**	**95th**
1	13.8	14.8	15.6	16.4	17.7	14.2	15.0	15.9	17.0	18.3
2	14.2	15.2	16.0	16.7	18.4	14.1	15.3	16.2	17.0	18.5
3	14.3	15.8	16.7	17.5	18.9	15.0	16.0	16.7	17.5	19.0
4	14.9	16.0	16.9	17.7	19.1	14.9	16.2	17.1	18.0	19.2
5	15.3	16.5	17.5	18.5	21.1	15.3	16.7	17.5	18.5	20.4
6	15.6	17.0	17.6	18.7	21.1	15.5	16.7	17.9	18.8	22.8
7	16.4	17.4	18.3	19.9	23.1	16.2	17.7	18.7	20.1	23.0
8	16.8	18.3	19.5	21.4	26.1	16.2	17.7	19.0	20.2	24.5
9	17.8	19.4	21.1	22.4	26.0	17.5	18.7	20.0	21.7	25.7
10	17.4	19.3	21.0	22.8	26.5	18.1	19.6	21.0	23.1	27.4
11	18.5	20.8	22.4	24.8	30.3	18.6	20.2	22.3	24.4	28.0
12	19.4	21.6	23.7	25.6	29.4	19.3	21.4	23.2	25.4	30.3
13	20.2	22.3	24.3	27.1	33.8	19.4	22.8	24.7	26.3	30.1
14	21.4	23.7	25.2	27.2	32.2	22.0	23.7	25.3	28.3	32.3
15	20.8	23.9	25.4	27.9	32.2	22.2	24.4	26.4	28.4	32.0
16	21.8	24.1	25.8	28.3	33.4	24.4	26.2	27.8	30.3	34.3
17	22.0	24.1	26.4	29.5	35.0	24.6	26.7	28.5	30.8	34.7
18	22.2	24.1	25.8	28.1	32.5	24.5	27.6	29.7	32.1	37.9
19-25	21.1	24.7	26.5	29.0	34.5	26.2	28.8	30.8	33.1	37.2
25-35	23.3	25.6	27.7	30.4	36.8	27.1	30.0	31.9	34.2	37.5
35-45	24.1	26.7	29.0	31.7	37.8	27.8	30.5	32.6	34.5	37.4
45-55	24.2	27.4	29.9	32.8	38.4	26.7	30.1	32.2	34.2	37.6
55-65	24.3	28.0	30.3	33.5	38.5	25.8	29.6	31.7	33.6	36.9
65-75	24.0	27.4	29.9	32.6	37.3	24.8	28.5	30.7	32.5	35.5

Data derived from the Health and Nutrition Examination Survey data of 1971-1974, using same population samples as those of the National Center for Health Statistics (NCHS) growth percentiles for children. Adapted from Frisancho, AR: New norms of upper limb fat and muscle areas for assessment of nutritional status, *Am J Clin Nutr* 34:2540, 1981.

Triceps Skinfold Percentiles (mm)

	Female percentiles					Male percentiles				
Age (yr)	5th	25th	50th	75th	95th	5th	25th	50th	75th	95th
1	6	8	10	12	16	6	8	10	12	16
2	6	9	10	12	16	6	8	10	12	15
3	7	9	11	12	15	6	8	10	11	15
4	7	8	10	12	16	6	8	9	11	14
5	6	8	10	12	18	6	8	9	11	15
6	6	8	10	12	16	5	7	8	10	16
7	6	9	11	13	18	5	7	9	12	17
8	6	9	12	15	24	5	7	8	10	16
9	8	10	13	16	22	6	7	10	13	18
10	7	10	12	17	27	6	8	10	14	21
11	7	10	13	18	28	6	8	11	16	24
12	8	11	14	18	27	6	8	11	14	28
13	8	12	15	21	30	5	7	10	14	26
14	9	13	16	21	28	4	7	9	14	24
15	8	12	17	21	32	4	6	8	11	24
16	10	15	18	22	31	4	6	8	12	22
17	10	13	19	24	37	5	6	8	12	19
18	10	15	18	22	30	4	6	9	13	24
19-25	10	14	18	24	34	4	7	10	15	22
25-35	10	16	21	27	37	5	8	12	16	24
35-45	12	18	23	29	38	5	8	12	16	23
45-55	12	20	25	30	40	6	8	12	15	25
55-65	12	20	25	31	38	5	8	11	14	22
65-75	12	18	24	29	36	4	8	11	15	22

Data derived from the Health and Nutrition Examination Survey data of 1971-1974, using same population samples as those of the National Center for Health Statistics (NCHS) growth percentiles for children. Adapted from Frisancho, AR: New norms of upper limb fat and muscle areas for assessment of nutritional status, *Am J Clin Nutr* 34:2540, 1981.

Mid–Upper-Arm Muscle Circumference Percentiles (cm)

	Female percentiles					Male percentiles				
Age (yr)	5th	25th	50th	75th	95th	5th	25th	50th	75th	95th
1	10.5	11.7	12.4	13.9	14.3	11.0	11.9	12.7	13.5	14.7
2	11.1	11.9	12.6	13.3	14.7	11.1	12.2	13.0	14.0	15.0
3	11.3	12.4	13.2	14.0	15.2	11.7	13.1	13.7	14.3	15.3
4	11.5	12.8	13.8	14.4	15.7	12.3	13.3	14.1	14.8	15.9
5	12.5	13.4	14.2	15.1	16.5	12.8	14.0	14.7	15.4	16.9
6	13.0	13.8	14.5	15.4	17.1	13.1	14.2	15.1	16.1	17.7
7	12.9	14.2	15.1	16.0	17.6	13.7	15.1	16.0	16.8	19.0
8	13.8	15.1	16.0	17.1	19.4	14.0	15.4	16.2	17.0	18.7
9	14.7	15.8	16.7	18.0	19.8	15.1	16.1	17.0	18.3	20.2
10	14.8	15.9	17.0	18.0	19.7	15.6	16.6	18.0	19.1	22.1
11	15.0	17.1	18.1	19.6	22.3	15.9	17.3	18.3	19.5	23.0
12	16.2	18.0	19.1	20.1	22.0	16.7	18.2	19.5	21.0	24.1
13	16.9	18.3	19.8	21.1	24.0	17.2	19.6	21.1	22.6	24.5
14	17.4	19.0	20.1	21.6	24.7	18.9	21.2	22.3	24.0	26.4
15	17.5	18.9	20.2	21.5	24.4	19.9	21.8	23.7	25.4	27.2
16	17.0	19.0	20.2	21.6	24.9	21.3	23.4	24.9	26.9	29.6
17	17.5	19.4	20.5	22.1	25.7	22.4	24.5	25.8	27.3	31.2
18	17.4	19.1	20.2	21.5	24.5	22.6	25.2	26.4	28.3	32.4
19-25	17.9	19.5	20.7	22.1	24.9	23.8	25.7	27.3	28.9	32.1
25-35	18.3	19.9	21.2	22.8	26.4	24.3	26.4	27.9	29.8	32.6
35-45	18.6	20.5	21.8	23.6	27.2	24.7	26.9	28.6	30.2	32.7
45-55	18.7	20.6	22.0	23.8	27.4	23.9	26.5	28.1	30.0	32.6
55-65	18.7	20.9	22.5	24.4	28.0	23.6	26.0	27.8	29.5	32.0
65-75	18.5	20.8	22.5	24.4	27.9	22.3	25.1	26.8	28.4	30.6

Values derived by formula calculation (see p. 461). Data derived from the Health and Nutrition Examination Survey data of 1971-1974, using same population samples as those of the National Center for Health Statistics (NCHS) growth percentiles for children. Adapted from Frisancho, AR: New norms of upper limb fat and muscle areas for assessment of nutritional status, *Am J Clin Nutr* 34:2540, 1981.

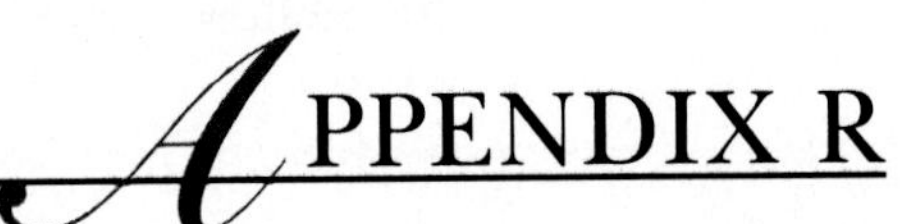

APPENDIX R

Normal Constituents of Blood and Urine in Adults

Normal Constituents of the Blood in the Adult

Physical measurements

Specific gravity		1.025-1.029
Viscosity (water as unity)		4.5
Bleeding time (capillary)	Minutes	1-3
Prothrombin time (plasma) (Quick)	Seconds	10-20
Sedimentation rate (Wintrobe method)		
Men	mm/hr	0-9
Women	mm/hr	0-20

Hemologic studies

Cell volume	%	39-50
Red blood cells	Million per mm^3	4.25-5.25
White blood cells	Per mm^3	5000-9000
Lymphocytes	%	25-30
Neutrophils	%	60-65
Monocytes	%	4-8
Eosinophils	%	0.5-4
Basophils	%	0-1.5
Platelets	Per mm^3	125,000-300,000

Proteins

Total protein (serum)	g/dl	6.5-7.5
Albumin (serum)	g/dl	4.5-5.5
Globulin (serum)	g/dl	1.5-2.5
Albumin: globulin ratio		1.8-2.5
Fibrinogen (plasma)	g/dl	0.2-0.5
Hemoglobin		
Males	g/dl	14-17
Females	g/dl	13-16

Nitrogen constituents

Nonprotein N (serum	mg/dl	20-36
(whole blood)	mg/dl	25-40
Urea (whole blood)	mg/dl	18-38
Urea N (whole blood)	mg/dl	8-18
Creatinine (whole blood)	mg/dl	1-2
Uric acid (whole blood)	mg/dl	2.5-5.0
Amino acid N (whole blood)	mg/dl	3-6

Carbohydrates and lipids

Glucose (whole blood)	mg/dl	70-90
Ketones—as acetone (whole blood)	mg/dl	1.5-2
Fats (total lipids) (serum)	mg/dl	570-820
Cholesterol (serum)	mg/dl	100-230
Bilirubin (serum)	mg/dl	0.1-0.25
Icteric index (serum)	units	4-6

Blood gases

CO_2 content (serum)	vol %	55-75
	mmol/L	(24.5-33.5)
CO_2 content (whole blood)	vol %	40-60
	mmol/L	(18.0-27.0)
Oxygen capacity (whole blood)		
Males	vol %	18.7-22.7
Females	vol %	17.0-21.0
Oxygen saturation		
Arterial blood	%	94-96
Venous blood	%	60-85

Acid-base constituents

Base, total fixed (serum)	mEq/L	142-150
Sodium (serum)	mg/dl	320-335
	mEq/L	(139-146)
Potassium (serum)	mg/dl	16-22
	mEq/L	(4.1-5.6)
Calcium (serum)	mg/dl	9.0-11.5
	mEq/L	(4.5-5.8)
Magnesium (serum)	mg/dl	1.0-3.0
	mEq/L	(1.0-2.5)
Phosphorus, inorganic (serum)	mg/dl	3.0-5.0
	mEq/L	(1.0-1.6)
Chlorides, expressed as Cl (serum)	mg/dl	352-383
	mEq/L	(99-108)
As NaCl (serum)	mg/dl	580-630
	mEq/L	(99-108)
Sulfates, inorganic as SO_4 (serum)	mg/dl	2.5-5.0
	mEq/L	(0.5-1.0)
Lactic acid (venous blood)	mg/dl	10-20
	mEq/L	(1.1-2.2)

Abbreviations and conversion factors:
dl = deciliter
ml = milliliter
µg = microgram

$$\text{mEq/L} = \frac{\text{mg/L}}{\text{Equivalent weight}}$$

$$\text{Equivalent weight} = \frac{\text{Atomic weight}}{\text{Valence of element}}$$

g = gram
mm^3 = cubic millimeter
mEq = milliequivalent

$$\text{mmol (millimole)/L} = \frac{\text{mg/L}}{\text{Molecular weight}}$$

vol % (volumes percent) = mmol/L × 2.24

Normal Constituents of the Blood in the Adult—cont'd

Acid-base constituents—cont'd

Serum protein base binding power	mEq/L	(15.5-18.0)
Base bicarbonate HCO_3 (serum)	mEq/L	(19-30)
pH (blood or plasma at 38° C)		7.3-7.45

Miscellaneous

Phosphatase (serum)	Bodansky units per deciliter	5
Iron (whole blood)	mg/dl	46-55
Ascorbic acid (whole blood)	mg/dl	0.75-1.50
Carotene (serum)	μg/dl	75-125

Normal Constituents of the Urine in the Adult

Urine constituents	**g/24 hr**
Total solids	55-70
Nitrogenous constituents	
Total nitrogen	10-17
Ammonia	0.5-1.0
Amino acid N	0.4-1
Creatine	None
Creatinine	1-1.5
Protein	None
Purine bases	0.016-0.060
Urea	20-35
Uric acid	0.5-0.7
Acetone bodies	0.003-0.015
Bile	None
Calcium	0.2-0.4
Chloride (as NaCl)	10-15
Glucose	None
Indican	0-0.030
Iron	0.001-0.005
Magnesium (as MgO)	0.15-0.30
Phosphate, total (as phosphoric acid)	2.5-3.5
Potassium (as K_2O)	2.0-3.0
Sodium (as Na_2O)	4.0-5.0
Sulfates, total (as sulfuric acid)	1.5-3.0
Physical measurements	
Specific gravity	1.010-1.025
Reaction (pH)	5.5-8.0
Volume (ml/24 hr)	800-1600

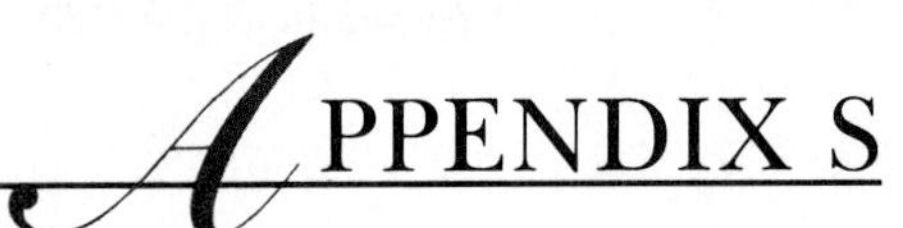

Appendix S

Exchange Lists for Meal Planning

Milk Exchange List

Skim milk (12 g carbohydrate, 8 g protein, 0 g fat, 90 kcal)

1 cup	Skin or nonfat milk (½% and 1%)
⅓ cup	Powdered (nonfat dry, before adding liquid)
½ cup	Canned, evaporated skim milk
1 cup	Buttermilk made from skim milk
1 cup	Yogurt made from skim milk (plain, unflavored)

Low-fat milk (12 g carbohydrate, 8 g protein, 5 g fat, 120 kcal)

1 cup	2% fat milk
1 cup	Plain nonfat yogurt (added milk solids)

Whole milk (12 g carbohydrate, 8 g protein, 8 g fat, 150 kcal)

1 cup	Whole milk
1 cup	Custard-style yogurt made from whole milk (plain, unflavored)

Vegetable Exchange List

(5 g carbohydrate, 2 g protein, 0 g fat, 25 kcal). 1 exchange equals ½ cup cooked vegetables or vegetable juice and 1 cup raw vegetables

Artichoke (½ medium)	Mushrooms (cooked)
Asparagus	Onions
Beans (green, wax, Italian)	Pea pods
Bean sprouts	Sauerkraut
Beets	Spinach (cooked)
Broccoli	Squash, summer, zucchini
Brussels sprouts	String beans (green, yellow)
Cabbage, cooked	Tomato
Carrots	Tomato juice
Cauliflower	Turnips
Eggplant	Vegetable juice
Green pepper	Zucchini (cooked)
Greens	

Fruit Exchange List

(15 g carbohydrate, 0 g protein, 0 g fat, 60 kcal). 1 fruit exchange equals:

1	Apple (2 in diameter)
4 rings	Dried apple
½ cup	Apple juice
½ cup	Applesauce (unsweetened)
½ cup	Apricots, canned
7 halves	Apricots, dried
4	Apricots, fresh
½	Banana, 9 in
¾ cup	Blackberries
¾ cup	Blueberries
1 cup	Raspberries
1¼ cup	Strawberries
⅓ melon	Cantaloupe (5 in diameter)
½ cup	Cherries, canned
12	Cherries (large, raw)
½ cup	Cider
⅓ cup	Cranberry juice cocktail
2½ medium	Dates
1½	Figs, dried
2	Figs, fresh (2 in diameter)
⅓ cup	Grape juice
½	Grapefruit
½ cup	Grapefruit juice
15	Grapes
⅛ melon	Honeydew melon (7 in diameter; cubes = 1 cup)
1	Kiwi (large)
¾ cup	Mandarin oranges
½ small	Mango
1 small	Nectarine (1½ in diameter)
1 small	Orange (2½ in diameter)
½ cup	Orange juice
½ cup or 2 halves	Peach, canned
1 medium or ¾ cup	Peach, fresh (2¾ in diameter)
½ cup or 2 halves	Pear, canned
1 small or ½ large	Pear, fresh
⅓ cup	Pineapple, canned
¾ cup	Pineapple, raw
½ cup	Pineapple juice
2	Plums (2 in diameter)
⅓ cup	Prune juice
3	Prunes, dried
2 tbsp	Raisins
2	Tangerine (2½ in diameter)
1¼ cups	Watermelon (cubes)

Starch/Bread Exchange List

(15 g carbohydrate, 3 g protein, 0 g fat, 80 kcal) 1 starch/bread exchange equals:

Bread

½ (1 oz)	Bagel, small
2 (⅔ oz)	Bread sticks (crisp, 4 in long, ½ in wide)
3 tbsp	Dried bread crumbs
½	English muffin
½ (1 oz)	Frankfurter bun
½ (1 oz)	Hamburger bun
½	Pita (6 in diameter)
1 (small)	Plain roll
1 slice	Raisin (unfrosted)
1 slice	Rye or pumpernickel
1	Tortilla (6 in diameter)
1 slice	White (including French and Italian)
1 slice	Whole wheat

Cereal/Grains/Pasta

½ cup	Bran flakes
½ cup	Cereal (cooked)
2½ tbsp	Cornmeal (dry)
2½ tbsp	Flour (dry)
3 tbsp	Grapenuts
¾ cup	Other ready-to-eat unsweetened cereal
½ cup	Pasta (cooked spaghetti, noodles, macaroni)
1½ cups	Puffed cereal (unfrosted)
⅓ cup	Rice or barley (cooked)
½ cup	Shredded wheat
3 tbsp	Wheat germ

Crackers/Snacks

8	Animal
3	Graham (2½-in square)
¾ oz	Matzoth(s) (4 × 6 in)
5 slices	Melba toast
24	Oyster
3 cups	Popcorn (popped with no added fat)
¾ oz	Pretzels
4	Rye crisp (2 × 3½ in)
6	Saltines

Dried Beans/Peas/Lentils

¼ cup	Baked beans
⅓ cup	Dried beans, such as kidney, white, split, blackeye (cooked)
⅓ cup	Lentils (cooked)

Starchy Vegetables

½ cup	Corn
1	Corn on the cob (6 inches)
½ cup	Lima beans
½ cup	Peas, green (canned or frozen)
½ cup	Potato, mashed
1 small	Potato, white (3 ounces baked)
1 cup	Winter squash, acorn or butternut
⅓ cup	Yam or sweet potato

Starch Group (with Fat)

1 starch/bread exchange
1 fat exchange

1	Biscuit (2½ in across)
1 (2 oz)	Corn bread (2-in cube)
6	Cracker, round butter type
10 (1½ oz)	French fries (2-3½ in)
1	Muffin, plain, small
2	Pancake (4 in diameter)
¼ cup	Stuffing, bread (prepared)
2	Taco shell (6 in across)
1	Waffle (4½ in square)
4-6 (1 oz)	Whole-wheat crackers (such as Triscuits)

Meat Exchange List

Lean (0 g carbohydrate, 7 g protein, 3 g fat, 55 kcal)

Beef	1 oz	Baby beef (lean), chipped beef, chuck, flank steak, tenderloin, plate ribs, round (bottom, top), all cuts rump, spare ribs, tripe
Cheese	1 oz	Cottage, farmer's, or pot (low-fat), grated parmesan
Fish	2 oz	Fresh or frozen, any type canned salmon, tuna, mackerel, crab, or lobster
Pork	1 oz	Leg (whole rump, center shank), ham (center slices), USDA good or choice grades such as round, sirloin, flank, and tenderloin
Poultry	1 oz	Chicken, turkey, Cornish hen (without skin)
Veal	1 oz	Leg, loin, rib, shank, shoulder, chops, roasts, all cuts except cutlets (ground or cubed)

Medium Fat (0 g carbohydrate, 7 g protein, 5 g fat, 75 kcal)

Beef	1 oz	All ground beef, roast (rib, chuck, rump), steak (cubed, porterhouse, T-bone), meat loaf
Cheese	¼ cup or 1 oz	Cottage (creamed), mozzarella (made with skim milk), ricotta, Neufchatel
Egg	1	Egg
Fish	¼ cup	Tuna (canned in oil); salmon (canned)
Lamb	1 oz	Leg, rib, sirloin, loin (roast and chops), shank, shoulder
Organ meat	1 oz	All types
Other	4 oz	Tofu
Pork	1 oz	Loin (all cuts tenderloin), chops, roast, Boston butt, cutlets

Poultry	1 oz	Capon, duck (domestic), goose, ground turkey, chicken with skin
Veal	1 oz	Cutlets

High Fat (0 g carbohydrate, 7 g protein, 8 g fat, 100 kcal)

Beef	1 oz	Brisket, corned beef (commercial), chuck (ground commercial), roasts (rib), steaks (club and rib); most USDA prime cuts of beef
Cheese	1 oz	All regular cheeses (American, blue, brick, Camembert, cheddar, Gouda, Limburger, Muenster, Swiss, Monterey), all processed cheeses
Cold cuts	1 oz	Bologna, salami, pimento loaf
Frankfurter	1 oz	Turkey, chicken
Lamb	1 oz	Patties (ground lamb)
Peanut butter	1 tbsp	
Pork	1 oz	Spare ribs, loin (back ribs), pork (ground), country-style ham, deviled ham, pork sausage
Sausage	1 oz	Polish, Italian

Fat Exchange List

(0 g carbohydrate, 0 g protein, 5 g fat, 45 kcal)

⅛ medium	Avocado
1 strip	Bacon, crisp
1 tsp	Butter, margarine
1 tbsp	Cream, heavy
2 tbsp	Cream, light
2 tbsp	Cream, sour
1 tbsp	Cream cheese
Dressing	
2 tsp	All varieties
	Mayonnaise type
1 tbsp	Gravy, meat
1 tbsp	Reduced kcalorie
Olives	10 small or 5 large
Nuts	
6	Almonds, whole, dry roasted
1 tbsp	Cashews, dry roasted
1 tbsp	Other
20 small or 10 large	Peanuts, Spanish, whole
10	Peanuts, Virginia, whole
2 large	Pecans, whole
2 tsp	Pumpkin seeds
1 tbsp	Seeds (pine, sunflower)
2 whole	Walnuts
Oil	
1 tsp	Corn, cottonseed, safflower, soy, sunflower, olive, peanut, canola

Free Foods

A free food is any food or drink that contains less than 20 kcal per serving. You can eat as much as you want of those items that have no serving size specified. You may eat two or three servings per day of those items that have a specific serving size. Be sure to spread them out through the day.

Drinks

Bouillon or broth without fat
Bouillon, low-sodium
Carbonated drinks, sugar-free
Carbonated water
Club soda
Cocoa powder, unsweetened (1 tbsp)
Coffee/tea
Drink mixes, sugar-free
Tonic water, sugar-free

Nonstick pan spray

Fruit

Cranberries, unsweetened (½ cup)
Rhubarb, unsweetened (½ cup)

Vegetables

(raw, 1 cup)
Cabbage
Celery
Chinese cabbage
Cucumber
Green onion
Hot peppers
Mushrooms (fresh)
Radishes
Zucchini

Salad greens

Endive
Escarole
Lettuce
Romaine
Spinach

Sweet substitutes

Candy, hard, sugar-free
Gelatin, sugar-free
Gum, sugar-free
Jam/jelly, sugar-free (2 tsp)
Pancake syrup, sugar-free (1-2 tbsp)
Sugar substitutes (saccharin, aspartame)
Whipped topping (2 tbsp)

Condiments

Catsup (1 tbsp)
Horseradish
Mustard
Pickles, dill, unsweetened
Salad dressing, low-kcalorie (2 tbsp)
Taco sauce (3 tbsp)
Vinegar

Seasonings

Basil (fresh)
Celery seeds
Cinnamon
Chili powder
Chives
Curry
Dill
Flavoring extracts (vanilla, almond, walnut, peppermint, butter, lemon, etc.)
Garlic
Garlic powder
Herbs
Hot pepper sauce
Lemon
Lemon juice
Lemon pepper
Lime
Lime juice
Mint
Onion powder
Oregano
Paprika
Pepper
Pimento
Soy sauce
Soy sauce, low-sodium (lite)
Spices
Wine, used in cooking (¼ cup)
Worcestershire sauce

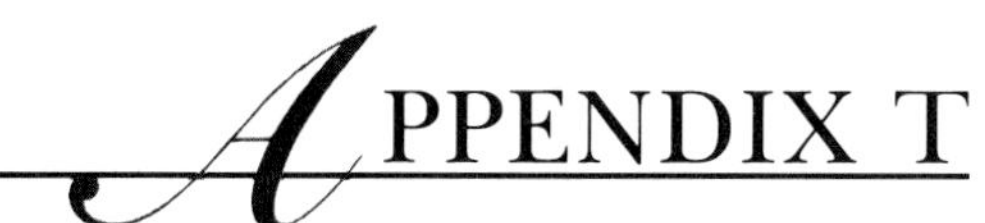

APPENDIX T

Dietary Guidelines for Americans

Eat a Variety of Foods

About 40 different known nutrients, and probably more as yet unknown factors, are needed to maintain health. No single food can supply all the essential nutrients in the amounts needed to maintain health. Thus the greater the variety of foods used, the less likely a person is to develop either a deficiency or an excess of any single nutrient. One way to ensure a varied balanced diet is to select foods each day from all the major food groups.

Maintain Healthy Weight

Excessive fatness is associated with some chronic disorders such as hypertension and diabetes, which in turn relate to heart disease. The healthy body weight, however, must be determined individually because many factors are involved, such as body composition (muscle/fat ratio), body metabolism, genetics, and physical activity.

Choose a Diet Low in Fat, Saturated Fat, and Cholesterol

Americans have traditionally consumed a high-fat diet. In some persons, excess fat leads to high levels of blood fats and cholesterol. Elevated blood levels of these fats and cholesterol are associated with a higher risk of coronary heart disease. Thus it is wise to reduce intake of fats in general, using them only in moderation.

Choose a Diet with Plenty of Vegetables, Fruits, and Grain Products

Increasing use of these foods will help supply more of the needed starches (complex carbohydrates) for energy, many essential nutrients, and necessary dietary fiber. Research indicates that certain types of dietary fiber may help control chronic bowel diseases, contribute to improved blood glucose management for persons with diabetes mellitus, and bind dietary cholesterol.

Use Sugars in Moderation

The major health hazard from eating too much sugar is tooth decay (dental caries). Contrary to popular opinion, however, too much sugar does not in itself cause diabetes. It can only contribute to poor control of diabetes in persons who have inherited the disease. Most Americans consume a relatively large amount of sugar, over 100 pounds per person per year, much of it in processed food products. Again, moderation is the key.

Use Salt and Sodium in Moderation

Our main source of dietary sodium is in ordinary table salt. Excessive salt is not healthy for anyone and certainly not for persons with hypertension. Many processed food products contain considerable amounts of salt and other sodium compounds, and many Americans use more salt in foods than they need. Thus it is wise to limit salt use in food preparation or at the table and to reduce the use of "salty" food products. This approach will lower individual salt tastes, which are learned habits and not biologic necessities. There is ample sodium as a natural mineral in foods to meet usual needs.

Drink Alcoholic Beverages in Moderation

Alcoholic beverages tend to be high in kcalories and low in other nutrients. Limited food intake may accompany excessive alcohol intake. Heavy drinking also contributes to chronic liver disease and some neurologic disorders, as well as some throat and neck cancers. Moreover, it is a major factor in highway deaths. Thus if alcohol is used at all, moderation is the key, and persons should *never* drink and drive.

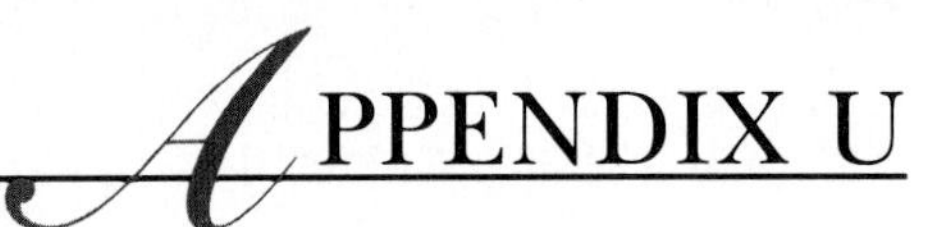

APPENDIX U

Recommended Nutrient Intakes for Canadians

Summary Examples of Recommended Nutrient Intake Based on Age and Body Weight Expressed as Daily Rates

Age	Sex	Energy (kcal)	Thiamin (mg)	Riboflavin (mg)	Niacin NE	n-3 PUFA (g)	n-6 PUFA (g)	Weight (kg)	Protein (g)	Vitamin A RE
0-4 months	Both	600	0.3	0.3	4	0.5	3	6.0	12*	400
5-12 months	Both	900	0.4	0.5	7	0.5	3	9.0	12	400
1 year	Both	1100	0.5	0.6	8	0.6	4	11	13	400
2-3 years	Both	1300	0.6	0.7	9	0.7	4	14	16	400
4-6 years	Both	1800	0.7	0.9	13	1.0	6	18	19	500
7-9 years	M	2200	0.9	1.1	16	1.2	7	25	26	700
	F	1900	0.8	1.0	14	1.0	6	25	26	700
10-12 years	M	2500	1.0	1.3	18	1.4	8	34	34	800
	F	2200	0.9	1.1	16	1.2	7	36	36	800
13-15 years	M	2800	1.1	1.4	20	1.5	9	50	49	900
	F	2200	0.9	1.1	16	1.2	7	48	46	800
16-18 years	M	3200	1.3	1.6	23	1.8	11	62	58	1000
	F	2100	0.8	1.1	15	1.2	7	53	47	800
19-24 years	M	3000	1.2	1.5	22	1.6	10	71	61	1000
	F	2100	0.8	1.1	15	1.2	7	58	50	800
25-49 years	M	2700	1.1	1.4	19	1.5	9	74	64	1000
	F	1900	0.8	1.0	14	1.1	7	59	51	800
50-74 years	M	2300	0.9	1.2	16	1.3	8	73	63	1000
	F	1800	0.8§	1.0§	14§	1.1§	7§	63	54	800
75+ years	M	2000	0.8	1.0	14	1.1	7	69	59	1000
	F‖	1700	0.8§	1.0§	14§	1.1§	7§	64	55	800
Pregnancy (additional)										
1st Trimester		100	0.1	0.1	0.11	0.05	0.3		5	0
2nd Trimester		300	0.1	0.3	0.22	0.16	0.9		20	0
3rd Trimester		300	0.1	0.3	0.22	0.16	0.9		24	0
Lactation (additional)		450	0.2	0.4	0.33	0.25	1.5		20	400

From Scientific Review Committee: Nutrition recommendations, *Health and Welfare,* Ottawa, 1990.

NE, Niacin equivalents; PUFA, polyunsaturated fatty acids; RE, retinol equivalents.

*Protein is assumed to be from breast milk and must be adjusted for infant formula.

†Infant formula with high phosphorus should contain 375 mg of calcium.

‡Breast milk is assumed to be the source of the mineral.

¶Smokers should increase vitamin C by 50%.

§Level below which intake should not fall.

‖Assumes moderate physical activity.

Vitamin D (μg)	Vitamin E (mg)	Vitamin C (mg)	Folate (μg)	Vitamin B_{12} (μg)	Calcium (mg)	Phosphorus (mg)	Magnesium (mg)	Iron (mg)	Iodine (μg)	Zinc (mg)
10	3	20	25	0.3	250†	150	20	0.3‡	30	2‡
10	3	20	40	0.4	400	200	32	7	40	3
10	3	20	40	0.5	500	300	40	6	55	4
5	4	20	50	0.6	550	350	50	6	65	4
5	5	25	70	0.8	600	400	65	8	85	5
2.5	7	25	90	1.0	700	500	100	8	110	7
2.5	6	25	90	1.0	700	500	100	8	95	7
2.5	8	25	120	1.0	900	700	130	8	125	9
2.5	7	25	130	1.0	1100	800	135	8	110	9
2.5	9	30	175	1.0	1100	900	185	10	160	12
2.5	7	30	170	1.0	1000	850	180	13	160	9
2.5	10	40¶	220	1.0	900	1000	230	10	160	12
2.5	7	30¶	190	1.0	700	850	200	12	160	9
2.5	10	40¶	220	1.0	800	1000	240	9	160	12
2.5	7	30¶	180	1.0	700	850	200	13	160	9
2.5	9	40¶	230	1.0	800	1000	250	9	160	12
2.5	6	30¶	185	1.0	700	850	200	13	160	9
5	7	40¶	230	1.0	800	1000	250	9	160	12
5	6	30¶	195	1.0	800	850	210	8	160	9
5	6	40¶	215	1.0	800	1000	230	9	160	12
5	5	30¶	200	1.0	800	850	210	8	160	9
2.5	2	0	200	1.2	500	200	15	0	25	6
2.5	2	10	200	1.2	500	200	45	5	25	6
2.5	2	10	200	1.2	500	200	45	10	25	6
2.5	3	25	100	0.2	500	200	65	0	50	6

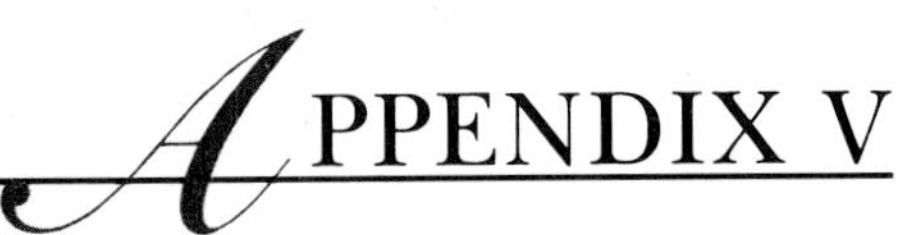

APPENDIX V

Guidelines for Nutritional Assessment and Care of Cystic Fibrosis

Step One: Calculation of Basal Metabolic Rate (BMR)

In cystic fibrosis care, if a patient fails to grow adequately while receiving kcalorie intake based on RDAs, use this table to calculate Basal Metabolic Rate (BMR) daily energy requirement.

World Health Organization Equations for Calculating Basal Metabolic Rate (kcal) from Body Weight (kg)

Age (years)	BMR (kcal) Females	BMR (kcal) Males
0-3	61.0 × (wt kg) − 51	60.9 × (wt kg) − 54
3-10	22.5 × (wt kg) + 499	22.7 × (wt kg) + 495
10-18	12.2 × (wt kg) + 746	17.5 × (wt kg) + 651
18-30	14.7 × (wt kg) + 496	15.3 × (wt kg) + 679
30-60	8.7 × (wt kg) + 829	11.6 × (wt kg) + 879

Adapted from World Health Organization: Energy and protein requirements, WHO Technical Report Series, Volume 924, No 724, 1985, Ramsey, BW et al: Nutritional assessment and management in cystic fibrosis, *Am J Clin Nutr* 55:108, 1992, and Cystic Fibrosis Foundation guidelines.

Step Two: Calculation of Daily Energy Expenditure (DEE) in Therapy

DEE = BMR × (AC + DC)

Abbreviations

DEE = daily energy expenditure (kcal)
BMR = basal metabolic rate (kcal)
AC = activity coefficient
DC = disease coefficient

Guidelines for AC and DC Values

Use the following tables to establish the appropriate activity coefficient and disease coefficient values.

Activity Coefficients (AC)

Activity level of patient	AC value
Confined to bed	1.3
Sedentary	1.5
Active	1.7

Disease Coefficients (DC)

Lung functioning level in cystic fibrosis	Forced air expiration volume in 1 second ($FEV_{1.0}$) (100% = normal FEV)	DC value
Close to normal lung function	>80%	0.0
Moderate lung disease	40%-79%	0.2
Severe lung disease	<40%	0.3
Very severe lung disease	<40%	0.5

Adapted from Ramsey BW et al: Nutritional assessment and management in cystic fibrosis, *Am J Clin Nutr* 55:108, 1992, and Cystic Fibrosis Foundation guidelines.

DEE Calculation

Determine the DEE for a school-age child with cystic fibrosis who is attending school, is relatively sedentary, and has a measured $FEV_{1.0}$ of 50% of predicted normal value.

DEE = BMR × (AC + DC)
= BMR × (1.5 + 0.2)
= BMR × 1.7

Step Three: Calculation of Daily Energy Requirement (DER) from Daily Energy Expenditure (DEE)

Calculation Method

1. Calculate the coefficient of fat absorption (CFA):

$$\text{CFA} = \frac{\text{Fat absorption (FA)}}{\text{Fat intake (FI)}} = \text{Fat absorption }\%^{*}$$

2. Use one of the following guideline formulas for DER:

$$\text{If CFA} > 0.93\text{, then DER} = \text{DEE}$$

or

$$\text{If CFA} = 0.93\text{, then DER} = \text{DEE} \times \frac{0.93}{\text{CFA}}$$

Abbreviations

CFA = coefficient of fat absorption
FA = fat absorption (kcal)
FI = fat intake (kcal)
DEE = daily energy expenditure (kcal)
DER = daily energy requirement (kcal)

*NOTE 1: The fat absorption % (CFA) is usually calculated in a clinical setting by medical laboratory analysis from a patient stool sample.
NOTE 2: If no laboratory analysis report is available, then use CFA = 0.85 as an approximation value in the DER calculation.
Adapted from Ramsey BW et al: Nutritional assessment and management in cystic fibrosis, *Am J Clin Nutr* 55:108, 1992, and Cystic Fibrosis Foundation guidelines.

DER Calculation Example

The fat absorption of a cystic fibrosis patient on enzyme therapy has been determined by laboratory analysis to be 78% of normal. Therefore, the CFA for this patient is 0.78. The DEE for this same patient is calculated to be 2000 kcal. Therefore, the DER for this patient is:

$$\text{DER} = \text{DEE} \times \frac{0.93}{\text{CFA}}$$

$$\text{DER} = 2000\text{ kcal} \times \frac{0.93}{0.78}$$

$$\text{DER} = 2384\text{ kcal/day}$$

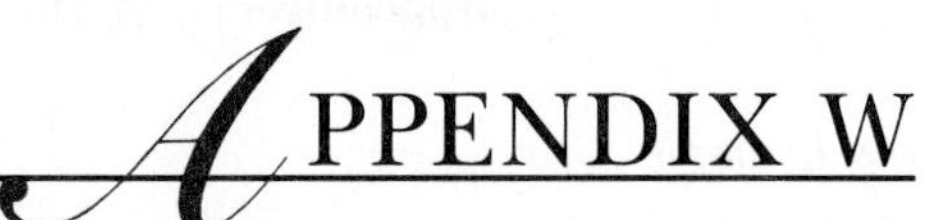

Diets for Nutritional Management of Renal Calculi

TABLE W–1

Low-Calcium Diet (approximately 400 mg calcium)

	Foods allowed	Foods not allowed
Beverage*	Carbonated beverage, coffee, tea	Chocolate-flavored drinks, milk, milk drinks
Bread	White, light rye bread, crackers	
Cereals	Refined cereals	Oatmeal, whole-grain cereals
Desserts	Cake, cookies, gelatin desserts, pastries, pudding, sherbets, all made without chocolate, milk or nuts; if egg yolk is used, it must be from one egg allowance	
Fat	Butter, cream, 2 tbsp/day; French dressing, margarine, salad oil, shortening	Cream (except in amount allowed), mayonnaise
Fruits	Canned, cooked, or fresh fruits or juice except rhubarb	Dried fruit, rhubarb
Meat, eggs	224 g (8 oz) daily of any meat, fowl, fish except clams, oysters, shrimp; not more than one egg daily, including those used in cooking	Clams, oysters, shrimp, cheese
Potato or substitute	Potato, hominy, macaroni, noodles, refined rice, spaghetti	Whole-grain rice
Soup	Broth, vegetable soup made from vegetables allowed	Bean or pea soup, cream or milk soup
Sweets	Honey, jam, jelly, sugar	
Vegetables	Any canned, cooked, fresh vegetables or juice except those listed	Dried beans, broccoli, green cabbage, celery, chard, collards, endive, greens, lettuce, lentils, okra, parsley, parsnips, dried peas, rutabagas
Miscellaneous	Herbs, pickles, popcorn, relishes, salt, spices, vinegar	Chocolate, cocoa, milk gravy, nuts, olives, white sauce

*Depending on calcium content of local water supply. In instances of high calcium content, distilled water may be indicated.

TABLE W–2

Low-Phosphorus Diet (approximately 1 g phosphorus and 40 g protein)

	Foods allowed	Foods not allowed
Milk	Not more than 1 cup daily; whole, skim, buttermilk or 3 tbsp powdered, including the amount used in cooking	
Beverages	Fruit juices, tea, coffee, carbonated drinks, Postum	Milk and milk drinks except as allowed
Bread	White only; enriched commercial, French, hard rolls, soda crackers, rusk	Rye and whole-grain breads, cornbread, biscuits, muffins, waffles
Cereals	Refined cereals, such as Cream of Wheat, Cream of Rice, rice, cornmeal, dry cereals, cornflakes, spaghetti, noodles	All whole-grain cereals
Desserts	Berry or fruit pies, cookies, cakes in average amounts; Jell-O, gelatin, angel food cake, sherbet, meringues made with egg whites, puddings if made with one egg or milk allowance	Desserts with milk and eggs, unless made with the daily allowance
Eggs	Not more than one egg daily, including those used in cooking; extra egg whites may be used	
Fats	Butter, margarine, oils, shortening	
Fruits	Fresh, frozen, canned, as desired	Dried fruits such as raisins, prunes, dates, figs, apricots
Meat	One large serving or two small servings daily of beef, lamb, veal, pork, rabbit, chicken, turkey	Fish, shellfish (crab, oyster, shrimp, lobster), dried and cured meats (bacon, ham, chipped beef), liver, kidney, sweetbreads, brains
Cheese	None	Avoid all cheese and cheese spreads
Vegetables	Potatoes as desired; at least two servings per day of any of the following: asparagus, carrots, beets, green beans, squash, lettuce, rutabagas, tomatoes, celery, peas, onions, cucumber, corn; no more than 1 serving daily of either cabbage, spinach, broccoli, cauliflower, brussels sprouts, artichokes	Dried vegetables such as peas, mushrooms, lima beans
Miscellaneous	Sugar, jams, jellies, syrups, salt, spices, seasonings; condiments in moderation	Chocolate, nuts, nut products such as peanut butter, cream sauces

Sample menu pattern

Breakfast	Lunch	Dinner
Fruit juice	Meat, 56 g (2 oz)	Meat, 56 g
Refined cereal	Potato	Potato
Egg	Vegetable	Vegetable
White toast	Salad	Salad
Butter	Bread, white	Bread, white
½ cup milk	Butter	Butter
Coffee or tea	½ cup milk	Dessert
	Dessert	Coffee or tea
	Coffee or tea	

TABLE W-3

Low-Calcium Test Diet (200 mg Calcium)

	Grams	Calcium (mg)
Breakfast		
Orange juice, fresh	100	19.00
Bread (toast), white	25	19.57
Butter	15	3.00
Rice Krispies	15	3.70
Cream, 20% butterfat	35	33.95
Sugar	7	0.00
Jam	20	2.00
Distilled water, coffee, or tea*		0.00
TOTAL		81.22
Lunch		
Beef steak, cooked	100	10.00
Potato	100	11.00
Tomatoes	100	11.00
Bread	25	19.57
Butter	15	3.00
Honey	20	1.00
Applesauce	20	1.00
Distilled water, coffee, or tea		0.00
TOTAL		56.57
Dinner		
Lamb chop, cooked	90	10.00
Potato	100	11.00
Frozen green peas	80	10.32
Bread	25	19.57
Butter	15	3.00
Jam	20	2.00
Peach sauce	100	5.00
Distilled water, coffee, or tea		0.00
TOTAL		60.89
TOTAL MILLIGRAMS CALCIUM		198.68

*Use distilled water only for cooking and for beverages.

TABLE W-4

Acid Ash Diet

The purpose of this diet is to furnish a well-balanced diet in which the total acid ash is greater than the total alkaline ash each day. It lists (1) unrestricted foods, (2) restricted foods, (3) foods not allowed, and (4) sample of a day's diet.

Unrestricted foods: Eat as much as desired of the following foods.

- Bread: any, preferably whole grain; crackers, rolls
- Cereals: any, preferably whole grain
- Desserts: angel food or sunshine cake; cookies made without baking powder or baking soda; cornstarch pudding, cranberry desserts, custards, gelatin desserts, ice cream, sherbet, plum or prune desserts; rice or tapioca pudding
- Fats: any, as butter, margarine, salad dressings, shortening, lard, salad oils, olive oil
- Fruits: cranberries, plums, prunes
- Meat, eggs, cheese; any meat, fish, or fowl, two servings daily; at least one egg daily
- Potato substitutes: corn, hominy, lentils, macaroni, noodles, rice, spaghetti, vermicelli
- Soup: broth as desired; other soups from foods allowed
- Sweets: cranberry or plum jelly; sugar, plain sugar candy
- Miscellaneous: cream sauce, gravy, peanut butter, peanuts, popcorn, salt, spices, vinegar, walnuts

Restricted foods: Do not eat any more than the amount allowed each day.

- Milk: 2 cups daily (may be used in other ways than as beverage)
- Cream: ⅓ cup or less daily
- Fruits: one serving of fruit daily (in addition to prunes, plums, cranberries); certain fruits listed under "Sample menu" are not allowed at any time
- Vegetables including potato: two servings daily; certain vegetables listed under "Foods not allowed" are not allowed at any time

Foods not allowed

- Carbonated beverages, such as ginger ale, cola, root beer
- Cakes or cookies made with baking powder or soda
- Fruits: dried apricots, bananas, dates, figs, raisins, rhubarb
- Vegetables: dried beans, beet greens, dandelion greens, carrots, chard, lima beans
- Sweets: chocolate or candies other than those under "Unrestricted foods"; syrups
- Miscellaneous: other nuts, olives, pickles

Sample menu

Breakfast	Lunch	Dinner
Grapefruit	Creamed chicken	Broth
Wheatena	Steamed rice	Roast beef, gravy
Scrambled eggs	Green beans	Buttered noodles
Toast, butter, plum jam	Stewed prunes	Sliced tomato
Coffee, cream, sugar	Bread, butter	Mayonnaise
	Milk	Vanilla ice cream
		Bread, butter

TABLE W–5

Low-Purine Diet (approximately 125 mg purine)

General directions

- During acute stages use only list 1.
- After acute stage subsides and for chronic conditions, use the following schedule:
  Two days a week, not consecutive, use list 1 entirely.
  The remaining days add foods from list 2 and 3, as indicated.
  Avoid list 4 entirely.
- Keep diet moderately low in fat.

Typical meal pattern

Breakfast	Lunch	Dinner
Fruit	Egg or cheese dish	Egg or cheese dish
Refined cereal and/or egg	Vegetables, as allowed (cooked or salad)	Cream of vegetable soup, if desired
White toast	Potato or substitute	Starch (potato or substitute)
Butter, 1 tsp	White bread	Colored vegetable, as allowed
Sugar	Butter, 1 tsp	White bread, butter, 1 tsp, if desired
Coffee	Fruit or simple dessert	Salad, as allowed
Milk, if desired	Milk	Fruit or simple dessert
		Milk

Food list 1: may be used as desired; foods that contain an insignificant amount of purine bodies

Beverages
- Carbonated
- Chocolate
- Cocoa
- Coffee
- Fruit juices
- Postum
- Tea

Butter*

Bread: white and crackers, cornbread

Cereals and cereal products
- Corn
- Rice
- Tapioca
- Refined wheat
- Macaroni
- Noodles

Cheese of all kinds*

Eggs

Fats of all kinds* (moderation)

Fruits of all kinds

Gelatin, Jell-O

Milk: buttermilk, evaporated, malted, sweet

Nuts of all kinds,* peanut butter*

Pies* (except mincemeat)

Sugar and sweets

Vegetables
- Artichokes
- Beets
- Beet greens
- Broccoli
- Brussels sprouts
- Cabbage
- Carrots
- Celery
- Corn
- Cucumber
- Eggplant
- Endive
- Kohlrabi
- Lettuce
- Okra
- Parsnips
- Potato, white and sweet
- Pumpkin
- Rutabagas
- Sauerkraut
- String beans
- Summer squash
- Swiss chard
- Tomato
- Turnips

*High in fat.

TABLE W–5

Low-Purine Diet (approximately 125 mg purine)—cont'd

Food list 2: one item four times a week; foods that contain a moderate amount (up to 75 mg) of purine bodies in 100 g serving

Asparagus	Finnan haddie	Mushrooms	Salmon
Bluefish	Ham	Mutton	Shad
Bouillon	Herring	Navy beans	Spinach
Cauliflower	Kidney beans	Oatmeal	Tripe
Chicken	Lima beans	Oysters	Tuna fish
Crab	Lobster	Peas	Whitefish

Food list 3: one item once a week; foods that contain a large amount (75-150 mg) of purine bodies in 100 g serving

Bacon	Duck	Perch	Sheep
Beef	Goose	Pheasant	Shellfish
Calf tongue	Halibut	Pigeon	Squab
Carp	Lentils	Pike	Trout
Chicken soup	Liver sausage	Pork	Turkey
Codfish	Meat soups	Quail	Veal
	Partridge	Rabbit	Venison

Food list 4: avoid entirely; foods that contain large amounts (150-1000 mg) of purine bodies in 100 g serving

Sweetbreads	825 mg	Liver (calf, beef)	233 mg	Meat extracts	160-400 mg
Anchovies	363 mg	Kidneys (beef)	200 mg	Gravies	Variable
Sardines (in oil)	295 mg	Brains	195 mg		

TABLE W–6

Low-Methionine Diet

	Foods allowed	Foods not allowed
Soup	Any soup made without meat stock or addition of milk	Rich meat soups, broths, canned soups made with meat broth
Meat or meat substitute	Peanut butter sandwich; spaghetti, or macaroni dish made without addition of meat, cheese, or milk; one serving per day: chicken, lamb, veal, beef, pork, crab, or bacon (3)	Fish and those not listed above
Beverages	Soy milk, tea, coffee	Milk in any form
Vegetables	Asparagus, artichoke, beans, beets, carrots, chicory, cucumber, eggplant, escarole, lettuce, onions, parsnips, potatoes, pumpkin, rhubarb, tomatoes, turnips	Those not listed as allowed
Fruits	Apples, apricots, bananas, berries, cherries, fruit cocktail, grapefruit, grapes, lemon juice, nectarines, oranges, peaches, pears, pineapple, plums, tangerines, watermelon, cantaloupe	Those not listed as allowed
Salads	Raw or cooked vegetable or fruit salad	
Cereals	Macaroni, spaghetti, noodles	
Bread	Whole wheat, rye, white	
Nuts	Peanuts	
Desserts	Fresh or cooked fruit, ices, fruit pies	
Eggs		In any form
Cheese		All varieties
Concentrated sweets	Sugar, jams, jellies, syrup, honey, hard candy	
Concentrated fats	Butter, margarine, cream	
Miscellaneous	Pepper, mustard, vinegar, garlic, oil, herbs, spices	

Meal pattern

Breakfast	Lunch	Dinner
1 cup fruit juice	1 serving soup	56 g (2 oz) meat
½ cup fruit	1 serving sandwich	1 med starch
1 slice toast	1 cup fruit	½ cup vegetable
1½ pats butter	240 ml (8 oz) soy milk*	1 serving salad
2 tsp jelly	3 tsp sugar	1 tbsp dressing
1 tbsp sugar	1 tbsp cream	1 slice bread
Beverage	Beverage	1 serving dessert
1 tbsp cream		1 tbsp sugar
		1 tbsp cream
		1½ pats butter
		Beverage

Sample menu

Breakfast	Lunch	Dinner
Orange juice	Vegetable soup, vegetarian	Chicken, roast
Applesauce	Peanut butter sandwich	Baked potato
Whole-wheat toast	Canned peaches	Artichoke
Butter	Soy milk*	Sliced tomatoes
Jelly	Sugar	French dressing
Sugar	Cream	Whole-wheat bread
Coffee	Coffee or tea	Fruit ice
Cream		Sugar
		Cream
		Butter
		Coffee or tea

Adapted from Smith DR, Kolb FO, and Harper HA: The management of cystinuria and cystine-stone disease, J Urol 81:61, 1959.
*Optional: use in children to include protein intake. Omit if urine calcium is elevated in adults.

APPENDIX X

Calculation Aids and Conversion Tables

More than 185 years ago a group of French scientists set up the metric system of weights and measures. Today, with refinements over years of use, it is called the "Systeme International" (SI). In 1975 our American Congress passed the Metric Conversion Act, which provides for conversion of our customary British/American system to the simpler metric system used by the rest of the world. We are now in the midst of this conversion, as evidenced by distance signs along highways and labels on many packaged foods in supermarkets. Here are a few conversion factors to help you make these transitions in your necessary calculations.

Metric System of Measurement

Like our money system, this is a simple decimal system based on units of 10. It is uniform and used internationally.

Weight units:	1 kilogram (kg)	=	1000 grams (gm or g)
	1 g	=	1000 milligrams (mg)
	1 mg	=	1000 micrograms (mcg or μg)
Length units:	1 meter (m)	=	100 centimeters (cm)
	1000 meters	=	1 kilometer (km)
Volume units:	1 liter (L)	=	1000 milliliters (ml)
	1 milliliter	=	1 cubic centimeter (cc)

Temperature units: Celcius (C) scale, based on 100 equal units between 0° C (freezing point of water) and 100° C (boiling point of water); this scale is used entirely in all scientific work.

Energy units:	Kilocalorie (kcal)	=	Amount of energy required to raise 1 kg water 1° C
	Kilojoule (kJ)	=	Amount of energy required to move 1 kg mass 1 m by a force of 1 newton
	1 kcal	=	4.184 kJ

In 1970 the American Institute of Nutrition's Committee on Nomenclature recommended that the term *kilojoule* (kJ) replace the kilocalorie (kcal). This change is gradually coming about.

British/American System of Measurement

Our customary system is a confusion of units with no uniform relationships. It is not a decimal system, but rather a jumbled collection of different units collected in usage and language over time. It is used mainly in America.

Weight units:	1 pound (lb)	=	16 ounces (oz)
Length units:	1 foot (ft)	=	12 inches (in)
	1 yard (yd)	=	3 feet (ft)
Volume units:	3 teaspoons (tsp)	=	1 tablespoon (tbsp)
	16 tbsp	=	1 cup
	1 cup	=	8 fluid ounces (fl oz)
	4 cups	=	1 quart (qt)
	5 cups	=	1 imperial quart (qt), Canada

Temperature units: Fahrenheit (F) scale, based on 180 equals units between 32° F (freezing point of water) and 212° F (boiling point of water) at standard atmospheric pressure

Conversions Between Measurement Systems

Weight:	1 oz	=	28.35 g (usually used as 28 or 30 g)
	2.2 lb	=	1 kg
Length:	1 in	=	2.54 cm
	1 ft	=	30.48 cm
	39.37 in	=	1 m
Volume:	1.06 qt	=	1 L
	0.85 imperial qt	=	1 L (Canada)

Temperature:	Boiling point of water	100° C	212° F
	Body temperature	37° C	98.6° F
	Freezing point of water	0° C	32° F

Interconversion formulas:

Fahrenheit temperature (°F) = $\frac{9}{5}$ (°C) + 32

Celsius temperature (°C) = $\frac{5}{9}$ (°F − 32)

Retinol Equivalents

The following definitions and equivalences that are internationally agreed on provide a basis for calculating retinol equivalent conversions.

Definitions: International units (IU) and retinol equivalents (RE) are defined as follows:

1 IU = 0.3 μg retinol (0.0003 mg)
1 IU = 0.6 μg beta-carotene (0.0006 mg)
1 RE = 6 μg retinol
1 RE = 6 μg beta-carotene
1 RE = 12 μg other provitamin A carotenoids
1 RE = 3.33 IU retinol
1 RE = 10 IU beta-carotene

Conversion formulas: On the basis of weight beta-carotene is $\frac{1}{2}$ as active as retinol; on the basis of structure the other provitamin carotenoids are $\frac{1}{4}$ as active as retinol. In addition, retinol is more completely absorbed in the intestine, whereas the provitamin carotenoids are much less well utilized, with an average absorption of about $\frac{1}{3}$. Therefore in overall activity beta-carotene is $\frac{1}{6}$ as active as retinol, and the other carotenoids are $\frac{1}{12}$ as active. These differences in utilization provide the basis for the 1:6:12 relationship shown in the equivalences given and in the following formulas for calculating retinol equivalents from values of vitamin A, beta-carotene, and other active carotenoids, expressed either as international units or micrograms:

If retinol and beta-carotene are given in micrograms:
Micrograms of retinol + (Micrograms of beta-carotene ÷ 6) = RE
If both are given as IU:
International units of retinol ÷ 3.33) + (International units of beta-carotene ÷ 10) = RE
If beta-carotene and other carotenoids are given in micrograms:
(Micrograms of beta-carotene ÷ 6) + (Micrograms of other carotenoids ÷ 12) = RE

Approximate Metric Conversions

When you know	Multiply by	To find
Ounces	28	Grams
Pounds	0.45	Kilograms
Length		
Inches	2.5	Centimeters
Feet	30	Centimeters
Yards	0.9	Meters
Miles	1.6	Kilometers
Volume		
Teaspoons	5	Millimeters
Tablespoons	15	Millimeters
Fluid ounces	30	Millimeters
Cups	0.24	Liters
Pints	0.47	Liters
Quarts	0.95	Liters
Temperature		
Fahrenheit temperature	$\frac{5}{9}$ (after subtracting 32)	Celsius temperature

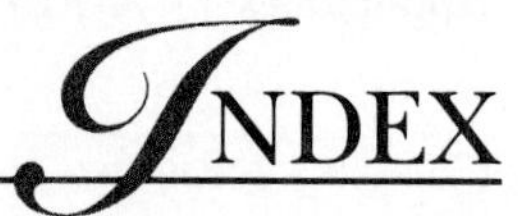

INDEX

B

C

D

Q

R

MEDIAN HEIGHTS AND WEIGHTS AND RECOMMENDED ENERGY INTAKE 10TH EDITION RDA

Category	Age (years) or Condition	Weight		Height		REE[a] (kcal/day)	Average Energy Allowance (kcal)		
		(kg)	(lb)	(cm)	(in)		Multiples of REE	Per kg	Per day[b]
Infants	0.0-0.5	6	13	60	24	320		108	650
	0.5-1.0	9	20	71	28	500		98	850
Children	1-3	13	29	90	56	740		102	1,300
	4-6	20	44	112	44	950		90	1,800
	7-10	28	62	132	52	1,130		70	2,000
Males	11-14	45	99	157	62	1,440	1.70	55	2,500
	15-18	66	145	176	69	1,760	1.67	45	3,000
	19-24	72	160	177	70	1,780	1.67	40	2,900
	25-50	79	174	176	70	1,800	1.60	37	2,900
	51+	77	170	173	68	1,530	1.50	30	2,300
Females	11-14	46	101	157	62	1,310	1.67	47	2,200
	15-18	55	120	163	64	1,370	1.60	40	2,200
	19-24	58	128	164	65	1,350	1.60	38	2,200
	25-50	63	138	163	64	1,380	1.55	36	2,200
	51+	65	143	160	63	1,280	1.50	30	1,900
Pregnant	1st Trimester								+0
	2nd Trimester								+300
	3rd Trimester								+300
Lactating	1st 6 months								+500
	2nd 6 months								+500

[a] Resting energy expenditure (REE); calculation based on FAO equations, then rounded. This is the same as RMR.
[b] Figure is rounded.

METROPOLITAN LIFE INSURANCE COMPANY HEIGHT-WEIGHT DATA, REVISED 1983

Height-Weight Tables for Adults (1983)

Height: Ft	In	WOMEN Frame* Small	Medium	Large	Height Ft	In	MEN Frame* Small	Medium	Large
4	10	102-111	109-121	118-131	5	2	128-134	131-141	138-150
4	11	103-113	111-123	120-134	5	3	130-136	133-143	140-153
5	0	104-115	113-126	122-137	5	4	132-138	135-145	142-156
5	1	106-118	115-129	125-140	5	5	134-140	137-148	144-160
5	2	108-121	118-132	128-143	5	6	136-142	139-151	146-164
5	3	111-124	121-135	131-147	5	7	138-145	142-154	149-168
5	4	114-127	124-138	134-151	5	8	140-148	145-157	152-172
5	5	117-130	127-141	137-155	5	9	142-151	148-160	155-176
5	6	120-133	130-144	140-159	5	10	144-154	151-163	158-180
5	7	113-136	133-147	143-163	5	11	146-157	154-166	161-184
5	8	126-139	136-150	146-167	6	0	149-160	157-170	164-188
5	9	129-142	139-153	149-170	6	1	152-164	160-174	168-192
5	10	132-145	142-156	152-173	6	2	155-168	164-178	172-197
5	11	135-148	156-159	155-176	6	3	158-172	167-182	176-202
6	0	138-151	148-162	158-179	6	4	162-176	171-187	181-207

Based on a weight-height mortality study conducted by the Society of Actuaries and the Association of Life Insurance Medical Directors of America, Metropolitan Life Insurance Company, revised 1983.

*Weights at ages 25 to 59 based on lowest mortality. Height includes 1-in heel. Weight for women includes 3 lb. for indoor clothing. Weight for men includes 5 lb. for indoor clothing. (see p. 347 for controversy surrounding the use and abuse of these tables over the years and Appendix K for determination of frame size.)